Molecular Biochemistry of Human Disease
Volume III

Author for Fundamentals of Clinical Diagnosis
George Feuer, Ph.D.
Professor
Departments of Clinical Biochemistry and
Pharmacology
Banting Institute
University of Toronto
Toronto, Canada

Author for Pathological Supplements
Felix A. de la Iglesia, M.D.
Vice President
Department of Pathology and Experimental
Toxicology
Warner-Lambert/Parke-Davis Pharmaceutical Research
Ann Arbor, Michigan

T0133934

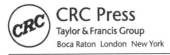

CRC Press
Taylor & Francis Group
Boca Raton London New York

CRC Press is an imprint of the
Taylor & Francis Group, an **informa** business

CRC Press
Taylor & Francis Group
6000 Broken Sound Parkway NW, Suite 300
Boca Raton, FL 33487-2742

Reissued 2019 by CRC Press

A Library of Congress record exists under LC control number:

Publisher's Note
The publisher has gone to great lengths to ensure the quality of this reprint but points out that some imperfections in the original copies may be apparent.

Disclaimer
The publisher has made every effort to trace copyright holders and welcomes correspondence from those they have been unable to contact.

ISBN 13: 978-0-367-26345-4 (hbk)
ISBN 13: 978-0-367-26348-5 (pbk)
ISBN 13: 978-0-429-29281-1 (ebk)

Visit the Taylor & Francis Web site at http://www.taylorandfrancis.com and the
CRC Press Web site at http://www.crcpress.com

PREFACE

The present volume is the final of this series where we attempted to bring to the medical scientific community an integrated view of the fundamentals of disease processes and clinical biochemical diagnoses. Basic medical knowledge is advancing at an accelerated pace due to significant progress in biotechnology and molecular biology. Many major breakthroughs are being accomplished at a steadfast rhythm in the diagnosis and treatment of diseases that were indurable until today. We foresee that in the near future, curative molecular control of many diseases will be easily achieved. Thus, an attempt to continue this series in view of such tremendous challenge would require the renewal of knowledge and efforts that are best recruited from the younger ranks of our scientific elite.

We hope that our message has been delivered and that in some way this series has been useful to eager students of all ages in all medical disciplines. The series was organized from a generalized viewpoint at elucidating the biochemical mechanisms of human disease, starting with basic disorders of metabolism through cellular alterations and integrated eventually in an organ-oriented approach. This last volume addresses this approach, covering inflammation, atherosclerosis, liver diseases, and central nervous system disorders.

Knowledge of inflammation has advanced significantly, amongst others in the area of mediators, mechanisms of cell injury, as well as better definition of the role of the diverse formed elements of the blood. The role of these diverse white cells in immune processes cannot be overemphasized due to recent advances in flowcitometry, immunocytochemistry, and monoclonal antibodies.

Atherosclerosis represents a major threat to the health and welfare of advanced societies and is expanding to cultures where this disease was not common barely a quarter of a decade ago. Recently, there has been a better definition of the pathogenesis of the disease, a better understanding of the role of receptors, a formal characterization of the risk factors in cariovascular disease. Furthermore, we witnessed the emerging protective value of high density lipoproteins in terms of coronary disease. At the time of this writing, we have evidence from the Helsinki Heart Study that myocardial infarction in a population at risk can be prevented by therapeutic intervention with gemfibrozil. This event is a landmark in the history of pharmacological control of disease, underlining the importance of the integrated biochemical and morphological approach to the study of various diseases.

The chapter devoted to liver diseases covers the highlights of important aspects of porphyrin metabolism, bile pigments, and jaundice. The role of various noxious agents, such as alcohol or other toxicants and drug-induced side effects will help the understanding of mechanisms in hepatic cell injury.

Diseases of the central nervous system reveal the molecular basis of many disorders. Epilepsy, migraine, and the role of excitatory peptides in these conditions is discussed. In addition, there are other discussions centered on metabolic and degenerative neuronal diseases, neurotoxicity, and alterations of memory and cognition.

As in the past, we have enjoyed the enthusiastic support of many colleagues and associates, and we wish to acknowledge Emmanuel Farber, John Kellen, Norbert Kerenyi, and Ross Cameron from the University of Toronto, Canada; Peter Ward and Robert Gray from the University of Michigan; Graham Smith, Peter Greaves, Robin Walker, and Chris Jobb from the Parke-Davis Research Institute in Toronto; Mary Carol Conroy and Mel Gluckman from the Pharmacology Department at Parke-Davis Research in Ann Arbor, MI. The support from Roger Westland and Anne Morrison for the review of structures and chemical nomenclature is also appreciated. In the same vein, we could not have completed this work without the unrelenting support of Kayla Tomsic, Debbie Earhart, and Priscilla Washburn. Mrs. Sonja Duda provided generous technical help in the compilation of references. We will be forever grateful to these individuals and apologize in case that a name was unintentionally omitted from mention.

It will be difficult to fill the void left in our daily toils after having completed this series. George has plans to develop a companion book for medical students; Felix is thinking about how to say no to him gracefully and getting a rusty fishing rod out of the closet.

George Feuer
Felix A. de la Iglesia

THE AUTHORS

George Feuer, Ph.D., C. Med. Sc., F.R.I.C., is Professor of Clinical Biochemistry and Professor of Pharmacology (Toxicology) in the Faculty of Medicine, at the University of Toronto, Canada. Dr. Feuer received his B.Sc. degree from University of Szeged, Hungary in 1943. He obtained his M.Sc. and Ph.D. (summa cum laude) degree in 1944 from the Department of Organic Chemistry and from the Department of Physical Chemistry, University of Szeged, respectively, and his C. Med. Sc. from the Hungarian Academy of Sciences, Budapest in 1952. He was appointed Assistant Professor of Organic Chemistry at the University of Szeged in 1945. He became an Associate Professor of Biochemistry at the University of Szeged in 1946 and at the University of Budapest in 1948, and became a Professor in 1950. He was appointed Head of the Department of Muscular- and Neurochemistry at the Hungarian Academy of Sciences in Budapest in 1953, and Head of Biochemistry at the Cancer Research Institute in Budapest in 1956. He left Hungary after the revolution in 1957 and became Senior Research Associate at the Department of Neurochemistry, Institute of Psychiatry, University of London, England in 1957, and Head of the Department of Biochemistry at the British Industrial Biology Research Association, Carshalton, England in 1963. He was appointed as Associate Professor of Clinical Biochemistry at the University of Toronto in 1968, Professor of Clinical Biochemistry in 1974, and Professor of Pharmacology (Toxicology) at the University of Toronto in 1980.

Among other awards, Dr. Feuer received an award from the Budapest County Council for research in chemical structures in 1945, and the Second Class Order of Merit of the Hungarian People's Republic for his scientific achievements in biochemistry in 1953. He was nominated for the Lucien Dautreband Prize, Fondation de Physiopathologie, Brussels, Belgium in 1976, and for the A. B. Wilson Prize, American Society of Cell Biology in 1983. He served as a member of the Medical Nobel Prize Committee in 1976.

Dr. Feuer is a member of the Canadian Biochemical Society, the Society of Toxicology of Canada, the New York Academy of Sciences, Fellow of the Royal Institute of Chemistry (England), the Society of Toxicology (U.S.), charter member International Society for the Study of Xenobiotics. He served as a member of the Editorial Board of Xenobiotica, Drug Metabolism and Drug Interactions and Élővilág; Reviewer of Modern Medicine of Canada and Medical Post.

Dr. Feuer has presented over 30 invited plenary lectures at international meetings, over 90 invited lectures at national and international meetings, and more than 250 guest lectures at universities, institutes, and public meetings including radio and television. He has published more than 300 research papers and reviews, and is author and co-author of 5 books. His current major interests include the molecular pathogenesis of hepatocarcinogenesis and related cachexia syndrome, and the oncostatic role of the pineal function in the development of malignant melanoma.

Felix A. de la Iglesia, M.D., is Vice President of Pathology and Experimental Toxicology at Warner-Lambert/Parke-Davis Pharmaceutical Research in Ann Arbor, Michigan, as well as Adjunct Professor of Toxicology at the School of Public Health and Research Scientist in the Department of Pathology, School of Medicine, University of Michigan, and Professor of Pathology, University of Toronto School of Medicine. He is a member of the Environmental Health Sciences Review Committee, External Consultant in Pathology and Toxicology to the National Institutes of Health, National Cancer Institute, and official expert in Pharmacology and Toxicology to the Ministries of Health of France and West Germany. In addition, he is Councilor and President of the Society of Toxicologic Pathologists and Past President of the Michigan Chapter of the Society of Toxicology. Born in 1939 in Argentina, he received his M.D. degree in 1964 from the National University of Cordoba,

Argentina, and completed postgraduate training in Experimental Pathology as Fellow of the Medical Research Council of Canada. In 1966, he joined the Warner-Lambert Research Institute of Canada in Ontario, and developed various research and administrative positions until becoming director of the institute. After moving to the U.S. in 1977, he became Director of Pathology and Experimental Toxicology until assuming his present position. His research interests are in the area of toxicodynamics of subcellular organelle changes in drug-induced hepatic injury, toxicological aspects of novel anticancer chemotherapeutic agents, and safety assessment of novel chemical entities leading to the development of therapeutic agents. A Diplomate of the Academy of Toxicological Sciences, his publications include more than 250 articles, and currently he is the Editor of *Toxicologic Pathology,* and an Editorial Board member of the journals *Toxicology and Applied Pharmacology, Drug Metabolism Reviews,* and *Toxicology.*

INTRODUCTION

In the course of recent decades a fundamentally new view has emerged in the analysis of the complexity of disease processes and their relationship to the regulation of cellular metabolism. It is now firmly established that many derangements of the normal structure and function of the organism stem from some impairment of the biochemical organization. Defects in normal biochemical processes proved to be the reason for the primary anomaly, even though they do not always result in immediate pathological conditions. However, when such biochemical changes persist they become irreversible and thus normal cells are progressively transformed into abnormal ones, resulting in pathological changes and clinical symptoms. Today, we understand a disease only if the impairment can be clearly identified with alterations of normal biochemical processes as recognized by various laboratory tests. Correlations between these biochemical tests and clinical manifestations provide key information on the basic etiology of human illness. The interpretation of clinical biochemical data is available for the diagnosis and at the same time this knowledge aids in management of the disease and in understanding the rationale behind drug therapy.

Although in many instances these interrelations have not yet been established, we now can consider that the task of correlating clinical signs and symptoms of diseases with laboratory data is unfinished, awaiting what further research will reveal about the connections between the manifestations of disease and impaired biochemical function. Clinical biochemistry has been growing steadily as new steps are discovered in the mechanisms of well-known diseases and new insights are being gained into the background and origin of abnormal biochemical processes. New methods are introduced in diagnosis, and new dugs are tested for therapy. Generally, there has been improved experience of disease mechanisms. Further progress in investigations of the biochemistry of human disease will disclose additional correlations, allowing us more knowledge of the primary biochemical lesions, which manifest in diseases of presently unknown origin or mechanism.

Although the title of this book might imply a wider academic scope, this book considers only basic problems regarding the correlation between altered biochemical processes and illness. Its purpose is to describe the development of abnormalities in biochemical reactions, as well as in the underlying mechanisms, and to illustrate how the action of drugs fits into reversing the changes of the progressing disorder caused by the derangement in normal reactions. Disease processes are usually complex; in these situations several interrelated systems function in an integrated manner. Although the main arguments of the book are based on biochemical information, an attempt is made to incorporate various other aspects originating from pathological and pharmacological studies into a uniform view. Considering the sick man as a unit, this work conveys an integrated picture of the biochemical changes associated with disease.

The primary aim of the book is to help medical, pharmacy, and advanced students in science to understand the growing importance of continuously progressing biochemical concepts in human disease. It may serve as a *vade mecum* for clinical biochemists to review the basis of their practical experience. At the same time it may also help physicians to brush up the clinical biochemistry learned during their years in medical school. Several excellent texts on general biochemistry are available; hence basic information will not be given in detail. However, there is reason to believe that many students and physicians as well would welcome a book in which the fundamental biochemistry underlying the course of disease is presented in an extended and readily understandable form. Thorough discussions on the interrelationships between organ, cell, or cellular organelle and disease, and more space than usual are devoted to the interpretation of the biochemical nature of human disease.

Essential knowledge of physiology, biochemistry, pathology, and pharmacology is assumed. The basic features of biochemistry, well described in standard textbooks, are omitted in order to focus the interest upon important issues of the relationships between impaired processes and disease. However, where necessary, limited background information is given to provide the reader with an introduction to the basis of a multitude of diseases with their various and often interrelated manifestations. At the same time more complex associations are also described and the defects in the molecular organization of the diseased cell or cellular organelle are discussed in depth. Relevant interactions with pharmacologically active substances, either produced by the body or applied by drug therapy, which may influence biochemical processes and the progress of disease are briefly mentioned. Essentials of diagnostic methods and interpretations are also presented.

In general, the basic philosophy of the book could be summarized as follows:

1. Most (if not all) diseases originate from an impairment of biochemical molecular mechanism of the organism.
2. Biochemical processes affected by the disease and manifested through pathological lesions, may be revealed by clinical biochemistry tests.
3. Based on this knowledge, the aim of therapy is to repair the damage.
4. The specific purpose of drug administration is to restore normal conditions: the action of drugs lies in reversing the clearly discernible changes which manifest in the biochemical mechanism.
5. Prolonged injury of the biochemical mechanism leads to irreversible alterations.

The subject matter includes:

1. General changes characteristic of cellular components
2. The mechanism whereby these changes alter homeostasis
3. Specialized changes occurring in individual diseases, associated with particular organs
4. Changes peculiar to unique situations, inborn errors, diseases of the newborn, and aging

The course of diseases is described as a continuous process similar to a flow sheet:

$$\text{Normal cell} \begin{array}{c} \nearrow \text{composition} \searrow \\ \searrow \text{structure} \nearrow \end{array} \text{biochemical process} \rightarrow$$

$$\text{impairment} \rightarrow \text{disease} \begin{array}{c} \nearrow \text{regeneration} \rightarrow \text{recovery} \\ \searrow \text{degeneration} \rightarrow \text{death} \end{array}$$

An understanding of the disease mechanism is essential for correct diagnosis and adequate therapy. This aim is presented in this book by summarizing our present knowledge on the molecular and cellular mechanisms of disease. This book is not comprehensive, because in several fields our knowledge is still fragmentary and no one could master all available information.

The various subjects have been arranged logically, starting from the participation of cellular elements in disease and continuing with disorders associated with a particular organ. The various topics may be read in sequence as they appear. Since, however, many biochemical findings accompanied by the progress of disease are not yet clearly understood, sometimes it may also be necessary to turn to earlier or later chapters. Hopefully, the background provided will be sufficiently clear to make it relatively easy to learn more about the various diseases from the general literature. A glossary of the essential terminology and normal ranges of various serum and urinary parameters are found in an Appendix in Volume III. Each chapter is followed by references, plus suggestions for further reading. It should be understood that in order to avoid an encyclopedic aggregation it was necessary to limit the number of these references, including only basic illustrative examples, mainly from the latest available reports. Perhaps many important contributions have been omitted in the text. Individual references are mentioned only when they are fairly recent, and the references from our laboratory only indicate our interest in various areas. We hope that the references will provide the interested reader with a starting point for further enquiry.

BASIC REFERENCE BOOKS

Biochemistry

Lehninger, A. L., *Biochemistry,* 2nd ed., Worth Publication, New York, 1975.

Montgomery, R., Dryer, R. L., Conway, T. W., and Spector, A. A., *Biochemistry: A Case-Oriented Approach,* 2nd ed., Mosby Company, New York, 1977.

Clinical Biochemistry

Thompson, R. H. S. and Wooton, I. D. P., *Biochemical Disorders in Human Disease,* 3rd ed., Academic Press, New York, 1970.

Zilva, J. F. and Pannall, P. R., *Clinical Chemistry in Diagnosis and Treatment,* 2nd ed., Year Book, Chicago, 1975.

Cantarow, A. and Trumper, C., *Clinical Biochemistry,* 7th ed., W. B. Saunders, Philadelphia, 1975.

Gray, C. H. and Howarth, D., *Clinical Chemical Pathology,* 8th ed., Burroughs-Wellcome Foundation, 1977.

Gornall, A. G., *Applied Biochemistry of Clinical Disorders,* 2nd ed., Harper & Row, New York, 1986.

Clinical Chemistry

Tietz, N.W., *Fundamentals of Clinical Chemistry,* 2nd ed., W. B. Saunders, Philadelphia, 1976.

Varley, T. R., *Practical Clinical Biochemistry,* 5th ed., Heinemann, New York, 1976.

Henry, J. B., *Todd-Sanford-Davidsohn: Clinical Diagnosis and Management,* 16th ed., W. B. Saunders, Philadelphia, 1979.

Brown, S. S., Mitchell, F. L., and Young, D. S., *Chemical Diagnosis of Disease,* Elsevier/North Holland, Amsterdam, 1979.

Disease

Stanbury, F. B., Wyngaarden, F. B., and Fredrickson, D. S., *The Metabolic Basis of Inherited Disease,* McGraw-Hill, New York, 1978.

Walter, J. B., *An Introduction to the Principles of Disease,* 2nd ed., W. B. Saunders, Philadlephia, 1982.

Riddell, R. H., Ed., *Pathology of Drug-Induced and Toxic Diseases,* Churchill Livingstone, London, 1982.

Robbins, S. L., Cotran, R. S., and Kumar, V., *Pathologic Basis of Disease,* 3rd ed., W. B. Saunders, Philadelphia, 1984.

Klaassen, C. D., Amdur, M. O., and Doull, J., *Casarett and Doull's Toxicology: The Basic Science of Poisons,* 3rd ed., Macmillan, New York, 1986.

MOLECULAR BIOCHEMISTRY
of
HUMAN DISEASE

Volume I

Basis of Abnormal Biochemical Mechanisms
Abnormalities of Protein Synthesis and Metabolism
Abnormalities of Lipid Synthesis and Metabolism
Abnormalities of Carbohydrate Synthesis and Metabolism
Abnormalities of Nucleic Acid and Purine or Pyrimidine
Synthesis and Metabolism

Volume II

Abnormalities of Water and Electrolyte Metabolism
Abnormalities of Trace Element Metabolism
Abnormalities of Cellular Organization
Glossary
Appendix

Volume III

Inflammation
Atherosclerosis
Liver Diseases
Diseases of the Nervous System

TABLE OF CONTENTS

Chapter 1

INFLAMMATION

I. INTRODUCTION

In health, an ordered interaction is maintained between cells, microcirculation, and extracellular fluid and such equilibrium is expressed as normal tissue homeostasis. Following injury, this homeostasis is disrupted and inflammation develops as a local reaction of the living tissue. Inflammation is the complex process by which the body responds to cellular damage; it attempts to localize, overcome, and eventually to repair this damage. The inflammatory process begins following a sublethal injury to tissue and ends with complete healing. Between the onset of injury and healing, a variety of cells are mobilized which undergo changes. Much of the inflammatory response is nonspecific and when it is turned on, all mechanisms operate at once. Inflammation also tends to prevent the dissemination of the lesion. If it is due to bacteria, the spread of the infection is blocked. Generally speaking, the more intense the reaction, the more likely is that the infection will be localized. The inflammatory process, essentially a defense mechanism, is aimed at preserving the viability of living tissues. While the inflammatory process is a beneficial response by the tissue, the processes associated with inflammation result in pain. Inflammation is quite a damaging event and sometimes leads not to healing, but to morbidity and death.[460]

Inflammation is the most common manifestation of disease, hence, it is one of the most important disorders and the most responsive to treatment. The widespread occurrence of inflammatory disorders stems from the fact that (1) many diseases are inflammatory in nature; (2) many secondary manifestations of basically noninflammatory diseases are also caused by primary inflammation processes (e.g., ulcer, cirrhosis); and (3) tissues dying from any cause often elicit an inflammatory reaction in the surrounding tissue. Therefore, signs of inflammation are present to some degree in nearly all diseases. In addition, inflammation is a normal and essential protective response against noxious stimuli that threaten the host to a certain extent, ranging from localized reactions to complex responses involving the whole organism.

Inflammatory reactions have four components: (1) trauma, (2) injury to local or ciculating cells, (3) release of inflammation mediators, and (4) tissue responses connected with the clinical signs and symptoms of the disease. Trauma causes cellular injury which leads to the adherence of inflammation mediators to the site of injury. These mediators in turn induce tissue responses responsible for the manifestation of the inflammatory process. In some instances, the trauma stimulates the production of inflammation mediators which act directly on the plasma and activate the kinin or complement system. Mediators can directly produce clinical signs such as erythema and burning sensation.

Acute inflammation is caused by the direct action of irritants (bacteria, chemicals, physical damage, irradiation, and many other causes), and the subsequent attempt by the body or tissue to remove the irritant and restore the homeostasis.[394] The first requisite for healing is the complete elimination of the harmful chemical or physical agent, or destruction of bacteria. Neither an inflammatory lesion nor a wound can heal if it still contains the corrosive chemical, a foreign body, or if it is infected. Dead fragments of tissue are removed through degradation by macrophages or by proteolysis. When this step has been accomplished, the process of healing can start, followed by sequential steps of repair. We use the word repair contemplating the fact that in this sense the human body has no replacement parts. If part of the kidney or any other organ is destroyed by inflammation, or another pathological process, the injured tissue is not replaced by new kidney tissue, but by scar

TABLE 1
Connective Tissue: Morphology and Composition

Cells	Fibers	Ground substance
Fibroblast	Collagen	Glycosaminoglycan
Chondroblast	Elastin	Hyaluronic acid
Osteoblast	Reticulin	Chondroitin
Odontoblast		Chondroitin sulfate A, B, C
Synovioblast		Dermatan sulfate
		Keratan sulfate
		Heparin
		Heparitin sulfate
		Proteoglycan
		Glycoprotein
		Soluble collagen
		Soluble elastin

Note: All connective tissue cells secrete collagen, elastin, reticulin, various glycosa-minoglycans (acid mucopolysaccharides), and glycoproteins.[25] Collagens have high glycine and lysine contents and two unique amino acids, hydroxyproline and hydroxylysine.[23,301] Reticulin contains a high percentage of collagen-like protein. Elastin is characterized by two specific amino acids, desmosine and isodesmosine, which have a ring structure and form bridges in a three-dimensional network.[361] Ground substance is heterogeneous and may arise locally or from the plasma.[383,461] The composition of the basement membrane is similar to the ground substance.[289]

tissue. With advancing age, degrading tissues can merely be replaced by scar tissue, which consists of strong and densely layered connective tissue fibers. Thus, connective tissue cannot substitute the original organ in the functional sense, and its composition reflects the change from tissues which possess diverse metabolic function and serve particular roles (Table 1).

Rheumatic diseases are characteristic examples of chronic inflammatory conditions. These chronic diseases appear as complex autoimmune processes affecting the connective tissue.[6] The changes differ from those of the controlled acute disease which is associated with a balanced proliferation of the connective tissue cells.[181] These diseases include rheumatoid arthritis, rheumatic fever, osteoarthritis, psoriasis, ankylosing spondylitis, and systemic lupus erythematosus among others. There are conditions connected with chronic inflammations involving single or multiple organ systems in the body.

Gout or gouty arthritis also belongs to the group of chronic inflammatory diseases, where abnormally high amounts of uric acid are present in the blood and often in the urine. When sodium urate concentration exceeds the solubility limits in the extracellular fluid, deposits are formed in tissues. Deposition of urate microcrystals in joints or adjacent tissues is followed by acute and chronic inflammatory response. The raised extracellular concentration of urate is due either to an enhanced metabolic production or to a reduced urinary clearance.

II. EFFECT OF INJURY ON THE CELL

Physical or chemical stimuli can disturb cellular homeostasis causing injury to the cell. Such disturbances may be transient and rapidly restored or adapted by the cell with no subsequent effects on homeostatic balance. In some instances, the disturbance may be more prolonged, and the cell responds with a series of structural and functional modifications before homeostasis is restored. However, when the integrated cell activity is irreversibly altered and cannot maintain homeostatic control, cell death results. Degradation of dead cells leads to necrosis. Necrosis represents autolytic reactions which break up the cell into individual components as a result of the action of endogenous hydrolytic enzymes predominantly localized in lysosomes. The necrotic process includes denaturation of proteins, modification of cell pH, and significant shifts in water content and electrolyte distribution.[457]

The primary effect of injury on the cell is the alteration of the normal relationship between cell membrane activities and cell energy metabolism. In mammalian cells, the cellular volume and electrolyte composition are regulated by the activity of membrane bound ATP-ases, usually regarded as membrane electrolyte pumps. These counteract with a tendency to reach equilibrium associated with the presence of negatively charged, nondiffusible macromolecules, predominantly proteins, which exist in both sides of the membrane.[337] If the membrane pump is impaired, the cellular electrolyte and water contents are increased to be equilibrated in both sides of the membrane.[385]

Complement lysis renders the membrane more permeable to ions, causing sodium influx and potassium efflux, and in turn stimulating Na^+/K^+-ATP-ase. This enzyme uses ATP and inorganic phosphate. ATP and inorganic phosphate enhance mitochondrial phosphorylation which uses up oxygen. If oxygen capacity is limited, the increased intracellular sodium ultimately causes inhibition of mitochondrial function and eventual disruption of cellular regulatory mechanisms. Should the sodium leak exhaust the handling capacity of the pump, the control of cell volume regulation is lost resulting in cellular swelling. Further changes in membrane permeability lead to loss of magnesium and influx of calcium. Calcium entry into the cell is associated with immediate structural changes, especially in sensitive tissues such as the heart.[526] The excess calcium is accumulated in mitochondria in the form of calcium phosphate precipitate.[184] The activity of Na^+/K^+-ATP-ase can also be modified by inhibitors such as ouabain, hypoxia, or metabolic changes that diminish oxidative phosphorylation and decrease ATP supply.[460] Anoxia or the presence of inhibition of the electron-transport system cause an acute reduction of ATP synthesis, and as a consequence, many metabolic processes become modified.

A. ACUTE CELL INJURY

The course of reactions in the cell to injury shows a sequence of changes in cellular organelles.[395,453] The initial response is dependent upon the causative physical, chemical, or microbiological agents evoking the different responses. Ultimately, however, the pathway of restitution to normal conditions or to final changes leading to necrosis is relatively independent from the nature of the injury. Thus, common patterns suggest that cellular organelles undergo similar changes during the inflammatory process.

Many stages can be defined in the process of acute cell injury. Following the effect of an injurious agent, the normal vascular perfusion of the cell is altered and oxygen intake is promptly reduced. Thus the initial cellular changes include decreased pO_2, the production of internal substrates is limited, and the removal of metabolites and other cell byproducts is decreased. This is rapidly continued by a decrease and consequent stoppage of respiratory processes which in turn cause a decreased intracellular ATP level. By way of a temporary compensation, the production of ATP is shifted to the glycolytic pathway.[262,513] This results in elevated lactate levels and an associated decrease in glycogen levels, increased rate of glycolysis, and lower intracellular pH. The fall in ATP concentration exerts a decrease in the activity of the electrolyte pump, and the concentration gradients for sodium, potassium, calcium, and magnesium are impaired leading to leakage of these ions. In later stages, the fall in ATP impairs ion transport across the cell membrane responsible for the maintenance of the normal extra- and intracellular equilibrium. The decreased pH also affects nuclear chromatin and nuclear RNA synthesis.[279]

Shortly after the onset of ischemic injury, mitochondria lose their matrix granules, the endoplasmic reticulum is dilated, and microvilli become distorted. These events can be

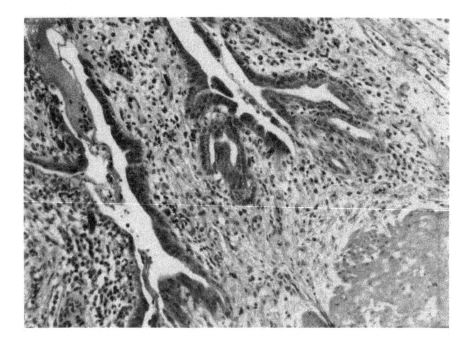

PLATE 1.   In chronic cholecystitis, deep Rokitansky-Aschoff sinuses are seen with chronic inflammatory cells infiltrating the stroma.

followed by electron microscopic studies. As the pH of the cell is lowered, a gradual decrease in the rate of glycolysis and fall in cellular ATP concentration occurs. This is reflected by decreased activities of many systems that require ATP such as electrolyte pump and protein synthesis. These changes are reversible at this point, but they become irreversible when enhanced permeability of mitochondrial inner membranes and swelling paralleled with influx of sodium and calcium content occur. The damage to the inner membrane is connected with release of phospholipids and fatty acids resulting from phospholipase action on these membranes.[45] In the endoplasmic reticulum, although ribosomes remain bound, the protein synthesis becomes defective. Changes in membrane stability are manifest by a whorl formation. These changes characterize toxic actions in the liver cell and in renal tubular cells.[399,459]

Irreversible changes become more evident in stages leading to necrosis. These changes are characterized by massive swelling of all mitochondria, marked increase in membrane permeability associated with leakage of proteins, cytosolic and membrane bound enzymes, and cofactors.[229] This stage is followed by rapid increase in the digestion of intracellular constituents associated with decreases in protein, RNA and DNA, and increases in free amino acids as well as acid soluble phosphates.

B. CHRONIC CELL INJURY

Some types of cell injury do not cause cell death, but induce prolonged changes which represent altered steady stages. In this state, interactions between cellular constituents and cell organelles can result in chronic cell injury which can also be reversible or irreversible. The morphological appearance of chronic inflammatory conditions is illustrated on Plates 1 and 2. Chronic inflammatory reactions can modify the cell structure (Plate 3).

In advanced lesions, the cell membrane shows diverse structural distortions. A variety of conditions modify the permeability of the cell membrane and influence membrane transport, including disorders of water and electrolyte movements and specific transport defects for various substrates. These membrane lesions can be congenital or acquired. Acquired lesions are often derived from toxic interactions. Aminoaciduria is associated with defects

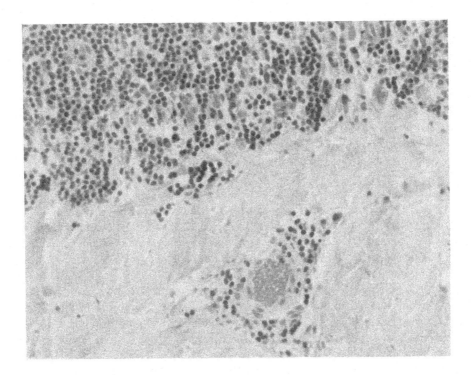

PLATE 2.   In chronic pericarditis, markedly thickened pericardium is seen with chronic inflammatory infiltrate.

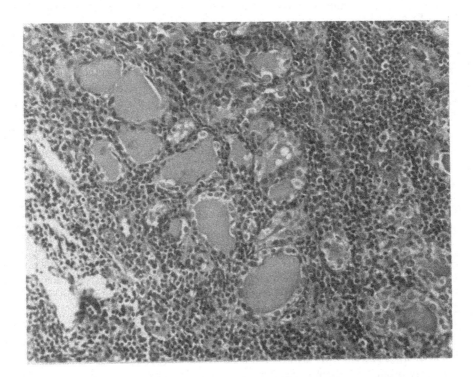

PLATE 3.   In subacute thyroiditis, the micrograph shows thyroid acini of varying size containing eosinophil colloid. Chronic inflammatory reaction is seen in the interacinar stroma.

in amino acid transport by the proximal tubular cells in the kidney.[71] Lead toxicity can cause membrane transport defects.[152] The erythrocyte membrane, especially, is very sensitive and shows cation transport defects in many disease conditions, such as various types of hemolytic anemias (sickle cell anemia, congenital hemolytic anemia), malaria, heavy metal poisoning, and digitalis poisoning. In cystic fibrosis and in syndromes related to burns, uremia, or shock, abnormalities of red cell transport have also been observed. In alcoholics, the so-called Zieve syndrome, plasma and erythrocyte membrane abnormalities are caused by changes in osmotic fragility due to abnormalities of membrane lipids.[271] Neoplasmic transformations and virus infections are associated with chronic modifications of the cell surface properties.[60,492]

Alterations in cell shape, particularly in the red cells, have been discussed in Volume II, Chapter 3. Myelin represents a special case, and changes in myelin occur in many disorders of the central and peripheral nervous systems, such as allergic encephalitis, neuritis, and multiple sclerosis,[266,375] and in axonal reactions appearing after traumatic or surgical interruption of central or peripheral axons. In cerebral edema, the myelin changes include separation of lamellae into granular vesicles and debris.

In chronic cell injury, many cellular cytoplasmic organelles show abnormalities. A variety of inflammatory factors induces dramatic changes involving the formation of a larger number of smaller mitochondria under some conditions and of a fewer number but larger mitochondria in others. Large mitochondria show irregular shape with disorganized cristae and paracrystalline inclusions in the inner compartment. The cause of megamitochondria production has been attributed to aging,[433] vitamin deficiency (vitamin E, riboflavin, thiamine),[283,447,521] essential fatty acid deficiency,[23] choline,[443] copper and iron deficiency,[90,516] alcoholism, and kidney hypertrophy.[230] The exact significance of these changes is not known, although in certain cases mitochondrial metabolism is reduced, whereas megamitochondria show normal function in some instances.

Inhibition of ferrochelatase activity localized only in mitochondria is connected with chronic lead toxicity.[161] Inhibition of this enzyme causes accumulation of iron pigments in mitochondria of the bone marrow. Lead poisoning also results in chronic mitochondrial lesion in kidney tubules, associated with the Fanconi syndrome due to intoxication.[3] Cardiac myopathy brought about by cobalt ingestion results in chronic defects of heart mitochondria involving pyruvate decarboxylase activity.

Among other cytoplasmic organelles, chronic cell injury causes numerous and diverse action on the endoplasmic reticulum. This organelle responds to injury with dilatation, and it is interrelated with increased sodium and decreased potassium content of the cell caused by malfunctioning of the sodium pump.[431,458] Further manifestations include changes in the hepatic endoplasmic reticulum membranes and associated ribosomes as a consequence of the action of toxic or carcinogenic chemicals. These lesions appear to be irreversible following the action of carcinogens. Various drugs, insecticides, pesticides, food additives, and carcinogenic compounds initiate the induction of endoplasmic reticulum membranes and increase enzyme and phospholipid synthesis. Toxic compounds cause concentric whorls and cluster formation, membrane lipid peroxidation, and membrane denaturation. During chronic injury, the Golgi apparatus is also dilated and fragmented. Details of subcellular membrane changes brought about by chronic effects are found in Volume II, Chapter 3.

Major changes associated with inflammation occur in lysosomes which contain various substances propagating the inflammatory response.[7,184,318,319,502,503] The mediator substances are then discharged and enzymes are also released, converting precursors to active mediators. The lysis of lysosomal membranes may happen through the detergent action of lysolecithins, which are essential components of membranes, or by the direct action of external labilizing agents, or by a selective intracellular rupture. Disruption of lysosomal membranes alone can produce an acute or chronic inflammatory reaction. Lysosomal enzymes may be released at sites where membrane-associated antigen-antibody complexes are formed. Secretion of specific lysosomal enzymes can also occur from macrophages during phagocytosis without marked membrane damage.

III. THE PHASES OF INFLAMMATION

There are two major phases in the mechanism of the inflammatory process. The first is the vascular phase which includes vasodilatation, increased vascular permeability and hyperemia, slow blood flow, stasis, and interior thrombosis. The second phase involves the formation of inflammatory exudates together with the release of mediators, edema, swelling, cellular infiltration, leukocytosis, and phagocytosis. Following these phases, the healing process starts, essentially by means of connective tissue proliferation.

Dilation and increased permeability of arterioles and venules show fundamental alterations underlying the inflammatory response. These vascular changes modify the cell structure and are associated with impairment of cell functions. As a response to altered cellular homeostasis, interrelated and organized dynamic biochemical processes are set in motion in successive phases to restore normal conditions. However, many steps of the inflammatory process may occur simultaneously.

A. VASCULAR CHANGES
1. Hyperemia and Blood Flow Impairment
Immediately following injury, hyperemia occurs and it is confined to the site of injury. Hyperemia is followed by a fall in blood velocity and, with mild injury, the development of stasis may take several hours. If the injury is severe, a complete standstill of the blood flow develops almost instantaneously. The vessels first affected are the small capillaries and venules in which the earliest change is seepage of plasma from the blood into the adjacent tissue and denser racking of the red cells. This change represents an increase in blood viscosity and accordingly, the blood flow gradually decreases until it stops completely. Thus, stasis appears to be the result of a severe injury to the blood-tissue barrier as a consequence of markedly increased permeability and rapid exudation of plasma. Platelets are the primary agents in the formation of hemostatic plugs arresting the bleeding from injured capillaries and venules. Quantitative defects in platelet formation or lack of their production can give rise to defective hemostasis.

2. Local Structural Changes
Many immediate structural changes occur at the local site of damage within a short time after injury. In the inflamed tissue we can see dilatation of small blood vessels and capillaries. As a consequence, there is a significant influx of blood into the area, containing great numbers of erythrocytes and leukocytes. In the dilated blood vessel the blood flow becomes slower and leukocytes adhere along the vessel walls. The accumulation of red cells is manifested clinically as erythema. The inflammatory response appears in a diphasic increase of vascular permeability and shows intravascular and extravascular changes (Figure 1). The fastest reaction is vasodilatation causing the permeability to increase at the level of the vascular wall. Small molecules leak out together with plasma fluid and enter the extravascular space in increasing amounts. The abnormal accumulation of fluid leads to edema. The peak of this immediate response is at about 30 min and progresses to a latent phase after about 2 h. Within 2 to 4 h, the vascular permeability becomes more marked and another wave of fluid loss occurs causing severe edema formation. This fluid carries large molecules from the plasma into the surrounding tissue including fibrinogen, which is transformed to fibrin in the course of the clotting process. During the initial period, polymorphonuclear leukocytes start invading the injured area. Examples of polymorphs infiltration are shown in Plates 4 to 7.

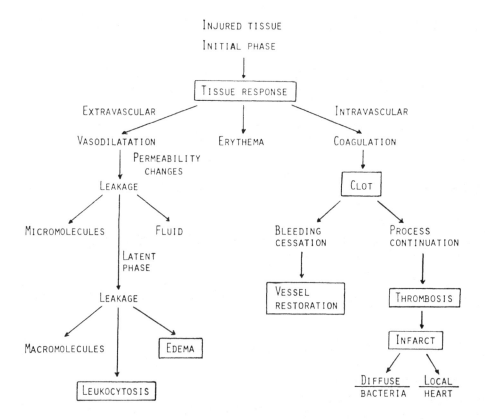

FIGURE 1.   Events occurring during the phases of acute inflammation. This flow chart shows the pathway of intra- and extravascular changes, and the formation of inflammatory exudate containing tissue fluid, micro- and macromolecules, leukocytes, and fragments or fluid derived form the agent causing tissue injury.

3. Blood Cell Migration

During the first stages of inflammation, polymorphonuclear leukocytes constitute the dominant cell type at the local tissue site. These cells are released from the bone marrow and their discharge is stimulated by factors originating from the site of injury (Figure 2). The nature of these factors has not been clearly identified. After the initial period of about 8 h the number of polymorphonuclear leukocytes decreases, and mononuclear cells collect in greater amounts. These cells are derived from circulating monocytes. The mechanism of release differs from that of polymorphonuclear cells. The bone marrow supplies the monocytes, but the release is induced directly by monocytogenic factors originating from lymph nodes. Following the inflammatory process, some materials from the site of injury enter the local lymph nodes causing hypertrophy of these small glands. These reactive, stimulated lymph nodes release transformed lymphocytes which produce several chemical substances essential for defensive processes. One of these factors is the monocytogenic factor stimulating the release of monocytes. When monocytes appear at the site of injury, they then initiate the release of the mitogenic factor from the lymphocytes. The mitogenic factor triggers off the process of proliferation and cell division at an accelerated rate. During chronic inflammation, the transformed lymphocytes are responsible for the initiation of the immune defense reaction.

The time course of erythrocyte and leukocyte accumulation and that of the biphasic increase of vascular permeability are different (Figure 3). Although the inflammatory response is biphasic, there are differences in the duration. The initial response lasts no longer than 2 h; the delayed response starts some time after 2 h and usually takes 10 to 12 h, but

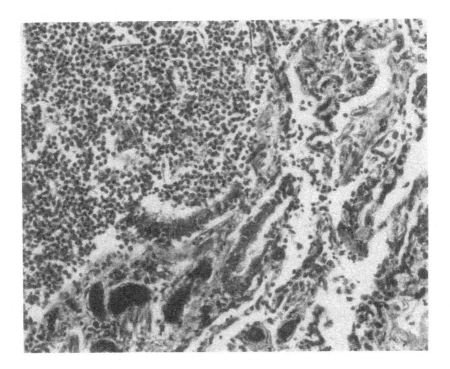

PLATE 4. In bronchopneumonia, dense collection of polymorphs are seen filling alveoli.

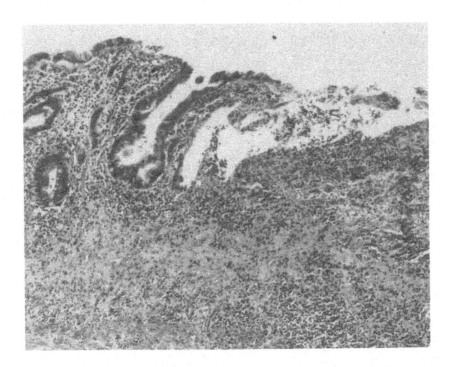

PLATE 5. In ulcerative colitis, the mucosa is ulcerated and densely infiltrated with polymorphs. The glands reveal reduced mucine secreting activity.

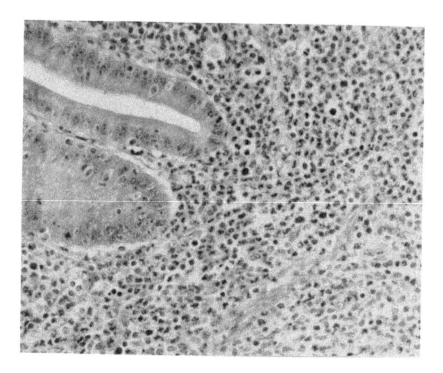

PLATE 6.   In acute diffuse suppurative appendicitis, the mucosa of the appendix is densely infiltrated by polymorphs.

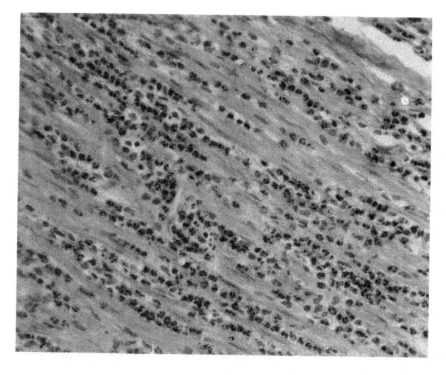

PLATE 7.   In acute diffuse appendicitis, the muscular layer shows dense polymorphonuclear infiltration.

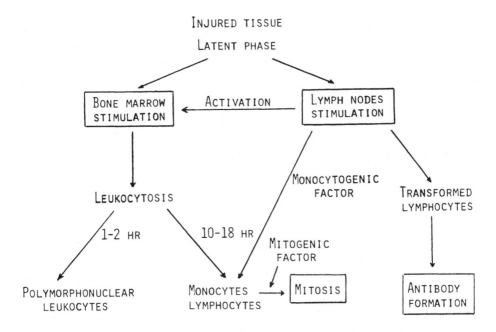

FIGURE 2.   The stages of inflammatory response. This chart illustrates the time course of changes in the type of leukocytes migrating to the site of injury, and the feedback of bone marrow stimulation characteristic of the acute phase; continued stimulation of this tissue and additional participation of lymph nodes, delayed phase; and potent stimulation of lymph nodes resulting in the restoration of the normal tissue or antibody formation, chronic phase.

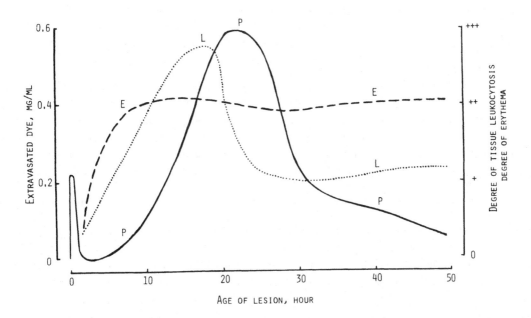

FIGURE 3.   Time course of changes in acute inflammation. The inflammatory reaction is produced in the skin of the guinea pig by UV irradiation. Differences are seen in the onset of these responses between vascular permeability, (P); erythema, (E); and leukocytosis, (L).

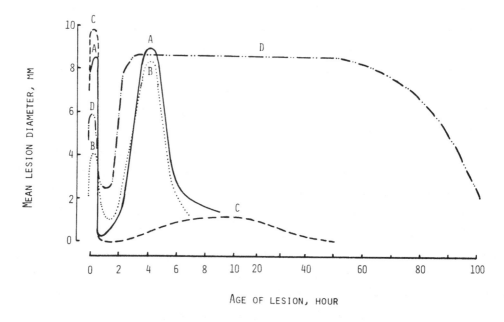

FIGURE 4.   Patterns of vascular permeability changes. These responses are induced by various types of injury in the skin of the guinea pig: (A) thermal injury, exposure to 54°C for 20 s; (B) acute bacterial infection; (C) chemical injury with xylol; (D) vibrio cholerae toxin.

it may be extended to over 90 h. The pattern of these responses is also related to the type of injury (Figure 4). Moreover, the nature of the irritant affects the tissue reaction, becoming apparent in permeability changes and intensity of leukocyte migration (Figure 5). The time difference has no influence on the action of leukocytes. Their adsorption to the vessel makes the vascular walls looser in texture and then leukocytes can pass through them into the neighboring tissue by means of diapedesis. Thus, a great number of leukocytes accumulate in the tissue immediately outside the vessels, setting in motion the attack action on bacteria and other irritants, mediated by phagocytosis and by release of the various chemicals which influence the function of many cell components.

The presence of leukocytes is also important as a primary response to bacteria. Polymorphonuclear leukocytes internalize bacteria which are slowly digested by phagocytosis. In addition, the serum contains antibacterial substances which paralyze the microorganism and enhances the task of the leukocytes. Antitoxic substances are also present which destroy the toxins secreted by the bacteria.

The degree and duration of the primary inflammatory response largely depends on the injuring microorganism and the nature of bacterial toxins. *Staphylococci* and some Gram-negative bacteria cause only small tissue injury, but elicit a very marked capillary response. These germs produce potent exotoxins which are secreted into injured cells and endotoxins which are intracellular. Both types of toxins can cause severe cell reactions in the infected host. On the other hand, *Mycobacterium tuberculosis* and similar organisms are not so irritant, and toxins produced are not so potent.

4. Thrombosis

Parallel with the extravascular events, changes take place within the vessels. The formation of intravascular clots in the inner lining of the vessel stops the loss of blood into surrounding tissue and therefore saves the tissue from further deterioration. There is a great similarity between the mechanisms involved in the formation of a hemostatic plug and a thrombus. A thrombus can be considered as the abnormal product of a normal mechanism leading to a deposit or mass formed from blood constituents on the surface of blood vessels.

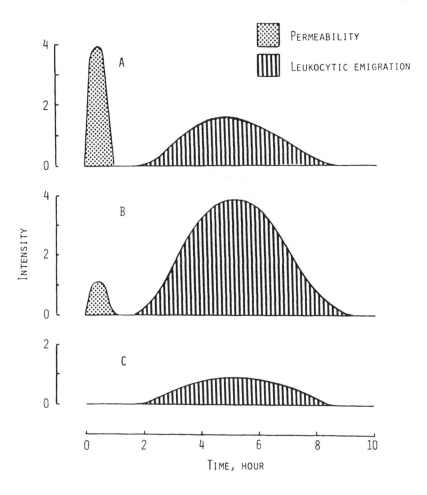

FIGURE 5. Effect of various intradermal irritations on initial inflammatory responses. The time course and degree of vascular permeability show differences following a single intradermal injection of (A) histamine, (B) serum, or (C) physiological saline solution.

Thrombi may be formed anywhere in the circulation, either in the capillaries, arteries, veins, or chambers of the heart. They are usually attached to the endothelial surface of the vessel or to the lining of the heart. A mural thrombus adheres only to one side of the vessel and the blood continues to flow past the thrombus. However, if the entire lumen of the vessel is sealed by the clot, the ensuing occlusive thrombosis leads to a complete cut-off of the blood supply to the tissue. Thus depending on the importance of the thrombosed vessel, this event will lead to the death of the organ. This process is the infarction which occurs after extensive thrombosis or embolus blocking the circulation in an end artery. Sometimes diffuse clot formation of small vessels throughout a whole organ can have fatal consequences. This situation occurs frequently in patients with bacteremia, as they stimulate the process of an extensive blood coagulation. Consequently, in organs such as the kidney or the lung, the microcirculation becomes plugged with clots causing a sudden loss of supply vital constituents and subsequent immediate deterioration of function. If the diffuse, multiple thrombosis is severe and involves the greater part of an organ, the patient may die from shock.

B. INFLAMMATORY EXUDATE

The inflammatory response is mediated by chemical substances affecting mainly the microcirculatory vessels. These substances are derived from leukocytes, serum, and tissue

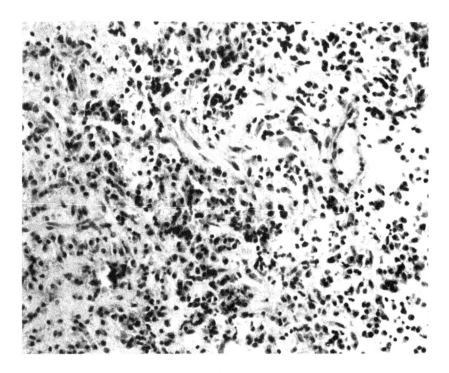

PLATE 8.   The micrograph shows inflammatory granulation tissue with lymphocytes, blood vessels, and several capillaries.

fluids, thereby forming the inflammatory exudate. The inflammatory exudate is responsible for swelling which is one of the cardinal features of inflammation.[265]

The swelling causes tension and pressure on the nerves of the inflamed area; this is the warning signal if a vital organ such as the heart is partially infarcted. The biphasic response of acute inflammatory processes is related to the production of different chemicals in the exudate.[453] These chemical mediators are histamine, the kinins, and prostaglandins.[46] The production of these compounds is associated with complex reactions involving a number of intermediate substances, the nature of which is not yet fully clear. The activation of the collagenase system has been suggested as triggering off the mechanism.[210] Other observations favor the view that stimulation of the complement system leads to the production of vasoactive factors. The role of this step as the trigger mechanism in acute inflammation has been considered.[101,102,144,515] An interaction between inflammatory cells, including granulocytes and lymphocytes, and blood vessels, is shown in Plate 8.

C. MEDIATORS

Inflammatory mediators are endogenous substances whose levels increase at the site of injury in association with the tissue response or structural damage. These mediators can be grouped into several categories according to their action: (1) direct acting mediators, such as histamine, serotonin, bradykinin, and prostaglandins which act through receptor binding; (2) lipid mediators (autocoids) and potent pharmacologically active substances; (3) lytic enzymes of plasma or cell origin which directly affect the integrity of the tissue and circulating cells; and (4) chemotactic factors which stimulate cell migration to the site of injury.

The inflammatory reactions result from the combined action of several mediators.[239] There are, however, specific differences between the various mediators.[38] One particular mediator may be more important for the whole process or for specific cellular organelles (Figure 6). The difference in the inflammatory response depends on the relative proportion of the different types of mediators released and on the duration of their release.

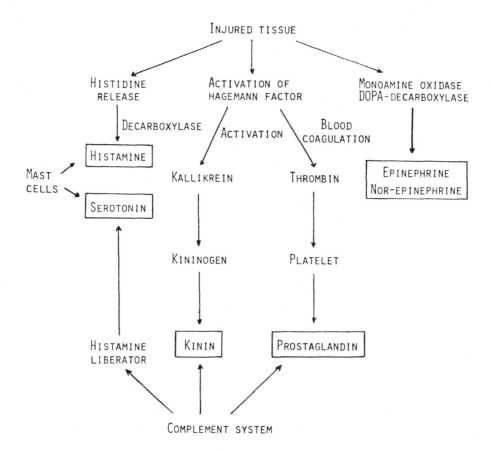

FIGURE 6. Release of mediators during acute inflammation. The immediate phase is triggered off by histidine and serotonin; the delayed phase by kinins and prostaglandins. The activation of kinins and prostaglandin-like substances and release of histamine activators in inflammation are also associated with the intact complement system. Through the vasodilatory action of these mediators, vascular permeability is increased and fluid and plasma molecules enter into the extracellular space. By the simultaneous discharge of inactivating enzymes, the vasoconstrictory effect of epinephrine and norepinephrine is eliminated.

Most chemical mediators of the acute inflammatory process have been highly purified, the chemical structures identified, and these compounds have been synthesized. Cell-derived mediators originate from various sources. Most cells contain preformed mediators in lysosomal or granular constituents, and they are released after cell stimulation or injury. Some mediators are common in many cell types, but many mediators are released only after a specific stimulation of a particular cell type, such as lymphokines or monokines.

D. VASOACTIVE AMINES
1. Histamine

The vasoactive amines, histamine and 5-hydroxytryptamine (serotonin), are relatively simple compounds and widely distributed in various tissues.[34,240,256,381,436,437] Histamine is the principal mediator of the inflammatory response to injury[438] and exerts both pro- and anti-inflammatory effects. Pharmacological actions, including alteration of the blood pressure, development of tissue edema, and effects on smooth muscle response, are shared with a variety and structurally unrelated compounds: serotonin, prostaglandins, and kinins. The involvement of these compounds is essential in the development of the inflammatory response.

Histamine is synthesized and stored mainly in mast cells. To a lesser extent, it is also

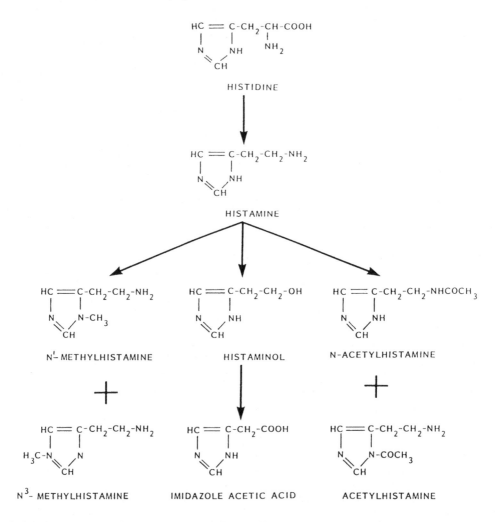

FIGURE 7.   Pathways of histamine synthesis and metabolism. The conversion of L-histidine to histamine is catalyzed by L-histidine decarboxylase (1). Histamine is metabolized by two alternative routes: histamine N-methyl transferase (2) or histaminase and monoamine oxidase (3). Methylimidazole acetic acid and imidazole acetic acid riboside have also been identified as minor metabolites. The relative importance of these pathways varies in different species. In man, ring N-methylation accounts for most of histamine loss; similarly, in dog, cat, and mouse, this is the major pathway. Rat metabolizes histamine by oxidation.[34]

formed from histidine by the action of histidine decarboxylase[277,403] (Figure 7). In the blood, the basophils are the predominant carriers of histamine, localized in cytoplasmic granules.[522] Mast cells and basophils also contain heparin. Histamine is bound to heparin by electrostatic forces through carboxylic groups and form a protein complex within these granules.[465] The major routes of metabolism involve methylation and oxidation,[404,523] and in man, the major metabolic route is ring N-methylation. Aspirin was found to inhibit imidazole acetic acid conjugation in therapeutic doses.[34]

Antihistamines prevent histamine binding to H_1 receptor sites. The stimulation of gastric acid secretion by histamine is an exception; in general, antihistamines do not block receptor binding of histamine to gastric H_2 receptors. Almost all antihistamines are alkyl substituted ethylamines[107] and inhibit physiological changes produced by histamine due to their structural similarity. The effect of antihistamines is greatest 1 h after administration, and their action is almost absent after 3 h.

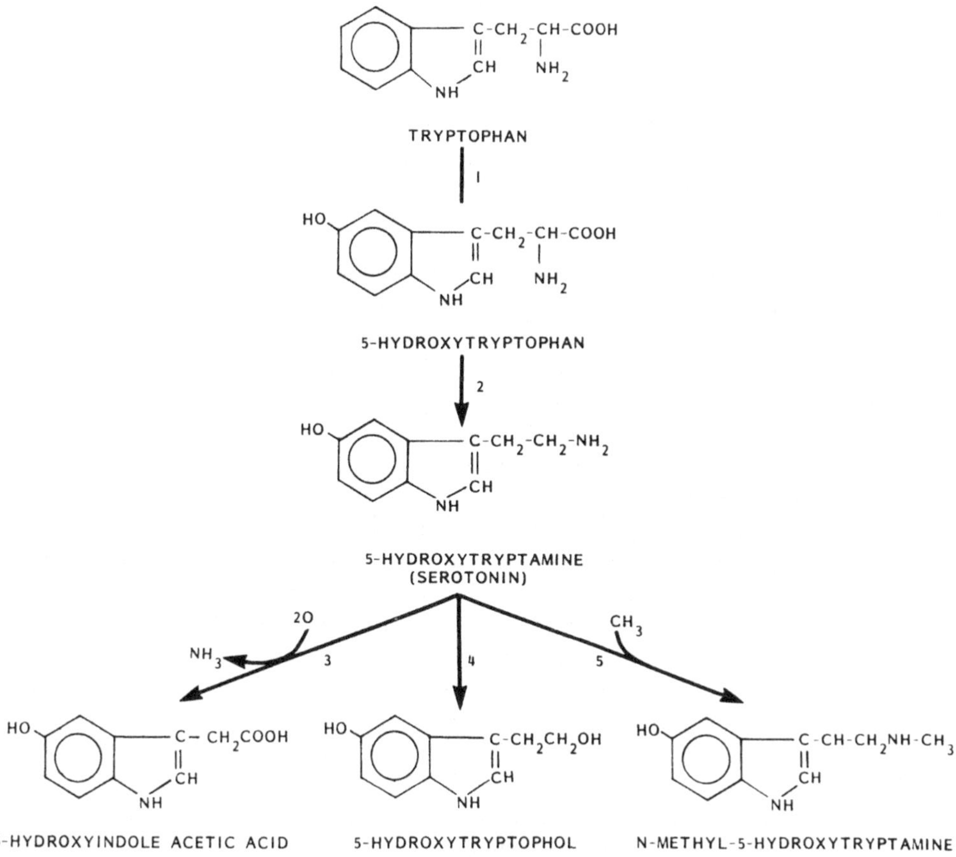

FIGURE 8. Pathways of 5-hydroxytryptamine (serotonin) synthesis and metabolism. Tryptophan is hydroxylated by hydroxylase (1) to form 5-hydroxytryptophan which is then decarboxylated by decarboxylase to 5-hydroxtryptamine (2). The most important route in the metabolism of 5-hydroxytryptamine is the degradation by monoamine oxidase (3) to 5-hydroxyindoleacetaldehyde, most of which is oxidized to 5-hydroxyindoleacetic acid. Some of the 5-hydroxyindoleacetaldehyde is reduced to 5-hydroxytryptophol by alcohol dehydrogenase (4), which is eliminated from the tissues as glucuronic acid and sulfuric acid conjugates. Minor pathway leads to methylated products (4). Little amount of 5-hydroxytryptamine is excreted in the urine in free form and some as conjugate.

2. Serotonin

5-Hydroxytryptamine occurs in a wide variety of tissues, and the most important localization is the gastrointestinal tract and brain, particularly associated with the enterochromaffin cells of the intestinal mucosa. Carcinoid tumors of these cells often contain very high concentrations of serotonin, and in the blood, serotonin is mainly bound to platelets. There are significant species differences in the histamine/serotonin content of mast cells; whereas histamine is a major vasoactive substance in man, rodent mast cells contain high serotonin levels.

Serotonin is derived from tryptophan which is first converted to 5-hydroxytryptophan and then decarboxylated to 5-hydroxytryptamine (Figure 8). Hydroxytryptamine is stored in the cells in inactive form and maintained at high concentration levels by active transport. It is located in large granules in the mast cells, adrenal medulla, intestinal mucosa, and in other sites.[139] Serotonin is also released by reserpine from its stores in the brain, platelets, and gastrointestinal tract. The release is relatively slow as compared to the liberation of histamine. The metabolism of 5-hydroxytryptamine follows several routes. The most important pathway is the degradation by monoamine oxidase leading to the main urinary metabolite 5-hydroxyindoleacetic acid.

$$\text{IgE} + \text{Ag} \longrightarrow \text{PROESTERASE} \xrightarrow[1]{\text{Co}^{++}} \text{ESTERASE} \xrightarrow{2} \text{ENERGY} \xrightarrow{3} \text{Ca}^{++} \xrightarrow{4} \text{HISTAMINE}$$

FIGURE 9.   Scheme of sequence of biochemical events involved in the antigen-induced release of histamine from human lung sensitized with immunoglobulin E. The process can be blocked by esterase inhibitors, such as diiso-propyl-fluorophosphate (1), inhibitors of energy production, such as 2-deoxyglucose (2), chelating agents (3), and cyclic AMP (4).[15,239]

Antagonists of 5-hydroxytryptamine exert competitive activity; different classes of antagonists can completely suppress its effects on intestinal and other smooth muscle.[224] Several lysergic acid derivatives have strong effects, the most powerful being lysergic acid diethylamide (LSD). Various antihistamines antagonize the action of 5-hydroxytryptamine on intestinal smooth muscle *in vitro*.[139,440]

3. Mechanism of Histamine and Serotonin Action

The release of histamine involves a cascading series of enzymatic reactions which are not clearly defined. Several of these steps are modulated by cyclic nucleotides, calcium flux, and microtubule control.[34] There are cellular membrane events in the release of mediators, and many stimuli involved have been identified.[290] The most studied conditions are the antigen-induced release, complement-mediated release, and physical stimuli.[350,351]

In antigen-induced release of histamine from mast cells or basophils, the initial step is connected with changes of the external surface of these cell membranes (Figure 9). Both the mast cell and basophilic leukocyte contain receptors specific for immunoglobulin E (IgE).[35,83,87] IgE combines with these cells through the Fc portion of the molecule.[49,83,219,221,222]

Histamine is released at the inflammatory site by two separate mechanisms; either from injured tissue or from mast cells and basophilic leukocytes. When the tissue is damaged, the injured cells release histidine into the exudate which is then immediately decarboxylated by histamine decarboxylase present in normal tissue.[403] This mechanism is responsible for a minor portion of the released histamine. The bulk of histamine is produced by mast cells present in connective tissue layers and concentrated in greatest number in the outer layer (adventitia) of blood vessels.[507] When a lesion occurs, the mast cells release their granular histamine content into the exudate by means of cell degranulation. Serotonin leaks out of the mast cells from the granules.[391] Both of these amines are vasoactive and cause dilatation and/or constriction of blood vessels, especially venules and arterioles. Histamine and serotonin produce the initial change in inflammation responsible for the local dilatation of the blood vessels.[186] In addition, they increase the size of interepithelial pores giving rise to small gaps between endothelial cells. Through these holes the cellular fluid and small molecules can readily and quickly penetrate into the extravascular space. The action is very rapid, reaching a peak at about 30 min following injury.

Mast cells are very sensitive to injury, and a variety of stimuli such as chemicals, bacterial toxins, ionizing radiation, heat, cold, or mechanical trauma can cause degranulation and release of the vasoactive amines. The exact mechanism whereby injury stimulates mast cell degranulation has not yet been solved. There are observations, however, that the activation of surface enzymes rich in amino acid N-terminals and the presence of free sulfhydryl groups are involved in this process.

During the period of acute response, blood vessel constrictors such as epinephrine and norepinephrine are inactivated.[342,414] The inactivation occurs through the actions of the enzymes monoamine oxidase and DOPA decarboxylase which are released from the injured cells. These enzymes block or inactivate the synthesis of epinephrine, and thus prevent vasoconstrictive action by these compounds.[15]

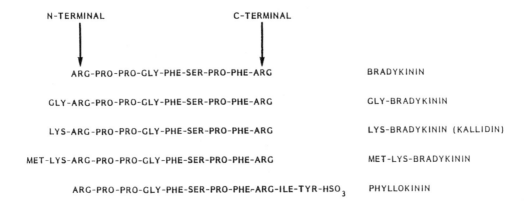

FIGURE 10.   Amino acid sequence of kinins. From a substrate in mammalian plasma, bradykinin, lysylbradykinin, and methionyllysyl-bradykinin are released by proteolytic action, trypsin, kallikrein, and acidification, respectively. Glycine-bradykinin is formed in wasp venom by trypsin. Phyllokinin was isolated from amphibian skin. Bradykinin and lysyl-bradykinin occur in human plasma.[255,402,512]

E. THE KININ-KALLIKREIN SYSTEM
1. Kinins

Kinins are mediators which appear during a late phase of inflammation and their action corresponds to the delayed response.[61,112,434] They play a major role in injury by participation in the increase of vascular permeability, edema formation, pain, and migration and extra-vascular accumulation of leukocytes. Kinins affect arterioles by markedly enhancing their permeability. The Hageman factor is also involved in this complex series of biochemical reactions, leading to blood coagulation.[160]

The kinins are straight chain small polypeptides; the prototype is a nonapeptide, bradykinin[88,115,364] (Figure 10). The other members of this group differ in one or two additional amino acids at the C- or N-terminal.[255,402,512] These polypeptides originate from the plasma and their production is related to lysosomal action. The kinins are produced by proteolytic and esterolytic enzymes (kininogenases)[113] acting on plasma glycoprotein substrates (kininogens).[44,164,166] Kininogenases include various kalikreins as well as trypsin, pepsin, and proteases in snake venoms and bacteria. Kininogenases can hydrolyze peptide bonds at the arginine carboxyl.

2. Kallikreins

These substances are widely distributed in the body occurring as inactive precursors or active substances. They have the greatest hydrolytic activity and substrate specificity and can be divided into plasma and tissue kallikreins.

Plasma kallikrein is a large molecule with a molecular weight of 97,000 Da.[167] It is an immunologically and physicochemically distinct molecule and exists as an inert precursor in the liver. Tissue kallikreins occur in many organs and can be found in secretions or excretions of glands, such as saliva, sweat, tears, pancreatic juice, feces, and urine. The various tissue kallkreins are distinct entities, but they are closely related. Molecular weights of homogeneous kallikreins from submaxillary gland, pancreas, and urine are 32,000, 33,300, and 36,300 Da, respectively.[132] They have different immunological and physicochemical characteristics and susceptibility to protease inhibitors.

Tissue kallikreins are present in active form in excretions or secretions, but they are usually inactive in the parent tissue as prekallikreins.[300,331,494] Prekallikreins are present in active form in the salivary gland; they are located in the secretory granules mainly at the apex of the serous cells. Prekallikreins are, however, inactive in the pancreas and confined to the zymogen granules of the acinar cells. They are activated by trypsin, which involves

TABLE 2
Relationship between Neutral Proteases Derived from Polymorphonuclear Neutrophils and Endogenous Protease Inhibitors[a]

Protease	Inhibitor	Source	Molecular weight ($\times 10^3$ dalton)
Elastase	α-Protease inhibitor	Liver	52
Cathepsin	α-Antichymotrypsin	Liver	68
Elastase	α-Macroglobulin	Liver	725
Cathepsin G		Macrophage	
Collagenase			
Elastase	Mucous proteinase inhibitor	Mucous epithelium	10
Cathepsin G			

[a]   Extracted from References 33, 133, 136, 194, 348, 349, 449, 456, and 510.

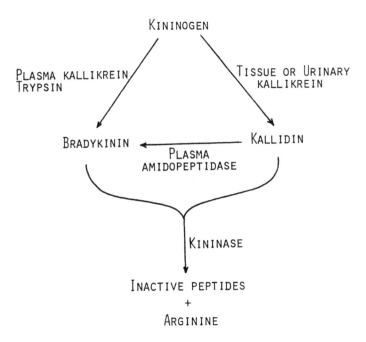

FIGURE 11.   Scheme of the interrelationships between kininogens, kinins, and their breakdown products.

only a minor modification of the molecule, possibly the removal of a steric hindrance from the active site for the substrate. Plasma prekallikreins are activated by the Hageman factor which is identical to factor XII of the blood coagulation system.[68,294,496] (Table 2).

3. Kininogens

Plasma kininogens are glycoproteins with various molecular weights. Until now only two groups of kininogens have been identified.[21,55,165,225,365] Low molecular weight (about 50,000 Da) kininogens I and II yield kallidin when treated with kallikrein isolated from human urine and bradykinin when treated with trypsin (Figure 11). High molecular weight kininogen A of about 200,000 Da, produces kallikrein when treated with urinary kallikrein, and bradykinin when treated with plasma kallikrein or trypsin. High molecular weight kininogen B is only affected by trypsin.

4. Mechanism of Action of the Kallikrein-Kinin System

The cascading events of kinin formation proceed along the following course. During the inflammatory process and due to the vascular injury, cathepsins are released from damaged lysosomes and these enzymes subsequently convert plasma protein-substrates to prekallikreins and kallikreinogen.[183,317] The latter is further converted to kallikrein. The Hageman or contact factor is also stimulated which activates kallikrein.[294] This is a trypsin-like plasma enzyme which, at low pH, cleaves the α_2-globulin polypeptide chain adjacent to a lysine radical to produce kinins (Figure 12).

In normal circumstances, kinins are present in the plasma in the form of inactive precursors. Following injury, a stimulus activates the kinin system, and through a series of biochemical reactions, potent specific compounds are produced; α-globulin is also present in the blood in the form of a precursor glycoprotein and cleavage first yields bradykinin. Kallikrein can also split the kininogen chain at other sites, resulting in two other kinins: lysyl-bradykinin and methionyl-lysylbradykinin. Some other kinins consisting of hexa- to decapeptides have also been identified; they are produced from larger molecules by hydrolysis. Finally, the enzyme kininase transforms these peptides into an inactive form. These kinins have similar biological actions. Methionyl-lysyl-bradykinin exerts a more prolonged effect, probably due to that this compound is more resistant to the metabolic action of kininase.

The proper role and mechanism of action of bradykinin in the inflammatory process has not yet been well clarified. Several functions have been suggested for these substances since they are potent vasodilators, promote leukocyte migration, lower blood pressure, and stimulate smooth muscle. Additionally, they play a role in local pain and part of the allergic reaction or function as local hormones that mediate defense reactions.

The production of kinins is associated with low pH which follows the waning of the acute histamine phase. When bradykinin accumulates in the inflammatory exudate, the marked increase in vascular permeability reoccurs. The migration of polymorphonuclear leukocytes potentiates kinin production probably by activating the plasma kinin generating system. When the pH of the exudate starts shifting to the range of pH 6 to 7, the activity of kininase increases; the kinin generating action of leukocytes diminishes, and the net result is that the kinin concentration decreases. As the action of kinins is worn off, the damaged cells are repaired, and vascular integrity is restored.[495]

F. LIPID MEDIATORS

Lipid mediators are synthesized and released by a wide variety of cell types, including neutrophilic, eosinophilic, and basophilic polymorphonuclear leukocytes, monocytes, mast cells, macrophages, and platelets. These lipid mediators can be grouped into two classes; (1) mediators derived from the arachidonic acid metabolism and (2) acetylated alkyl phosphoglycerides. These mediators and related compounds are now classified as autacoids rather than as mediators. Autacoids represent highly potent pharmacological agents previously described as autopharmacological agents or local hormones.

1. Prostaglandins

Recent studies have shown that prostaglandins are mediators of inflammation, inducing many signs such as erythema, fever, vasodilatation, increased vascular permeability, and induction of pain.[46,54,363] Prostaglandins have been found in several types of inflammatory processes. Substances which antagonize their action or inhibit their synthesis reduce the intensity of inflammation. Prostaglandins act synergistically with other mediators in producing edema. Nonsteroidal anti-inflammatory drugs inhibit prostaglandin, prostacycline, and thromboxane production, whereas antipyretic drugs inhibit prostaglandin generation.[122,123,162]

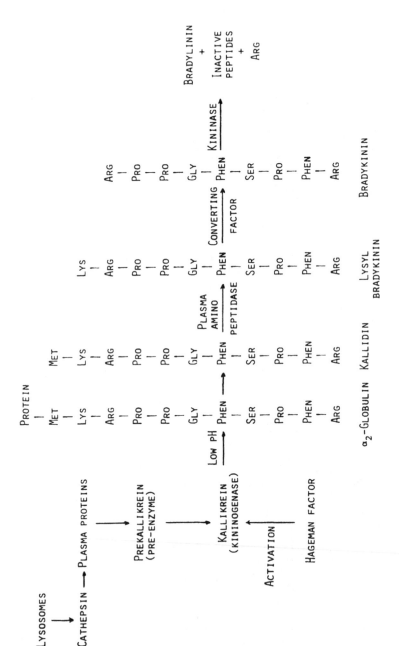

FIGURE 12.   Formation of kinins during the inflammatory process. Sequential activation of various plasma proteolytic and aminopeptidase activities converts α_2-globulin to bradykinin. Further breakdown leads to inactive peptides.

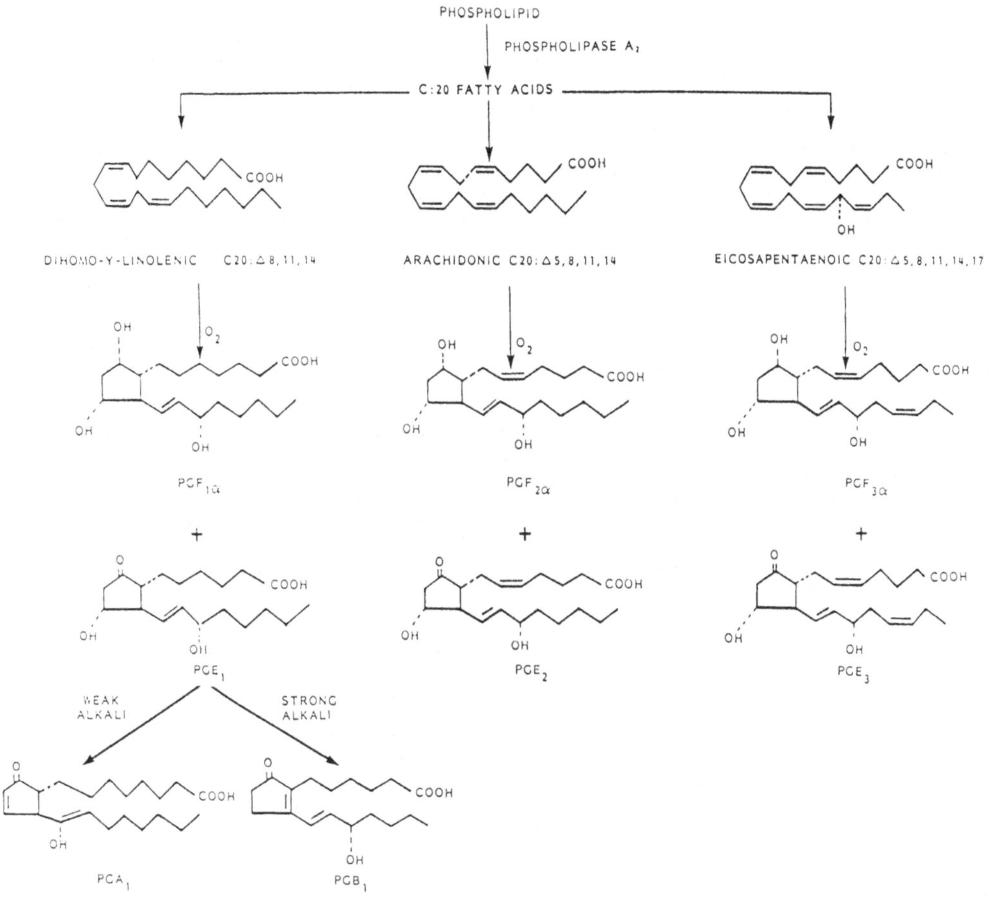

FIGURE 13. Biochemical pathways of prostaglandin synthesis.

There are vascular effects of prostaglandins which differ from the action of other mediators. Their action is sustained, and they counteract the vasoconstriction caused by angiotensin or noradrenaline. The induction of erythema by prostaglandins in cutaneous vessels is long-lasting, sometimes up to 10 h, showing that the duration of release is prolonged.[123] The vasodilator action on other vascular beds, however, only lasts for a few minutes.[200,423] Prostaglandins are released locally, and their effect can be reduced by anti-inflammatory drugs. Prostaglandins elicit direct action on the microvasculature, but not through the release of other endogenous substances such as histamine or serotonin. Swelling (edema) and vasodilatation caused by prostaglandins do not respond to antihistaminics. Parallel with the appearance of prostaglandins, histamine, kinin, and serotonin are also released, correlating with the infiltration of the exudate by leukocytes and tissue responses.

Possible mechanisms involved in the production of prostaglandins during acute inflammation are the liberation of unsaturated fatty acids by phospholipase, cyclization, and conversion of these substances to prostaglandins by the prostaglandin synthetase enzyme. The precursors of prostaglandins are essential fatty acids such as arachidonic acid, eicosapentaenoic acid, or dihomo-γ-linolenic acid (Figure 13). These are released from the cell membrane by membrane-bound phospholipase A_2. From this precursor, and through cyclic endoperoxide intermediates, prostaglandins are formed.[168,345,514] Phospholipase A_2 is released from lysosomes during phagocytosis by leukocytes (Figure 14). Prostaglandins are also derived from platelets, and there is an association between the release of prostaglandins and phospholipases.[171] The production of prostaglandins can be inhibited by nonsteroidal anti-

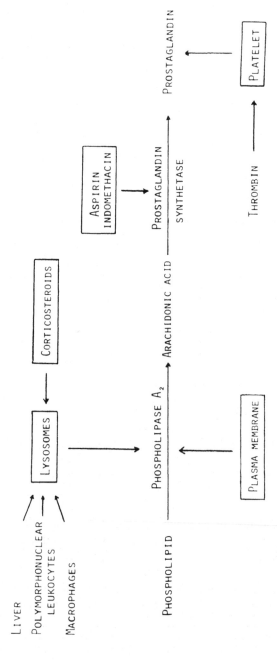

FIGURE 14.   Mechanism of prostaglandin production and release in tissues. During phagocytosis, phospholipase A₂ is released from the lysosomes of leukocytes engaged in phagocytosis. Phospholipase acts on polyunsaturated fatty acids, particularly on arachidonic acid producing prostaglandins. Corticosteroids inhibit the damage to lysosomal membranes in the phagocytosing cell, and the liberation of phospholipase A₂ thus prevent the action of microorganisms. In contrast, nonsteroidal anti-inflammatory agents have limited effects on phagocytic cells. They inhibit prostaglandin synthesis by blocking cyclooxygenase, thus preventing the transformation of arachidonic acid to prostaglandin and thromboxanes (c.f. Figure 16). These inflammatory substances mediate vascular reactivity and platelet aggregation.

inflammatory drugs such as aspirin or indomethacin.[128] Probably these drugs are inhibitors of the cyclooxygenase cycle. There are differences between sensitivity and anti-inflammatory action of aspirin-like drugs in prostaglandin synthetase activity from various tissues.[128] Hydrocortisone and synthetic anti-inflammatory steroids inhibit prostaglandin release from intact cells, tissues, and organs, but do not inhibit conversion of arachidonic acid to prostaglandins by microsomal cyclooxygenase. This implies a direct interaction of corticosteroids with biomembranes, which might either impair the supply of endogenous substitutes for prostaglandin synthesis or inhibit the transport of these compounds through membranes.[162]

Prostaglandins exert a great variety of physiological actions, but the chemical basis still remains unresolved.[306,314] Prostaglandins have been inplicated in both the induction and in the relief of inflammation. In the process of inflammation, when polymorphonuclear leukocytes migrate into the inflamed area, leukocytes release lysosomal phospholipase A_2, which in turn hydrolyzes phospholipids and produces polyunsaturated fatty acids, precursors of prostaglandins. The effect of prostaglandins on the inflammatory response is reinforced by the release of polyunsaturated fatty acids. Some prostaglandins, such as prostaglandin E_1, mimic cyclic AMP action in their effects on the cell. This led to the proposal that prostaglandins mediate the synthesis of cyclic AMP in response to the binding of a hormone to the cell surface. Prostaglandins may cross the cell membrane and cause allosteric activation of adenylate cyclase.[242] Prostaglandin E_2 often shows opposite physiological effects, and it may function in different ways. It has been established that cyclic AMP can suppress inflammation, and prostaglandin E_2 can also exert similar effects. While prostaglandin E relieves asthma, prostaglandins induce allergic responses. However, the opposite actions may be true; prostaglandins E regulate cyclic AMP levels, whereas prostaglandins F regulate cyclic GMP content. In turn, the cellular response to certain stimuli is dependent on the relative cyclic AMP and cyclic GMP concentrations inside the cell.

The foregoing indicates that prostaglandins have a complex role in inflammation (Figure 15). These compounds may provide a balance in inflammatory processes since they are able to mediate or suppress the inflammatory response. Prostaglandins may reduce the inflammatory response through a balance which occurs locally between the concentrations of prostaglandins E and F. The aggregation of platelets is enhanced by prostaglandin E_2 and inhibited by prostaglandin E_1. Prostaglandin E_1 or E_2 induce increased vascular permeability in the skin, and prostaglandin $F_{2\alpha}$ causes an inhibition. The formation of these compounds follows a common pathway until the final stages (Figure 13). Since there is no interconversion between prostaglandin E and F, the local control of the inflammatory reactions may, therefore, depend on the preferential biosynthesis of one or another type of prostaglandins.

2. Other Arachidonic Acid-Derived Mediators

Some fatty acid compounds are precursors of prostaglandins synthesis and derive from the transformation of prostaglandins.[169,172,250,359,366,422,445] When prostaglandins are produced, the 20-carbon atom polyenoic acids are hydrolyzed from fatty acid-containing phosphoglycerides by phopholipase A_2. This hydrolytic enzyme is specific for the *sn*-2 position of the phospholipid. A microsomal enzyme system converts the released polyenoic fatty acids to prostaglandin. Prostaglandin synthetase is the term commonly used for a microsomal complex of enzymes which transforms arachidonic acid and related substrates to a variety of oxygenated products. The precise function of these products depends on the tissue. In platelets, thromboxane A_2 is the primary derivative, whereas in the aorta, mainly prostacyclin is formed.[471] In the sequence, the first enzymatic reaction is catalyzed by prostaglandin cyclooxygenase which is common to all tissues.[263]

During this process, O_2-requiring cyclooxygenase or lipoxygenase produce potent peroxy acids[47] (Figure 16), and in some tissues, including the lung and platelets, prostaglandins are transformed to nonprostaglandin products. One of these is a labile hemiacetal derivative

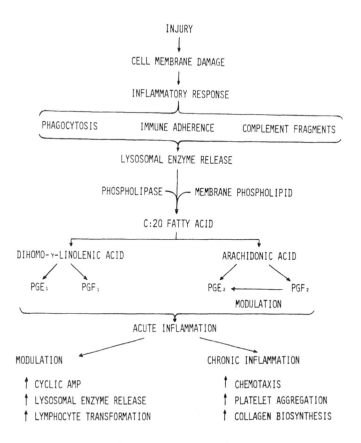

FIGURE 15.   Action of prostaglandins in the inflammatory response. Prostaglandin synthesis occurs in the damaged tissue at the site of inflammation. Prostaglandins then produce the cardinal signs of this condition: they increase local vascular permeability and induce vasodilatation. These effects can potentiate the actions of other mediators such as histamine and bradykinin. The modulations of acute inflammation involves an increase of cyclic AMP production, lysosomal enzyme release, and lymphocyte transformation. Effects on chemotaxis, platelet aggregation, and collagen biosynthesis are also connected with chronic conditions.

thromboxane A which can be further converted to thromboxane B.[335] A biochemical characteristic of prostaglandins and other arachidonic acid-derived mediators is rapid catabolism. Many arachidonic acid derivatives arise by β- or ω-oxidation and reduction, and the distribution of these metabolic products shows variations among species. The catabolism is especially active in the lungs, and prostaglandins and their derivatives entering the bloodstream are removed by simple transport process through the lungs.

An important arachidonic acid intermediate is prostacyclin, which has been even considered as a hormone with therapeutic potential.[468] Prostaglandin endoperoxides, thromboxane A_2, and prostacyclin are unstable, but have potent and sometimes opposing biological activities. Cyclic endoperoxides, thromboxanes, and prostacyclin are produced by the catalytic action of cyclooxygenase.[173] Lipoxygenase enzymes convert arachidonic acid to hydroperoxy acids and leukotrienes (Figure 16). The 5- or 12-lipoxygenases have been identified in platelet, lung, leukocytes, blood vessels, and epicardium, but like cyclooxygenase, it is probably present in all tissues.[114,468]

3. Acetylated Alkyl Phosphoglycerides

Acetylated alkyl phosphoglycerides represent a novel class of lipid autacoids. They exert

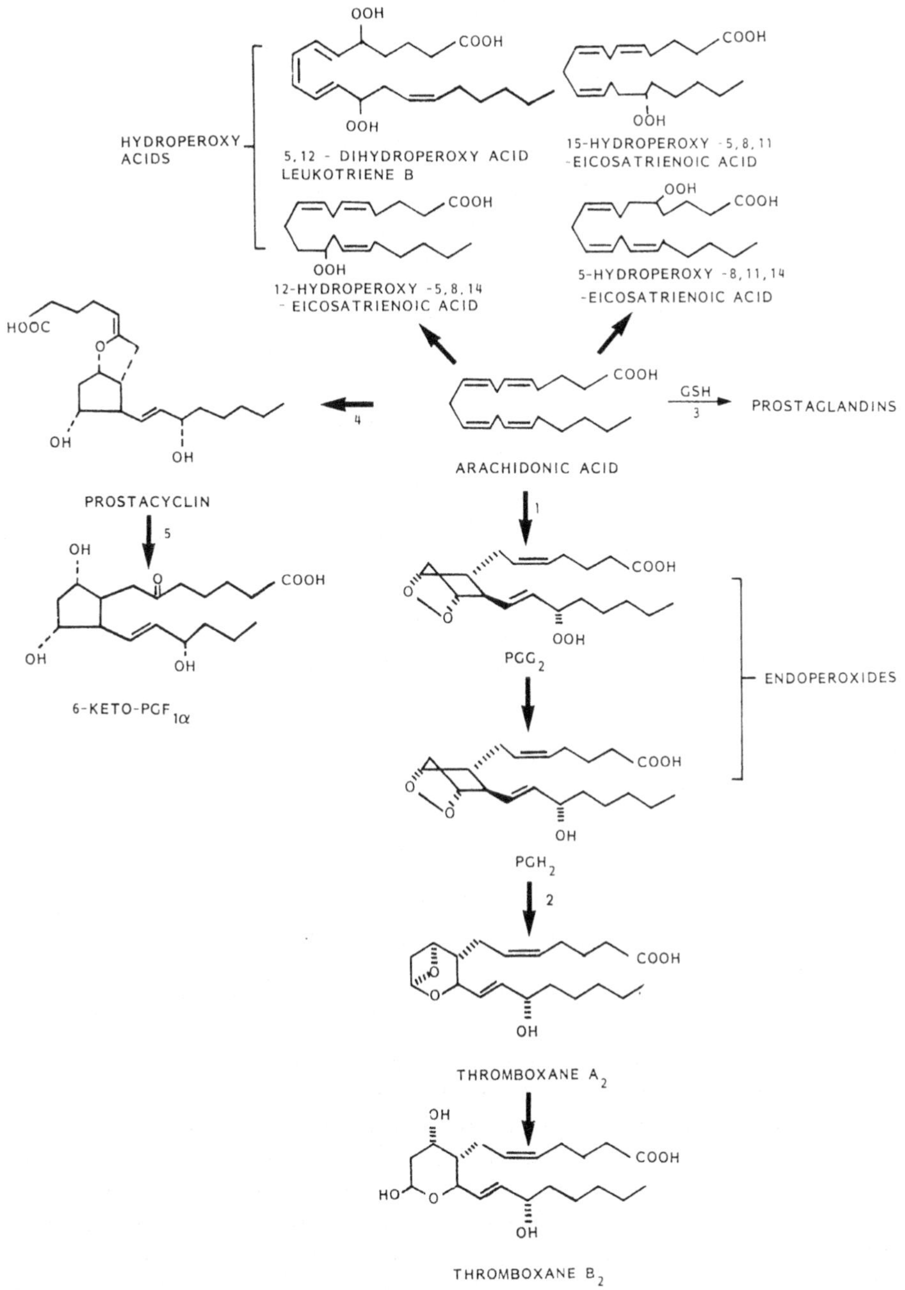

FIGURE 16. Biochemical pathways of arachidonic acid-derived mediators. During the process of phagocytosis membrane derived C:20 fatty acid derivatives are formed including endoperoxides, thromboxanes, and prostacyclin.[250] Furthermore, arachidonic acid is converted to hydroperoxy acids.[47] When a phagocytic cell encounters a particle phospholipase, activation leads to arachidonic acid liberation from the cell membrane. The oxidative transformation of arachidonic acid gives rise to endoperoxides catalyzed by cyclooxygenase (1). Through several isomerase reactions (2) these compounds are converted to thromboxanes.[335] From arachidonic, series of prostaglandins are also produced (3). Some of these reactions involve the participation of glutathione. Arachidonic acid is the precursor of prostacyclin (4) which is fairly unstable and converted (5) to a stable metabolite, 6-keto-prostaglandin F_1.[366] In several systems endoperoxides, prostaglandins and thromboxanes show proinflammatory actions. Formation of hydroperoxy acids may have an important role in leukocyte functions.[47]

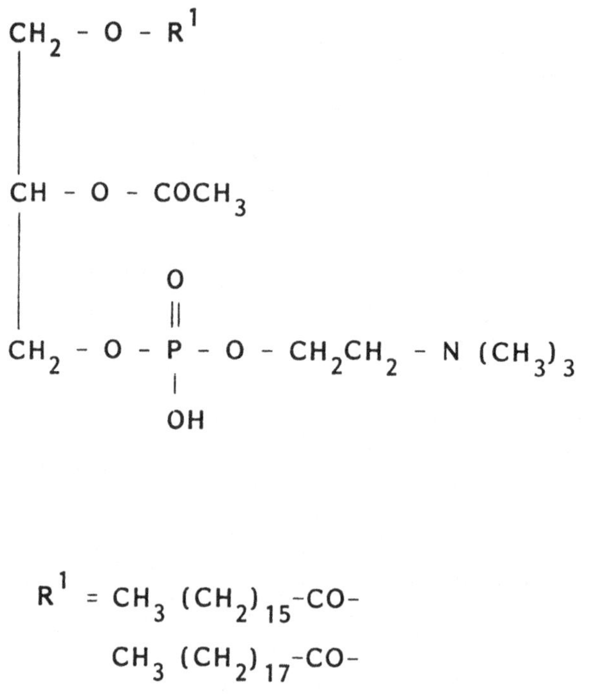

$$CH_2 - O - R^1$$

$$CH - O - COCH_3$$

$$CH_2 - O - \overset{\overset{\displaystyle O}{\|}}{\underset{\underset{\displaystyle OH}{|}}{P}} - O - CH_2CH_2 - N(CH_3)_3$$

$$R^1 = CH_3(CH_2)_{15}-CO-$$

$$CH_3(CH_2)_{17}-CO-$$

FIGURE 17. The chemical structure of acetylated alkyl phosphoglycerides.

potent pharmacologic and inflammatory properties. They are produced by a variety of inflammatory cells.[369,370] Among these autacoids two compounds have been isolated and synthesized: 1-O-hexadecyl- and 1-O-octadecyl-2-acetyl-sn-glyceryl-3-phosphorylcholine (AGEPC, Figure 17). *In vivo* and *in vitro* studies have shown the ability of these substances to stimulate human platelets[304] and polymorphonuclear neutrophils.[416] AGEPC is also capable of inducing many well-known signs of acute inflammation.[368,369,370] Intravenous infusions of microgram amounts of AGEPC into experimental animals produce all the pathological signs of IgE-induced systemic anaphylactic shock.[367] AGEPC also stimulates neutrophil aggregation, secretion of azurophilic and specific granule enzymes, and chemotaxis, showing vasoactive properties and inducing smooth muscle contraction. The AGEPC substance also induces enhanced vascular permeability about 1 to 10,000 times greater extent than histamine or leukotriene D or E,[215,216] and about 100 to 1000 times more potent than either serotonin or bradykinin.[115,436] Among various analogs, different in the polar head group, only 3-phosphoryl-N-monomethyl-ethanolamine and 3-phosphoryl-N,N-dimethylethanolamine show similar sensitivity to AGEPC.[215] It causes erythema and edema in skin and produces transient, severe burning pain.[371]

4. Role of Lipids in Neutrophil Activation

Polymorphonuclear neutrophils have highly specialized primary functions: phagocytosis, destruction, and digestion of microorganisms. If the neutrophil functions are defective, recurrent infections become frequent. At the site of inflammation, neutrophils release their granular contents, and active oxidants and arachidonic acid derivatives (prostaglandins, leukotrienes, thromboxanes, and 5-hydroxy-peroxyeicosatetraenoic acid) are released which are responsible for the initiation and amplification of the inflammatory response and for the destruction of tissues surrounding the inflamed area.[501]

The responses of neutrophils are connected with various ligands such as chemotactic peptides, immune complexes, complement components, and lectins, which react with specific receptors of plasma membranes. This ligand reaction activates cell responses such as chemotaxis, aggregation, phagocytosis, degranulation, and generation of active oxidants containing superoxide (O_2-). The specific receptors are embedded in the lipid bilayers of the plasmalemma. Membrane phospholipids do not serve only as inert matrix for membrane proteins and barrier to water-soluble compounds, but as substrates for dynamic interactions between protein and lipid membrane constituents.[417] Treatment of the membrane with surface active agents such as deoxycholate, saponin, and digitonin, stimulates a respiratory burst similar to phagocytosis.[390] Addition of phospholipase C to neutrophils also causes a respiratory burst.[247] These treatments modify the lipoprotein structure of the plasma membrane, and this change represents a stimulus for cell activation.

A series of steps are involved in the activation of neutrophils resulting in the change of the lipoprotein structure: (1) binding of the ligand with the receptor, (2) translocation of Ca^{2+} ions across the plasmalemma, (3) activation of membrane-bound adenylate cyclase enzyme, (4) release of arachidonic acid and its metabolism through cyclooxygenase and lipoxygenase pathways, and (5) fusion of the granule membrane with the plasmalemma. The enhanced entry of Ca^{2+} into the cell causes changes in phospholipid metabolism, including an increase in the transformation of phosphatidylinositol to diglyceride, phosphorylation to phosphatidic acid, and synthesis of phosphatidyl inositol.[174,232,233,308,500] The translocation of Ca^{2+} in lipid bilayers is connected with phosphatidic acid, oxidized trienoic acids, and increased levels of cyclic AMP.[56,140,430,478]

G. INFLAMMATORY PLASMA PROTEINS

The sources of most inflammatory proteins and peptides are the several different types of leukocytes. These cells contain many potentially harmful substances within their cytoplasm clustered in granules which are released into the surrounding inflamed tissue and appear in the circulation as various plasma proteins. There are five groups: (1) proteases, antiproteases, and oxidizing enzymes; (2) blood coagulation system; (3) complement systems; (4) kallikrein-kinin system; and (5) the fibrinolytic system. In this section only the role of proteases, antiproteases, and oxidants during inflammation in tissue injury will be discussed. The kallikrein-kinin system has protein components, but the active mediators are relatively small peptides derived from proteins of this system.

In the course of acute inflammation, polymorphonuclear neutrophils or, in the case of chronic reactions, monocytes and macrophages accumulate at the site of injury and liberate various proteases into the surrounding connective tissue.[360,412,472] Polymorphonuclear neutrophils contain both acid and neutral proteases, and these enzymes can cause damage to connective tissue structures.[412] Neutral proteases determine more likely the extent of the extracellular damage. The polymorphonuclear leukocyte-derived neutral proteases are stored in specific granules and include elastase, collagenase, cathepsin G, and a serine-protease, an enzyme with trypsin-like action. Mononuclear phagocytes secrete neutral proteases which also decompose macromolecules of connective tissues.[510] Macrophage neutral proteases are secreted by stimulated cells and include procollagenase, elastase (which is different from the polymorphonuclear neutrophil enzyme), and plasminogen activator.[506] These enzymes degrade connective tissue targets which include Types I, II, III, and IV collagen, amorphous elastin and associated microfibrils, and matrix proteoglycans.

There is, however, a system of protease inhibitors in tissue fluids which can protect connective tissue macromolecules against the action of proteases released from leukocytes.[194,349,456] These antiproteases include α_1-M.S.T.-proteinase inhibitor (α_1-antitrypsin), α_1-antichymotrypsin,[348] α_2-macroglobulin, and a mucous proteinase inhibitor. The interac-

TABLE 3
Constituents of Neutrophil Granules[a]

Enzymes	Proteases	Cathepsin, collagenase, elastase, leukoprotease, histonase
	Lipases	Acid lipase, phospholipase, sphingomyelinase, glucocerebrosidase
	Esterases	Aryl sulphatase, acid phosphatase, alkaline phosphatase
	Oxidases	NADH-oxidase, NADPH-oxidase, peroxidase
	Carbohydrases	β-Glucuronidase, β-galactosidase, α-glucosidase, α-mannosidase, N-acetyl-β-glucosaminidase, lysozyme
	Nucleases	Nucleotidase, ribonuclease, deoxyribonuclease
Macromolecules		Cationic proteins, lactoferrin, mucopolysaccharides

[a] Compiled from References 42, 226, 324, 346, and 417.

tion between the endogenous inhibitors of inflammatory cell proteases and the antiproteases is presented in Table 3. The α_1-proteinase inhibitor is one of the most important components of the antiprotease system in man, responsible for more than 90% of the inhibitory capacity of normal human serum for regulating neutrophil elastase action.[449] The second important inhibitor is the mucous proteinase inhibitor which is not present in the circulation, but is secreted locally by the mucous epithelium of selected organs. This antiprotease inhibits the action of the polymorphonuclear neutrophil-derived elastase. Protease inhibitors in tissue fluids provide a protective role for connective tissue macromolecules against the attack of phagocyte-derived proteases. It is essential that a local balance between inflammatory cell proteases, circulating antiproteases and mucus, exercise control of the degree of tissue damage brought about by the inflammatory process.[27]

The balance between proteases and antiproteases is further modulated by oxidation processes.[31,33,158,159] The α_1-proteinase inhibitor and the mucous inhibitor both are susceptible to inactivation by oxidants.[63] In the case of the α_1-proteinase inhibitor, this is connected with the oxidation of methionine residues in or near the active site of the antiprotease.[234] Reactive oxygen species are formed by polymorphonuclear neutrophils, macrophages, and monocytes and released into the extracellular space. Simultaneously with this process, enzymes are also discharged that inactivate mucous proteinase and α_1-proteinase inhibitors. Various oxidants produced by the halide system and myeloperoxidase-H_2O_2 systems of polymorphonuclear leukocytes and monocytes can also destroy the activity of these inhibitors. Due to the oxidation processes which eliminate the effects of α_1-proteinase and mucous proteinase inhibitors, the most effective endogenous protease regulators, particularly the potent polymorphonuclear monocyte elastase, may remain free. Thus, the protease released at the site of inflammation acts on collagen, elastin, and proteoglycan if the concentrations of oxidizing substances are high enough.[158] The impairment of balance of interaction between proteases, antiproteases, and oxidants may result in tissue injury (Figure 18).

Polymorphonuclear neutrophil elastase can hydrolyze a variety of proteins; it solubilizes elastin, cartilage proteoglycan, and several types of collagen molecules. The elastase cleaves Types I and II collagens at the nonhelical teleopeptide region of the molecules which contains the intermolecular cross-links. The resultant depolymerization facilitates further nonspecific proteolytic action. Types III and IV collagens are hydrolyzed by the polymorphonuclear neutrophil elastase across the helical portion of the tropocollagen portion. In addition to these structural tissue components, a variety of important proteins present at the inflammatory sites can also be destroyed by elastase, such as intermediates of the kallikrein-kinin system, complement system, clotting and fibrinolytic cascades, and immunoglobulins.[26,133] Cathepsin G shows chymotrypsin-like properties, and it attacks the microfibrillar components of the elastic fiber, proteoglycan molecules, and certain components of the complement, clotting, and fibrinolytic systems.

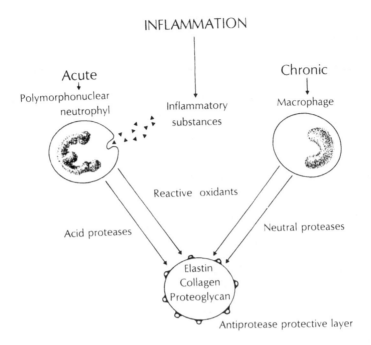

FIGURE 18. Schematic representation of plasma protein participation in the inflammatory process. At the site of inflammation, tissue is injured and proteases, antiproteases, and reactive oxidants interact to regulate the degree of connective tissue destruction.

IV. MECHANISM OF INJURED TISSUE CLEARANCE

Depending on the cause of injury, the damaged tissue is infiltrated with the exudate containing neutrophils, lymphocytes, and macrophages associated with increased fluid and protein accumulations such as albumin, fibrinogen, fibrin, acute phase proteins, glycoproteins, and immunoglobulins. The various conditions include (1) the adherence of eosinophils and neutrophils during immediate hypersensitivity; (2) neutrophils in heat, ultraviolet (UV) radiation, or *Staphylococcus aureus,* and *Streptococcus pyogenes*-induced skin injury, reaching a peak within 3 to 20 h; (3) macrophages in tuberculin sensitization, reaching a vascular permeability peak within 24 h; and (4) macrophages in dinitrochlorobenzene sensitization reaching a peak within 24 to 48 h.[322]

The outcome of tissue injury therefore depends on the nature and duration of the injurious agent, on the type of tissue injured, and on the extent of damage. Complete restoration to normal conditions usually occurs following mild chemical or physical injury of brief duration or when the infection caused by a microorganism leads to little destruction.[218]

A. PHAGOCYTOSIS

The major mechanism of removal of foreign matter or dead tissue by neutrophils and macrophages is by ingestion. This process represents phagocytosis and has several phases such as (1) chemotaxis, (2) recognition and attachment, (3) ingestion and phagosome formation, (4) degranulation, (5) increased oxidation, and (6) destruction of microorganism and digestion. The first phase in the process of clearing is the directional movement of phagocytic cells toward debris or bacteria which is essential in surface contact and recognition. The migration of phagocytes is dependent on microfilaments containing myosin and actin.[524]

Several low molecular weight peptides have been characterized to possess chemotactic

TABLE 4
Enzyme Content of Lysomal Granules[22,29]

Class of enzymes	Azurophil granules	Specific granules
Neutral proteases	Elastase	Collagenase
	Cathepsin G	
	Third serine proteinase	
	Chemotactic factor,	
	generating protease	
	Kininogen activator	
Acid hydrolases	Cathepsin D	
	Cathepsin B	
	β-Glucuronidase	
	α-Mannosidase	
	β-Glycerophosphatase	
	N-Acetyl-β-glucosaminidase	
	Acid lipase	
	Acid ribonuclease	
	Acid deoxyribonuclease	
	Arylamidase	
	Myeloperoxidase	Lysozyme
	Lysozyme	
Other proteins	Phagocytin	Lactoferrin
		Alkaline phosphatase

activity. These include C3a, C5a, and the trimolecular complex C567, which are produced from the activation of the complement cascade by antibody-coated bacteria.[435] These factors may be formed by the complement pathway or directly activated by bacterial proteases and breakdown products of collagen, fibrin, or cells.[206,398,487] Activation of the Hageman factor and the plasminogen proactivator also produces chemotactic factors.[244] Mast cells release a tetrapeptide chemotactic factor with the sequence VAL–GLY–SER–GLU or ALA–GLY–SER–GLU from eosinophils.[149,253] The interaction of a specific antigen with T lymphocytes leads to the production of lymphokines. Some of these agents have chemo-hemotactic activity for lymphocytes, neutrophils, eosinophils, and monocytes.[387]

In the next phase, phagocytes recognize the area of damaged tissue. Specific antibodies coat bacteria which are mainly IgG$_1$ and IgG$_3$ with intact Fc and Fab portions.[214,373] This process is called opsonization. C reactive proteins, α- and β-globulins, C3a- and C5a-peptide fragments also exert coating ability.[206,441] Tuftsin, a tetrapeptide with the amino acid sequence THR–LYS–PRO–ARG, also acts on phagocytes.[332] Tuftsin is a natural macrophage activator and exerts immunogenic, antineoplastic, and other effects. Following the association, the particles become attached to neutrophils by receptors for the Fc region of IgG.[409]

Ingestion and phagosome formation is an energy-dependent process and requires Ca^{2+} and Mg^{2+}, while the role of cyclic AMP is questioned.[394] Phagocytes extend pseudopodia around the attached particles; these then become fused and encased in a phagocytotic vacuole or phagosome. The phagosome moves away from the cell membrane and further fuses with cytoplasmic granules.[441] The migrating pseudopodia contain a rich network of microfilaments containing actin and myosin which interact with microtubules during ingestion.

After endocytosis, the phagosomes are combined with neutrophil or macrophage granules. These are the primary lysosomes which release their enzyme content to the phagocytic vacuoles and become secondary lysosomes.[193] In the case of neutrophils the primary granules are rich in lysosomal enzymes such as acid hydrolases, neutral proteinases, and various other enzymes which destroy microorganisms (Table 4). During the degranulation process some of the secondary lysosomes may fuse with additional primary lysosomes producing a single phagocytic vacuole. Some secondary lysosomes may form a residual body after releasing

TABLE 5
Blood Coagulation Factors

Name and synonyms	International nomenclature
Fibrinogen	Factor I
Prothrombin	Factor II
Tissue thromboplastin	Factor III
Calcium	Factor IV
Prothrombin accelerator proaccelerin, AC globulin, labile factors	Factor V
Serum prothrombin conversion accelerator, autoprothrombin I, stable factor	Factor VII
Antihemophilic globulin, von Willebrand factor	Factor VIII
Plasma thromboplastin component, autoprothrombin II, Christmas factor	Factor IX
Stuart-Prower factor	Factor X
Plasma thromboplastin antedecent	Factor XI
Hageman factor	Factor XII
Fibrin stabilizing factor	Factor XIII
Prekallikrein, Fletcher factor	
Kininogens, Fitzgerald factor	

their enzymes. This body contains indigestible material which may be eliminated from the cell. Lysosomal granules may also be discharged from the cell during the ingestion phase. Completely degraded materials diffuse through the membrane into the cytoplasm from secondary lysosomes.

The degranulation is associated with a strong respiratory process which generates highly reactive agents. The respiratory burst increases oxygen uptake, hydrogen peroxide (H_2O_2) and superoxide (O_2-) production, and hexose monophosphate shunt.[17,19] NADPH represents the electron donor, and the enzyme responsible for these catalytic activities is localized on the plasma membrane. The enhanced respiration produces many oxidizing agents which are used by phagocytes for the destruction of microorganisms. Part of the microbial killing system is oxygen-dependent and functions with H_2O_2 and myeloperoxidase, superoxide, hydroxyl radicals, and singlet oxygen.[17] The antimicrobial potency of H_2O_2 is increased by myeloperoxidase. Superoxide is produced during phagocytosis. Singlet oxygen (l_{O_2}) is also formed during the enhanced respiration as an end-product of the myeloperoxidase reaction. The latter is different from the atmospheric oxygen in electron distribution around the two oxygen nuclei.

Oxygen-independent systems also participate in the elimination of microbial infection. These systems involve the production of acidic environment, cationic proteins, lysozyme, and lactoferrin. The pH of the phagocytic vacuoles is low probably due to lactic acid formation. The acid pH enhances the activity of many enzymes. Lysozyme exerts its microbicidal action by hydrolyzing glycosidic bonds. The function of the bacteriostatic lactoferrin is connected with retardation of bacterial growth by binding essential iron.[22]

B. LYSOSOMAL DIGESTION

Lysosomal enzymes are associated with intracellular digestive functions in phagocytic cells. Neutrophil leukocytes and macrophage granules are the major sources of lysosomal enzymes in the inflammatory response. The lysosomal enzymes degrade all types of macromolecules, such as proteins, peptides, carbohydrates, nucleic acids and lipids. Some of these enzymes are presented in Table 5, showing the similarity with enzymes occurring in neutrophil granules (Table 4). All cathepsins have broad substrate specificity and occur in multiple forms with identical catalytic activity.[22] Elastase and cathepsin G stimulate lymphocytes and initiate antibody production.[475] Neutral lysosomal proteases cleave C and C5 fragments into active chemotactic agents[488] and activate kininogen to bradykinin and plasminogen to plasmin.[193] Neutrophil leukocytes contain collagenases which split GLY–ILE or GLY–LEU bonds in collagen, yielding smaller peptide fragments which are further degraded by elastase, cathepsin B, or metalloproteinase enzymes.[30,268,324]

Neutral and acid lipases and phospholipases are also present in lysosomal granules. During phagocytosis of *Escherichia coli*, granulocyte phospholipase A2 degrades phospholipids in the bacterial wall, and the fatty acids produced are incorporated into granulocyte lipids.[117] The degradation of microbial lipids is dependent on the accessibility of the lipid rather than their composition.[493] Various lysosomal enzymes degrade nucleic acids and glycoproteins and hydrolyze phosphate or sulfate esters, such as acid phosphatases and arylsulfatases.[29,493] The slow reacting substance of anaphylaxis released from mast cells is inactivated by arylsulfatase B present in eosinophils.[493]

During inflammation, the degree of tissue damage is partly related to the balance between the activity of leukocytic lysosomal enzymes and antienzyme factors. Various tissues possess endogenous protease inhibitors, and plasma contains antiproteases which have major roles in diminishing the inflammatory response in several diseases.[464] The various antiproteases include α_1-antitrypsin, antichymotrypsin, α_2-macroglobulin, and β_1-anticollagenase. These inhibitors are glycoproteins with molecular weights ranging from 40,000 Da for β_1-anticollagenase, 47,500 to 55,000 Da for α_1-antitrypsin, and 725,000 to 820,000 Da for α_2-macroglobulin. Antiproteases are produced predominantly in the liver, and α_1-antitrypsin and α_2-macroglobulin bind proteases such as collagenase, neutrophil elastase, and kallikrein. α_1-Antitrypsin also inactivates the fibrinolytic action of neutrophils at neutral pH, while the activity is sharply reduced below pH 5. In inflammatory exudates, its action is inhibited by lactic acid produced by neutrophiles.[226,264]

α_1-Macroglobulin accumulates in extracellular fluids such as ascitic fluid where it complexes with proteases and in the exudate of inflamed joints.[347,419] In experimental arthritis, changes in the joints are associated with increased serum levels of α_2-macroglobulin;[273] however, in most other diseases α_2-macroglobulin shows no change in plasma. In rheumatoid arthritis, collagenase-α_2-macroglobulin complexes are present in the synovial fluid representing protective reaction against inflammation.[505] Antichymotrypsin behaves as an acute phase reactant after myocardial infarction and acute bacterial infection,[14] and while its concentration in bronchial secretions is high, this may represent a local defense role.[396]

C. LYMPHATICS DRAINAGE

The role of lymphatics is cardinal in the resolution of the inflammatory response by representing an effective route for the elimination of excess interstitial fluid, macromolecules, cell debris, and removing toxic agents or involving microorganisms. Antigen transport to lymph nodes is necessary for the development of effective immunity.

Following a mild lesion caused by bacteria, chemicals, or heat, the lymphatics dilate and open junctions are established between endothelial cells with subsequent increased permeability to blood cells and macromolecules. These changes are associated with the effects of edema fluid affecting anchoring filaments attached to the lymphatic wall.[65] Inflammation causes a 10- to 20-fold increase in lymph flow and raises the protein concentration from 1 to 2 g/dl to 5g or more as a result of increased accumulation of proteins and cell debris in the interstitial tissue due to proteolytic enzyme activity. The lymphatics contain many enzymes which originated from injured tissue. Large molecules produced by enzyme action also increase the osmolarity of the interstitial fluid, particularly following bacterial injury or burns. In the case of thermal lesion, lymphatic drainage reaches a maximum in the first hour.[384]

V. CAUSES OF INADEQUATE CLEARANCE

When the injurious agent is not destroyed or digested by the phagocytic system, or if there is a defect in the function of the phagocytic cells or in lymphatic drainage, clearance becomes inadequate. There are many agents which are not cleared adequately. These are mostly exogenous inert materials (asbestos, silica, talc or carbon particles, iron, barium, and beryllium), endogenous particles (urate crystals, hair, and bone), bacteria with capsules or an outer coat which are resistant to phagocytic action and digestion *(M. tuberculosis, M. leprae, Brucella, Listeria monocytogenes)*, viruses (measles, herpes, poxviruses), rickettsia *(R. rickettsi)*, protozoa *(toxoplasma, leishmania)*, and fungi *(Cryptococcus neoformans)*.

A. EXOGENOUS AGENTS
1. Microorganisms

The action of tubercle bacilli *(M. tuberculosis)* is the classic example where the digestion and destruction of the bacteria is slow. When they are inhaled into the alveoli they are processed by macrophages with varying enzyme content and killing capacity.[339] Lysosomal lipases remove the outer lipid coat of the tubercle bacilli and then lysozyme and other enzymes destroy the remaining mucopeptide structure. If the killing capacity of macrophages is inadequate, the tubercle bacilli multiply within alveolar macrophages. Following the death of these macrophages, enzymes and bacteria are released which in turn are digested by other macrophages. Ultimately, the tubercle bacilli are destroyed by monocytes activated by T-lymphocyte products (lymphokines).[93] The interplay between macrophages and tubercle bacilli causes local tissue necrosis and eventual fibrosis, where enzymes released from macrophages are involved in the initiation of fibrosis.[6]

Many bacteria kill phagocytes such as the pathogenic streptococci and staphylococci. In *Streptococcus* infection the production of streptolysin O destroys the polymorph neutrophil granules by osmotic force. Antiphagocytic substances are also present on bacterial surfaces, such as polysaccharide capsules (pneumococci, *Haemophilus influenzae, Klebsiella pneumoniae*) or specific proteins (protein A: *Staphylococcus aureus;* protein M: streptococci). Protein A from *S. aureus* inhibits phagocytosis and becomes bound to the Fc portion of IgG, hence inhibits binding to the Fc surface receptors of neutrophils.[311]

2. Particles

Insoluble particles are cleared inadequately by cells participating in the inflammatory response and produce fibrosis or granulomatous lesions. Inhaled silica particles with a diameter of less than 10μm produce changes in the lung when they are inhaled. These particles are phagocytozed by alveolar macrophages. Some macrophages clear silica up the respiratory bronchioles and trachea; although many cells pass through the hilum into the lymphatics. Since silica particles are toxic, they kill the cells and induce fibrosis around lymphatics and in lymph nodes.[5]

B. DEFECTS OF PHAGOCYTOSIS

Several clinical syndromes are associated with defects in phagocytic function. These are connected with (1) disorders of chemotaxis and mobility, (2) disorders of attachment, ingestion, and degranulation, (3) deficiencies of endogenous protease inhibitors, (4) deficiencies of fibrin degradation, and (5) failure of lymphatic drainage.

There are conditions when the inflammatory cells are mobilized and transported to the site of infection quite poorly due to defects in the cells, to the presence of inhibitors of movement, or to deficiencies in chemotactic factors.[394] These cellular abnormalities characterize the Chediak-Higashi syndrome, where macrophages and neutrophils show defective chemotaxis. This condition is connected with recurrent infections.[75] The basic abnormality in this condition is attributed to faulty microtubule assembly. Job's syndrome with recurrent staphylococcal abscesses shows high serum IgE levels, and in chronic eczema, neutrophils show faulty chemotaxis.[191] Monocyte chemotaxis is defective in Wiskott-Aldrich syndrome,[11] leukemia,[362] and melanoma.[432] Abnormal actin has been found in neutrophils from patients with recurrent infections.[442] This may indicate that the cause of these abnormalities is due to a fault of the cytoskeletal proteins, causing a failure to clear the causative microorganisms.

In several diseases, serum inhibitors of phagocytic mobility have been found, as in rheumatoid arthritis,[321] diabetes mellitus,[320] hepatic cirrhosis,[98] and chronic granulomatous disease,[489] where immune complexes may inhibit neutrophil chemotaxis. Several drugs also decrease chemotaxis; colchicine and corticosteroids are among these.

Defective chemotaxis may also be due to impaired synthesis of chemotactic factors. Various components of the complement also play a part as endogenous chemotactic factors. Genetic deficiencies in the synthesis of these components are associated with recurrent infections.[206] Such deficiencies have been described in C1r, C2, C3, and C5 components.[509] In case of homozygous C3 deficiency, recurrent pneumonia, impetigo, and otitis media are often manifest, and supplementation of C3 factor to the serum can correct this impairment.[10]

C. DEFECTS OF INGESTION, DEGRANULATION, AND BACTERIAL CELL KILLING

In some disorders the attachment of the particles of microorganisms to neutrophils or mononuclear phagocytes is inadequate due to an abnormalitity in the complement system or to lack of antibodies. Low serum levels of C3 or failure of activation of C3 to C3b is connected with recurrent infections. Defective serum opsonic activity has been described in newborns with low C3 and C5 levels and in patients with hepatic cirrhosis, acute glomerulonephritis, systemic lupus erythematosus, postsplenectomy, and increased catabolism of C3 component.[442] In these cases, usually very virulent bacteria such as *Streptococci, Pneumococci*, and *Haemophilus influenzae* are responsible for the recurrent infection.

Defects in the ingestion phase of phagocytosis are related to immune complexes which block the degradation of opsonized particles. Impaired degranulation occurs in the Chediak-Higashi syndrome, where the fusion of phagosomes with the giant cytoplasmic granules in monocytes or neutrophils is defective,[518] leading to impairment of myeloperoxidase and bacterial killing. Enzyme defects in the oxidative killing mechanism can also occur in early childhood in chronic granulomatous disease, and consequently, the clearance of pyogenic microorganism is faulty, resulting in serious recurrent bacterial infections, such as pneumonia, osteomyelitis, and liver abscesses.[209] These infections are difficult to treat and heal slowly, often resulting in granulomata of the skin and lymph nodes.

In chronic granulomatous disease, the basic defect resides in the ability of phagocytes to initiate the respiratory burst due to lack of NADPH oxidase, which is responsible for the primary oxygen consuming process.[17,18,196] The result of this defect is a failure of the cells to generate O_2- or H_2O_2 and to activate the myeloperoxidase-halide system.[89]

There are certain bacteria which are phagocytozed, but not killed intracelullarly such as *E. coli* and *S. aureus*. These bacteria are catalase-positive and serious infections caused by these bacteria are fairly common, in contrast to the catalase-negative bacteria, such as *Streptococci* and *Pneumococci,* which produce H_2O_2. Neutrophils cannot provide H_2O_2, but can kill bacteria in chronic granulomatous disease using H_2O_2 supplied by other sources. Staphylococci and pneumococci produce their own H_2O_2, and thus, these catalase-negative bacteria contribute to their own destruction by providing sufficient H_2O_2 inside the phagocytic vacuole. Catalase destroys the small amounts of H_2O_2 in catalase-positive bacteria thus preventing their own death.[89,394] Catalase-positive bacteria also survive within neutrophils for relatively long periods and can cause widespread infection when transported throughout the body.[199]

Absolute deficiency of glucose-6-phosphate dehydrogenase is also associated with symptoms of chronic granulomatous disease. The clinical manifestation of this condition is similar to the disease induced by bacteria, although the onset of infectious lesions mostly occurs in late childhood or adolescence.[20,156] The microorganisms involved are *E. coli, S. aureus* and *K. pneumoniae.* The lack of H_2O_2 causes the persistence of pyogenic microorganisms and chronic infection.[20] In contrast to chronic granulomatous condition and glucose 6-phosphate dehydrogenase deficiency, patients with myeloperoxidase deficiency rarely develop infections. The phagocytes of myeloperoxidase-deficient patients show a characteristic bactericidal abnormality *in vitro.* There is a delay in bacteria killing, but by about 4 h almost all ingested microorganisms are killed.[17,18]

1. Protease Inhibitor Deficiency

Endogenous protease inhibitors modulate the extent and degree of tissue damage in inflammation. In genetically determined α_1-antitrypsin deficiency, pulmonary emphysema develops as a result of uncontrolled digestion of lung tissue due to proteolytic enzymes released from macrophages and neutrophils. Elastase is the major enzyme responsible for the damage.[227] These patients may also have a chemotactic factor inactivator deficiency. The latter blood components inactivate C3a, C5a, and C567 complex and bacterial chemotactic factors. Lack of chemotactic factor inactivator may contribute to tissue proteolysis by enhancing the adherence of neutrophils to the injured lung mediated by enhanced chemotactic activity.

The degradation of fibrin and removal of breakdown products are necessary during the inflammatory process. Fibrin is present in the initial step and also provides a framework for fibrosis to take place during healing. Persistence of fibrin in pleurisy causes extensive fibrosis and adhesions between pleural surfaces. Fibrin degradation products in the Bowman's space of the glomerulus may also lead to proliferation of the epithelial cells and crescentic glomerulonephritis with ultimate fibrosis.[72]

D. CONSEQUENCES OF ABNORMAL CLEARANCE

Inadequate clearance of injurious agents can lead to suppuration, chronic inflammation, fibrosis, amyloidosis, and autoimmunity. Failure of destruction and clearance of pyogenic microorganisms during the early stages of inflammation result in a purulent exudate characterized by living and dead neutrophils, living and dead microorganisms, and cell debris. When this exudate is localized to a focal site, it represents an abscess. Many microorganisms induce suppuration, such as *E. coli,* gonococci, streptococci, and meningococci. Turpentine also induces a suppurative reaction,[218] and a large number of neutrophils releases significant amounts of proteolytic enzymes causing tissue injury and cell death.

Insoluble particles such as silica, asbestos, and suture material if not cleared rapidly, produce fibrosis. Pathogenic organisms such as tubercle bacilli within a focus of chronic infection also encapsulate by fibrosis. Chronic inflammation represents protracted tissue damage and continuing infiltration of macrophages, lymphocytes, and plasma cells. The presence of lymphocytes and plasma cells indicates an immunological reaction. Either T or B lymphocytes play important roles in chronic inflammation, and the immune response usually develops against the injurious agent persisting in the tissues. In some situations, however, immune reactivity may result against the modified components of the host's own tissue.[146] Examples of chronic inflammation where lymphocytes and macrophages exert an essential role include chronic hepatitis, chronic pyelonephritis, rheumatoid arthritis, and ulcerative colitis.

Macrophages may be activated by particles such as silica or asbestos, bacterial cell walls and endotoxins, antigen-antibody complexes, the complement cleavage product C3b, and lymphokines derived from T lymphocytes. A range of mediators are secreted which kill bacteria, attract more phagocytes into the lesion, and initiate fibrosis and repair. Sensitized T lymphocytes react with specific antigens and liberate lymphokines which activate macrophages to kill intracellular bacteria, viruses, and fungi. The activated macrophages secrete neutral proteinases to degrade collagen, elastin, and proteoglycan, to cleave C3, and to activate plasminogen. The complement components (C3a, C5a, C567) are chemotactic for macrophages, while plasminogen leads to the production of plasmin, which degrades fibrin. Fibrin degradation products and some lymphokins are also chemotactic for macrophages; thus more phagocytes are released into chronic lesions.

Amyloidosis repesents a long-term failure of clearance of many agents causing chronic inflammation, such as in chronic osteomyelitis, rheumatoid arthritis, tuberculosis, ulcerative colitis, and leprosy. Amyloid is a fibrillar protein which differs in composition depending on the nature of the precursor. In secondary amyloidosis the amyloid A produced has a unique amino acid sequence derived by lysosomal enzyme action from a serum protein called serum A-related protein. This protein is normally present in low concentration in normal serum, but elevated in infectious or rheumatoid arthritis.[145]

VI. PARTICIPATION OF SUBCELLULAR ORGANELLES

The course of cellular reactions to injury shows a sequence of changes in cytoplasmic organelles. The initial response is dependent upon the causative physical, chemical, or microbiological agents evoking different responses. Ultimately, however, the pattern of either restituting the normal conditions or that of final changes leading to necrosis is relatively independent from the nature of the injury. These common patterns suggest that cellular organelles undergo similar changes during the inflammatory process.

A. MITOCHONDRIA

The initial intracellular changes involve the mitochondria, endoplasmic reticulum, and lysosomes. Injury interferes with the normal perfusion of the cell, and oxygen intake is promptly reduced. The production of internal substrates is limited, and the removal of metabolites and other cell byproducts is decreased. A reduced respiration associated with impaired mitochondrial function in turn decreases the intracellular ATP level, and by way of a temporary compensation, the production of ATP is shifted to the glycolytic pathway.[262,513] This results in an elevated lactate level and associated decrease in pH and glycogen. In latter stages, the fall in ATP impairs the activity of ion transport across the cell membrane responsible for the maintenance of the normal extra- and intracellular milieu. In advanced lesions, the cell membranes show some structural distortion. The deranged mitochondrial function is also accompanied by loss of matrix granules, and increased permeability of mitochondrial inner membranes is followed by swelling resulting in structural damage.

B. ENDOPLASMIC RETICULUM

The endoplasmic reticulum responds to injury with dilatation, interrelated with increased sodium and decreased potassium content of the cell caused by malfunctioning of the sodium pump.[431,458]

C. LYSOSOMES

Major changes associated with inflammation occur in lysosomes.[7,8,184,318,319,502,503] These organelles contain several substances propagating the inflammatory response which are discharged, including enzymes which when released, convert precursors to active mediators. The lysis of lysosomal membranes may occur due to the detergent action of lysolecithins which are essential components of membranes, or by the direct action of external labilizing agents, or by a selective intracellular rupture. The latter effects have already been discussed previously. Disruption of lysosomal membranes alone can produce acute or chronic inflammatory reactions. Lysosomal enzymes may be released at sites where membrane-associated antigen-antibody complexes are formed. Secretion of specific lysosomal enzymes can also occur from macrophages during phagocytosis without marked membrane damage.[29]

VII. PARTICIPATION OF FORMED ELEMENTS

A. NEUTROPHIL LEUKOCYTES

1. Mechanisms of Action

Neutrophils are also recognized as polymorphonuclear leukocytes or granulocytes. These terms are not sufficiently specific since they equally include neutrophils, eosinophils and basophils. In man and in many species, neutrophils indicate clearly the specific type of cell involved in inflammation.[192] Neutrophils contain large number of cytoplasmic granules, with many enzymes and other constituents (Table 4). During inflammation oxygen and glucose uptake, lactic acid production is increased in relationship with the activation of cytoplasmic oxidases, especially NADH oxidase.[378] Hydrogen peroxide is produced, and the peroxide operates through the glutathione cycle or the ascorbic acid oxidation-reduction system which converts NADPH to NADP, driving in turn the enhanced hexose monophosphate shunt.[97] When neutrophil activity is increased, the metabolism and turnover of neutral lipids and phospholipids is also markedly enhanced. Combination of arachidonic acid metabolites and platelet activating factors brings about neutrophil degranulation.[346] Nonsteroidal anti-inflammatory agents also modify neutrophil activity.[246] During inflammation due to bacterial infection, neutrophils undertake several activities: (1) sticking to capillary endothelium in the inflamed area, (2) migration, (3) traversing the vessel wall into the tissues, (4) chemotaxis and attachment to the microorganisms (5) phagocytosis and incorporation of the invading bacteria, (6) degranulation, (7) bactericidal action, and (8) digestion of the engulfed bacterial particles. During acute inflammation, neutrophils play also an important role in the deposition of platelets.[22,223]

The net surface charge of neutrophil membrane is negative, caused in part by the presence of sialic acid in the membrane. Under certain conditions, neutrophils have a tendency to stick to various surfaces or to stick to one another forming clumps. Factors involved in this process are plasma proteins, particularly fibrinogen and divalent cations.[9] These leukocytes can move along blood vessel walls or in tissues, usually moving in a zig-zag pattern and sending out new pseudopodia in a random fashion. Neutrophil movement varies depending on the physical and chemical nature of the environment, and under ideal conditions, these cells can travel 35 to 40 μm/min.[103] Neutrophils penetrate through capillaries or venules by squeezing themselves through small openings in the vessel wall, usually at the junctions between endothelial cells.[127]

Chemotaxis is probably related to the existence of a concentration gradient surrounding the chemotactic particle. Various substances, (e.g., bacterial factors) released by cells and complement fragments exert influences on chemotaxis.[525] When contact is established between a neutrophil and a small particle, the particle is internalized by the process of phagocytosis. There are two stages in neutrophil phagocytosis: attachment and ingestion. The cell membrane and particle or bacterium unite closely and no extracellular fluid is engulfed. In some cases, some of the surrounding medium is incorporated into the leukocyte along with the particle; this process is called "piggy back" phagocytosis.[401] During this process, serum substances act on the surfaces of bacteria by simple absorption and render them more susceptible for phagocytosis to take place. These serum substances are similar to antibodies or complements and collectively are named opsonins.[429] Part of the serum effect is due to colloid osmotic action and inactivation of toxic substances present in trace amounts. Phagocytosis by neutrophils is efficient over a pH range from 6 to 8 and is independent on the presence of oxygen in the environment; divalent cations seem to be necessary.

Following ingestion of bacteria neutrophils are degranulated. Hydrolytic enzymes are released from a granule-bound state to a soluble form into a pouch within the leukocyte.[79] The lysis of granules, leading to the discharge of hydrolases, is controlled to the extent to degrade engulfed material without digesting adjacent cytoplasm or nuclear structures at the same time. Neutrophils also exert bactericidal action associated with various metabolic products which have antibacterial effects including lactic acid and other organic acids, aldehydes, antibacterial proteins (lyzozyme, lactoferrin, cationic proteins), and the hydrogen peroxide-peroxidase system. Finally, depending on the nature of the engulfed particle, the ultimate fate is slow digestion. Within an hour macromolecular components such as proteins, nucleic acids, and complex lipids are broken down into smaller molecules to be used by the neutrophil for its own metabolic need or to be excreted from the cell.[77] Neutrophils can digest many biological materials, containing enzymes capable of degrading various types of polymers.[136] Inert materials such as carbon or polystyrene particles may remain unchanged for a long period within the cell.

2. Abnormalities of Neutrophil Leukocytes

Neutrophils protect the host against microbial invasion. In this host resistance, several steps are involved: production of neutrophils from bone marrow stem cells, maturation, release into circulation, sticking to vessel walls, mobility, migration into tissues, chemotaxis, phagocytosis degranulation, and digestion. Interference or abnormalities in any of these steps results in functional deficits. There are conditions where neutrophils are reduced in number or even absent. Individuals afflicted with agranulocytosis have greatly enhanced susceptibility to infection and sepsis. Application of excessive amounts of certain adrenal corticosteroids, cytotoxic drugs, or massive irradiation disturb the availability of neutrophils as well as their action on antibody formation. If these conditions suppress the production of neutrophils in the bone marrow, the circulating and tissue levels fall after the bone marrow pool is depleted. In a condition called cyclic neutropenia, the synthesis of neutrophils is intermittently inadequate due to a defect of the feedback regulatory mechanism that controls normal neutrophil production and function.[87] Tumor promotors split centrosomes in polymorphonuclear neutrophils,[405] and in breast cancer lysosomal enzymes of neutrophils show significant differences.[42] Tetracyclin suppresses the production of migration inhibitory factors in humans, and thus the action of this antibiotic contributes to the bactericidal action of neutrophils.[137]

In some forms of chronic granulocytic leukemia, neutrophil production and maturation are stopped at the myelocyte stage, and thus large numbers of immature cells are present in the bloodstream. Since these cells are morphologically and functionally immature, individuals suffering from this disorder have increased susceptibility to infections.[52] The high susceptibility to certain forms of bacterial sepsis of the renal medulla is connected with a delayed or inadequate influx of neutrophils during the inflammatory response. High salt concentration in the peritubular fluid or ammonia produced in the kidney may impair the migratory or phagocytic capacity of neutrophils.[70,386] Membrane fluidizers can affect the number and affinity of chemotactic receptors on polymorphonuclear leukocytes.[454] Chemotactic peptides induce changes in the cytosolic Ca^{2+} content of neutrophils from patients with chronic granulomatous disease.[272] Threadworm infection causes intense cellular responses in humans.[141]

Several congenital abnormalities in neutrophil structure or functions have been described.[260,410] In some lipid storage diseases, neutrophils show an inability to degrade certain phospholipids. In Gaucher's disease, neutrophils have low levels of glucocerebroside-clearing activity, and patients with Niemann-Pick's disease are unable to break down sphingomyelin normally.[241] Defective nuclear maturation occurs in the so-called Pegler-Huet neutrophils showing incompletely segmented nuclei. Inherited abnormalities also occur in neutrophil cytoplasmic structures.[260] In chronic granulomatous disease characterized by recurrent sepsis and widespread granulomatous inflammation,[197] the number of neutrophils is within normal range and exert normal function related to chemotaxis and phagocytosis. However, these neutrophils fail to kill certain bacteria due to a metabolic defect, connected with no increase in oxygen consumption and shunt activity, which occur normally after phagocytosis in normal neutrophils. This lack of bactericidal action is essentially a result of reduced or absent production of hydrogen peroxide, a factor active on its own or in conjunction with myeloperoxidase or other cofactors in killing bacteria.[291] Subnormal activities of NADH oxidase, glucose 6-phosphate dehydrogenase, and glutathione peroxidase have also been reported.[36,198]

In other genetically determined diseases of neutrophils there is an absence of peroxidase or glucose 6-phosphate dehydrogenase.[84,270]

B. MONONUCLEAR PHAGOCYTES
1. Macrophage Formation

Heterogenous tissue macrophages derive from bone marrow precursor stem cells.[106,471] The earliest mononuclear phagocytes produced are the promonocytes which by division give rise to monocytes. After a short maturation period in the bone marrow, they are released into the peripheral blood. Once in the circulation, monocytes represent only a small fraction of the blood-borne white cells. These cells disappear from the circulation with a half-life of 22 h, and in inflammatory conditions they migrate into tissues as macrophages.[470] Under stress or disease conditions, cells resembling typical macrophages may be present in the circulation in small numbers. These cells may enter through the thoracic duct. Dislodged Kupffer cells, representing macrophages of the liver, may also be present in the blood for a short period. Endotoxins have significant effects on macrophage lysosomal enzyme release in several liver disorders.[448] Oxygen radical scavengers protect alveolar macrophages from hyperoxic damage.[175] In contrast, ammonium chloride, zymosan, and tunicamycin affect the biosynthesis and transport of lysosomal enzymes in human macrophages.[220]

Intracellular levels of acid hydrolases represent the most important enzymatic correlate of mononuclear phagocyte maturation.[439] Enzymes packaged in the lysosomes of macrophages[57] are given in Table 5. The membrane-bound acid hydrolases exist in latent form within the membrane.[150] Enzymatic activity is markedly enhanced by agents which disrupt the integrity of the lysosomal membrane, thus allowing substrate-enzyme interactions. Levels of lysosomal enzymes differ among macrophage populations, and in general, they are greater in more mature or activated cells. At the same time during maturation of the macrophage and as acid hydrolases accumulate within the cell, there is a concomitant increase in the number of cytoplasmic granules or dense bodies which have the properties of lysosomes.[338]

2. Endocytosis

The ability of macrophages to internalize exogenous substances is highly developed, constituting a versatile function in inflammation.[78] A wide range of molecules can be sequestered and concentrated in the macrophage cytoplasm. The term phagocytosis is strictly used for the uptake of particles, and the term pinocytosis for when soluble molecules are incorporated.[341] The process of particle ingestion can be separated into two distinct phases and was described earlier. These phases are continuous and overlapping, but in some instances can be clearly separated. Macrophages take up both particulate and soluble exogenous molecules to a greater extent than many other tissue cells with similar activities.[299,341,374] Moveover, macrophages have a much wider spectrum of molecules, which it can internalize, than neutrophilic leukocytes. In particular, macrophages can ingest particles smaller than 0.1 μm as well as soluble molecules, whereas neutrophils are ineffective in this range. During the process of endocytosis, exogenous molecules are sequestered within vacuoles derived from the plasma membrane. These are transferred to the perinuclear area. In this

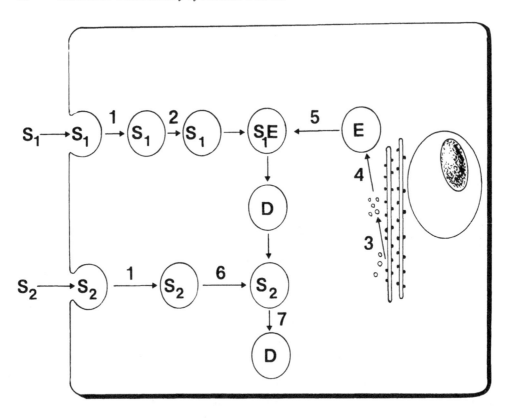

FIGURE 19.   Mechanism of endocytosis. Exogenous substances (S) are sequestered within vacuoles derived from the plasma membrane (1) and transported into the vicinity of the nucleus (2). Proteins, including hydrolytic enzymes (E), are produced by the endoplasmic reticulum (3) and transferred to the Golgi complex where they are incorporated into primary lysosomes (4). Fusion of primary lysosomes with endocytic vacuoles results in secondary lysosomes (5) where exogenous substances and hydrolytic enzymes are mixed. Secondary lysosomes or digestive bodies (D) may be more condensed and can incorporate exogenous substances by pinocytosis (6) to produce larger phagocytic vacuoles converting it to a digestive body (7).

area of the cytoplasm, newly synthesized proteins, including hydrolytic enzymes, are produced by the endoplasmic reticulum and transferred to the Golgi complex with subsequent packing into Golgi-derived vesicles or into primary lysosomes. Fusion of primary lysosomes with endocytic vacuoles produces secondary lysosomes or digestive bodies where exogenous substrates are mixed with hydrolases. Secondary lysosomes may take up more exogenous substrates derived from pinocytosis (Figure 19).

There are a number of substances that stimulate pinocytotic activity of macrophages *in vitro*;[80,411] these include various anionic molecules, such as dextransulfate, bicarboxylic amino acids (L-glutamic acid, L-aspartic acid), hyaluronic acid, heparin, or chondroitin sulfate C. Some of these agents are found in the inflammatory exudate and may play a cumulative role in stimulating macrophages during inflammation. Fe^{3+} affects phagocytic and metabolic activity of human polymorphonuclear leukocytes in the presence of various ligands.[467] Air pollutants alter the oxidative metabolism and phagocytic capacity of pulmonary alveolar macrophages,[389] and testicular macrophages show hormonal responsiveness.[533]

In contrast to stimulatory actions, X-irradiation and certain drugs cause a decrease of macrophage activity. Following the exposure of experimental animals to sublethal doses of X-rays, the production of circulating monocytes is drastically diminished.[470,475] The effect of irradiation is due to damage to the bone marrow precursors such as promonocytes. Within a day or two the number of monocytes falls to low levels together with other white cells and platelets and requires several weeks to return to normal levels. Macrophages already present in the tissues are relatively resistant to ionizing radiation.

In animal experiments, large doses of corticosteroids decrease the number of mononuclear phagocytes entering the site of the inflammatory lesion, but do not alter the number of macrophages present in the tissue.[76,452] The effect steroids on sequestration of the monocyte is probably a lytic action. The depleted circulating pool influences the number of cells arriving at the inflammatory site associated with enhanced susceptibility to infection. On the other hand, macrophage receptors for bacterial cell wall sugars are the possible determinants of susceptibility and may be representing the product of immune response genes.[498]

C. PLATELETS

1. Platelet Aggregation

Platelets are characteristic cells which play an important role when blood vessels are injured. Since inflammation occurs as a response to tissue injury, the hemostatic function of platelets can be considered as part of the inflammatory process.[504] Platelets do not play a central role in inflammation, but modify the course of the inflammatory response by releasing pharmacologically active substances. This release can be modulated by nonsteroidal anti-inflammatory drugs.

Platelets circulate normally through the endothelium-lined blood vessels as disk-shaped cells or cell fragments. In platelet storage, white blood cells play an important role.[151] When the vessels are injured and the endothelium is damaged, the platelets come in contact with other elements of the vascular wall and initiate a series of processes leading to the formation of the hemostatic plug or to the production of a potentially dangerous thrombus.[53,111] Adhesion of platelets to the vessel wall is the first event in the inflammatory process followed by aggregation and consolidation of the platelet mass with release of certain constituents.[78] EDTA inhibits clumping.[400]

Platelet aggregation is ADP dependent and stimulated by contact with microfibrils or exposure to thrombin.[135,313] Exogenous epinephrine stimulates α-receptors on platelets.[451] The platelet aggregation induced by any of these agents can be prevented by EDTA, indicating that bivalent cations are involved in the process. Aggregation of platelets is a phenomenon absent in patients with a rare congenital hemorrhagic disease, known as thrombasthenia,[529] and can be modified by drugs[91,120] and other conditions.[37,62,116,195,275,353,358] There are differences in the effect of certain drugs on platelets from normal or thrombasthenia patients.[267] In leukemic children, sequential changes develop following treatment with L-asparaginase, prednisone, or vincristine.[372]

In thrombocytopenia, platelets interact with antigen-antibody complexes. Thrombocytopenia of the newborn can be characterized by failure of production, increased utilization, and destruction or abnormal dilution.[13] Certain drugs can induce this disease by inducing antibodies which subsequently react with the free drug to produce the complex.[418] Further, the complex is taken up by platelets and destroys them. Circulating antiplatelet antibodies have been demonstrated in idiopathic thrombocytopenia and in systemic lupus erythematosus.[208]

In von Willebrand's disease, platelets interact with antihemophylic globulin (Factor VIII);[310] this factor also affects the adhesion of platelets to human artery endothelium.[425] Factor VIII-related antigen increases platelet adhesion to collagen.[1] Antiplatelet antibodies have been detected in patients with idiopathic thrombocytopenic purpura, systemic lupus erythematosus, and in other clinical disorders.[249]

2. Release Mechanisms

Adhesion of platelets to collagen and other stimuli induce the release of ADP and other constituents from platelets. These stimuli include (1) particulate materials (collagen, antigen-antibody complexes), (2) enzymes (thrombin, trypsin), and (3) low molecular weight compounds (ADP, epinephrine).[204] The action of thrombin and collagen is to release serotonin from platelets. ADP and epinephrine produce two waves of platelet aggregation; the second wave is connected with the release of ADP, ATP, and serotonin, and under some conditions certain platelet enzymes are also discharged. Thrombin releases selective hydrolytic enzymes present in the α-granules, such as β-glucuronidase, cathepsin, and β-N-acetylglucosaminidase. Only small amounts of acid phosphatases are released from platelet granules, and cytoplasmic or mitochondrial enzymes are not discharged from platelets.[201,202a] The release process in hemostasis is very rapid and needs ATP derived from glycolysis or from oxidative phosphorylation. Changes occur in membrane phospholipid distribution during platelet activation,[39] and myosin phosphorylation may be involved in the initiation of this process.[92] Hypertension and the ratio of total cholesterol to HDL cholesterol and kallikrein excretion are related to platelet aggregation.[276]

A number of investigations described the role of agents and factors involved in inhibition of platelet aggregation and release. Among these, chelating agents bind calcium ions and thus prevent aggregation. Release of ADP or epinephrine is coupled with primary ADP-induced platelet aggregation. Substances which inhibit release also block aggregation. Adenosine, dibutyryl cyclic AMP, SH-group reactive substances can act on both processes. Elevation of cyclic AMP within platelets by stimulation of adenyl cyclase or inhibition of phosphodiesterase also inhibit release or aggregation brought about by collagen, epinephrine, or ADP.[466,530]

D. MAST CELLS
1. Normal and Neoplastic Mast Cells

The thymus and the spleen are the main sites where mast cells are produced; fixed undifferentiated mesenchymal cells represent the main source of mast cells.[207,208,418] Mast cells proliferate by mitosis[4,142] and are mainly formed in loose connective tissue. Thus, their presence in various tissues and organs has been correlated with tissue collagen content. Bone and cartilage do not contain mast cells, but the surrounding dense layers of connective tissue, the perichondrium and periosteum, possess a fair number of mast cells. Parenchymatous organs such as kidney, liver, and adrenals have relatively low connective tissue content, and mast cells are rare in these organs. In ovaries, testes, spleen, pancreas, lymph glands, salivary glands, and heart, mast cells occur more frequently. In organs rich in connective tissue, large numbers of mast cells are found, such as lung, mammary gland, and prostate. Mast cells are numerous in the digestive tract, serous membranes, and skin. Normal human skin contains between 2000 and 7500 mast cells/cm^3 depending on the region.[235]

Mast cell proliferation or hyperplasia is rather common in a wide variety of conditions. Mast cell neoplasias are relatively rare. In experiments using mice, mast cell proliferation occurs in the skin after painting with 3-methylcholanthrene. It is not clear whether the increase in numbers of mast cells is a hyperplastic reaction associated with the production of skin cancer or the result of a direct response to the carcinogen representing true neoplastic proliferation.[86] Morphologically, hyperplastic mast cells are not significantly different from normal mast cells. In contrast, neoplastic mast cells may show the general characteristics of neoplastic cells such as polymorphism, decreased number and distribution of cytoplasmic granules, increased nucleus size and large nucleoli, frequent mitosis, and sometimes the presence of giant multinucleated cells.

Mast cells contain various mucopolysacharides. Heparin is the major constituent, but various amounts of chondroitin sulfate, heparin monosulfate, and hyaluronic acid are also present. Histamine is formed in the mast cell from histidine by decarboxylation. Normal and neoplastic mast cells not only synthesize histamine, but also take up this amine by passive process.[96] The exogenous histamine is bound to the mast granules. The degranulation and histamine release induced by releasing agents are enzymatic processes requiring energy and are blocked by inhibitors.[130,131] There are chemicals which affect degranulation and release by mechanisms which alter the membrane integrity of the mast cell. Serotonin and heparin also reside in the granules. Serotonin and histamine may be synthesized in the cytoplasm and stored in granules in inactive form.[168]

2. Mast Cells in Disease

During acute inflammation, the disappearance of mast cells is preceded by degranulation. In this process histamine, heparin, some enzymes, and occasionally serotonin are discharged from intact mast cells into the surrounding ground substance of connective tissue. This release, as an important feature of acute inflammation, is connected with some stages including hyperemia, increased vascular permeability, edema, and initiation of the repair processes. Mast cells are invariably increased in chronic inflammatory processes and are particularly numerous in the connective tissue bordering neoplasia. Mast cells may participate in defense reactions against tumor cells by interfering with cell division. This role is connected with the release of heparin which is an inhibitor of mitosis,[278] possibly through an interaction with the metabolism of nucleoproteins.[357] In cancer of the cervix, a close association was found between mast cells and mitotic tumor cells.[153]

In methylcholanthrene-induced experimental carcinogenesis, mast cells are involved in the promotion phase.[380] It has been suggested that in the process of skin tumor formation, mucopolysaccharides derived from mast cells may play an inhibitory role by restoring permeability of the connective tissue to normal.[86] In subcutaneous Walker's carcinoma, the initial phase is more rapid in rats with depleted mast cells than in controls.[126] Local serotonin injections inhibit subsequent growth, while heparin and histamine are ineffective. In the defensive role of mast cells in tumor growth serotonin may be the inhibitory factor.

E. LYMPHOCYTES

1. Origin and Classification

Lymphocytes are the major constituents of normal lymph nodes, white pulp of the spleen, and unencapsulated lymphoid tissue from the lungs and alimentary tract. In normal blood, lymphocytes constitute the large portion of leukocytes and are predominant in lymph.[528] Many conditions modify lymphocyte production and destruction, including various drugs, aging, radiation therapy, and several diseases.[16,69,88,163,252,257,280,284,298,312,334,413,420,421,446,450,463,497] These conditions also alter lymphocyte composition.[333,455] The mitogenic response of normal lymphocytes is suppressed by serum factors from patients with testicular germ cell tumors.[479] Lymphocytes are prominent in the bone marrow, intestinal submucosa, and in tissues during chronic inflammation. Lymphocytes are divided into three groups with respect to size: small (nuclear diameter range 6 to 8 μm), medium (6 to 10 μm), and large (>10 μm). Small lymphocytes are further subdivided into two species, both derived from precursors in the bone marrow, but during their extramedullary development they acquire distinct properties such as thymus-dependent, or T lymphocytes and thymus-independent, or B lymphocytes. These lymphocytes operate separately or together in a broad range of immunological system disorders. Large and medium size lymphocytes are proliferating rapidly, small lymphocytes are rarely divided. Some small lymphocytes can survive for an exceptionally long time in man. The mechanism of lymphocyte activation is associated with the internal activity of the immune system.[85] Patients given large doses of ionizing irradiation show some years later that small lymphocytes differentiate and divide under the influence of phytohemagglutinin.[340] Many investigations established that one of the major functions of lymphocytes is their participation in the immune responses.[12]

2. Molecular Mediators in Lymphocytes

When lymphocytes are exposed to antigen many pharmacologically active substances have been detected in the medium.[302] Some of these molecules inhibit the migration of macrophages, some are cytotoxic to target cells,[154,155] chemotactic for leukocytes,[486,490] and mitogenic for nonsensitive lymphocytes.[154,527]

Certain infectious diseases, especially those caused by intracellular parasites, are not controlled by serum antibodies. Although parasites sequestered within cells are inaccessible to antibodies, the body defends itself against infections by mechanisms associated with delayed-type hypersensitivity. Specific sets of lymphocytes are involved in this protection against infection. These lymphocytes are present in the spleen, thoracic duct, or peritoneal cavity and exert their protective influence through mononuclear phagocytes with the help of molecular mediators.[261,303] Reacting lymphocytes release a chemotactic agent which finds its way into an infective focus and influence the disposition of monocytes within lesions. A similar factor from immune lymphocytes may stimulate metabolic activity and enhance microbicidal action of migrating phagocytes.[147] The formation of immunoglobulins by circulating lymphocytes is related to this process.[469]

F. COMPLEMENT SYSTEM

It has been generally established that human complement can be separated into several proteins with hemolytic activities required for immune-lytic reactions.[323,336,481] The complement system and inactivation of complement components play an important role in the inflammatory process. Components or fragments of the complement can induce changes in cell membranes and in vascular permeability. These mechanisms are also related to systems involved in kinin formation or coagulation. Certain complement-mediated reactions are connected with hypersensitivity diseases and with basic reactions that become manifest in organ transplantation and in tumor immunity.

The interaction of proteins of the complement system in an organized cascading order results in a variety of biological phenomena, which include the release of vasoactive peptides, the attraction of polymorphonuclear, neutrophils, increase of phagocytosis, and disruption of cell membranes. During the inflammatory process, by releasing histamine from mast cells, the complement system causes increased capillary permeability, edema, and contraction of smooth muscle. In histamine-independent reactions, it causes directed migration of polymorphonuclear neutrophils, opsonization of particles or membranes to facilitate contact with phagocytic cells, and contraction of specialized muscles such as the rat uterus or guinea pig ileum. The complement system also takes part in the initiation of the blood coagulation process by immune complexes.

The most important events in the complement system lead to the activation of Cl or C3 and possibly C8. In these processes, antibody-dependent and antibody-independent mechanisms participate. C5 component is essential in the production of fragments that are important in the inflammatory processes via histamine release or chemotaxis. Two specific peptides derived from C3 and C5 components can induce histamine release, smooth muscle contraction, and chemotactic activity. These peptides of the complement system are referred to as C3a and C5a anaphylatoxin.[476]

In rheumatoid arthritis, in which significant inflammation persists, materials which are normally rapidly removed from the circulation remain stagnant in the joints, including aggregated γ-globulin[426] and breakdown products of the complement system.[531] In rheumatoid effusions, there is a decrease in synovial fluid total hemolytic complement activity. Particularly, C2, C3, and C4 components are depressed,[392] and the trimolecular complex of C5, C6, and C7 is present.[491] This could result from (1) a selective destruction of a single or several components of complement inhibitors, or (2) an increased activity of complement inhibitors, or (3) an enhanced metabolism of the late acting components of the complement system through an alternate pathway. There is evidence that an alternate pathway of complement metabolism is activated in the rheumatoid joint.[148]

VIII. MECHANISM OF FEVER PRODUCTION

Elevation of the body temperature or fever is the most common manifestation of inflammation. This elevation is caused generally by an alteration in the central nervous regulation of body temperature. In a few instances, increased temperature may be associated with a direct activation of a peripheral mechanism which enhances heat production or diminishes heat loss, i.e., hyperthyroidism or pheochromocytoma. Hyperthermia during exercise, in the postovulatory phase of the menstrual cycle, or at the beginning of menopause are not considered fever.

The maintenance of normal body temperature is controlled by a complex set of reactions and feedback mechanisms associated with the production and dissipation of body heat. These reactions are triggered by the hypothalamus as a response to stimuli received from thermoreceptors. These receptors are present abundantly in the skin and possibly in the hypothalamus itself, in the spinal cord, and in the viscera. An interaction between the peripheral and central mechanisms determines the response of the body to internal or external environmental temperature changes. The temperature of the blood flowing through the hypothalamus appears to be the most important factor in the initiation of heat changes. The thermostatic set point of this organ in man reacts very sensitively to changes as small as a fraction of 1°. When the temperature of the blood perfusing the hypothalamus is raised, there is loss of heat via vasodilation, perspiration, and panting. During fever, hypothalamic temperature regulation is still obtained, but at a higher baseline level.

Inflammation is connected with the release of pyrogenic products derived from bacteria, viruses and fungi, or from the destruction of cellular organelles. In the case of infection by bacteria or viruses, two mechanisms have been considered recently in the pathogenesis of fever in inflammatory reaction. One is based on the release of endogenous pyrogen substances from cells, and the other is related to pharmacological mediation. An indirect hyperthermia also exists which is connected with the mobilization of endogenous pyrogens from the tissues by the microorganism. However, in the case of bacterial or viral infections the production of endotoxins and their secretion into the cell are probably the major factors contributing to the manifestation of fever. Various pyrogens can be detected in the circulation and can exert direct effects on the regulatory centers of the hypothalamus.

It is not known whether bacterial endotoxins can also act directly on the hypothalamus producing fever, but it is evident that much of their pyrogenic action is mediated by fever-inducing endogenous substances. In a variety of experimental fevers, the rise of temperature is produced by circulating endogenous pyrogens which are different from the initially injected agents. In spite of the different etiology of the fever in different species, the pyrogens are structurally similar. These molecules have direct and immediate action on the thermoregulatory center. The elaboration of a circulating pyrogen of endogenous origin suggests a common pathway for the pathogenesis of fever during inflammation.

Endogenous pyrogen substances are also released from polymorphonuclear leukocytes. Granulocytes in the normal human blood contain little or no detectable pyrogen, but leukocytes present in the inflammatory exudate cause fever.

Besides inflammation, clinical conditions accompanied by fever are hypersensitivity, tissue necrosis and malignancy, and others. The mechanisms of fever production associated with neoplasia is unknown; it is possible that certain tumor cells synthesize endogenous pyrogens. The sequence of events participating in the mechanism of increased body temperature in different diseases may be diverse, since a variety of activators and cell types, endogenous and exogenous pyrogens, and regulating factors may be present in varying amounts. The interrelationship between these factors is probably complex and their release from the host by the infectious agent can be envisaged in many ways (Figure 20).

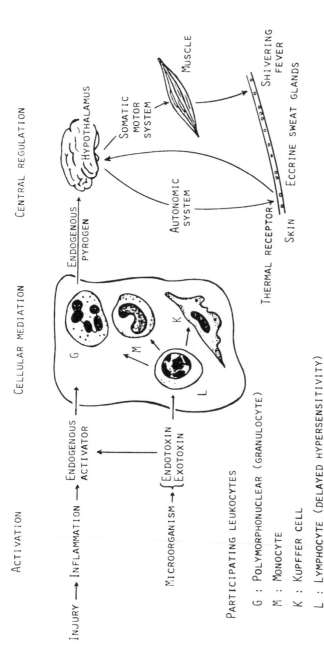

FIGURE 20.   Scheme of pathways participating in the pathogenesis of fever. These include activation leading to the release of endogenous pyrogen, cellular mediation, and central feedback regulation. The infectious agent can directly evoke an inflammatory response by releasing exotoxins or endotoxins by being phagocytozed or indirectly by activating endogenous activators, which in turn produce endogenous pyrogens. The central regulation is connected to peripheral receptors by the autonomic nervous system, however, the physiological pathway of fever sensation is relayed by the somatic motor system.

A. BACTERIAL ENDOTOXINS

Endotoxins constitute part of the cell wall and form the O-antigen in Gram-negative bacteria. The presence of these endotoxins in Gram-positive bacteria and in other micro-organisms has not yet been confirmed.

These bacterial endotoxins are macromolecular lipopolysaccharide substances containing complex polysaccharides, phosphate and lipid, with molecular weights ranging from 10^5 to 10^6 Da. The endotoxin molecule is made up of three regions: (1) central polysaccharide core consisting of at least five sugar molecules, including 2-keto-3-deoxyoctonic acid combined with phosphate radicals and ethanolamine; (2) lipid is attached to the centrum by an acid-labile bond through 2-keto-3-deoxyoctonic acid; and (3) O-antigen-specific side chains responsible for the immunological specificity.[205,281,344,520] Smaller fragments of the lipopolysaccharide unit with a molecular weight of 10^5 Da or lower may show strong pyrogenic potency. Ethanolamine and phosphate are retained during degradation of this substance, and endotoxins cause fever production highly sensitive to dosage.

From the beginning of inflammation there is a lag period before the onset of hyperthermia. In experimental animals following the intravenous inoculation of moderate doses of endotoxin, this delay is about 20 to 30 min and develops during the latency period leukopenia. With increased amounts of endotoxin, the fever response shows a biphasic character associated with progressive leukocytosis. The latency period between the release of endotoxin and the onset of fever suggests that in the case of Gram-negative bacteria, endotoxins exert their action by liberating endogenous substances from the host cells.

The pyrogenic lipopolysaccharide endotoxin is absent in the cell wall of Gram-positive bacteria, and therefore, their fever-inducing action is different. Sufficient doses of Gram-positive bacteria produce a biphasic febrile reaction after a delay of 45 to 60 min. This latency is longer than the delayed action of endotoxins (Figure 21). It seems that Gram-positive bacteria are pyrogenic by themselves due to their capacity to be phagocytozed and accordingly, they provoke a profound inflammatory reaction at extravascular sites by releasing endogenous pyrogens into the circulation. The nature of pyrogenic factors isolated from Gram-positive bacteria differs from those of Gram-negatives. A primarily intracellular and group-specific pyrogen and several extracellular substances have been isolated from Gram-positive bacteria. These are different from each other in antigen response and also distinct chemically from the endotoxins of Gram-negative bacteria; they are mucopeptides rather than lipopolysaccharides.

B. VIRAL ENDOTOXINS

In viral infections, the pyrogenic substances are closely associated with the viral particle. The latent period before the onset of the febrile response is 1 to 2 h, and the fever is accompanied by a progressive and prolonged leukopenia. At present little is known about the chemical nature of specific factors in viruses which cause fever; a carbohydrate fraction seems to be responsible for the action.

C. LEUKOCYTE PYROGENS

Several types of mononuclear cells are involved in the production of endogenous pyrogens. The release of these substances from different granulocytes in the exudate during inflammation causes hyperthermia. The release of these pyrogens is followed by the action of various irritants (bacterial infections: pneumococcal peritonitis, streptococcal skin lesions, or pharyngitis; Gram-positive organisms: viruses, particulate substances, and antigens). The mechanism of the pyrogen production from leukocytes is associated with an activation by the irritants.

The process of cell activation leading to pyrogen release probably begins with an interaction of the inducing agent with leukocytes followed by an alteration of the cell mem-

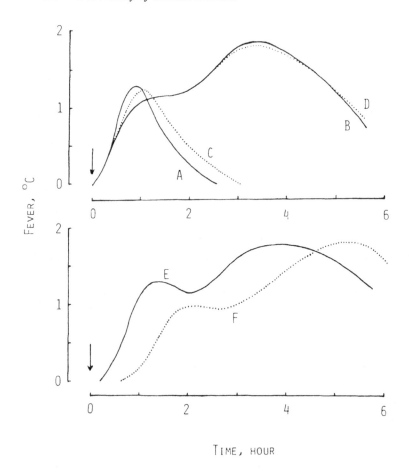

FIGURE 21. Time course of fever production following various endogenous and exogenous pyrogens. Endogenous pyrogens: (A) leukocytes (5×10^7), (B) leukocytes 1×10^9, (C) serum endogenous pyrogen low dose, (D) high dose. Exogenous pyrogens: (E) Gram-negative bacterial endotoxin, (F) Gram-positive cells, colloidal particles, viruses. The latency period shows differences, and the biphasic response is marked only in larger doses.

brane. The pyrogen producing leukocytes contain a nonpyrogenic precursor which is converted to the effective agent through an enzymatic step. The activation represents either an increased enzyme or precursor synthesis.

The action of the endogenous pyrogen is mediated through the anterior hypothalamus where thermosensitive neurons are located. The precise way these neurons are affected has not yet been revealed. Changes in local concentrations of prostaglandins or monoamines and ionic balance have been postulated in the process.

Leukocyte pyrogens are produced by several types of cells in man. They may derive from basic proteins of lysosomes or polymorphonuclear leukocytes. These substances are polypeptides with a molecular weight of 10 to 20×10^3 Da, and probably contain small amounts of carbohydrate and lipid. These polypeptides are destroyed by alkali, and the presence of free sulfhydryl groups seems to be essential for pyrogenic activity. The chemical identification of these substances indicate a clear differentiation from bacterial endotoxins. Leukocyte pyrogens are also very potent and in nanogram quantities can elevate body temperature significantly. Several experimental models have established that monocytes and macrophages also provide endogenous pyrogens. Kupfer cells can also be activated by various microbial agents to produce pyrogens in the liver.

D. PHARMACOLOGICAL SUBSTANCES

Many pharmacological agents can cause elevations of body temperature, including epinephrine, norepinephrine, or serotonin. The effect of epinephrine and norepinephrine may be related to direct vasoconstriction of peripheral vessels. These amines may play a role in the fever associated with pheochromocytoma. Investigations on the action of endogenous pyrogens revealed that in the hypothalamus their pyrogenic effect is mediated by norepinephrine stored locally. On the other hand, serotonin seems to be necessary for the cooling effect.

Several steroids and bile acids which belong to the epi-stereoisomer series (5β-H ring structure) possess pyrogenic activity. The effect of these steroid metabolites is associated with a variety of clinical fevers. Their mechanism of action has not yet been revealed, but it is unlikely that they act directly on the thermoregulatory center. The pyrogenic activity of various related compounds shows correlations with the steric configuration of steroids or bile acids and with the presence of a hydroxyl group. Some experiments revealed that steroid fever is accompanied by a pronounced leukocytosis, a consequence of granulocyte mobilization from the bone marrow. These steroids may, therefore, initiate the release of endogenous pyrogens.

Among these steroids a metabolite, etiocholanolone, has been shown to induce fever in human subjects.[248,258,519] Etiocholanolone is derived from either testosterone, Δ4-androstene-3,17,-dione or dehydroepiandrosterone (Figure 22), and it probably originates from the testes and adrenal cortex. Etiocholanolone has no hormonal activity; it is excreted into the urine in free form and conjugated with glucuronic acid. Etiocholanolone is pyrogenic to humans only in its unconjugated form and in amounts that are known to be produced under physiological circumstances. Androsterone, which is formed in parallel with etiocholanolone, is only slightly pyrogenic. This steroid contains the allo ring structure.

Etiocholanolone is highly inflammatory at the injection site and the fever produced by this compound can be abolished by cortisol if injected together with etiocholanolone. Aspirin elicits only a slight suppressing action. The inhibitory effect of cortisol suggests an interaction between these steroids at the cellular level *in situ* in the subsequent fever response. The action of etiocholanolone is probably mediated through the labilization of lysosomes and release of endogenous pyrogens.

Prostaglandins are involved in the pathogenesis of fever; small doses of prostaglandin E_1 or E_2 injected into the cerebral ventricles of experimental animals induce a pronounced hyperthermic response. Other prostaglandins such as $F_2\alpha$ have no pyrogenic action. Antipyretic drugs (aspirin, sodium salicylate, indomethacin, and acetaminophen) suppress the effect of prostaglandins. It has been suggested that these drugs inhibit the synthesis of the pyrogens at the site of inflammation or might act by interfering with the production of prostaglandin in the hypothalamus. Differences in the effect of drugs might be related to a different sensitivity of hypothalamic prostaglandin synthetase to any drug. Some antipyretic drugs such as paracetamol do not inhibit the febrile response of prostaglandin, which indicates that prostaglandins may play a role as neurohumoral transmitters in fever production.

IX. REACTION OF THE BLOOD CIRCULATION TO INJURY

A. FACTORS INVOLVED IN THROMBOSIS AND HEMOSTASIS
1. Blood Coagulation

Blood coagulation is involved in the processes of inflammation and tissue repair, in hemostasis and thrombosis, and in the production or activation of chemotactic factors that cause pain and factors that influence the permeability and contraction of blood vessels.

The end-point of blood coagulation is the transformation of fibrinogen to fibrin by the action of thrombin.[40,67,160,245] This can be divided into two systems based on the mechanisms

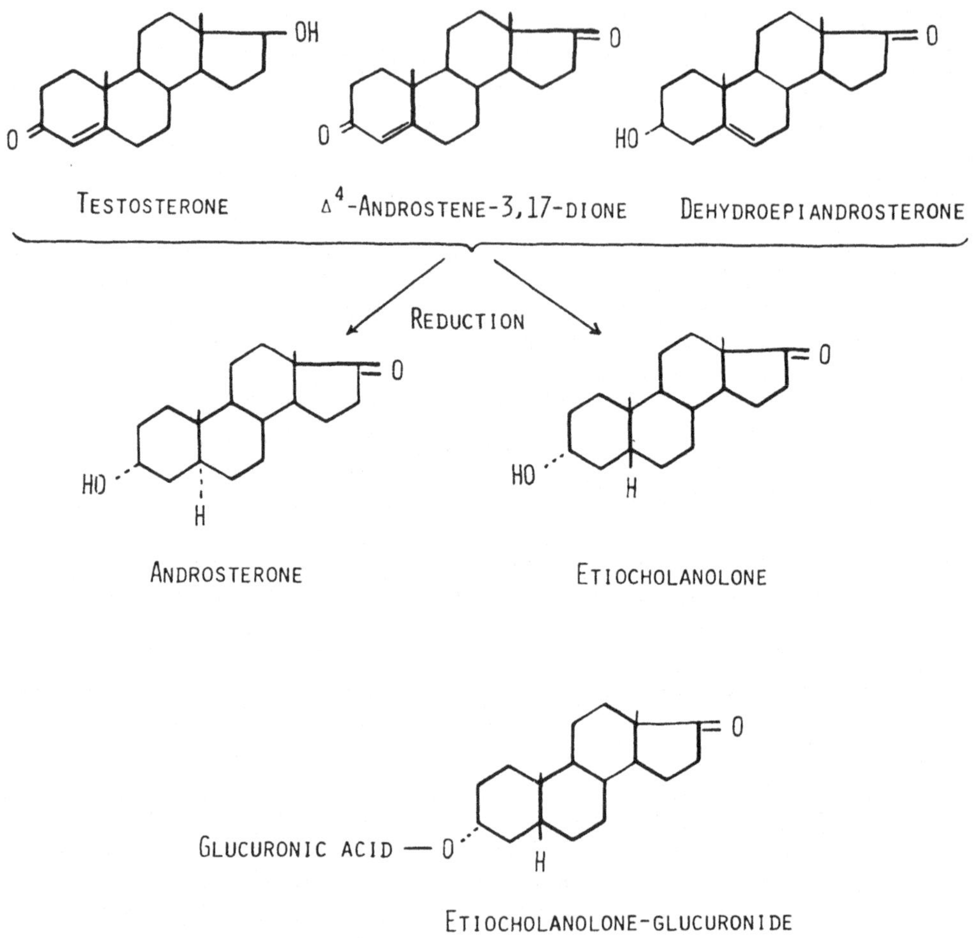

FIGURE 22.   Mechanism of etiocholanolone synthesis.

by which thrombin is formed from prothrombin. According to the extrinsic mechanism, tissue thromboplastin is derived from the injured cells, and it converts prothrombin to thrombin in the presence of several factors (Table 4) such as calcium, Factor VII, Factor V, and Factor X (Figure 23). In the intrinsic mechanism, blood generates an activating agent that rapidly transforms prothrombin to thrombin using calcium, platelets, Factor XII, Factor XI, Factor IX, Factor VIII, Factor V, and Factor X.[40] The thrombin so formed then activates the conversion of fibrinogen to fibrin.

Factors involved in fibrin formation which promote coagulation are the procoagulants. In addition to these activating factors, there are a number of inhibitors that can limit these reactions and thus the extent of fibrin formation. These are the anticoagulants.

2. Thrombin-Fibrinogen Reaction

The transformation of blood from fluid state into gel is connected with the production of an interwoven network of insoluble fibrin from fibrinogen. Human fibrinogen is a dimer protein constituted from three pairs of chains joined by disulfide bridges[316] with a molecular weight approximating 340,000 Da and a structure described as $(A\alpha, B\beta, \gamma)_2$ where $A\alpha$, $B\beta$, and γ represent fibrinopeptides A, B, and C, respectively. The stability of fibrinogen is associated with the negatively charged amino terminal regions of the $A\alpha$ and $B\beta$ chains. The coagulation takes place in two distinct stages.[105,293] The first stage is enzymatic, thrombin

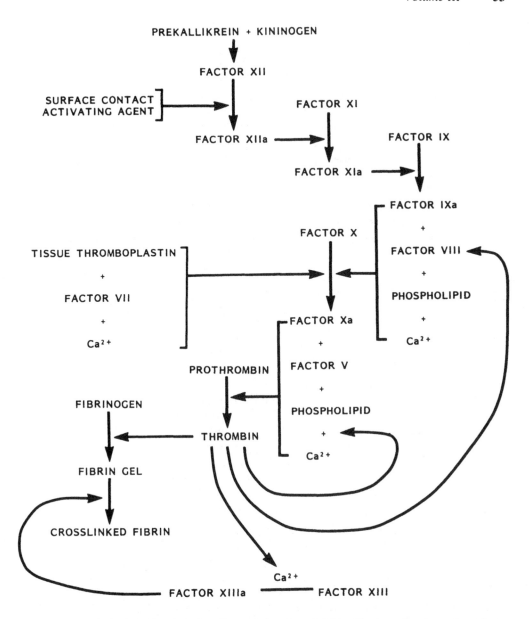

FIGURE 23.   Mechanism of blood clotting. The extrinsic pathway is initiated by tissue thromboplastin, while the intrinsic pathway is connected with surface contact or other activating agents. Collagen and antigen-antibody complexes represent such contact surfaces. The various steps in this cascade of coagulation indicate the formation of active forms of various clotting factors.

cleaves four arginyl-glycine bonds of fibrinogen and by releasing fibrinopeptides, fibrin is formed that can be represented by the formula $(\alpha\beta\gamma)_2$. Two other peptides are also released, AP and Y; these are analogs to fibrinopeptide A. Peptides released from fibrinogen, particularly fibrinopeptide B, enhance the response of smooth muscle to various stimuli. The second stage is the polymerization of fibrin.[43] During this stage, fibrin monomers aggregate to form the matrix of the clot. Fibrinopeptide A is necessary for the initiation of polymerization, and it is released more rapidly than fibrinopeptide B. The release of the latter takes place simultaneously with polymerization.

Plasma contains a fibrin stabilizing factor (Factor XIII) which is activated by thrombin and calcium ions to Factor XIIIa (Figure 23). This then catalyzes the production of a γ–Glu–ε–Lys bond between glutamine and lysine side chains of neighboring fibrin molecules. Intermolecular γ–γ linkages are formed rapidly followed by a slower production of α–α cross-linkages.[105,125] Subjects with a defect in Factor XIII cannot produce firm cross-links and they have a tendency to bleeding, poor wound healing, and easy bruising.[2]

Fibrinogen-fibrin transformation occurs continuously to some extent in the circulating blood. Altered fibrinogen has been found in the blood of patients with clinical conditions associated with intravascular thrombosis. This altered fibrinogen is partially converted to fibrin. During this conversion some of its fibrinopeptide A is lost, and it is called cryofibrinogen or cryoprofibrin because it precipitates in the cold from heparinized blood.[59,343]

3. Thrombin Formation

Thrombin with a molecular weight of 34,000 to 40,000 Da, is not present in detectable amounts in normal blood. It is formed from its precursor, prothrombin of 65,000 to 74,000 Da molecular weight. Prothrombin is an α-globulin and forms a single polypeptide chain; recently, its structure has been established.[288] Thrombin is composed of two polypeptide chains connected by a disulfide bridge.[187] The transformation of prothrombin to thrombin by Factor Xa is very rapid in the presence of Factor Va phospholipid and calcium ions. This reaction is part of a series of processes called the coagulation cascade [285] (Figure 22). Contact of the blood with activating substances or surfaces, such as glass, activates Factor XII. This factor activates Factor XI, which in turn activates Factor IX. Activated Factor IX, in association with Factor VIII, phospholipid, and calcium ions, activates Factor X. This factor then causes the conversion of prothrombin to thrombin. Some of these activation processes are intrinsically related to limited proteolysis.

Calcium binding sites on Factor X and prothrombin are involved in the binding of these molecules to phospholipid.[189] The binding of clotting factors to the phospholipid facilitates the enzyme reaction. Platelets are important in the intrinsic pathway of blood clotting, since they provide most phospholipid to which these coagulation factors can be attached. Substances such as collagen and thrombin induce the release reaction from platelets which makes a phospholipoprotein platelet factor available on the surface of platelets.[231]

Platelet aggregation may play an important role in the initiation of coagulation. Factors that induce platelet aggregation also accelerate clotting in platelet-rich plasma.[177,330] Platelets exposed to ADP can activate Factor XII and when platelets interact with collagen, Factor XI is activated even in the blood of Factor XII-deficient patients. The activated coagulation factors from the platelet membrane are protected from destruction by naturally occurring inhibitors present in plasma.[483]

There is a complex relationship among the activation of Factor XII, activation of Factor XI, formation of plasmin, formation of kallikrein, and the effect of high-molecular weight kininogen (Figure 23). Subjects with prekallikrein deficiency elicit no special symptoms, but their blood exerts a prolonged clotting time *in vitro*. They show a defective surface-mediated activation of fibrinolysis and defective permeability enhancement.[397,499] In this disease condition kallikrein accelerates the activation of Factor XII and Factor VII, and enhances the conversion of kininogen to bradykinin.[245] A defect in kininogen production is due to the deficiency of high-molecular weight kininogen, and it prolongs clotting time *in vitro*, with an impaired generation of the vascular permeability factor. Various steps involved in blood coagulation and vascular alterations are presented in a scheme (Figure 24).

4. Anticoagulant Factors

These factors represent important checks to the coagulation process. Without the action of these substances a simple injury can produce events leading to widespread intravascular coagulation that would be disastrous for the organism. Several plasma proteins have been identified that can inhibit proteolytic enzymes, and under some circumstances can act as

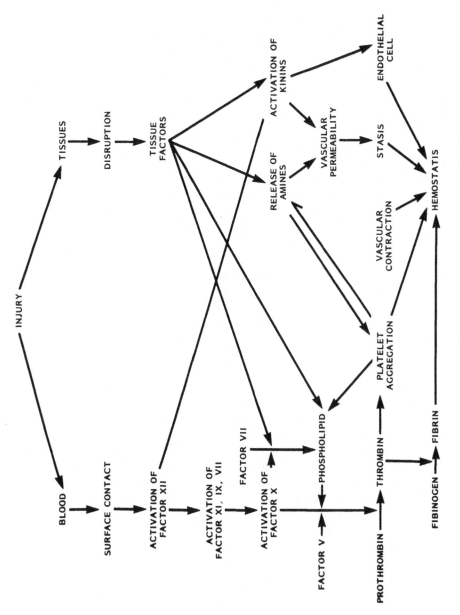

FIGURE 24.   Schematic presentation of blood coagulation and vascular changes following injury. In addition to this scheme, surface contact may cause platelet aggregation, and tissue disruption and may also cause vascular contraction directly.

anticoagulants. These proteins comprise about 20% of the globulin faction and include α-antitrypsin, $α_2$-macroglobulin, Cl-inactivator, and antithrombin III exerting a serine-esterase inhibitor action.[180,406]

The $α_1$-antitrypsin acts against thrombin, activated Factor XI, and in a limited way, against the action of kallikrein.[134,138,185] The action of $α_2$-macroglobulin is predominantly connected with its binding to proteins. It forms complexes with plasmin, kallikrein, thrombin, and chymotrypsin, and the complex formation does not prevent the complex from being active against the usual substrates of these enzymes. Some proteolytic activity still remains present, and when $α_2$-macroglobulin-enzyme complexes are formed they are rapidly cleared from the circulation.[180] It seems that in the binding between $α_2$-macroglobulin and the enzyme the active site is not fully blocked, and therefore the enzyme is able to degrade some substances.[179] The role of $α_2$-macroglobulin is complex. When it binds to a protease, (1) the substrate specificity of the proteolytic enzyme is modified; (2) the activity of the bound protease is preserved, but the effect of other plasma inhibitors are minimized; and (3) the complex is rapidly cleared from the circulation. The inhibitory action of $α_2$-macroglobulin is related to the size of the substrate. The higher the molecular weight of the substrate, the greater is the extent of inhibition.

The inhibitor of the first activated component of complement (Cl inactivator) inhibits both the coagulant action of activated Factor XII and the ability of this factor to initiate the conversion of prekallikrein to kallikrein.[408] The effect of this inhibitor is less important than $α_2$-antitrypsin.

5. Plasmin

Fibrin in the blood clot is comparatively stable; under certain circumstances, however, it is lysed rapidly. The rapid lysis is not associated with increased proteolytic activity of the tissues or leukocytes, but it is the result of the activation of a proenzyme, the plasminogen activator in the blood itself. Plasminogen is converted to a proteolytic enzyme called plasmin or fibrinolysin. Plasminogen is present in the blood, in lymph, in some other body fluids and tissues, and in exudates in certain conditions. Plasminogen is a protein constituted as a single polypeptide chain with a molecular weight of 81,000 to 92,000 Da. Plasmin contains two chains connected by a disulfide bond, with a molecular weight of about 73,000 to 84,000. The conversion of plasminogen to plasmin due to the cleavage of a single bond resulting in the active molecule and the release of a peptide from the NH_2-terminus of the molecule, weighing 8000 Da.[379,382]

Three major mechanisms are considered to function in plasmin production: (1) specific activators convert plasminogen to plasmin such as urokinase, streptokinase, and other tissue plasminogen activators; (2) nonspecific activation which mediate directly the conversion such as trypsin; and (3) inert proactivator which is converted to a plasminogen activator.[532] Most tissues contain substances that activate plasminogen, but the most significant source resides in the walls of the blood vessels.

Urokinase is a proteolytic enzyme isolated from urine, it activates plasminogen by cleaving a Arg–Val bond and produces active plasmin.[444,474] Urokinase may derive directly from the kidney or may be formed elsewhere in the body and excreted into the urine. Cultured human kidney cells and cultures from other cell types also produce urokinase.[28] Streptokinase forms an active complex with plasminogen; subsequently, plasmin complexes are produced by cleaving the Arg–Val bond. At the end of the process, the streptokinase in the complex is fragmented.[24,295,296,377,382] Other agents also increase fibrinolytic activity in the blood, including vasoactive substances (vasopressin and epinephrine), anabolic steroid hormones, hypoglycemic drugs (tolbutamide), bacterial pyrogens, and several hydrotropic agents (urethane and urea).[24,305,482]

In addition to the effects on fibrinogen and fibrin, plasmin also digests other proteins such as several coagulation factors (Factor V and Factor VIII) (Table 2), growth hormone, ACTH, and glucagon. Plasmin can activate and fragment Factor XII, and activated Factor XII in time can enhance plasmin formation.[243] Plasmin can also activate various complement components (C5 and C3) and release a chemotactic factor.[377,484,485]

The activation of plasminogen to plasmin is controlled in the blood by some inhibitors.[178,407,408] There are two classes of inhibitors: (1) inhibitors of plasminogen activation and (2) inhibitors of plasmin action. Inhibitors of plasminogen activation are present in plasma and placental tissue. They inhibit urokinase, and subsequently, plasminogen activator is released from the vessel wall. Plasmin is inhibited by α_1-antitrypsin, α_2-macroglobulin, Cl inactivator, and antithrombin III. α_1-Macroglobulin is the most potent and probably modifies the proteolytic activity of the plasmin by forming a high molecular weight complex. In the inhibitory action of antithrombin III, heparin plays a part by rapid acceleration of the process.[180,190]

6. Hemostasis and Platelets

Platelets are the fundamental elements involved in the formation of a hemostatic plug from circulating blood. When the wall of the vessel is injured, platelets adhere to structures of the subendothelial layer which includes collagen, some types of basement membrane, and the microfibrils around elastin.[32,231,325] Platelets accumulate around the injured endothelial cells, or if the endothelium is exposed, they adhere to thrombin.[118] Collagen causes a release of the granular content of platelets.[32] The structural feature of collagen interactions with platelets include enhanced affinity between platelets and collagen and subsequent adherence, platelet spreading, and activation of arachidonic acid metabolism leading to thromboxane A_2 synthesis, platelet aggregation, and finally, discharge of platelet granules. Part of the polypeptide chain of the monomeric collagen is required for the platelet-collagen association which initiates the arachidonate pathway.[307]

When platelets interact with collagen they are stimulated to release their granular contents.[203] There are three types of granulars: (1) amine storage granules, containing ATP, ADP, epinephrine, serotonin, pyrophosphate, divalent cations (Ca^{2+}, Mg^{2+}), and antiplasmin; (2) lysosomal granules containing acid hydrolases; and (3) α-granules, containing fibrinogen, and a factor that increases vessel wall permeability.[282] Antiheparin factor and glycosaminoglycans are present in both amine storage granules and α-granules. The content of amine storage granules is discharged slowly by low concentrations of thrombin or collagen, but higher concentrations are necessary to release the content of the lysosomal granules.

Agents that initiate discharge of platelet granule contents also activate processes leading to various oxidation products from arachidonic acid.[427,428,462] Some intermediates can cause aggregation independent from ADP.[259,287,329] Among these, thromboxane A_2, prostaglandin G_2, and prostaglandin H_2 are strong aggregating agents. These agents also activate phospholipase A_2 which hydrolyzes the ester bond between phospholipid and arachidonate. When platelets undergo the discharge reaction, phospholipoproteins also become available on the surface, which is required in certain steps of the coagulation sequence (Figure 24).

Platelet aggregation can also be induced by various proteolytic enzymes (trypsin, elastase, plasmin, papain, and pronase), snake venoms, vasoactive substances (serotonin, vasopressin, epinephrine, and norepinephrine), viruses, bacteria (endotoxins), antigen-antibody complexes, platelet antibodies, fatty acids, (particularly saturated, but also some of the long-chain unsaturated fatty acids), and foreign particles.[328,356] Some of these agents act through the release reactions stimulating the production of prostaglandin endoperoxides, thromboxane A_2, prostaglandin G_2, and prostaglandin H_2.

7. Inhibitors of Platelet Aggregation

A variety of substances inhibit platelet reactions.[66,228,327,388] These include (1) inhibition of the primary phase of ADP-induced aggregation, (2) conversion of platelet arachidonate to prostaglandin endoperoxides, prostaglandin G_2, and H_2, and thromboxane A_2, (3) adherence of platelet to surfaces, (4) release reaction, and (5) interaction of platelets with components of the coagulation process.

The major inhibitory effects of anti-inflammatory drugs (aspirin, indomethacin, phenylbutazone) are related to the inhibition of the synthesis of labile aggregating substances derived from arachidonate. These agents inhibit the cyclooxygenase enzyme that converts arachidonate to prostaglandin endoperoxides and thromboxane A_2. They inhibit the second phase of aggregation induced by ADP or epinephrine. Aggregation and release brought about by collagen, bacteria, viruses, or α-globulin-coated surfaces can also be inhibited by non-steroidal anti-inflammatory drugs[327] and uricosuric agents. The effect of aspirin is different from the other drugs; 4 to 7 d after administration, it is still effective on platelet reactions. This is probably due to an irreversible acetylation of cyclooxygenase.

Various compounds increase cyclic-AMP concentration in platelets and inhibit the primary phase of ADP-induced aggregation. These include prostaglandin E_1, a potent stimulator of adenylate cyclase. Inhibition of phosphodiesterases also results in raised cyclic-AMP levels, and prototype inhibitors are methyl xanthines and pyrimidopyrimidine derivatives. However, in these cases higher concentrations are required.

AMP, ATP, adenosine, and their analogs can also block the primary phase of ADP-induced platelet aggregation.[182] These effects may be related to competition, since AMP and ATP may compete with ADP for the binding sites on platelet surface.[286,355] Adenosine as a precursor enhances cyclic AMP synthesis. AMP also inhibits nucleoside diphosphate kinase, present on the platelet surface, which reacts with ADP.

Heparin inhibits the action of thrombin on platelets, α-adrenergic blocking agents (dihydroergotamine and phentolamine), and also inhibits epinephrine-induced aggregation. Many other drugs such as antihistamines, antidepressants, tranquilizers, antiserotonin drugs, and penicillin, and related antibiotics interfere with platelet reactions.[328]

B. MECHANISMS OF HEMOSTASIS
1. Normal Hemostasis

Due to the number and frequency of injuries to vessels, hemostasis is of great importance to the organism. Hemorrhage occurs from an injured vessel if there is an opening in the wall which is large enough to let the blood flow out from the vessel into the exterior surface or into a cavity or tissue space where the blood pressure is lower than that in the vessel. Bleeding can be stopped if a pressure-resisting mass is formed which blocks the opening or if the pressure difference between the vascular lumen and the outside is controlled. These conditions can be achieved if external pressure is applied, the pressure in the vessel is reduced, or sufficient blood accumulates and hematoma is formed in the perivascular tissue space. Within the vessel, blood pressure may be reduced by active contraction of the vessels and diversion of the blood through passing vessels, or by a general fall of blood pressure.

Three types of wounds can be distinguished. (1) Small arteries or veins and arterioles or venules are transected. In this case, in normal subjects, the hemostatic mechanism is adequate to prevent excessive loss of blood. (2) If medium-sized arteries or veins are damaged, fatal blood loss may occur. Vessel contractions, fall in blood pressure, and the hemostatic mechanism may be adequate to arrest bleeding. (3) In large artery or vein damage, the problem is the same as in medium-size vessels, but fatal blood loss occurs almost invariably. The hemostatic mechanism is inadequate to stop bleeding in this type of injury. However, puncture wounds to large vessels are usually followed by contractions of the vessel wall around the site of injury and by formation of a hemostatic plug containing a mass of blood elements.

During normal hemostasis, the vascular injury produces an initial change in the characteristics of the vessel surface, causing the platelets to accumulate. In smaller vessels, the main stimulus for this process is the exposure of subendothelial tissues, in particular basement membrane of collagen. In large arteries, the microfibrils associated with elastin also provide a surface where platelets aggregate. The exposure to subendothelial tissues activates the intrinsic pathway of the coagulation mechanism and the release of thromboplastin from the damaged tissue. Traces of thrombin adhere to the endothelium and subendothelial structures. Coating with thrombin enhances the adherance of platelets to these structures. The exposure to collagen exerts several actions, and when platelets are attached to collagen, ADP is released causing platelet clumping. Collagen can activate Factor XII and the interaction with platelets and plasma proteins can lead to the activation of Factor XI. Additional ADP is released from the injured tissues and possibly from erythrocytes. Labile prostaglandin endoperoxides and thromboxane A_2 are formed from platelet arachidonate during collagen-induced aggregation and release. These substances also enhance platelet accumulation and release of platelet granule contents.

The mass of platelets represents the focus for the initiation of coagulation.[95] This clump or mass is formed initially to arrest bleeding from an injured vessel. It also protects the activated clotting factors from inactivation by plasma inhibitors and catalyzes the coagulation reactions that lead to the formation of thrombin. Traces of thrombin may cause the release of more platelet ADP and mobilizes arachidonate which induces further platelet aggregation. Platelet aggregation in turn enhances clotting activity and release of vasoactive compounds.[315] In addition, thrombin accelerates clotting through the action of Factors V and VIII. These effects include the formation of sufficient thrombin from the plasma and the production of fibrin adjacent to the periphery of the platelet mass. Fibrin is mainly responsible for the stabilization of the initial platelet aggregate and for making it impermeable to blood.

During the following 20 h, the intitial platelet aggregate is gradually transformed into a firm mass.[211,212,236] There is a gradual increase in the amount of fibrin around the platelets at the periphery of the mass. Platelets in the center separate from each other as a result of deaggregation, possibly due to the loss or removal of aggregating substances. Plasma penetrates between the separated platelets, and the space becomes filled with fibrin formed from fibrinogen. Platelets degenerate, and some are phagocytozed by polymorphonuclear leukocytes and mononuclear cells. Eventually, a fibrin rich mass is formed with residual platelet debris scattered between the fibrin shreds.

The accumulation of various components of hemostasis is controlled in several ways. (1) ADP is quickly transformed to AMP which limits the extent of platelet aggregation; this process contributes to the breakdown of platelet aggregates. (2) The active aggregating agents formed from arachidonate have a very short half-life lasting no more than a few minutes. (3) Anticoagulants present in blood neutralize thrombin and other intermediates of the clotting process.[41] (4) Fibrin adsorbs thrombin and limits the diffusion of the platelet-fibrin mass into the surrounding blood. In normal circumstances, there is a balance between factors promoting the growth of the hemostatic plug and those limiting the extent of growth. This balance is controlled to achieve arrest of bleeding, thus the extension of bleeding throughout the vascular tree is prevented. The role of fibrinolysis in limiting the size of the clot is not known. It has, however, an importance in the removal of fibrin during the breakdown process.

2. Abnormalities of Hemostasis

Significant changes in blood coagulation and fibrinolytic systems occur in many disease states and conversely, changes in blood coagulation and fibrinolytic systems lead to certain disease manifestations.[473,480] The coagulation system responds to stress, shock, and trauma in a dynamic fashion. Partial thromboplastin times were found shortened in fractures,[51] fat embolism, hemorrhagic shock,[393] and combat casualties.[424] During the acute period of cerebrovascular disease and acute shock, partial thromboplastin times are shortened, while platelet adhesiveness and blood fibrinogen are increased.[94,119] It has also been found that in certain conditions the fibrinolytic response is defective, such as in arteriosclerosis, acute and chronic thromboembolism, hyperlipemia, and vasculitis.[100]

Several conditions are followed by changes in plasma fibrinogen concentration and these include stress, shock, trauma, and surgical interventions. Fibrinogen increases following surgery and various types of injury, such as hemorrhagic and traumatic shock and post-fracture. A transient decrease in fibrinogen has been reported postoperatively and after burns.

Following shock or trauma, the fibrinolytic system is activated. A prompt and transient increase occurs during hemorrhagic shock with a decrease of plasminogen. Profibrinolysin becomes depleted indicating its conversion to fibrinolysin. In humans dying of shock, there is evidence of disseminated intravascular coagulation,[176] most frequently in venules and glomerular tufts of kidneys, pancreatic venules, alveolar capillaries of the myocardium, and portal branches of the liver and cerebral vessels. Massive hemorrhages initate coagulation, which is responsible for the increased catabolic rate of fibrinogen. In disseminated intravascular coagulation, the physiologic equilibrium of procoagulant and anticoagulant factors is disturbed. Bacterial endotoxins, antigen-antibody complexes, hypoxia, proteolytic actions, and endothelial damage, among other factors can lead to this condition.

The activation of the fibrinolytic system is triggered by (1) direct activation of prothrombin by proteolytic enzymes such as trypsin or thrombin, (2) stimulation of the prothrombin activation system by release of tissue extract into the blood, and (3) stimulation of the intrinsic prothrombin activation system through the contact phase of blood clotting. Pathologically, the disseminated intravascular coagulation is characterized by the presence of thrombi in the microcirculation. The localization of the thrombi in various organs depends on the severity of intravascular clotting, the potency and portal entry of the coagulant substance into the circulation, the activation of inhibition of the fibrinolytic system, the stimulation of α-adrenergic receptors sites in the kidney, the filtration mechanism in the glomerulus, and the ability of the reticuloendothelial system to clear fibrin and its degradation products.

The disseminated intravascular coagulation syndrome occurs in acute form in obstetrical accidents: placental absorption, amniotic fluid embolism, and dead fetus syndrome; in acute intravascular hemolysis due to incompatible blood transfusion; in antigen-antibody reaction occurring in graft rejection; in bacterial infections such as pseudomonas sepsis and meningoccemia; viral, proteal, rickettsial, and urinary infections; and in various shock states. Disseminated intravascular coagulation is also associated with chronic forms of many diseases, such as toxemia of pregnancy, allergic vasculitis, giant hemangioma, paroxsysmal nocturnal hemoglobinuria, and malignancy.[297,352]

The clinical manifestation of coagulation disorders is connected with the consumption of platelets and coagulation factors during intravascular thrombosis leading to bleeding, hypotension, and shock. The localization of the thrombi is dependent on the areas of stasis in the vascular system as well as from the release of vasoactive substances. In the acute phase, pulmonary thrombosis causes shock, purpura is formed in the skin vessels and hematemesis in the gastrointestinal tract or melena. Following the acute phase, organ necrosis manifests presented as renal cortical necrosis, and connected with kidney, adrenal, or pituitary failure.

3. Deficiency Disorders of Hemostasis

Coagulation disorders include abnormalities of fibrinogen production and metabolism. There are two types: afibrinogenemia or impaired conversion of fibrinogen to fibrin.[376] Subjects with congenital absence of fibrinogen have a severe bleeding tendency. These patients are not able to synthesize any fibrinogen-like material. There are a number of individuals whose plasma contains fibrinogen-like substance that coagulate upon the effects of thrombin, but it is abnormally slow. These individuals have a mild bleeding tendency, and some have impaired wound healing or cerebrovascular disease.[50] Investigations on these fibrinogens revealed an abnormality in the amino acid sequence of the protein stucture, which is probably responsible for the delayed response to thrombin. In some patients with afibrinogenemia, ADP-induced platelet aggregation is decreased.[326]

Hemorrhagic syndromes are connected with inherited defects of coagulation factors (Table 2). In these disorders the defect is mainly due to the synthesis of an abnormal protein rather than the lack of production.[376] Deficiences of Factors VII, VIII, and IX are the most frequently occurring disease conditions. Both defects are related to extrinsic and intrinsic pathways of coagulation[89,157] Factor VIII and Factor IX deficiencies are X chromosome-linked disorders, and they are mainly found in males. The management of Factor VIII inhibitors in nonhemophilic patients seems to be essential.[157] Hereditary antithrombin III deficiency is connected with venous thrombosis.[309] In certain conditions, such as colon adenocarcinoma, the production of acquired factors has been observed.[81]

In Factor VII-deficient patients the extrinsic pathway of coagulation is abnormal.[237] There is a defect in the synthesis of thrombin and fibrin which represents the third step of the hemostatic plug formation. The primary plug forms in a normal period of time, and these plugs have normal amounts of fibrin around the periphery of platelet aggregates, making them stable and impermeable to the blood. When the primary plug is dislodged several hours after it has formed, the new plug formation is inadequate to arrest bleeding rapidly in Factor VII-deficient patients. The plug formed is irregular and has an increased number of channels. Hemorrhagic symptoms occur in these subjects only when levels of Factor VII are extremely low, indicating that the extrinsic mechanism of clotting is not critical for primary hemostasis.

In contrast, marked abnormalities are present in patients with Factor VIII or Factor IX deficiency representing the congenital defects in intrinsic pathway of coagulation.[104,212,237] Injury of a small artery or vein leads to the formation of a platelet mass within a normal time, but the plug is unstable. Within a few minutes of the primary arrest of bleeding, it is renewed, sometimes because part of the plug is dislodged. Bleeding may again be temporarily stopped, but it may take 20 to 30 min before the hemorrhage is finally arrested. Skin wounds in patients with hemophilia A (Factor-VIII deficiency) contain platelet masses, but they are greatly deficient in fibrin. This condition represents defects in the intrinsic mechanisms of clotting; although a primary platelet mass is formed, it leads to an unstable clot. Another problem in these cases is the formation of a new clot if the old one is dislodged. In Factor-VIII deficient subjects, if the primary clot is removed 24 h after its formation, a new one does not form, and only small aggregates of loosely packed platelets adhere near the open ends of the severed vessels.[237] These subjects bleed continuously until external measures are applied. Thus subjects with Factor VIII deficiency show defective formation of the primary clot and more abnormalities in the formation of the secondary plug. Since the initial platelet plug is unstable and its transformation to a fibrin mass is very slow, hemophiliacs are more vulnerable to the action of a hemostatic plug being dislodged than normal subjects.

There are some subjects with Factor XIII deficiency.[108] This deficiency is hereditary and patients with this disorder often severely hemorrhage after an injury, and they also show defective wound healing. In some of these individuals an inactive protein related to Factor XIII has been demonstrated.

Factor X deficiency disease has also been described, and individuals with this deficiency have a bleeding tendency similar to that of classic hemophilia.[99,143] The congenital defect of Factor II (thrombin) is very rare. Most of the individuals with this disorder have 2 to 10% prothrombin activity, and the susceptibility to bleeding shows some parallelism to the level of prothrombin.[238,251,415] Factor XI and Factor XII deficiencies have also been observed. Deficiency of Factor XI is a relatively uncommon disorder and is manifested as a hemorrhagic disorder. The hemorrhagic tendency is, however, much less severe than in hemophilia.[129] Congenital deficiency of Factor V is also rare, and the associated bleeding tendency is only moderately severe.[354]

X. NUTRITIONAL ELEMENTS IN WOUND HEALING

Wound healing is the key to the recovery from any injury. The orderly sequence of events in wound healing is one of the most important hemeostatic controls of the body defenses. For these programmed events to take place, the tissues must be adequately nourished. The most important factor is vitamin C and other nutrients include vitamin A, members of the vitamin B complex, zinc, and other trace elements.

A. VITAMIN C

This compound is essential for collagen production and is concentrated in the tissues of healing wounds, where it affects the hydroxylation of proteins.[73] This process requires molecular oxygen with the production of free hydroxy radicals. NADH:monodehydroascorbic acid transhydrogenase is a flavoprotein that catalyzes proton transfer from NADH to the ascorbic acid radical to form reduced ascorbic acid.

Hydroxyproline is an important constituent of collagen. The formation of this compound by hydroxylation is also catalyzed by NADH:monodehydroascorbic acid transdehydrogenase. First, proline is incorporated into the collagen and becomes hydroxylated after the peptide chain is produced.[217] Similarly to proline, lysine is also incorporated into the collagen and subsequently hydroxylated to hydroxylysine. The hydroxylation of these two compounds represents a key step in collagen synthesis. Hydroxyproline and hydroxylysine take part in cross-linking of peptide chains which are necessary for the collagen molecule to become finally assembled into a typical triple helix. Besides ascorbic acid and molecular oxygen, the hydroxylation process requires ferrous iron and α-ketoglutarate.

B. VITAMIN B COMPLEX

Most components of the vitamin B complex are related to intrinsic metabolic processes within the cell. Deficiencies of these vitamins cause a reduction in the rate of wound healing. Investigations have shown that vitamin B_{12} increases tensile strength of the wounds in experimental animals.[124] Folinic acid enhances wound healing, especially during the first few days.[82] In pyridoxine and riboflavin deficient animals, there is significantly decreased healing.[48] Pyridoxine administration, however, to normal animals does not cause any improvements,[58] whereas D-panthenol stimulates wound healing.[64]

C. VITAMIN A

This vitamin is essential for epithelial growth, with stimulatory effects on the basal cells of the epidermis.[517] In vitamin A deficiency, the epithelial surfaces show the early and most serious changes. Experimental studies have revealed the effects of vitamin A and hydrocortisone on β-glucuronidase activity of healing wounds. Glucuronidase activity is increased in the skin of the wounded area; it is further raised by vitamin A during the first 7 d of healing and is depressed by corticosterone.[292] It is likely that the effect of vitamin A is related to the lability of lysosomal enzymes by a lysing effect on the membrane, thus making the contained hydrolytic enzymes available, whereas corticosterone increases membrane stability.[121]

The retardation of wound healing by salicylates is reversed by vitamin A.[109] In the absence of aspirin, vitamin A promotes healing and enhances mucopolysaccharide formation in granulation tissue. The administration of aspirin suppresses mucopolysaccharide formation and inflammation, and both effects are reversed by vitamin A. Various vitamin A derivatives including retinol (vitamin A alcohol) and retinyl acetate or retinoic acid (vitamin A acid) all promote skin wound healing. These compounds also reverse the inhibitory action of aspirin or sodium salicylate. Retinoic acid counteracts the inhibition exerted by the local application and hydrocortisone or oral administration of prednisone.[231] β-Carotene shows similar effectiveness as vitamin A in reversing the effects of glucocorticoids in wound healing.[483]

D. VITAMIN K

The action of this vitamin group shows similarity to that of glucocorticoids. They are effective against chronic inflammation, but ineffective in acute inflammation.[534,535,536] Vitamin K_1 (phylloquinone) and vitamin K_3 prevent the development of granulomata.

E. VITAMIN E

This compound is considered a lysosomal stabilizer[110] and an anti-inflammatory agent. Vitamin E is also an antioxidant and inhibits the accumulation of peroxides thus preventing free radical damage to tissues. Generally, vitamin E stabilizes biological membranes and maintains their integrity, however, it does not prevent the wound healing retardation brought about by glucocorticoids. Vitamin E shows a similar effect to corticoids, and vitamin A reverses its action. It may be the significance of vitamin E is to control and reduce undesirable excess scar formation.

F. PROTEINS

Experimental studies have shown that the healing process of surface wounds is markedly prolonged by protein deficiency, and the deficiency can be reversed by the administration of DL-methionine.[499] In patients DL-methionine is also effective, whereas other amino acids, lysine, valine, or tryptophane do not exert similar effects to methionine despite that lysine represents an important constituent of collagen. Although there is a greater nitrogen retention when methionine is fed, the protein sulfur is more important than protein nitrogen in the promotion of wound healing. In protein-deficient animals, there is a lack of mucopolysaccharides and impaired collagen production in wounds; methionine restores the synthesis of both compounds. When methionine and vitamin C are given together they are more effective than either compound given alone. Lysine deficiency exerts only a moderate effect on wound healing.[245] In this case the epithelial regeneration is prompt, and there is no difference in mucopolysaccharide synthesis. Lysine deficiency reduces the ability of fibroblasts to synthesize proteins. Moreover, the structure of fibroblasts is modified in lysine deficient animals, resulting in decreased production of collagen precursors and mature collagen, and as a result, the scar becomes porous.

G. TRACE METALS

In certain conditions, lower serum zinc levels are found in patients suffering from inflammation, infection, or acute and chronic glomerulonephritis. Deficiency of zinc can affect wound healing.[180,269] Immediately after injury there is rapid accumulation of zinc in skin wounds, lasting for about 12 d when zinc levels fall to those in intact skin. This may suggest that traces of zinc are important in the early phases of wound healing, when collagen precursors and collagen are formed. In surgical patients, altered zinc level may result due to reduced food intake, particularly in malnourished patients or in patients maintained on prolonged parenteral fluid therapy. There is a significant zinc deficiency in severely burned patients. Administration of zinc (200 mg three times daily) increases wound healing by about 60%. Cells which are farthest removed from blood vessels are the most affected by zinc deficiency.[508] There is an inverse relationship between the pH of the wound and the tissue zinc concentrations, indicating a possible metabolic mechanism responsible for the

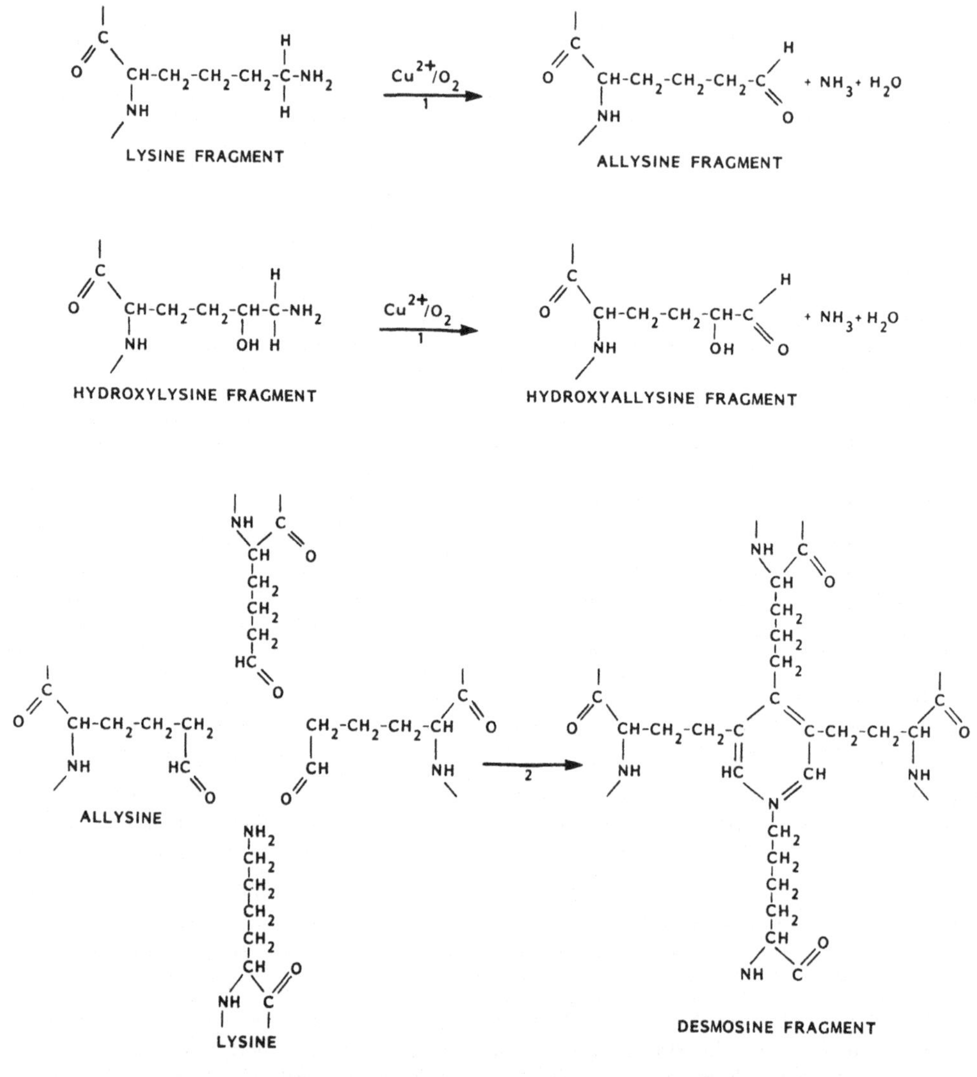

FIGURE 25.   Primary stages of tissue collagen synthesis. Lysine and hydroxylysine fragments of precursor enzymes are oxidized in the presence of Cu^{2+} ions (1) to form allysine or hydroxyallysine fragments. Condensation reactions (2) combine allysine and hydroxyallysine fragments with lysine residues to produce desmosine and hydroxydesmosine fragments, respectively, representing the formation of cross-linkages.

accumulation of this trace element in the wound.[274] Zinc also stabilizes lysosomal membranes, and its effect may be related to the synthesis of collagen precursor proteins.[74]

In addition to zinc, manganese, copper, chromium, and selenium are also necessary for normal growth and development.[406] Trace amounts of copper may be required for the normal function of fibroblasts, and copper also plays a role in elastin formation, probably in relation to the activity of amine oxidase. Copper and pyridoxine (a coenzyme) deficiency prevents the transformation of lysine residues of elastin into desmosine and isodesmosine derivatives necessary for cross-linkages in the elastin molecule (Figure 25). Manganese is mostly concentrated in mitochondria, and it may play a part in the metabolic activity of these subcellular organelles, affecting the activity of cells involved in wound healing.

XI. LABORATORY DIAGNOSIS OF INFLAMMATION

There are differences in the systemic response to injury between the acute and chronic phases of inflammation. In acute inflammation the characteristic signs are increased metabolism and temperature, elevated leukocyte count (mainly polymorphonuclear leukocytes), enhanced erythrocyte sedimentation rate, increased synthesis of serum α-globulins and fibrinogen; decreased albumin level, and release of cytoplasmic enzymes into the serum. In contrast, in chronic inflammatory conditions, some changes occurring in the acute phase cannot be easily diagnosed; the erythrocyte sedimentation rate may be enhanced, and a positive skin test may indicate the presence of a viable microorganism responsible for the chronic infection. However, other changes are characteristic: negative nitrogen balance associated with weight loss and possibly cachexia, leukocytosis in the peripheral blood (mainly lymphocytes and mononuclear leukocytes), and increased antibody production.

A. LEUKOCYTE COUNTS

The white cell count of peripheral blood plays an important part in the diagnosis of inflammation. In health, the normal leukocyte count ranges between 4000 and 10,000/mm^3 and is made up of 65% polymorphonuclear leukocytes, 30% lymphocytes, and 5% monocytes. When an acute inflammatory process is present, such as in burns or infections, the total white cell count can range from 20,000 to 25,000/mm^3 with more than 90% polymorphonuclear leukocytes. During chronic infection, mainly lymphocytes and monocytes account for the white elements that are present in the peripheral blood. In leukemia the white cell count often exceeds 40,000/mm^3.

B. ERYTHROCYTE SEDIMENTATION RATE

During acute inflammation, the sedimentation rate of red blood cells is enhanced, a parameter change that may not be apparent in chronic disease. However, decreased erythrocyte number can be seen in chronic inflammation because of reduced production in the bone marrow.

During the inflammatory process, fluid leaks out from the capillaries into the tissue, and plasma proteins remain behind in the vessels. The increased protein coats the red cells making them clump together. This clumping process causes an increase in the normal settling out of red cells, i.e., the sedimentation of these relatively dense particles in the fluid medium. If the blood of a healthy individual is treated with heparin to prevent coagulation, the erythrocytes settle out very slowly. In contrast, if the blood of a patient with acute or chronic inflammation is allowed to stand, the erythrocytes will settle very rapidly, being heavier than the plasma density. Red blood cells are normally kept in suspension by the colloid action of serum proteins, particularly albumins. The relative amounts and composition of serum proteins are altered in disease, thus the colloid stability is interfered with resulting in accelerated sedimentation rate of erythrocytes. In addition, the sedimentation rate is faster when the particles in the blood are larger, as is the case of red blood cell clumping in inflammation.

The measurement of erythrocyte sedimentation rate is a simple but non-specific procedure. Increased sedimentation rates are seen, however, in nearly all inflammatory diseases and in other conditions such as advanced cancer or tuberculosis. The erythrocyte sedimentation rate is often more affected by secondary complications such as pneumonia, pleurisy, thrombophlebitis, or arthritis, rather than by the primary disease. However, the test for erythrocyte sedimentation rate may lead to important secondary observations. The appearance of the plasma in the sedimentation tube and the presence of a pathological cell aggregation may yield valuable supplementary information. The color of the plasma can indicate various specific changes: golden yellow hemolysis may represent a drug side effect; unusually clear-iron deficiency is connected with anemia; straw color is connected with pernicious anemia; and dark yellow is related to jaundice. The clarity of the plasma can also provide some diagnostic value in specifying the origin of the inflammatory processes: cloudy, indicates diabetes or nephrosis owing to lipid increase and/or release of proteins, or lipoproteins; white cells on the top layer may reflect leukemia.

C. SERUM PROTEINS

Serum proteins show changes in both acute and chronic inflammatory disorders. In acute inflammation, serum albumin is decreased, and α_1- and α_2-globulins are increased, representing increased synthesis or release of glycoproteins which are required as substrates and enzymes for kinin formation. Mucoproteins and various reactive proteins are produced by the liver in response to acute injury. In chronic inflammation, an increase in γ-globulin is representative, indicating enhanced antibody synthesis (Figure 26).

Circulating antibodies appear particularly in virus diseases. These antibodies can be detected by means of a variety of agglutination, precipitation, and complement fixation tests. These tests frequently reveal the presence of a specific infecting agent which is useful for determining the best course of therapy. The application of these different tests is not only essential to diagnose the cause of the inflammatory condition, but also serves as a guide on the progress of drug or other therapy.

D. SERUM ENZYMES

An increased level of serum enzymes usually indicates an acute inflammatory condition. An individual who has developed an acute liver disorder or who just suffered a myocardial infarct usually shows markedly increased serum transaminases, lactic dehydrogenase, γ-glutamyl transpeptidase, and in the case of myocardial injury, elevation of creatinine phosphokinase. These enzymes are released from damaged cells into the circulation. They and other enzymes may be elevated in the blood following injury to a variety of organs including the lung, kidney, pancreas and others. If increased serum enzymes are found in individuals with a chronic inflammatory disease, this usually represents an acute flare-up. Enzyme changes are often the only biochemical abnormalities which can be detected. In rapidly growing malignant tumors, there is an abnormally high activity of lactic dehydrogenase which is sometimes the first biochemical sign of disease.[188] Genetic polymorphism sometimes leads to the production of abnormal peptides. This occurs occasionally in cancer patients presenting abnormal lactate dehydrogenase bands on electrophoresis. Determination of lactic dehydrogenase isoenzymes gives certain indication of the tissue origin and may reflect the course of disease (Figure 27).

XII. ACTION OF ANTI-INFLAMMATORY DRUGS

Anti-inflammatory drugs are used to inhibit or reverse changes caused by the inflammation and ensuing tissue response, counteracting the effect of substances which potentiate the onset of the various phases. In the broadest sense, anti-inflammation agents can include antibiotics, anticoagulants, antimetabolites, proteolytic enzymes, antikinins, antihistamines, monoamine oxidase inhibitors, steroids, stabilizers of lysosomes, and suppressors of antibody formation. The action of these drugs of varying structure and pharmacological effects can be correlated with various processes taking place during inflammation (Figure 28).

Antibiotic therapy is applied to combat excess pathogens initiating the inflammatory response, and anticoagulants are used to reduce the intensity of blood coagulation in particular cases where it can lead to extensive vascular thrombosis and necrosis of capillaries and small vessels. After cardiac infarct or phlebitis, these drugs are given to prevent further expansion of inflammation and thrombosis of the damaged heart or peripheral muscle. The administration of these drugs is monitored with great care since bleeding tendency can increase.

Proteolytic enzymes, particularly trypsin in combination with chymotrypsin, have been used locally for the prevention and treatment of inflammatory states, and these enzymes are

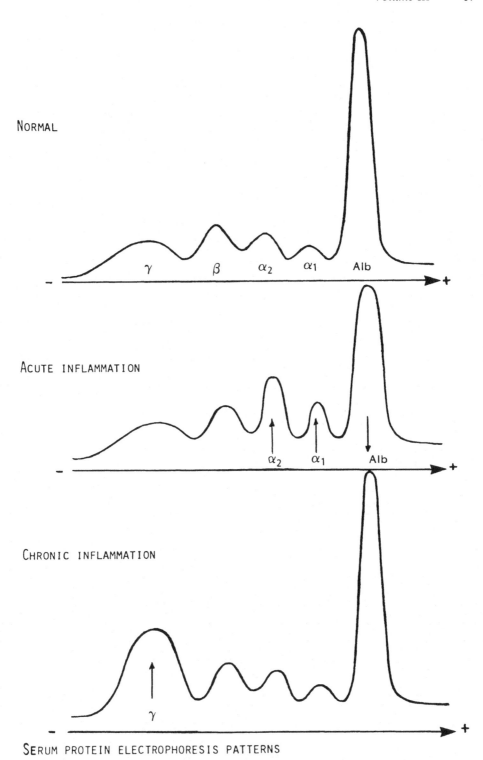

FIGURE 26. Alterations in serum protein electrophoresis pattern in inflammation. During the acute disease the decrease in albumin and increase in α_1- and α_2-globulins are the nonspecific changes. In the chronic disease γ-globulin is elevated representing the increased production of circulating antibodies.

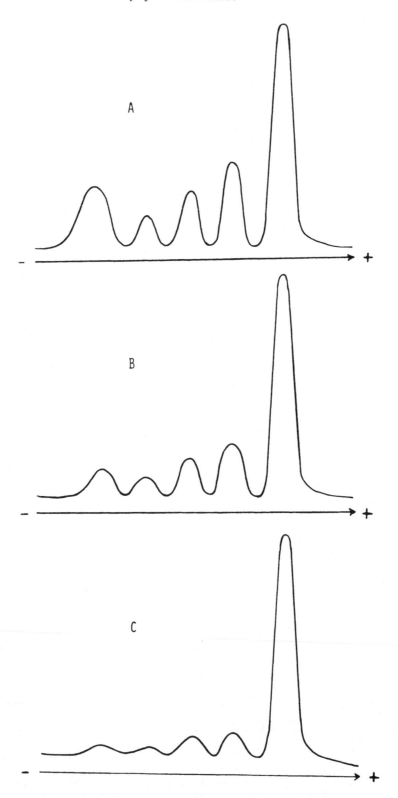

FIGURE 27.   Alterations in serum lactic dehydrogenase pattern with rapidly growing malignant teratoma. Increased total level was (A) first observed, (B) 4 months later, and (C) 5 months later. The individual isoenzymes show significant variations.

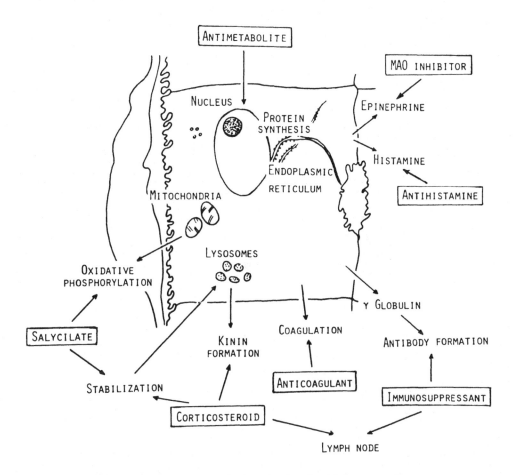

FIGURE 28.   Possible mechanism of action of anti-inflammatory drugs.

rapidly inactivated when injected into closed cavities. A number of other proteolytic enzymes, such as elastase, papain (papase, ananase), bromelains, and fibrinuclease, have been applied also for the prevention and treatment of a variety of inflammatory conditions. The topical application of these substances will remove clotted blood and necrotic tissue from the surface of wounds and ulcers.

In the early phases of inflammation, the increased vascular permeability is induced by histamine. Immediately after symptoms become evident, this can be reversed by antihistamine drugs. Such therapy is useful during the acute inflammatory phases and is effective to reduce allergic inflammation. The vasodilatation is counteracted by the vasoconstrictive effect of epinephrine and norepinephrine. However, the activity of these amines is short-lived due to the release of monoamine oxidase released from injured cells. Monoamine oxidase inhibitors can block the enzyme activity, and the action of epinephrine on micro-circulation is restored. This diminishes the severity of the inflammatory response, and subsequently, the normal vascular permeability is reestablished with reduced edema formation.

The onset of tissue swelling and pain is probably mediated by kinins and prostaglandins. The effect of salicylates (aspirin) in reducing these symptoms is probably related to their ability to inactivate kinins by preventing the activation of kallikrein. These drugs may exert part of their anti-inflammatory effect by rendering lysosomal membranes more stable and less permeable, thus blocking the release of proteolytic enzymes and hydrolases. Salicylates do not affect bradykinin synthesis or inhibit the formation of kallikrein nor do they antagonize

ENDOTHELIAL CELL   PLATELET

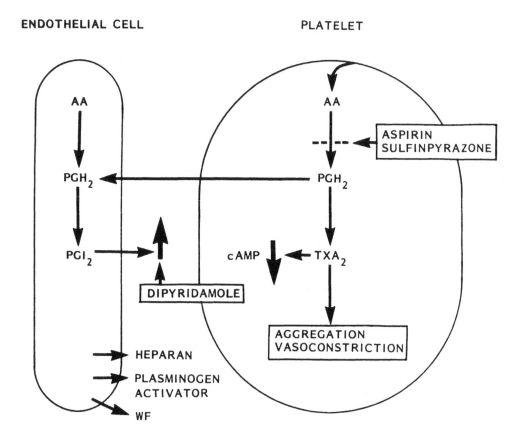

FIGURE 29. Possible action of drugs on platelet-endothelial cell interplay. The platelet releases thromboxane A_2 (TXA_2) which causes aggregation and vasoconstriction. The endothelial cell releases prostacyclin (PGI_2) which antagonizes the effects of thromboxane. Aspirin and sulfinpyrazone inhibit prostaglandin and thromboxane synthesis from arachidonic acid (AA). Dipyridamole enhances prostacyclin effect. The endothelial cell contains other hemostasis modulating factors such as tissue plasminogen activator, heparin, and von Willebrand factor (WF).[111,310]

histamine or serotonin. The antirheumatic effect of salicylates is related to the inflammatory component of this disease,[511] suppressing the clinical signs, and in some cases even improving the histological picture. Subsequent damage, cardiac lesions, and other visceral changes are unaffected by salicylates. The mechanism of action of aspirin is related to the inhibition of prostaglandin synthesis (Figure 28), and the anti-inflammatory effect of adrenocortical steroids is associated with the stabilization of lysosomal membranes.

The nonsteroid acidic anti-inflammatory drugs (aspirin, phenylbutazone, flufenamic acid, indomethacin) inhibit several biochemical reactions, such as hydrolysis of proteins by proteolytic enzymes resembling trypsin, biosynthesis of histamine by histidine decarboxylase, and mitochondrial processes, including oxidative phosphorylation (Figure 29). Nonacidic derivatives of these drugs, such as salicylamide *N*-arylanthranilamides, and the amide of indomethacin are ineffective anti-inflammatory agents. These compounds elicit no inhibitory activity against enzyme reactions. Whereas the biochemical reactions are dissimilar, it has been shown that a common radical, an ε-amino group of a lysine residue of the protein involved in the process, is essential in the enzyme-substrate interaction. The lysine ε-amino group belongs either to the protein substrate or to part of the enzyme protein. The acidic nonsteroid drugs form anions and become bound to the lysyl ε-amino group of the enzyme protein. Through this binding these agents interfere with the enzyme reactions that require the presence of these free ε-amino groups. Reactions dependent on such an amino group include the specific effect of trypsin-like proteolytic activity which occurs at a peptide bond adjacent to a lysine residue. Binding of pyridoxal phosphate as coenzyme of decarboxylase are necessary to histamine biosynthesis and mitochondrial oxidative phosphorylation.

Apparently, there are common sites of action between the acidic inflammatory drugs and various steroids such as the stabilization of lysosomal membranes.[8] There are also relevant differences between the two groups of compounds. In many cases, corticosteroids stimulate enzyme systems which are inhibited by the acidic non-steroidal drugs. In general, salicylates and derivatives inhibit the exudative rather than the proliferative phase of inflammation, whereas corticosteroids have an enhancing action on proliferation.

Several chronic inflammatory conditions are associated with the production of circulating antibodies, and thus, this process is intrinsically associated with the perpetuation of the inflammation process. In many cases, antibody-antigen reactions may result in the precipitation of various complex structures which themselves can induce an active, acute inflammatory response. Accordingly, suppression of the antibody production may interrupt this cycle. Corticosteroids decrease the proliferation of lymphocytes by a direct action on lymphoid tissue, inhibiting protein synthesis, and specifically, antibody production. While tissue responses to inflammation are improved by steroid therapy, agents or conditions causing the chronic disorder are still present. Recently, very potent antimetabolites frequently applied in cancer chemotherapy are being found to inhibit antibody formation by lymphocytes. These chemotherapeutic agents block nucleic acid synthesis, DNA replication, and the role of transfer RNA in synthesizing proteins. This inhibitory action leads to a generalized decreased production of antibodies and proteolytic enzymes which participate in mediator synthesis. Given the drastic nature of these effects, treatment is confined to situations where first line therapy has not been effective and when risk/benefit assessments point heavily toward the patient's welfare.

REFERENCES

1. **Aihara, M., Cooper, H. A., and Wagner, R. H.,** Platelet-collagen interactions: increase in rate of adhesion of fixed washed platelets by factor VIII-related antigen, *Blood,* 63, 495, 1984.
2. **Alami, S. Y., Hampton, J. W., Race, G. J., and Speer, R. J.,** Fibrin stabilizing factor (Factor XIII), *Am. J. Med.,* 44, 1, 1968.
3. **Albahary, C.,** Lead and hemopoiesis. The mechanism and consequences of the erythropathy of occupational lead poisoning, *Am. J. Med.,* 52, 367, 1972.
4. **Allen, A. M.,** Deoxyribonucleic acid synthesis and mitosis in mast cells of the rat, *Lab. Invest.,* 11, 188, 1962.
5. **Allison, A. C.,** Lysosomes in pathology, in *Recent Advances in Histopathology,* Anthony, P. P. and Woolf, N., Eds., Churchill Livingstone, Edinburgh, 1978, 68.
6. **Allison, A. C., Ferluga, J., Prydz, H., and Schorlemmer, H. U.,** The role of macrophage activation in chronic inflammation, *Agents Actions,* 8, 27, 1978.
7. **Allison, A. C., Harington, J. S., and Birbeck, M.,** An examination of the cytotoxic effects of silica on macrophages, *J. Exp. Med.,* 124, 141, 1966.
8. **Allison, A. C., Magnus, I. A., and Young, M. R.,** Role of lysosomes and of cell membranes in photosensitization, *Nature (London),* 209, 874, 1966.
9. **Allison, F., Jr., Lancaster, M. G., and Crosthwaite, J. L.,** Studies on the pathogenesis of acute inflammation. V. An assessement of factors that influence in vitro the phagocytic and adhesive properties of leukocytes obtained from rabbit peritoneal exudate, *Am. J. Pathol.,* 43, 775, 1963.
10. **Alper, C. A., Colten, H. R., Rosen, F. S., Rabson, A. R., Macnab, G. M., and Gear, J. S.,** Homozygous deficiency of C3 in a patient with repeated infections, *Lancet,* 2, 1179, 1972.
11. **Altman, L. C., Synderman, R., and Blaese, R. M.,** Abnormalities of chemotactic lymphokine synthesis and mononuclear leukocyte chemotaxis in Wiskott-Aldrich syndrome, *J. Clin. Invest.,* 54, 486, 1974.
12. **Aman, P., Gordon, J., and Klein, G.,** TPA activation and differentiation of human peripheral B lymphocytes, *Immunology,* 51, 27, 1984.
13. **Andrew, M. and Kelton, J.,** Neonatal thrombocytopenia, *Clin. Perinatol,* 11, 359, 1984.

14. **Aronsen, K. F., Ekelund, G., Kindmark, C. O., and Laurell, C. B.,** Sequential changes of plasma proteins after surgical trauma, *Scand. J. Clin. Lab. Invest.,* 29(Suppl. 124), 127, 1972.
15. **Assem, E. S. K. and Schild, H. O.,** Inhibition by sympathomimetic amines of histamine release by antigen in passively sensitized human lung, *Nature (London),* 224, 1028, 1969.
16. **Astle, C. M. and Harrison, D. E.,** Effects of marrow donor and recipient age on immune responses, *J. Immunol.,* 132, 673, 1984.
17. **Babior, B. M.,** Oxygen-dependent microbial killing by phagocytes. Part I, *N. Engl. J. Med.,* 298, 659, 1978.
18. **Babior, B. M.,** Oxygen-dependent microbial killing by phagocytes. Part 2, *N. Engl. J. Med.,* 298, 721, 1978.
19. **Badwey, J. A., Curnutte, J. T., and Karnovsky, M. L.,** The enzyme of granulocytes that produces superoxide and peroxide. An elusive pimpernel, *N. Engl. J. Med.,* 300, 1157, 1979.
20. **Baehner, R. L., Johnston, R. B., Jr., and Nathan, D. G.,** Comparative study of the metabolic and bactericidal characteristics of severely glucose-6-phosphate dehydrogenase deficient polymorphonuclear leukocytes and leukocytes from children with chronic granulomatous disease, *J. Reticuloendothel. Soc.,* 12, 150, 1972.
21. **Bagdasarian, A., Talamo, R. C., and Colman, R. W.,** Isolation of high molecular weight activators of human plasma prekallikrein, *J. Biol. Chem.,* 248, 3456, 1973.
22. **Baggiolini, M., Bretz U., Dewald, B., and Feigenson, M. E.,** The polymorphonuclear leukocyte, *Agents Actions,* 18, 3, 1978.
23. **Bailey, E., Taylor, C. B., and Bartley, W.,** Turnover of mitochondrial components of normal and essential fatty acid-deficient rats, *Biochem. J.,* 104, 1026, 1967.
24. **Bajaj, S. P. and Castellino, F. J.,** Activation of human plasminogen by equimolar levels of streptokinase, *J. Biol. Chem.,* 252, 492, 1977.
25. **Balazs, E. A., Ed.,** *Chemistry and Molecular Biology of the Intercellular Matrix,* Vol. 1, Academic Press, New York, 1970.
26. **Banda, M. J. and Werb, Z.,** Macrophage elastase degradation of immunoglobulins regulate binding to macrophage Fc receptors. Part 1, *Fed. Proc.,* 39, 799, 1980.
27. **Banda, M. J., Clark, E. J., and Werb, Z.,** Limited proteolysis by macrophage elastase inactivates human alpha-1-proteinase inhibitor, *J. Exp. Med.,* 152, 1563, 1980.
28. **Barlow, G. H.,** Urinary and kidney cell plasminogen activator (urokinase), *Methods Enzymol.,* 45, 239, 1976.
29. **Barrett, A. J.,** Properties of lysosomal enzymes, in *Lysosomes in Biology and Pathology,* Vol. 2, Dingle, J. T. and Fell, H. B., Eds., North-Holland, Amsterdam, 1969, 245.
30. **Barrett, A. J.,** The possible role of neutrophil proteinases in damage to articular cartilage, *Agents Actions,* 8, 11, 1978.
31. **Baugh, R. J. and Travis, J.,** Human leukocyte granule elastase: rapid isolation and characterization, *Biochemistry,* 15, 836, 1976.
32. **Baumgartner, H. R., Muggli, R., Tschopp, T. B., and Turitto, V. T.,** Platelet adhesion, release and aggregation in flowing blood: effects of surface properties and platelet function, *Thromb. Haemostasis,* 35, 124, 1976.
33. **Beatty, K., Bieth, J., and Travis, J.,** Kinetics of association of serine proteinases with native and oxidized α-1-proteinase inhibitor and α-1-antichymotrypsin, *J. Biol. Chem.,* 255, 3931, 1980.
34. **Beaven, M. A.,** Histamine, *N. Engl. J. Med.,* 294, 320, 1976.
35. **Becker, K. E., Ishizaka, T., Metzger, H., Ishizaka, K., and Grimley, P. M.,** Surface IgE on human basophils during histamine release, *J. Exp. Med.,* 138, 394, 1973.
36. **Bellanti, J. A., Cantz, B. E., and Schlegel, R. J.,** Accelerated decay of glucose 6-phosphate dehydrogenase activity in chronic granulomatous disease, *Pediatr. Res.,* 4, 405, 1970.
37. **Bellucci, S., Tobelem, G., and Caen, J. P.,** Inherited platelet disorders, *Prog. Hematol.,* 13, 223, 1983.
38. **Beer, D. J., Matloff, S. M., and Rocklin, R. E.,** The influence of histamine on immune and inflammatory responses, *Adv. Immunol.,* 35, 209, 1984.
39. **Bevers, E. M., Comfurius, P., and Zwaal, F. A.,** Changes in membrane phospholipid distribution during platelet activation, *Biochem. Biophys. Acta,* 736, 57, 1983.
40. **Biggs, R. and Denson, K. W. E.,** Natural and pathological inhibitors of blood coagulation, in *Human Blood Coagulation, Haemostasis and Thrombosis,* 4th ed. Biggs, R., Ed., Blackwell Scientific, Oxford, 1972, 133.
41. **Bischof, P., Meisser, A., Haenggeli, L., Reber, G., Bouvier, C., Béguin, F., Herrmann, W. L., and Sizonenko, P. C.,** Pregnancy-associated plasma protein-A (Papp-A) inhibits thrombin-induced coagulation of plasma, *Thromb. Res.,* 32, 45, 1983.
42. **Blicharski, J., Lisiewicz, J., and Moszczynski, P.,** Lysosomal enzymes of neutrophils in women with breast cancer, *Folia Histochem. Cytochem.,* 21, 195, 1983.
43. **Blombäck, B., Hogg, D. H., Gardlund, B., Hessel, B., and Kudryk, B.,** Fibrinogen and fibrin formation, *Thromb. Res.,* 8 (Suppl. 2), 329, 1976.

44. **Bock, P. E. and Shore, J. D.**, Protein-protein interactions in contact activation of blood coagulation. Characterization of fluorescein-labeled human high molecular weight kininogen-light chain as a probe, *J. Biol. Chem.*, 258, 15079, 1983.
45. **Boime, I., Smith, E. E., and Hunter, F. E., Jr.**, Stability of oxidative phosphorylation and structural changes of mitochondria in ischemic rat liver, *Arch. Biochem. Biophys.*, 128, 704, 1968.
46. **Bomalaski, J. S., Williamson, P. K., and Zurier, R. B.**, Prostaglandins and the inflammatory response, *Clin. Lab Med.*, 3, 695, 1983.
47. **Borgeat, P. and Samuelsson, B.**, Arachidonic acid metabolism in polymorphonuclear leukocytes: effects of ionophore A 23187, *Proc. Natl. Acad. Sci. U.S.A.*, 76, 2148, 1979.
48. **Bosse, M. D. and Axelrod, A. E.**, Wound healing in rats with biotin, pyridoxin or riboflavin deficiencies, *Proc. Soc. Exp. Biol. Med.*, 67, 418, 1948.
49. **Bourne, H. R., Lichtenstein, L. M., and Melmon, K. L.**, Pharmacologic control of allergic histamine release in vitro: evidence for an inhibiting role of 3'5'-adenosine monophosphate in human leukocytes, *J. Immunol.*, 108, 695, 1972.
50. **Boysen, G., Boss, A. H., Odum, N., and Olsen, J. S.**, Prolongation of bleeding time and inhibition of platelet aggregation by low-dose acetylsalicylic acid in patients with cerebrovascular disease, *Stroke*, 15, 241, 1984.
51. **Bradford, D. S., Foster, R. R., and Nossel, H. L.**, Coagulation alterations, hypoxemia, and fat embolism in fracture patients, *J. Trauma*, 10, 307, 1970.
52. **Brandt, L.**, Studies on the phagocytic activity of neutrophilic leucocytes, *Scand. J. Haematol.*, Suppl. 2, 1, 1967.
53. **Brinkhous, K. M.**, Report of the subcommittee on Human Factor VIII and IX preparations, *Thromb. Diath. Haemorrh.*, Suppl. 39, 413, 1970.
54. **Brocklehurst, W. E.**, Role of kinins and prostaglandins in inflammation, *Proc. R. Soc. Med.*, 64, 4, 1971.
55. **Brocklehurst, W. E. and Mawr, G. E.**, The purification of a kininogen from human plasma, *Br. J. Pharmacol.*, 27, 256, 1966.
56. **Broekman, M. J., Ward, J. W., and Marcus, A. J.**, Phospholipid metabolism in stimulated human platelets: changes in phosphatidylinositol, phosphatidic acid and lysophospholipids, *J. Clin. Invest.*, 66, 275, 1980.
57. **Brown, J. A. and Swank, R. T.**, Subcellular redistribution of newly synthesized macrophage lysosomal enzymes. Correlation between delivery to the lysosomes and maturation, *J. Biol. Chem.*, 258, 15323, 1983.
58. **Brown, S. O., Sorg, V., and Jones, J. T.**, Burn healing in rats maintained on diets containing different levels of pyridoxine, *Tex. Rep. Biol. Med.*, 20, 562, 1962.
59. **Budzynski, A. Z., and Marder, V. J.**, Determination of human fibrinopeptide A by radioimmunoassay in purified systems and in the blood, *Thromb. Diath. Haemorrh.*, 34, 709, 1975.
60. **Burger, M. M.**, Surface changes in transformed cells detected by lectins, *Fed. Proc.*, 32, 91, 1973.
61. **Burrowes, C. E., Movat, H. Z., and Soltay, M. J.**, The kinin system of human plasma. IV. The action of plasmin, *Proc. Soc. Exp. Biol. Med.*, 138, 959, 1971.
62. **Carlsson, I. and Wennmalm, A.**, Platelet aggregability in smoking and non-smoking subjects, *Clin. Physiol.*, 3, 565, 1983.
63. **Carp, H. and Janoff, A.**, Inactivation of bronchial mucous proteinase inhibitor by cigarette smoke and phagocyte-derived oxidants, *Exp. Lung Res.*, 1, 225, 1980.
64. **Casadio, S., Mantegani, A., Coppi, G., and Pala, G.**, On the healing properties of esters of D-panthenol with terpene acids with particular reference to D-pantothenyl trifarnesylacetate, *Arzneim. Forsch.*, 17, 1122, 1967.
65. **Casley-Smith, J. R.**, The lymphatic system in inflammation, in *The Inflammatory Process*, Vol. 2, Zweifach, B. W., Grant, L., and McClusky, R. T., Eds., Academic Press, New York, 1973, 161.
66. **Cazenave, J.-P., Packham, M. A., Guccione, M. A., and Mustard, J. F.**, Inibition of platelet adherence to a collagen-coated surface by nonsteroidal anti-inflammatory drugs, pyrimido-pyrimidine and tricyclic compounds, and lidocaine, *J. Lab. Clin. Med.*, 83, 797, 1974.
67. **Chan, J. Y. C., Habal, F. M., Burrowes, C. E., and Movat, H. Z.**, Interaction between factor XII (Hageman factor), high molecular weight kininogen and prekallikrein, *Thromb. Res.*, 9, 423, 1976.
68. **Chan, J. Y. C., Burrowes, C. E., and Movat, H. Z.**, Surface activation of factor XII (Hageman factor) — critical role of high molecular weight kininogen and another potentiator, *Agents Actions*, 8, 65, 1978.
69. **Cherayil, G. D.**, Sialic acid and fatty acid concentrations in lymphocytes, red blood cells and plasma from patients with multiple sclerosis, *J. Neurol. Sci.*, 63, 1, 1984.
70. **Chernew, I. and Braude, A. I.**, Depression of phagocytosis by solutes in concentrations found in the kidney and urine, *J. Clin. Invest.*, 41, 1945, 1962.
71. **Christensen, H. N., Handlogten, M. E., and Thomas, E. L.**, Na plus-facilitated reactions of neutral amino acids with a cationic amino acid transport system, *Proc. Natl. Acad. Sci. U.S.A.*, 63, 948, 1969.

72. **Churg, J., Morita, T., and Suzuki, Y.**, Glomerulonephritis with fibrin and crescent formation, in *Glomerulo-nephritis, Morphology, Natural History, and Treatment*, Part 2, Kincaid-Smith, P., Mathew, T. H., and Lovell Becker, E., Eds., (Perspectives in Nephrology and Hypertension, Vol. 1), John Wiley & Sons, New York, 1973, 677.

73. **Chvapil, M.**, Disruption of healed scars in scurvy — the result of disequilibrium in collagen metabolism, *Plast. Reconstr. Surg.*, 57, 376, 1976.

74. **Chvapil, M. and Zukoski, C. F.**, New concept on the mechanisms of the biological effect of zinc, in *Clinical Applications of Zinc Metabolism*, Pories, W. J., Ed., Charles C Thomas, Springfield, 1974, 67.

75. **Clark, R. A. and Kimball, H. R.**, Defective granulocyte chemotaxis in Chediak-Higashi syndrome, *J. Clin. Invest.*, 50, 2645, 1971.

76. **Cohn, Z. A.**, Determinants of infection in the peritoneal cavity. III. The action of selected inhibitors on the fate of *Staphylococcus aureus* in the mouse, *Yale J. Biol. Med.*, 35, 48, 1962.

77. **Cohn, Z. A.**, The fate of bacteria within phagocytic cells. II. The modification of intracellular degradation, *J. Exp. Med.*, 117, 43, 1963.

78. **Cohn, Z. A.**, The macrophage-versatile element of inflammation, *Harvey Lect.*, 77, 63, 1981-82.

79. **Cohn, Z. A. and Hirsch, J. G.**, The influence of phagocytosis on the intracellular distribution of granule-associated components of polymorphonuclear leukocytes, *J. Exp. Med.*, 112, 1015, 1960.

80. **Cohn, Z. A. and Parks, E.**, The regulation of pinocytosis in mouse macrophages. IV. The immunological induction of pinocytic vesicles, secondary lysosomes, and hydrolytic enzymes, *J. Exp. Med.*, 125, 1091, 1967.

81. **Collins, H. W. and Gonzalez, M. F.**, Acquired factor IX inhibitor in a patient with adenocarcinoma of the colon, *Acta Haematol*, 71, 49, 1984.

82. **Calnan, J. and Davies, A.**, The effect of methotrexate (amethopterin) on wound healing, an experimental study, *Br. J. Cancer*, 19, 505, 1965.

83. **Conrad, D. H., Basin, H., Sehon, A. H., and Froese, A.**, Binding parameters of the interaction between rat IgE and rat mast cell receptors, *J. Immunol.*, 114, 1688, 1975.

84. **Cooper, M. R., DeChatelet, L. R., McCall, C. E., LaVia, M. F., Spurr, C. L., and Baehner, R. L.**, Complete deficiency of leukocyte glucose-6-phosphate dehydrogenase with defective bactericidal activity, *J. Clin. Invest.*, 51, 769, 1972.

85. **Coutinho, A., Bandeira, A., Björklund, M., Forni, L., Forsgren, S., Freitas, A. A., Gullberg, M., Holmberg, D., et al.**, From the mechanisms of lymphocyte activation to internal activity in the immune system, *Ann. Immunol. (Paris)*, 134D, 93, 1983.

86. **Cramer, W. and Simpson, W. L.**, Mast cells in experimental skin carcinogenesis, *Cancer Res.*, 4, 601, 1944.

87. **Cronkite, E. P. and Vincent, P. C.**, Granulocytopoiesis, in *Hemopoietic Cellular Proliferation*, Stohlman, F., Jr., Ed., Grune & Stratton, New York, 1970, 211.

88. **Cupps, T. R., Edgar, L. C., Thomas, C. A., and Fauci, A. S.**, Multiple mechanisms of B cell immunoregulation in man after administration of *in vivo* corticosteroids, *J. Immunol.*, 132, 170, 1984.

89. **Curnutte, J. T., Whitten, D. M., and Babior, B. M.**, Defective superoxide production by granulocytes from patients with chronic granulomatous disease, *N. Engl. J. Med.*, 290, 593, 1974.

90. **Dallman, P. R. and Goodman, J. R.**, Enlargement of mitochondrial compartment in iron and copper deficiency, *Blood*, 35, 496, 1970.

91. **D'Andrea, G., Toldo, M., Cananzi, A., and Ferro-Milone, F.**, Study of platelet activation in migraine: control by low doses of aspirin, *Stroke*, 15, 271, 1984.

92. **Daniel, J. L., Molish, I. R., Rigmaiden, M., and Stewart, G.**, Evidence for a role of myosin phosphorylation in the initiation of the platelet shape response, *J. Biol. Chem.*, 259, 9826, 1984.

93. **Dannenberg, A. M.**, Macrophages in inflammation and infection, *N. Engl. J. Med.*, 293, 489, 1975.

94. **Danta, G.**, Second phase platelet aggregation induced by adenosine diphosphate in patients with cerebral vascular disease and in control subjects, *Thromb. Diath. Haemorrh.*, 23, 159, 1970.

95. **Davis, T. M. E. and Bown, E.**, Analysis of platelet aggregation using particle collision theory, *Am. J. Physiol.*, 245, R776, 1983.

96. **Day, M. and Stockbridge, A.**, The effect of drugs on the uptake of amines by mast cells, *Br. J. Pharmacol. Chemother.*, 23, 405, 1964.

97. **DeChatelet, L. R., Cooper, M. R., and McCall, C. E.**, Stimulation of the hexose monophosphate shunt in human neutrophiles by ascorbic acid: mechanism of action, *Antimicrob. Agents Chemother.*, 1, 12, 1972.

98. **DeMeo, A. N. and Anderson, B. R.**, Defective chemotaxis associated with a serum inhibitor in cirrhotic patients, *N. Engl. J. Med.*, 286, 735, 1972.

99. **Denson, K. W. E., Lurie, A., De Cataldo, F., and Mannucci, P. M.**, The factor-X defect: recognition of abnormal forms of factor X, *Br. J. Haematol.*, 18, 317, 1970.

100. **De Takats, G.**, Heparin tolerance revisited, *Surgery*, 70, 318, 1971.

101. **Di Rosa, M., Giroud, J. P. and Willoughby, D. A.**, Studies on the mediators of the acute inflammatory response induced in rats in different sites by carrageenan and turpentine, *J. Pathol.*, 104, 15, 1971.

102. **Di Rosa, M., Papadimitriou, J. M., and Willoughby, D. A.,** A histopathological and pharmacological analysis of the mode of action of nonsteroidal anti-inflammatory drugs, *J. Pathol.,* 105, 239, 1971.
103. **Dittrich, H.,** Physiology of neutrophils, in *The Physiology and Pathology of Leukocytes,* Braunsteiner, H. and Zucker-Franklin, D., Eds., Grune & Stratton, New York, 1962, 130.
104. **Dodds, W. J.,** Hereditary and acquired hemorrhagic disorders in animals, in *Progress in Hemostasis and Thrombosis,* Vol. 2, Spaet, T. H., Eds., Grune & Stratton, New York, 1974, 215.
105. **Doolittle, R. F.,** Structural aspects of the fibrinogen to fibrin conversion, *Adv. Protein Chem.,* 27, 1, 1973.
106. **Dougherty, G. J. and McBride, W. H.,** Macrophage heterogeneity, *J. Clin. Lab. Immunol.,* 14, 1, 1984.
107. **Douglas, W. W.,** Histamine and antihistamines; 5-hydroxytryptamine and antagonists, in *The Pharmacological Basis of Therapeutics,* 4th Ed., Goodman, L. S. and Gilman, A., Eds., MacMillan, New York, 1970, chap. 29, p. 621.
108. **Duckert, F.,** Le facteur 13 et la protéine 13, *Nouv. Rev. Fr. Hematol.,* 10, 685, 1970.
109. **Ehrlich, H. P. and Tarver, H.,** Effects of beta-carotene, vitamin A, and glucocorticoids on collagen synthesis in wounds, *Proc. Soc. Exp. Biol. Med.,* 137, 936, 1971.
110. **Ehrlich, H. P., Tarver, H. and Hunt, T. K.,** Inhibitory effects of vitamin E on collagen synthesis and wound repair, *Ann. Surg.,* 175, 235, 1972.
111. **Eichner, E. R.,** Platelets, carotids and coronaries; critique on antithrombotic role of antiplatelet agents, exercise, and certain diets. *Am. J. Med.,* 77, 513, 1984.
112. **Eisen, V. and Glanville, K. L. A.,** Separation of kinin-forming factors in human plasma, *Br. J. Exp. Pathol.,* 50, 427, 1969.
113. **Eisen, V. and Vogt, W.,** Plasma kininogenases and their activators, in *Handbook of Experimental Pharmakology,* Vol. 25, Erdös, E., Ed., Springer-Verlag, Berlin, 1970, 82.
114. **Ellis, E. F., Oelz, O., Roberts, L. J., II, Payne, N. A., Sweetman, B. J., Nies, A. S., and Oates, J. A.,** Coronary arterial smooth muscle contraction by a substance released from platelets: evidence that it is thromboxane A_2, *Science,* 193, 1135, 1976.
115. **Elliott, D. F., Horton, E. W., and Lewis, G. P.,** Actions of pure bradykinin, *J. Physiol. (London),* 153, 473, 1960.
116. **Elliott, J. M.,** Platelet receptor binding studies in affective disorders, *J. Allective Disord.,* 6, 219, 1984.
117. **Elsbach, P., Goldman, J., and Patriarca, P.,** Phospholipid metabolism by phagocyte cells. VI. Observations on the fate of phospholipids of granulocytes and ingested *Escherichia coli* during phagocytosis, *Biochim. Biophys. Acta,* 280, 33, 1972.
118. **Essien, E. M., Cazenave, J.-P., Moore, S., and Mustard, J. F.,** Effect of heparin and thrombin on platelet adherence to the surface of rabbit aorta, *Thromb. Res.,* 13, 69, 1978.
119. **Ettinger, M. G., Kusonoki, R., and Fujishima, H.,** Stroke: U.S. and Japan; blood coagulation studies, *Geriatrics,* 24, 116, 1969.
120. **Fedder, I. L., Holme, S., Vlasses, P. H., Ferguson, R. K., and Murphy, S.,** Effect of intravenous carbenicillin, cefoxitin and cefamandole on ADP-induced platelet aggregation and shape change, *Thromb. Res.,* 32, 215, 1983.
121. **Fell, H. B. and Thomas, L.,** The influence of hydrocortisone on the action of excess vitamin A on limb bone rudiments in culture, *J. Exp. Med.,* 114, 343, 1961.
122. **Ferreira, S. H., Lorenzetti, B. B., and Correa, M. A.,** Central peripheral antianalgesic action of aspirin-like drugs, *Eur. J. Pharmacol.,* 53, 39, 1978.
123. **Ferreira, S. H., Nakamura, M., and de Abreu Castro, M. S.,** The hyperalgesic effects of prostacyclin and PGE_2, *Prostaglandins,* 16, 31, 1978.
124. **Findlay, C. W., Jr.,** Effect of vitamin B_{12} on wound healing, *Proc. Soc. Exp. Biol. Med.,* 82, 492, 1953.
125. **Finlayson, J. S.,** Crosslinking of fibrin, *Semin. Throm. Hemostas.,* 1, 33, 1974.
126. **Fisher, E. R. and Fisher, B.,** Role of mast cells in tumor growth, *Arch. Pathol.,* 79, 185, 1965.
127. **Florey, H. W. and Grant, L H.,** Leucocyte migration from small blood vessels stimulated with ultraviolet light: an electron-microscope study, *J. Pathol. Bacteriol.,* 82, 13, 1961.
128. **Flower, R. J. and Blackwell, G. J.,** The importance of phospholipase A_2 in prostaglandin biosynthesis, *Biochem. Pharmacol.,* 25, 285, 1976.
129. **Forbes, C. D. and Ratnoff, O. D.,** Studies on plasma thromboplastin antecedent (factor XI), PTA deficiency and inhibition of PTA by plasma: pharmacologic inhibitors and specific antiserum, *J. Lab. Clin. Med.,* 79, 113, 1972.
130. **Fredholm, B. and Haegermark, Ö.,** Histamine release from rat mast cells induced by a mast cell degranulating fraction in bee venom, *Acta Physiol. Scand.,* 69, 304, 1967.
131. **Fredholm, B. and Haegermark, Ö.,** Studies on the histamine releasing effect of bee venom fractions and compound 48-80 on skin and lung tissue of the rat, *Acta. Physiol. Scand.,* 76, 288, 1969.
132. **Fritz, H., Eckert, I., and Werle, E.,** Isolierung und Charakterisierung von sialinsäurehaltigem und sialinsäurefreiem Kallikrein aus Schweinepankreas, *Hoppe-Seyler's Z. Physiol. Chem.,* 348, 1120, 1967.
133. **Fritz, H., Schiessler, H., and Geiger, R.,** Naturally occurring low molecular weight inhibitors of neutral proteinases from PMN-granulocytes and of kallikreins, *Agents Actions,* 8, 57, 1978.

134. **Fritz, H., Wunderer, G., Kummer, K., Heimburger, N., and Werle, E.,** Alpha 1-antitrypsin und c-1-Inaktivator: progressiv-Inhibitoren für Serum Kallikreine von Mensch und Schwein, *Hoppe-Seyler's Z. Physiol. Chem.,* 353, 906, 1972.

135. **Gaarder, A., Jonsen, J., Laland, S., Hellem, A., and Owren, P. A.,** Adenosine diphosphate in red cells as a factor in the adhesiveness of human blood platelets, *Nature (London),* 192, 531, 1961.

136. **Gadek, J. E., Fells, G. A., Wright, D. G., and Crystal, R. G.,** Human neutrophil elastase functions as a type III collagen "collagenase", *Biochem. Biophys. Res. Commun.,* 95, 1815, 1980.

137. **Ganguly, R., Pennock, D., and Kluge, R. M.,** Suppression of the production of migration inhibitory factor in humans by tetracycline, *J. Infect, Dis.,* 148, 611, 1983.

138. **Gans, H. and Tan, B. H.,** Alpha 1-antitrypsin, an inhibitor for thrombin and plasmin, *Clin. Chim. Acta,* 17, 111, 1967.

139. **Garattini, S. and Valselli, L.,** Serotonin, Elsevier, Amsterdam, 1965.

140. **Garcia-Sainz, J. A., Hoffman, B. B., Li, S.-Y., Lefkowitz, R. J., and Fain, J. N.,** Role of alpha adrenoceptors in the turnover of phosphatidylinositol and of $alpha_2$ adrenoceptors in the regulation of cyclic AMP accumulation of hamster adipocytes, *Life Sci.,* 27, 953, 1980.

141. **Genta, R. M., Ottesen, E. A., Neva, F. A., Walzer, P. D., Tanowitz, H. B., and Wittner, M.,** Cellular responses in human strongyloidasis, *Am. J. Trop. Med. Hyg.,* 32, 990, 1983.

142. **Ginsburg, H. and Lagunoff, D.,** The in-vitro differentiation of mast cells. Cultures of cells from immunized mouse lymph nodes and thoracic duct lymph on fibroblast monolayers, *J. Cell. Biol.,* 35, 685, 1967.

143. **Girolami, A., Molaro, G., Lazzarin, M., Scarpa, R., and Brunetti, A.,** A "new" congenital haemorrhagic condition due to the presence of an abnormal factor X (factor X Friuli): study of a large kindred, *Br. J. Haematol.,* 19, 179, 1970.

144. **Giroud, J. P. and Willoughby, D. A.,** The interrelations of complement and a prostaglandin-like substance in acute inflammation, *J. Pathol.,* 101, 241, 1970.

145. **Glenner, G. G. and Page, D. L.,** Amyloid, amyloidosis and amyloidgenesis, *Int. Rev. Exp. Pathol.,* 15, 1, 1976.

146. **Glynn, L. E.,** Pathology, pathogenesis and aetiology of rheumatoid arthritis, *Ann. Rheum. Dis.,* 31, 412, 1972.

147. **Godal, T., Rees, R. J. W., and Lamvik, J. O.,** Lymphocyte-mediated modification of blood-derived macrophage function in vitro; inhibition of growth of intracellular mycobacteria with lymphokines, *Clin. Exp. Immunol.,* 8, 625, 1971.

148. **Goetze, O., Zvaifler, N. J., and Müller-Eberhard, H. J.,** Evidence for complement activation by the C3 activator system in rheumatoid arthritis, *Arthritis Rheum.,* 15, 111, 1972.

149. **Goetzl, E. J. and Austen, K. F.,** Purification and synthesis of eosinophilotactic tetrapeptides of human lung tissue: identification as eosinophil chemotactic factor of anaphylaxis, *Proc. Natl. Acad. Sci. U.S.A.,* 72, 4123, 1975.

150. **Goldstein, E.,** Hydrolytic enzymes of alveolar macrophages, *Rev. Infect. Dis.,* 5, 1078, 1983.

151. **Gottschall, J. L., Johnston, V. L., Rzad, L., Anderson, A. J., and Aster, R. H.,** Importance of white blood cells in platelet storage, *Vox Sang.,* 47, 101, 1984.

152. **Goyer, R. A.,** The renal tubule in lead poisoning, I. In mitochondrial swelling and aminociduria, *Lab. Invest.,* 19, 71, 1968.

153. **Graham, R. M. and Graham, J. B.,** Mast cells and cancer of the cervix, *Surg. Gynecol. Obstet.,* 123, 3, 1966.

154. **Granger, G. A.,** Mechanisms of lymphocyte-induced cell and tissue destruction in vitro, *Am. J. Pathol.,* 60, 469, 1970.

155. **Granger, G. A., Shacks, S. J., Williams, T. W., and Kolb, W. P.,** Lymphocyte in vitro cytotoxicity: specific release of lymphotoxin-like materials from tuberculin-sensitive lymphoid cells, *Nature (London),* 221, 1155, 1969.

156. **Gray, G. R., Stamatoyannopoulos, G., Naiman, S. C., Kliman, M. R., Klebanoff, S. J., Austin, T., Yoshida, A., and Robinson, G. C. F.,** Neutrophil dysfunction, chronic granulomatous disease and nonspherocytic haemolytic anaemia caused by complete deficiency of glucose-6-phosphate dehydrogenase, *Lancet,* 2, 530, 1973.

157. **Green, D.,** The management of factor VIII inhibitors in nonhemophilic patients, *Prog. Clin. Biol. Res.,* 150, 337, 1984.

158. **Greenwald, R. A. and Moy, W. W.,** Inhibition of collagen gelation by action of the superoxide radical, *Arthritis Rheum.,* 22, 251, 1979.

159. **Greenwald, R. A. and Moy, W. W.,** Effect of oxygen-derived free radicals on hyaluronic acid, *Arthritis Rheum.,* 23, 455, 1980.

160. **Griffin, J. H. and Cochrane, C. G.,** Mechanism for the involvement of high molecular weight kininogen in surface-dependent reactions of Hageman factor, *Proc. Natl. Acad. Sci. U.S.A.,* 73, 2554, 1976.

161. **Grinstein, M., Bannerman, R. M., and Moore, C. V.,** The utilization of protoporphyrin 9 in heme synthesis, *Blood,* 14, 476, 1959.

162. **Gryglewski, R. J.,** Steroid hormones, anti-inflammatory steroids and prostaglandins, *Pharmacol. Res. Commun.*, 8, 337, 1976.

163. **Guha Thakurta, S., De, M., and Chowdhury, J. R.,** Effect of radiotherapy on lymphocyte subpopulations in patients with carcinoma of the breast and uterine cervix, *Indian J. Med. Res.*, 78 Suppl., 46, 1983.

164. **Habal, F. M. and Movat, H. Z.,** Kininogens of human plasma, *Semin. Thromb. Hemostasis*, 3, 27, 1976.

165. **Habermann, E.,** Enzymatic kinin release from kininogen and from low-molecular compounds, in *Hypotensive Peptides*, Erdös, E. G., Back, N., and Sicuteri, F., Eds., Springer-Verlag, New York, 1966, 116.

166. **Habermann, E.,** Kininogens, in *Handbook of Experimental Pharmakology*, Erdös, E. G., Ed., Springer-Verlag, Berlin, 1970, 250.

167. **Habermann, E. G. and Klett, W.,** Reinigung und einige Eigenschaften eines Kallikreins aus Schweineserum, *Biochem. Z.*, 346, 133, 1966.

168. **Hagen, P.,** Biosynthesis and storage of histamine, heparin and 5-hydroxytryptamine in the mast cell, *Can. J. Biochem. Physiol.*, 39, 639, 1961.

169. **Hamberg, M. and Samuelsson, B.,** Detection and isolation of an endoperoxide intermediate in prostaglandin biosynthesis, *Proc. Natl. Acad. Sci. U.S.A.*, 70, 899, 1973.

170. **Hamberg, M. and Samuelsson, B.,** Prostaglandin endoperoxides. VII. Novel transformations of arachidonic acid in guinea-pig lungs, *Biochem. Biophys. Res. Commun.*, 61, 942, 1974.

171. **Hamberg, M. and Samuelsson, B.,** Prostaglandin endoperoxides. Novel transformation of arachidonic acid in human platelets, *Proc. Natl. Acad. Sci. U.S.A.*, 71, 3400, 1974.

172. **Hamberg, M., Svensson, J., Wakabayashi, T., and Samuelsson, B.,** Isolation and structure of two prostaglandin endoperoxides that cause platelet aggregation, *Proc. Natl. Acad. Sci. U.S.A.*, 71, 345, 1974.

173. **Hamberg, M., Svensson, J., and Samuelsson, B.,** Thromboxanes: a new group of biologically active compounds derived from prostaglandin endoperoxides, *Proc. Natl. Acad. Sci. U.S.A.*, 72, 2994, 1975.

174. **Hanley, M. R., Lee, C. M., Jones, L. M., and Michell, R. H.,** Similar effects of substance P and related peptides on salivation and on phosphatidylinositol turnover in rat salivary glands, *Mol. Pharmacol.*, 18, 78, 1980.

175. **Harada, R. N., Vatter, A. E., and Repine, J. E.,** Oxygen radical scavengers protect alveolar macrophages from hyperoxic injury in vitro, *Am. Rev. Respir. Dis.*, 128, 761, 1983.

176. **Hardaway, R. M.,** *Syndromes of disseminated intravascular coagulation*, Charles C Thomas, Springfield, IL, 1966.

177. **Hardisty, R. M. and Hutton, R. A.,** Platelet aggregation and the availability of platelet factor 3, *Br. J. Haematol.*, 12, 764, 1966.

178. **Harpel, P. C.,** Studies on human plasma alpha-2-macroglobulin-enzyme interactions. Evidence for proteolytic modification of the subunit chain structure, *J. Exp. Med.*, 138, 508, 1973.

179. **Harpel, P. C. and Mosesson, M. W.,** Degradation of human fibrinogen by plasma alpha-2-macroglobulin-enzyme complexes, *J. Clin. Invest*, 52, 2175, 1973.

180. **Harpel, P. C. and Rosenberg, R. D.,** α2-Macroglobulin and antithrombin-heparin cofactor: modulators of hemostatic and inflammatory reactions, in *Progress in Hemostasis and Thrombosis*, Vol. 3, Spaet, T. H., Ed., Grune & Stratton, New York, 1976, 145.

181. **Harris, E. D., Jr., Vater, C. A., Mainardi, C. L., and Werb, Z.,** Cellular control of collagen breakdown in rheumatoid arthritis, *Agents Actions*, 8, 36, 1978.

182. **Haslam, R. J. and Lynham, J. A.,** Activation and inhibition of blood platelet adenylate cyclase by adenosine or by 2-chloroadenosine, *Life Sci.*, 11, 1143, 1972.

183. **Hawkins, D.,** Neutrophilic leukocytes in immunologic reactions: evidence for the selective release of lysosomal constituents, *J. Immunol*, 108, 310, 1972.

184. **Hawkins, H. K., Ericsson, J. L. E., Biberfeld, P., and Trump, B. F.,** Lysosome and phagosome stability in lethal cell injury. Morphologic tracer studies in cell injury due to inhibition of energy metabolism, immune cytolysis and photosensitization, *Am. J. Pathol.*, 68, 255, 1972.

185. **Heck, L. W. and Kaplan, A. P.,** Substrates of Hageman factor. I. Isolation and characterization of human factor XI (PTA) and inhibition of the activated enzyme by alpha-1-antitrypsin, *J. Exp. Med.*, 140, 1615, 1974.

186. **Heitz, D. C. and Brody, M. J.,** Possible mechanism of histamine release during active vasodilatation, *Am. J. Physiol.*, 228, 1351, 1975.

187. **Heldebrant, C. M., Butkowski, R. J., Bajaj, S. P., and Mann, K. G.,** The activation of prothrombin. II. Partial reactions, physical and chemical characterization of the intermediates of activation, *J. Biol. Chem.*, 248, 7149, 1973.

188. **Henderson, A. R., Ahmad, D., and McKenzie, D.,** Increased synthesis of lactate dehydrogenase "H" subunit by a malignant tumor, *Clin. Chem.*, 20, 1466, 1974.

189. **Henriksen, R. A. and Jackson, C. M.,** Cooperative calcium binding by the phospholipid binding region of bovine prothrombin: a requirement for intact disulfide bridges, *Arch. Biochem. Biophys.*, 170, 149, 1975.

190. **Highsmith, R. F. and Rosenberg, R. D.,** The inhibition of human plasmin by human antithrombin-heparin cofactor, *J. Biol. Chem.*, 249, 4335, 1974.

191. **Hill, H. R., Ochs, H. D., Quie, P. G., Clark, R. A., Pabst, H. F., Klebanoff, S. J., and Wedgwood, R. J.,** Defect in neutrophil granulocyte chemotaxis in Job's syndrome of recurrent 'cold' staphylococcal abscesses, *Lancet,* 2, 617, 1974.

192. **Hirsch, J. G.,** Neutrophil leukocytes, in *The Inflammatory Process,* Vol. 1, 2nd ed., Zweifach, B. W., Grant, L., and McCluskey, R. T., Eds., Academic Press, New York, 1974, 411.

193. **Hirschhorn, R.,** Lysosomal mechanism in the inflammatory process, in *The Inflammatory Process,* Vol. 1, 2nd ed., Zweifach, B. W., Grant, L., and McCluskey, R. T., Eds., Academic Press, New York, 1974, 259.

194. **Hochstrasser, K.,** Low molecular weight proteinase inhibitors in the respiratory tract. Biochemistry and function, in *Biochemistry, Pathology and Genetics of Pulmonary Emphysema,* Sadoul, P. and Bignon, J., Eds., Pergamon Press, Oxford, 1980.

195. **Hoffman, D. R., Hajdu, J., and Snyder, F.,** Cytotoxicity of platelet activating factor and related alkyl-phospholipid analogs in human leukemia cells, polymorphonuclear neutrophils, and skin fibroblasts, *Blood,* 63, 545, 1984.

196. **Hohn, D. C. and Lehrer, R. I.,** NADPH oxidase deficiency in X-linked chronic granulomatous disease, *J. Clin. Invest.,* 55, 707, 1975.

197. **Holmes, B., Page, A. R., and Good, R. A.,** Studies of the metabolic activity of leukocytes from patients with a genetic abnormality of phagocytic function, *J. Clin. Invest.,* 46, 1422, 1967.

198. **Holmes, B., Park, B. H., Maliwista, S. E., Quie, P. G., Nelson, D. L., and Good, R. A.,** Chronic granulomatous disease in females. A deficiency of leukocyte glutathione peroxidase. *N. Engl. J. Med.,* 283, 217, 1970.

199. **Holmes, B., Quie, P. G., Windhorst, D. B., and Good, R. A.,** Fatal granulomatous disease of childhood. An inborn abnormality of phagocytic function, *Lancet,* 1, 1225, 1966.

200. **Holmes, S. W., Horton, E. W., and Main, I. H. M.,** The effect of prostaglandin E₁ on responses of smooth muscle catecholamines, angiotensin and vasopressin, *Br. J. Pharmacol. Chemother.,* 21, 538, 1963.

201. **Holmsen, H. and Day, H. J.,** The selectivity of the thrombin-induced platelet release reaction: subcellular localization of released and retained constituents, *J. Lab. Clin. Med.,* 75, 840, 1970.

202. **Holmsen, H., Day, H. J., and Storm, E.,** Adenine nucleotide metabolism of blood platelets. VI. Subcellular localization of nucleotide pools with different functions in platelet release reaction, *Biochim. Biophys. Acta,* 186, 254, 1969.

203. **Holmsen, H., Day, H. J., and Stormorken, H.,** The blood platelet release reaction, *Scand. J. Haematol.,* Suppl. 8, 1, 1969.

204. **Holmsen, H., Whaun, J., and Day, H. J.,** Inhibition by lanthanum ions of ADP-induced platelet aggregation, *Experientia,* 27, 451, 1971.

205. **Horecker, B. L.,** The biosynthesis of bacterial polysaccharides, *Annu. Rev. Microbiol.,* 20, 253, 1966.

206. **Hoskings, C. S., Fitzgerald, M. G., and Shelton, M. J.,** The immunological investigation of children with recurrent infections, *Aust. Paediatr. J.,* 14(Suppl.), 1, 1978.

207. **Hottendorf, G. H., Nielsen, S. W., and Kenyon, A. J.,** Ribonucleic acid in canine mast cell granules and the possible interrelation of mast cells and plasma cells, *Pathol. Vet.,* 3, 178, 1966.

208. **Hottendorf, G. H., Nielsen, S. W., and Kenyon, A. J.,** Plasma mast cells, *Nature (London),* 212, 829, 1966.

209. **Houck, J. C., Ed.,** Chemical messengers of the inflammatory process, in *Handbook of Inflammation,* Elsevier/North Holland, Amsterdam, 1979.

210. **Houck, J. C., Barnes, S. G., and Chang, C.,** Products of collagenolysis: an important mediator of cell infiltration during inflammation, in *Immunopathology of Inflammation,* Forscher, B. K. and Houck, J. C., Eds., (Int. Congr. Ser., No. 229), Excerpta Medica, Amsterdam, 1971, 39.

211. **Hovig, T., Dodds, W. J., Rowsell, H. C., and Mustard, J. F.,** The transformation of hemostatic platelet plugs in normal and Factor IX deficient dogs, *Am. J. Pathol.,* 53, 355, 1968.

212. **Hovig, T., Roswell, H. C., Dodds, W. J., Jørgensen, L., and Mustard, J. F.,** Experimental hemostasis in normal dogs and dogs with congenital disorders of blood coagulation, *Blood,* 30, 636, 1967.

213. **Huang, T. W., Lagunoff, D., and Benditt, E. P.,** Nonaggregative adherence of platelets to basal lamina in vitro, *Lab. Invest.,* 31, 156, 1974.

214. **Huber, H. and Fudenberg, H. H.,** Receptor sites of human monocytes for IgG, *Int. Arch. Allergy Appl. Immunol.,* 34(1), 18, 1968.

215. **Humphrey, D. M., McManus, L. M., Hanahan, D. J., and Pinckard, R. N.,** Vasoactive properties of 1-O-alkyl-2-acetyl-sn-glyceryl-3-phosphorylcholine and analogues, *Lab. Invest.,* 46, 422, 1982.

216. **Humphrey, D. M., Pinckard, R. N., McManus, L. M., and Hanahan, D. J.,** Intradermal neutrophil infiltrates induced by 1-O-alkyl-2-acetyl-sn-glyceryl-3-phosphorylcholine (AGEPC), *Fed. Proc.,* 40, 1003, 1981.

217. **Hunt, T. K.,** Control of wound healing with cortisone and vitamin A, in *The Ultrastructure of Collagen,* Longacre, J. J., Ed., Charles C Thomas, Springfield, IL, 1976, 497.

218. **Hurley, J. V.,** The sequence of early events, in *Inflammation,* Vane, J. R. and Ferreira, S. H., Eds., Vol.50/I Chap., 2 Springer-Verlag, Berlin, 1978, 26.

219. **Ignarro, L. J. and Columbo, C.** Enzyme release from polymorphonuclear leukocyte lysosomes: regulation by autonomic drugs and cyclic nucleotides, *Science*, 180, 1181, 1973.

220. **Imort, M., Zühlsdorf, M., Feige, U., Hasilik, A., and von Figura, K.,** Biosynthesis and transport of lysosomal enzymes in human monocytes and macrophages. Effects of ammonium chloride, zymosan and tunicamycin, *Biochem. J.*, 214, 671, 1983.

221. **Ishizaka, T., Ishizaka, K., Orange, R. P., and Austen, K. F.,** The capacity of human immunogobulin E to mediate the release of histamine and slow-reacting substance of anaphylaxis (SRS-A) from monkey lung, *J. Immunol*, 104, 335, 1970.

222. **Ishizaka, T., Ishizaka, K., and Tomioka, H.,** Release of histamine and slow-reacting substance of anaphylaxis (SRS-A) by IgE-anti-IgE reactions on monkey mast cells, *J. Immunol.*, 108, 513, 1972.

223. **Issekutz, A. C., Ripley, M., and Jackson, J. R.,** Role of neutrophils in the deposition of platelets during acute inflammation, *Lab. Invest.*, 49, 716, 1983.

224. **Jacob, J.,** *Les antagonistes de la serotonine. Actualité's pharmacologiques*, Masson, Paris, 1960.

225. **Jacobsen, S. amd Kriz, M.,** Some data on two purified kininogens from human plasma, *Br. J. Pharmacol.*, 29, 25, 1967.

226. **Janoff, A.,** Neutrophil proteases in inflammation, *Annu. Rev. Med.*, 23, 177, 1972.

227. **Janoff, A., Sloan, B., Weinbaum, G., Damiano, V., Sandhaus, R. A., Elias, J., and Kimbel, P.,** Experimental emphysema induced with purified human neutrophil elastase: tissue localization of the instilled protease, *Am. Rev. Respir. Dis.*, 115, 461, 1977.

228. **Jenkins, C. S. P., Packham, M. A., Guccione, M. A., and Mustard, J. F.,** Modification of platelet adherence to protein-coated surfaces, *J. Lab. Clin. Med.*, 81, 280, 1973.

229. **Jennings, R. B., Herdson, P. B., and Sommers, H. M.,** Structural and functional abnormalities in mitochondria isolated from ischemic dog myocardium, *Lab. Invest.*, 20, 548, 1969.

230. **Johnson, H. A. and Amendola, F.,** Mitochondrial proliferation in compensatory growth of the kidney, *Am. J. Pathol.*, 54, 35, 1969.

231. **Joist, J. H., Dolezel, G., Lloyd, J. V., and Mustard, J. F.,** Phospholipid transfer between plasma and platelets in vitro, *Blood*, 48, 199, 1976.

232. **Jones, L. M., Cockcroft, S., and Michell, R. H.,** Stimulation of phosphatidylinositol turnover in various tissues by cholinergic and adrenergic agonists, by histamine and by caerulein, *Biochem. J.*, 182, 669, 1979.

233. **Roberts, M. L. and Tennes, K. A.,** Receptor interactions in stimulation of hydrolysis of inositol phospholipids. *Eur. J. Pharmac.*, 109, 293, 1985.

234. **Johnson, D. and Travis, J.,** The oxidative inactivation of human alpha-1-proteinase inhibitor: further evidence for methionine at the reactive center, *J. Biol. Chem.*, 254, 4022, 1979.

235. **Johnson, H. H., Jr.,** Variations in histamine levels in guines pig skin related to skin region; age (or weight); and time after death of the animal, *J. Invest. Dermatol.*, 27, 159, 1956.

236. **Jørgensen, L. and Borchgrevink, C. F.,** The platelet plug in normal persons. II. The histological appearance of the plug in the secondary bleeding time test, *Acta Pathol. Microbiol. Scand.*, 57, 427, 1963.

237. **Jørgensen, L. and Borchgrevink, C. F.,** The haemostatic mechanism in patients with haemorrhagic diseases. A histological study of wounds made for primary and secondary bleeding time tests, *Acta Pathol. Microbiol. Scand.*, 60, 55, 1964.

238. **Josso, F., Lavernge, J. M., and Soulier, J. P.,** Les dysprothrombinémies constitutionnelles et aeguises, *Nouv. Rev. Fr. Hematol.*, 10, 633, 1970.

239. **Kaliner, M. and Austen, F.,** A sequence of biological events in the antigen induced release of chemical mediator from sensitized human lung tissue. *J. Exp. Med.*, 138, 1077, 1973.

240. **Kaliner, M. and Austen, K. F.,** Cyclic AMP, ATP, and reversed anaphylactic histamine release from rat mast cells, *J. Immunol.*, 112, 664, 1974.

241. **Kampine, J. P., Brady, R. O., Kanfer, J. N., Feld, M., and Shapiro, D.,** Diagnosis of Gaucher's disease and Niemann-Pick disease with small samples of venous blood, *Science*, 155, 86, 1967.

242. **Kantor, H. S., Tao, P., and Kiefer, H. C.,** Kinetic evidence for the presence of two prostaglandin receptor sites regulating the activity of intestinal adenylate cyclase sensitive to Escherichia coli enterotoxin, *Proc. Natl. Acad. Sci. U.S.A.*, 71, 1317, 1974.

243. **Kaplan, A. P. and Austen, K. F.,** A prealbumin activator of prekallikrein II. Derivation of activators prekallikrein from active Hageman factor by digestion with plasmin, *J. Exp. Med.*, 133, 696, 1971.

244. **Kaplan, A. P., Goetzl, E. J., and Austen, K. F.,** The fibrinolytic pathway of human plasma. II. The generation of chemotactic activity by activation of plasminogen proactivator, *J. Clin. Invest.*, 52, 2591, 1973.

245. **Kaplan, A. P., Meier, H. L., and Mandle, R., Jr.,** The Hageman factor dependent pathways of coagulation, fibrinolysis, and kiningeneration, *Thromb. Hemostas.*, 3, 1, 1976.

246. **Kaplan, H. B., Edelson, H. S., Korchak, H. M., Given, W. P., Abramson, S., and Weissmann, G.,** Effects of non-steroidal anti-inflammatory agents on human neutrophil functions in vitro and in vivo, *Biochem. Pharmacol.*, 33, 371, 1984.

247. **Kaplan, S. S., Finch, S. C., and Basford, R. E.,** Polymorphonuclear leukocyte activation: effects of phospholipase C, *Proc. Soc. Exp. Biol.*, 140, 540, 1972.

248. **Kappas, A., Hellman, L., Fukushima, D. K., and Gallagher, T. F.,** The pyrogenic effect of etiocholanolone (3α-hydroxyetiocholane-17-one), *J. Clin. Endocrinol. Metab.*, 17, 451, 1957.

249. **Karpatkin, S., Strick, N., Karpatkin, M. B., and Siskind, G. W.,** Cumulative experience in the detection of antiplatelet antibody in 234 patients with idiopathic thrombocytopenic purpura, systemic lupus erythematosus and other clinical disorders, *Am. J. Med.*, 52, 776, 1972.

250. **Katler, E. and Weissmann, G.,** Steroids, aspirin and inflammation, *Inflammation*, 2, 295, 1977.

251. **Kattlove, H. E., Shapiro, S. S., and Spivack, M.,** Hereditary prothrombin deficiency, *N. Engl. J. Med.*, 282, 57, 1970.

252. **Katz, P., Zaytoun, A. M., and Lee, J. H., Jr.,** The effects of in vivo hydrocortisone on lymphocyte-mediated cytotoxicity, *Arthritis Rheum.*, 27, 72, 1984.

253. **Kay, A. B., Stechschulte, D. J., and Austen, K. F.,** An eosinophil leukocyte chemotactic factor of anaphylaxis, *J. Exp. Med.*, 133, 602, 1971.

254. **Kefalides, N. A. and Denduchis, B.,** Structural components of epithelial and endothelial basement membranes, *Biochemistry*, 8, 4613, 1969.

255. **Kellermeyer, R. W. and Graham, R. C., Jr.,** Kinins-possible physiologic and pathologic roles in man, *N. Engl. J. Med.*, 279, 754, 1968.

256. **Kelly, M. T., Martin, R. R., and White, A.,** Mediators of histamine release from human platelets, lymphocytes and granulocytes, *J. Clin. Invest.*, 50, 1044, 1971.

257. **Kennes, B., Brohée, D., and Neve, P.,** Lymphocyte activation. V. Acquisition of response to T cell growth factor and production of growth factors by mitogen-stimulated lymphocytes, *Mech. Ageing Dev.*, 23, 103, 1983.

258. **Kimball, H. R., Vogel, J. M., Perry, S., and Wolff, S. M.,** Quantitative aspects of pyrogenic and hematologic responses to etiocholanolone in man, *J. Lab. Clin. Med.*, 69, 415, 1967.

259. **Kinlough-Rathbone, R. L., Reimers, H. J., Mustard, J. F., and Packham, M. A.,** Sodium arachidonate can induce platelet shape change and aggregation which are independent of the release reaction, *Science*, 192, 1011, 1976.

260. **Klebanoff, S. J.,** Intraleukocytic microbicidal defects, *Annu. Rev. Med.*, 22, 39, 1971.

261. **Koster, F. T., McGregor, D. D., and Mackaness, G. B.,** The mediator of cellular immunity. II. Migration of immunologically committed lymphocytes into inflammatory exudates, *J. Exp. Med.*, 133, 400, 1971.

262. **Kübler, W. and Spieckermann, P. G.,** Regulation of glycolysis in the ischemic and the anoxic myocardium, *J. Mol. Cell. Cardiol.*, 1, 351, 1970.

263. **Kuehl, F. A., Egan, R. W., and Humes, J. L.,** Prostaglandin cyclooxygenase, *Prog. Lipid Res.*, 20, 97, 1981.

264. **Kueppers, F. and Bearn, A. G.,** A possible experimental approach to the association of hereditary alpha-1-antitrypsin deficiency and pulmonary emphysema, *Proc. Soc. Exp. Biol. Med.*, 121, 1207, 1966.

265. **Kurihara, A., Ohuchi, K., and Tsurufuji, S.,** Reduction by dexamethasone of chemotactic activity in inflammatory exudates, *Eur. J. Pharmacol.*, 101, 11, 1984.

266. **Lampert, P. W. and Schochet, S. S., Jr.,** Demyelination and remyelination in lead neuropathy. Electron microscopic studies, *J. Neuropathol. Exp. Neurol.*, 27, 527, 1968.

267. **Langer, B. G., Gonnella, P. A., and Nachmias, V. T.,** Alpha-actinin and vinculin in normal and thrombasthenic platelets, *Blood*, 63, 606, 1984.

268. **Lazarus, G. S., Daniels, J. R., Brown, R. S., Bladen, H. A., and Fullmer, H. M.,** Degradation of collagen by a human granulocyte collagenolytic system, *J. Clin. Invest.*, 47, 2622, 1968.

269. **Lee, P. W. R., Green, M. A., Long, W. B., III, and Gill, W.,** Zinc and wound healing, *Surg. Gynecol. Obstet.*, 143, 549, 1976.

270. **Lehrer, R. I. and Cline, J. J.,** Leukocyte myeloperoxidase deficiency and disseminated candidiasis: the role of myeloperoxidase in resistance to Candida infection, *J. Clin. Invest.*, 48, 1478, 1969.

271. **Lessin, L. S., Jensen, W. N., and Klug, P.,** Ultrastructure of the normal and hemoglobinophathic red blood cell membrane. Freeze-etching an stereoscan electron microscopic studies, *Arch. Intern. Med.*, 129, 306, 1972.

272. **Lew, P. D., Wollheim, C., Seger, R. A., and Pozzan, T.,** Cytosolic free calcium changes induced by chemotactic peptide in neutrophils from patients with chronic granulomatous disease, *Blood*, 63, 231, 1984.

273. **Lewis, D. A.,** Endogenous anti-inflammatory proteins, *Biochem. Pharmacol.*, 26, 693, 1977.

274. **Lichti, E. L., Turner, M., Hensel, J. H., and DeWeese, M. S.,** Wound fluid zinc levels during tissue repair; sequential determination by means of surgically implanted teflon cylinders, *Am. J. Surg.*, 121, 665, 1971.

275. **Liithje, J. and Ogilvie, A.,** Diadenosine triphosphate mediates human platelet aggregation by liberation of ADP, *Biochem. Biophys. Res. Commun.*, 118, 704, 1984.

276. **Lin, J. H., Shiigai, T., and Takeuchi, J.,** Relation of family history of hypertension to platelet aggregation, ratio of total cholesterol to HDL cholesterol and urinary kallikrein excretion, *Bull. Tokyo Med. Dent. Univ.*, 31, 13, 1984.

277. **Lindell, S. E. and Westling, H.,** Histamine metabolism in man, in *Handbook of Experimental Pharmakology*, Vol. 18, Part 1, Eichler, O. and Farrah, A., Eds., Springer-Verlag, Berlin, 1966, 734.

278. **Lippman, M.,** The growth-inhibitory action of heparin on the Ehrlich ascites tumor in mice, *Cancer Res.,* 176, 11, 1957.

279. **Littau, V. C., Alfrey, V. G., Frenster, J. H., and Mirsky, A. E.,** Active and inactive regions of nuclear chromatin as revealed by electron microscope autoradiography, *Proc. Natl. Sci. U.S.A.,* 52, 93, 1964.

280. **Lüderitz, O., Staub, A. M., and Westphal, O.,** Immunochemistry of O and R antigens of Salmonella and related Enterobacteriaceae, *Bacteriol. Rev.,* 30, 192, 1966.

281. **Lumio, J., Welin, M. G., Hirvonen, P., and Weber, T.,** Lymphocyte subpopulations and reactivity during and after infectious mononucleosis, *Med. Biol.,* 61, 208, 1983.

282. **Lüscher, E. F. and Käser-Glanzmann, R.,** Platelet heperain-neutralizing factor (platelet factor 4), *Thromb. Diath. Haemorrh.,* 33, 66, 1975.

283. **Luse, S. A., Burch, H. B., and Hunter, F. E.,** Ultrastructural and enzymatic changes in the liver of the riboflavin deficient rat, in *Electron Microscopy,* Proc. Int. 5th Congr. Electron Microscopy, Vol. 2, Breese, S. S., Jr., Ed., Academic Press, New York, 1962, 5.

284. **Maca, R. D.,** The effects of prostaglandins on the proliferation of cultured human T lymphocytes, *Immunopharmacology,* 6, 267, 1983.

285. **MacFarlane, R. G.,** An enzyme cascade in the blood clotting mechanism, and its function as a biochemical amplifier, *Nature (London),* 202, 498, 1964.

286. **MacFarlane, D. E. and Mills, D. C. B.,** The effect of ATP on platelets: evidence against the central role of released ADP in primary aggregation, *Blood,* 46, 309, 1975.

287. **MacFarlane, D. E., Walsh, P. N., Mills, D. C. B., Holmsen, H., and Day, H. J.,** The role of thrombin in ADP-induced platelet aggregation and release: a critical evaluation, *Br. J. Haematol.,* 30, 457, 1975.

288. **Magnusson, S., Sottrup-Jensen, L., Petersen, T. E., and Claeys, H.,** The primary structure of prothrombin, the role of vitamin K in blood coagulation and a thrombin catalyzed "negative feed-back" control mechanism for limiting the activation of prothrombin, in *Prothrombin and Related Coagulation Factors,* (Boerhaave Ser. Postgrad. Med. Educ. No. 10), Hemker, H. C. and Veltkamp, J. J., Eds., Leiden Univ. Press, Leiden, 1975, 25.

289. **Mahieu, P. and Winand, R. J.,** Chemical structure of tubular and glomerular basement membranes of human kidney. Isolation, purification, carbohydrate and amino acid composition., *Eur. J. Biochem.,* 12, 410, 1970.

290. **Majno, G., Gilmore, V., and Leventhal, M.,** On the mechanism of vascular leakage caused by histamine type mediators. A microscopic study in vivo, *Circ. Res.,* 21, 833, 1967.

291. **Mandell, G. L. and Hook, E. W.,** Leucocyte bactericidal activity in chronic granulomatous disease: correlation of bacterial hydrogen peroxide production and susceptibility to intracellular killing, *J. Bacteriol.,* 100, 531, 1969.

292. **Manning, J. P. and DiPasquale, G.,** The effect of vitamin A and hydrocortisone on the normal alkaline phosphatase response to skin wounding in rats, *J. Invest. Dermatol.,* 49, 225, 1967.

293. **Marder, V. J.,** The structure-function relationship of fibrinogen, *Thromb. Diath. Haemorrh. (Suppl.),* 54, 135, 1973.

294. **Margolis, J.,** The mode of action of Hageman factor in the release of plasma kinin, *J. Physiol.,* 151, 238, 1960.

295. **Markus, G., Evers, J. L., and Hobika, G. H.,** Activator activities of the transient forms of the human plasminogen-streptokinase complex during its proteolytic conversion to the stable activator complex, *J. Biol. Chem.,* 251, 6495, 1976.

296. **Markus, G., Kohga, S., Camiolo, S. M., Madeja, J. M., Ambrus, J. L., and Karakousis, C.,** Plasminogen activators in human malignant melanoma, *J. Natl. Cancer Inst.,* 72, 1213, 1984.

297. **Mari, G., Marassi, A., and DiCarlo, V.,** Protein C: a new plasma protein related to postoperative hypercoagulability, *Ital. J. Surg. Sci.,* 14, 9, 1984.

298. **Mastro, A. M.,** Phorbol ester tumor promoters and lymphocyte proliferation, *Cell Biol. Int. Rep.,* 7, 881, 1983.

299. **Mauël, J.,** Microbicidal mechanisms of macrophages, *Curr. Probl. Clin. Biochem.,* 13, 180, 1983.

300. **McConnell, D. J.,** Inhibitors of kallikrein in human plasma, *J. Clin. Invest.,* 51, 1611, 1972.

301. **McCullagh, K. A. and Balian, G.,** Collagen characterization and cell transformation in human atherosclerosis, *Nature (London),* 258, 73, 1975.

302. **McGregor, D. D. and Mackaness, G. B.,** Lymphocytes, in *The Inflammatory Process,* 2nd ed., Vol. 1, Zweifach, B. W., Grant, L., and McCluskey, R. T., Eds., Academic Press, New York, 1974, 1.

303. **McGregor, D. D., Koster, F. T., and Mackaness, G. B.,** The mediator of cellular immunity. I. The life-span and circulation dynamics of the immunologically committed lymphocyte, *J. Exp. Med.,* 133, 389, 1971.

304. **McManus, L. M., Hanahan, D. J., and Pinckard, R. N.,** Human platelet stimulation by acetyl glyceryl ether phosphorylcholine (AGEPC), *J. Clin. Invest.,* 67, 903, 1981.

305. **McNicol, G. P. and Douglas, S. A.,** The fibrinolytic enzyme system, in *Human Blood Coagulation, Haemostasis and Thrombosis,* 4th ed., Biggs, R., Ed., Blackwell Scientific, Oxford, 1972, 361.

306. **Melby, C. L.,** Inhibition of prostaglandin synthesis: a possible mechanism for stress-induced hypertension, *Med. Hypotheses,* 10, 445, 1983.
307. **Michaeli, D. and Swanson, A. L.,** Localization of the platelet-activation site in mammalian collagen type I, *Fed. Proc.,* 35, 332, 1976.
308. **Michell, R. H.,** Inositol phospholipids in membrane function, *Trends Biochem. Sci.,* 4, 128, 1979.
309. **Michiels, J. J. and Van Vliet, H. H.,** Hereditary antithrombin III deficiency and venous thrombosis, *Neth. J. Med.,* 27, 226, 1984.
310. **Miller, J. L., Boselli, B. D., and Kupinski, J. M.,** In vivo interaction of von Willebrand factor with platelets following cryoprecipitate transfusion in platelet-type von Willebrand's disease, *Blood,* 63, 226, 1984.
311. **Mims, C. A.,** *The Pathogenesis of Infectious Disease,* 2nd ed., Academic Press, London, 1982.
312. **Miwa, H.,** Identification and prognostic implication of tumor infiltrating lymphocytes — a review, *Acta Med. Okayama,* 38, 215, 1984.
313. **Morgenstern, E. and Reimers, H. J.,** The platelet contacts during aggregation, *Blut,* 48, 81, 1984.
314. **Moore, T. C.,** The modulation by prostaglandins of increases in lymphocyte traffic induced by bradykinin, *Immunology,* 51, 455, 1984.
315. **Moorehead, M. T., Westengard, J. C., and Bull, B. S.,** Platelet involvement in the activated coagulation time of heparinized blood, *Anesth. Analg.,* 63, 394, 1984.
316. **Mosesson, M. W. and Finlayson, J. S.,** The search for the structure of fibrinogen, in *Progress in Hemostasis and Thrombosis,* Vol. 3, Spaet, T. H., Ed., Grune & Stratton, New York, 1976, 61.
317. **Movat, H. Z.,** The plasma kallikrein-kinin system and its interrelationship with other components of the blood, in *Handbook of Experimental Pharmakology,* Suppl. Vol. 25, Erdös, E. G., Ed., Springer-Verlag, Berlin, 1979, 1.
318. **Movat, H. Z., Macmorine, D. R., and Takeuchi, Y.,** The role of PMN-leukocyte lysosomes in tissue injury, inflammation and hypersensitivity. 8. Mode of action and properties of vascular permeability factors released by PMN-leukocytes during ''in vitro'' phagocytosis, *Int. Arch. Allergy Appl. Immunol.,* 40, 218, 1971.
319. **Movat, H. Z., Uriuhara, T., Takeuchi, Y., Macmorine, D. R., and Burke, J. S.,** The role of PMN-leukocyte lysosomes in tissue injury, inflammation and hypersensitivity. VII. Liberation of vascular permeability factors from PMN-Leukocytes during ''in vitro'' phagocytosis, *Int. Arch. Allergy Appl. Immunol.,* 40, 197, 1971.
320. **Mowat, A. G. and Baum, J.,** Chemotaxis of polymorphonuclear leukocytes from patients with diabetes mellitus, *N. Engl. J. Med.,* 284, 621, 1971.
321. **Mowat, A. G. and Baum, J.,** Chemotaxis of polymorphonuclear leukocytes from patients with rheumatoid arthritis, *J. Clin. Invest.,* 50, 2541, 1971.
322. **Muller, H. K.,,** Mechanisms of clearing injured tissue, in *Tissue Repair and Regeneration,* (Handbook of Inflammation) Glynn, L. E., Ed., Elsevier/North-Holland, Amsterdam, V3, 145, 1981.
323. **Müller-Eberhard, H. J.,** Chemistry and reaction mechanisms of complement, *Adv. Immunol.,* 8, 1, 1968.
324. **Murphy, G., Reynolds, J. J., Bretz, U., and Baggiolini, M.,** Collagenase is a component of the specific granules of human neutrophil leucocytes, *Biochem. J.,* 162, 195, 1977.
325. **Mustard, J. F., Kinlough-Rathbone, R. L., and Packham, M. A.,** Recent status of research in the pathogenesis of thrombosis, *Thromb. Diath. Haemorrh. Suppl.,* 59, 157, 1974.
326. **Mustard, J. F. and Packham, M. A.,** Factors influencing platelet function: adhesion, release and aggregation, *Pharmacol. Rev.,* 22, 97, 1970.
327. **Mustard, J. F. and Packham, M. A.,** Platelets, thrombosis and drugs, *Drugs,* 9, 19, 1975.
328. **Mustard, J. F. and Packham, M. A.,** The reaction of the blood to injury, in *Inflammation, Immunity and Hypersensitivity,* 2nd ed., Movat, H. Z., Ed., Harper & Row, Hagerstown-New York, 1979, 557.
329. **Mustard, J. F., Packham, M. A., Perry, D. W., Guccione, M. A., and Kinlough-Rathbone, R. L.,** Enzyme activities on the platelet surface in relation to the action of adenosine diphosphate, in *Biochemistry and Pharmacology of Platelets,* Ciba Foundation Symposium 35 (NS), Elsevier, New York, 1975, 47.
330. **Mustard, J. F., Rowsell, H. C., Lotz, F., Hegardt, B., and Murphy, E. A.,** The effect of adenine nucleotides on thrombus formation, platelet count, and blood coagulation, *Exp. Mol. Pathol.,* 5, 43, 1966.
331. **Nagasawa, S. and Nakayasu, T.,** Enzymatic and chemical cleavages of human kininogens, in *Chemistry and Biology of the Kallikrein-Kinin System In Health and Disease,* Pisano, J. J. and Austen, K. F., Eds., Fogarty Internat. Center Proc. No. 27, U.S. Government Printing Office, Washington, D. C., 1976, 139.
332. **Najjar, V. A. and Nishioka, K.,** ''Tuftsin'': a natural phagocytosis-stimulating peptide, *Nature (London),* 228, 672, 1970.
333. **Nardiello, S., Russo, M., Pizzella, T., and Galanti, B.,** Different levels of lymphocyte adenosine deaminase in active and inactive forms of chronic liver disease, *J. Clin. Lab. Immunol.,* 11, 177, 1983.
334. **Nathaniel, D. and Mellors, A.,** Mitogen effects on lipid metabolism during lymphocyte activation, *Mol. Immunol.,* 20, 1259, 1983.

335. **Needleman, P., Moncada, S., Bunting, S., Vane, J. R., Hamberg, M., and Samuelsson, B.,** Identification of an enzyme in platelet microsomes which generates thromboxane A_2 from prostaglandin endoperoxides, *Nature (London),* 261, 558, 1976.

336. **Nelson, R. A.,** The complement system, in *The Inflammatory Process,* 2nd ed., Vol. 3, Zweifach, B. W., Grant, L., and McCluskey, R. T., Eds., Academic Press, New York, 1974, 37.

337. **Netter, H.,** Physicochemical principles of vital processes, in *Theoretical Biochemistry,* Ottaway, L. H. and Irvine, F. M., Eds., Oliver and Boyd, Edinburgh, 1969, 38.

338. **Nichols, B. A., Bainton, D. F., and Farquhar, M. G.,** Differentiation of monocytes. Origin, nature and fate of their azurophil granules, *J. Cell Biol.,* 50, 498, 1971.

339. **Nogueira, N.,** Intracellular mechanisms of killing, *Contemp. Top. Immunobiol.,* 12, 53, 1984.

340. **Norman, A., Sasaki, M. S., Ottoman, R. E., and Fingerhut, A. G.,** Lymphocyte lifetime in women, *Science,* 147, 745, 1965.

341. **North, R. J.,** The suppression of cell-mediated immunity to infection by an antibiotic drug. Further evidence that migrant macrophages express immunity, *J. Exp. Med.,* 132, 535, 1970.

342. **Northover, B. J. and Subramanian, G.,** Some inhibitors of histamine-induced and formaldehyde-induced inflammation in mice, *Br. J. Pharmacol. Chemother.,* 16, 163, 1961.

343. **Nossel, H. L.,** Radioimmunoassay of fibrinopeptides in relation to intravascular coagulation and thrombosis, *N. Engl. J. Med.,* 295, 428, 1976.

344. **Nowotny, A.,** Molecular aspects of endotoxic reactions, *Bacteriol. Rev.,* 33, 72, 1969.

345. **Nugteren, D. and Hazelhof, E.,** Isolation and properties of intermediates in prostaglandin biosynthesis, *Biochim. Biophys. Acta,* 325, 448, 1973.

346. **O'Flaherty, J. T., Wykle, R. L., Thomas, M. J., and McCall, C. E.,** Neutrophil degranulation responses to combinations of arachidonate metabolites and platelet-activating factor, *Res. Commun. Chem. Pathol. Pharmacol.,* 43, 3, 1984.

347. **Ohlsson, K.,** Interaction between endogenous proteases and plasma protease inhibitors in vitro and in vivo, in *Bayer Symposium V. Proteinase Inhibitors,* Fritz, H., Tschesche, H., Greene, L. J., and Truscheit, E., Eds., Springer-Verlag, Berlin, 1974, 96.

348. **Ohlsson, K. and Akesson, U.,** Alpha 1-antichymotrypsin interaction with cationic proteins from granulocytes, *Clin. Chim. Acta,* 73, 285, 1976.

349. **Ohlsson, K. and Olsson, I.,** Neutral proteases of human granulocytes. III. Interaction between human granulocyte elastase and plasma protease inhibitors., *Scand. J. Clin. Lab. Invest.,* 34, 349, 1974.

350. **Orange, R. P., Austen, W. G., and Austen, K. F.,** Immunological release of histamine and slow-reacting substance of anaphylaxis from human lung. I. Modulation by agents influencing cellular levels of cyclic $3',5'$-adenosine monophosphate, *J. Exp. Med.,* 134(Suppl. 136), 1971.

351. **Orange, R. P., Kaliner, M. A., Laraia, P. J., and Austen, K. F.,** Immunological release of histamine and slow reacting substance of anaphylaxis from human lung. II. Influence of cellular levels of cyclic AMP, *Fed. Proc.,* 30, 1725, 1971.

352. **Osterud, B. and Due, J., Jr.,** Blood coagulation in patients with benign and malignant tumours before and after surgery; special reference to thromboplastin generation in monocytes. *Scand. J. Haematol.,* 32, 258, 1984.

353. **Otsuki, Y., Kondo, T., Shio, H., Kameyama, M., and Koyama, T.,** Platelet aggregability in cerebral thrombosis — analysed for vessel stenosis, *Stroke,* 14, 368, 1983.

354. **Owren, P. A.,** Coagulation of blood; investigations on new clotting factor, *Acta Med. Scand.,* 128(Suppl. 194), 1, 1947.

355. **Packham, M. A., Ardlie, N. G., and Mustard, J. F.,** Effect of adenine compounds on platelet aggregation, *Am. J. Physiol.,* 217, 1009, 1969.

356. **Packham, M. A., Kinlough-Rathbone, R. L., Reimers, H. J., Scott, S., and Mustard, J. F.,** Mechanisms of platelet aggregation independent of adenosine diphosphate, in *Prostaglandins in Hematology,* International Symposium on Prostaglandins in Hematology, Philadelphia, 1976, (Monogr. Physiol. Soc. Philadelphia). Silver, M. J., Smith, J. B., and Kocsis, J. J., Eds., Spectrum Publications, New York, 3, 1977, 247.

357. **Paff, G. H., Sugiura, H. T., Bocher, C. A., and Roth, J. S.,** The probable mechanism of heparin inhibition of mitosis, *Anat. Rec.,* 114, 499, 1952.

358. **Pales, J. L., Lopez, A., and Vidal, S.,** Effect of polyamines on platelet aggregation, *Scand. J. Haematol.,* 32, 241, 1984.

359. **Panganamala, R. V., Gillespie, A. C., and Merola, A. J.,** Assay of prostacyclin synthesis in intact aorta by aqueous sampling, *Prostaglandins,* 21, 1, 1981.

360. **Panrucker, D. E. and Lorscheider, F. L.,** Synthesis of acute-phase alpha 2-macroglobulin during inflammation and pregnancy, *Ann. N.Y. Acad. Sci.,* 417, 117, 1984.

361. **Partridge, S. M., Thomas, J., and Elsden, D. F.,** Structure and metabolism of elastin and resilin; nature of the cross-linkages in elastin, in *Structure and Function of Connective and Skeletal Tissue,* Jackson, S. F., Ed., Butterworths, London, 1965, 88.

362. **Perillie, P. E. and Finch, S. C.,** The local exudative cellular response in leukaemia, *J. Clin. Invest.,* 39, 1353, 1960.
363. **Pickles, V. R.,** The prostaglandins, *Biol. Rev. Cambridge Philos. Soc.,* 42, 614, 1967.
364. **Pierce, J. V.,** Structural features of plasma kinins and kininogens, *Fed. Proc.,* 27, 52, 1968.
365. **Pierce, J. V. and Webster, M. E.,** The purification and some properties of two different kallidinogens from human plasma, in *Hypotensive Peptides,* Erdös, E. G., Back, N., and Sicuteri, F., Eds., Springer-Verlag, New York, 1966, 130.
366. **Pifer, D. D., Cagen, L. M., and Chesney, C. M.,** Stability of prostaglandin I_2 in human blood, *Prostaglandins,* 21, 165, 1981.
367. **Pinckard, R. N., Farr, R. S., and Hanahan, D. J.,** Physicochemical and functional identity of rabbit platelet-activating factor (PAF) released in vivo during IgE anaphylaxis with PAF released in vitro from IgE sensitized basophils, *J. Immunol.,* 123, 1847, 1979.
368. **Pinckard, R. N., McManus, L. M., Demopoulos, C. A., Halonen, M., Clark, P. O., Shaw, J. O., Kniker, W. T., and Hanahan, D. J.,** Molecular pathobiology of acetyl glyceryl ether phosphorylcholine (AGEPC): evidence for the structural and functional identify with platelet-activating factor, *J. Reticuloendothel. Soc.,* 28 (Suppl.), 95, 1980.
369. **Pinckard, R. N., McManus, L. M., Halonen, M., and Hanahan, D. J.,** Immunopharmacology of acetyl glyceryl ether phosphorylcholine (AGEPC), in *Immunopharmacology of the Lung,* (Long Biol. Health Dis. 19), Newball, H. H., Ed., Marcel Dekker, New York, 1983, 73.
370. **Pinckard, R. N., McManus, L. M., and Hanahan, D. J.,** Chemistry and biology of acetyl glyceryl ether phosphorylcholine (platelet-activating factor), *Adv. Inflammation Res.,* 4, 147, 1982.
371. **Pinckard, R. N., McManus, L. M., O'Rourke, R. A., Crawford, M. H., and Hanahan, D. J.,** Intravascular and cardiovascular effects of acetyl glyceryl ether phosphorylcholine (AGEPC) infusion in the baboon, *Clin. Res.,* 28, 358A, 1980.
372. **Pui, C. H., Jackson, C. W., Chesney, C., Lyles, S. A., Bowman, W. P., Abromowitch, M., and Simone, J. V.,** Sequential changes in platelet function and coagulation in leukemic children treated with L-asparaginase, prednisone and vincristine, *J. Clin. Oncol.,* 1, 380, 1983.
373. **Quie, P. G.,** Bactericidal function of human polymorphonuclear leukocytes, *Pediatrics,* 50, 264, 1972.
374. **Rabinovitch, M.,** Phagocytosis: the engulfment stage, *Semin. Hematol.,* 5, 134, 1968.
375. **Raine, C. S., Wisniewski, H., and Prineas, J.,** An ultrastructural study of experimental demyelination and remyelination. II. Chronic experimental allergic encephalomyelitis in the peripheral nervous system, *Lab. Invest.,* 21, 316, 1969.
376. **Ratnoff, O. D.,** The molecular basis of hereditary clotting disorders, in *Progress in Hemostasis and Thrombosis,* Vol. 1, Spaet, T. H., Ed., Grune & Stratton, New York, 1972, 39.
377. **Ratnoff, O. D. and Naff, G. B.,** The conversion of C'ls to C'l esterase by plasmin and trypsin, *J. Exp. Med.,* 125, 337, 1967.
378. **Reed, P. W.,** Glutathione and the hexose monophosphate shunt in phagocytizing and hydrogen peroxide-treated rat leukocytes, *J. Biol. Chem.,* 244, 2459, 1969.
379. **Rickli, E. E.,** The activation mechanism of human plasminogen, *Thromb. Diath. Haemorrh.,* 34, 386, 1975.
380. **Riley, J. F.,** Mast cells and cancer in the skin of mice, *Lancet,* 2, 1457, 1966.
381. **Riley, J. F. and West, G. B.,** The presence of histamine in tissue mast cells, *J. Physiol. (London),* 120, 528, 1953.
382. **Robbins, K. S. and Summaria, L.,** Plasminogen and plasmin, *Methods Enzymol.,* 45, 257, 1976.
383. **Robert, L., Kadar, A., and Robert, B.,** The macromolecules of the intercellular matrix of the arterial wall: collagen, elastin proteoglycans and glycoproteins, *Adv. Exp. Med. Biol.,* 43, 85, 1973.
384. **Roberts, J. C. and Courtice, F. C.,** Measurements of protein leakage in the acute and recovery stages of a thermal injury, *Aust. J. Exp. Biol. Med. Sci.,* 47, 421, 1969.
385. **Robinson, J. D.,** Regulating ion pumps to control cell volume, *J. Theor. Biol.,* 19, 90, 1968.
386. **Rocha, H. and Fekety, F. R., Jr.,** Acute inflammation in the renal cortex and medulla following thermal injury, *J. Exp. Med.,* 119, 131, 1964.
387. **Rocklin, R. E.,** Mediators of cellular immunity, their nature and assay, *J. Invest. Dermatol.,* 67, 372, 1976.
388. **Rome, L. H., Lands, W. E. M., Roth, G. J., and Majerus, P. W.,** Aspirin as a quantitative acetylating reagent for the fatty acid oxygenase that forms prostaglandins, *Prostaglandins,* 11, 23, 1976.
389. **Romert, L., Bernson, V., and Pettersson, B.,** Effects of air pollutants on the oxidative metabolism and phagocytic capacity of pulmonary alveolar macrophages, *J. Toxicol. Environ. Health,* 12, 417, 1983.
390. **Rossi, F. and Zatti, M.,** Mechanism of the respiratory stimulation in saponine-treated leukocytes; the KCN-insensitive oxidation of NADPH, *Biochim. Biophys. Acta,* 153, 296, 1968.
391. **Rowley, D. A. and Benditt, E. P.,** 5-Hydroxytryptamine and histamine as mediators of vascular injury produced by agents which damage mast cells in rats, *J. Exptl. Med.,* 103, 399, 1956.
392. **Ruddy, S. and Austen, K. F.,** The complement system in rheumatoid synovitis. I. An analysis of complement component activities in rheumatoid synovial fluids, *Arthritis Rheum.,* 13, 713, 1970.

393. **Rutherford, R. B., West, R. L., and Hardaway, R. M.,** III. Coagulation changes during experimental hemorrhagic shock; clotting activity, contribution of splanchnic circulation and acidosis as controlled by THAM, *Ann. Surg.,* 164, 203, 1966.

394. **Ryan, G. B. and Majno, G.,** Acute inflammation. A review, *Am. J. Pathol.,* 86, 185, 1977.

395. **Ryan, U.S. and Ryan, J. W.,** Endothelial cells and inflammation, *Clin. Lab. Med.,* 3, 577, 1983.

396. **Ryley, H. C. and Brogan, T. D.,** Quantitative immunoelectrophoretic analysis of the plasma proteins in the sol phase of sputum from patients with chronic bronchitis, *J. Clin. Pathol.,* 26, 852, 1973.

397. **Saito, H., Ratnoff, O. D., and Donaldson, V. H.,** Defective activation of clotting, fibrinolytic, and permeability-enhancing systems in human Fletcher trait plasma, *Circ. Res.,* 34, 641, 1974.

398. **Sandberg, A. L., Snyderman, R., Frank, M. M., and Osler, A. G.,** Production of chemotactic activity by guinea pig immunoglobulins following activation of the C3 complement shunt pathway, *J. Immunol.,* 108, 1227, 1972.

399. **Sarma, D. S. R., Reid, I. M., Verney, E., and Sidransky, H.,** Studies on the nature of attachment of ribosomes to membranes in liver. I. Influence of ethionine, sparsomycin, CCl_4, and puromycin on membrane-bound polyribosomal disaggregation and on detachment of membrane-bound ribosomes from membranes, *Lab. Invest.,* 27, 39, 1972.

400. **Savage, R. A.,** Pseudoleukocytosis due to EDTA-induced platelet clumping, *Am. J. Clin. Pathol.,* 81, 317, 1984.

401. **Sbarra, A. J., Shirley, W., and Bardawil, W. A.,** "Piggy-back" phagocytosis, *Nature (London),* 194, 255, 1962.

402. **Schachter, M.,** Kallikreins and kinins, *Physiol. Rev.,* 49, 509, 1969.

403. **Schayer, R. W.,** Induced synthesis of histamine, microcirculatory regulation and the mechanism of action of the adrenal glucocorticoid hormones, *Progr. Allergy,* 7, 187, 1963.

404. **Schayer, R. W.,** Enzymic formation of histamine from histidine, in *Handbook of Experimental Pharmakology,* Vol. 18, Part 1, Eichler, O. and Farah, A., Eds., Springer-Verlag, Berlin, 1966, 688.

405. **Schliwa, M., Pryzwansky, K. B., and Borisy, G. G.,** Tumor promoter-induced centrosome splitting in human polymorphonuclear leukocytes, *Eur. J. Cell Biol.,* 32, 75, 1983.

406. **Schreiber, A. D.,** Plasma inhibitors of the Hageman factor dependent pathways, *Semin. Thromb. Hemostas.,* 3, 43, 1976.

407. **Schreiber, A. D., Kaplan, A. P., and Austen, K. F.,** Plasma inhibitors of the components of the fibrinolytic pathway in man, *J. Clin. Invest.,* 52, 1394, 1973.

408. **Schreiber, A. D., Kaplan, A. P., and Austen, K. F.,** Inhibition by ClINH of Hageman factor fragment activation of coagulation, fibrinolysis, and kinin generation, *J. Clin. Invest.,* 52, 1402, 1973b.

409. **Scribner, D. J. and Fahrney, D.,** Neutrophil receptors for IgG and complement: their roles in the attachment and ingestion phases of phagocytosis, *J. Immunol,* 116, 892, 1976.

410. **Seger, R.,** Inborn errors of oxygen-dependent microbial killing by neutrophils, *Ergeb. Inn. Med. Kinderheilkd.,* 51, 29, 1984.

411. **Seljelid, R., Silverstein, S. C., and Cohn, Z. A.,** The effect of poly-L-lysine on the uptake of reovirus double-stranded RNA in macrophages in vitro, *J. Cell Biol.,* 57, 484, 1973.

412. **Senior, R. M. and Campbell, E. J.,** Neutral proteinases from human inflammatory cells. A critical review of their role in extracellular matrix degradation, *Clin. Lab. Med.,* 3, 645, 1983.

413. **Seon, B. K.,** Specific killing of human T-leukemic cells by immunotoxins prepared with ricin A chain and monoclonal anti-human T-cell leukemia antibodies, *Cancer Res.,* 44, 259, 1984.

414. **Setnikar, I., Salvaterra, M., and Temelcou, O.,** Antiphlogistic activity of iproniazid, *Br. J. Pharmacol. Chemotherap.,* 14, 484, 1959.

415. **Shapiro, S. S., Martinez, J., and Holburn, R.,** Congenital dysprothrombinemia: an inherited structural disorder of human prothrombin, *J. Clin. Invest.,* 48, 2251, 1969.

416. **Shaw, J. O., Pinckard, R. N., Ferrigni, K. S., McManus, L. M., and Hanahan, D. J.,** Activation of human neutrophils with 1-0-hexadecyl/octadecyl-2-acetyl-sn-glyceryl-3-phosphorylcholine (platelet-activating factor), *J. Immunol.,* 127, 1250, 1981.

417. **Shinitzky, M.,** *Physical Chemical Aspects of Cell Surface Events in Cellular Regulation,* DeLisi, C. and Blumenthal, R., Eds., Elsevier, Amsterdam, 1979, 173.

418. **Shulman, N. R.,** A mechanism of cell destruction in individuals sensitized to foreign antigens and its implications in autoimmunity. Combined clinical staff conference at the National Institute of Health, *Ann. Intern. Med.,* 60, 506, 1964.

419. **Shtacher, G., Maayan, R., and Feinstein, G.,** Proteinase inhibitors in human synovial fluid, *Biochim. Biophys. Acta,* 303, 138, 1973.

420. **Si, L., Whiteside, T. L., Schade, R. R., and Van Thiel, D.,** Lymphocyte subsets studied with monoclonal antibodies in liver tissues of patients with alcoholic liver disease, *Alcoholism,* 7, 431, 1983.

421. **Si, L. S., Whiteside, T. L., Schade, R. R., and Van Thiel, D. H.,** Studies of lymphocyte subpopulations in the liver tissue and blood of patients with chronic active hepatitis (CAH), *J. Clin. Immunol.,* 3, 408, 1983.

422. **Siegel, M. I., McConnell, R. T., Bonser, R. W., and Cuatrecasas, P.,** The production of 5-HETE and leukotriene B in rat neutrophils from carrageenan pleural exudates, *Prostaglandins,* 21, 123, 1981.
423. **Siggins, G. R.,** Prostaglandins and the microvascular system: physiological and histochemical correlations, in *Prostaglandins in Cellular Biology,* Ramwell, P. W. and Pharriss, B. B., Eds., Plenum Press, New York, 1972, 451.
424. **Simmons, R. L., Collins, J. A., Heisterkamp, C. A., III, Mills, D. E., Andren, R., and Phillips, L. L.,** Coagulation disorders in combat casualties, I. Acute changes after wounding. II. Effects of massive transfusion. III. Postresuscitative changes, *Ann. Surg.,* 169, 455, 1969.
425. **Sixma, J. J., Sakariassen, K. S., Beeser-Visser, N. H., Ottenhof-Rovers, M., and Bolhuis, P. A.,** Adhesion of platelets to human artery subendothelium: effect of factor VIII-von Willebrand factor of various multimeric composition, *Blood,* 63, 128, 1984.
426. **Sliwinski, A. J. and Zvaifler, N. J.,** The removal of aggregated and nonaggregated autologous gamma globulin from rheumatoid joints, *Arthritis Rheum.,* 12, 504, 1969.
427. **Smith, J. B., Ingerman, C., Kocsis, J. J., and Silver, M. J.,** Formation of prostaglandins during the aggregation of human blood platelets, *J. Clin. Invest.,* 52, 965, 1973.
428. **Smith, J. B., Ingerman, C. M., and Silver, M. J.,** Prostaglandins and precursors in platelet function, in *Biochemistry and Pharmacology of Platelets,* Ciba Foundation Symposium 35, (NS), Elsevier, New York, 1975, 207.
429. **Smith, M. R. and Wood, W. B., Jr.,** Heat labile opsonins to pneumococcus. I. Participation of complement, *J. Exp. Med.,* 130, 1209, 1969.
430. **Smolen, J. E., Korchak, H. M., Serhan, C. N., and Weissmann, G.,** The relative roles of extracellular and intracellular calcium in lysosomal enzyme release and superoxide anion generation by human polymorphonuclear leukocytes, *J. Cell Biol.,* 87, 303, 1980.
431. **Smuckler, E. A. and Benditt, E. P.,** Studies on carbon tetrachloride intoxication. III., A subcellular defect in protein synthesis, *Biochemistry,* 4, 671, 1965.
432. **Snyderman, R., Dickson, J., Meadows, L., and Pike, M.,** Deficient monocyte chemotactic responsiveness in humans with cancer, *Clin. Res.,* 22, 430A, 1974.
433. **Sohal, R. S., McCarthy, J. L., and Allison, V. F.,** The formation of ''giant'' mitochondria in the fibrillar flight muscles of the house fly, *Musca domestica,* L., *J. Ultrastruct. Res.,* 39, 484, 1972.
434. **Soltay, M. J., Movat, H. Z., and Özge-Anwar, A. H.,** The kinin system of human plasma. V. The probable derivation of pre-kallikrein activator from activated Hageman factor (XXIa), *Proc. Soc. Exp. Biol. Med.,* 138, 952, 1971.
435. **Sorkin, E., Stecher, V. J., and Borel, J. F.,** Chemotaxis of leukocytes and inflammation, *Ser. Haematol.,* 3, 131, 1970.
436. **Sparrow, E. M. and Wilhelm, D. L.,** Species differences in susceptibility to capillary permeability factors: histamine 5-hydroxytryptamine and compound 48/80, *J. Physiol. (London),* 137, 51, 1957.
437. **Spector, W. G. and Willoughby, D. A.,** Vasoactive amines in acute inflammation, *Ann. N.Y. Acad. Sci.,* 116, 839, 1964.
438. **Spector, W. G. and Willoughby, D. A.,** *The Pharmacology of Inflammation,* Grune & Stratton, New York, 1968.
439. **Steinman, R. M. and Cohn, Z. A.,** The interaction of particulate horseradish peroxidase (HRP) — anti HRP immune complexes with mouse peritoneal macrophages in vitro, *J. Cell Biol.,* 55, 616, 1972.
440. **Stone, C. A., Wenger, H. C., Ludden, C. T., Stavorski, J. M., and Ross, C. A.,** Antiserotonin-antihistaminic properties of cyproheptadine, *J. Pharmacol. Exp. Ther.,* 131, 73, 1961.
441. **Stossel, T. P.** Phagocytosis. Part I. *N. Engl. J. Med.,* 290, 717, 1974; Part II, 290, 774, 1974; and Part III, 290, 833, 1974.
442. **Stossel, T. P.,** How do phagocytes eat?, *Ann. Intern. Med.,* 89, 398, 1978.
443. **Sugioka, G., Porta, E. A., and Hartroft, W. S.,** Early changes in livers of rats fed choline-deficient diets at four levels of protein, *Am. J. Pathol.,* 57, 431, 1969.
444. **Summaria, L., Boreisha, I. G., Arzadon, L., and Robbins, K. C.,** Activation of human Glu-plasminogen to Glu-plasmin by urokinase in presence of plasmin inhibitors. Streptomyces leupeptin and human plasma alpha$_1$-antitrypsin and antithrombin III (plus heparin), *J. Biol. Chem.,* 252, 3945, 1977.
445. **Svensson, J., Hamberg, M., and Samuelsson, B.,** Prostaglandin endoperoxides. IX. Characterization of rabbit aorta contracting substance (RCS) from guinea pig lung and human platelets, *Acta Physiol. Scand.,* 94, 222, 1975.
446. **Takatsuji, T., Takekoshi, H., and Sasaki, M. S.,** Induction of chromosome aberrations by 4.9 MeV protons in human lymphocytes, *Int. J. Radiat. Biol.,* 44, 553, 1983.
447. **Tandler, B., Erlandson, R. A., Smith, A. L., and Wynder, E. L.,** Riboflavin and mouse hepatic cell structure and function. II. Division of mitochondria during recovery from simple deficiency, *J. Cell Biol.,* 41, 477, 1969.
448. **Tanner, A. R., Keyhani, A. H., and Wright, R.,** The influence of endotoxin in vitro on hepatic macrophage lysosomal enzyme release in different rat models of hepatic injury, *Liver,* 3, 151, 1983.

449. **Tegner, H.,** Quantitation of human granulocyte protease inhibitors in non-purulent bronchial lavage fluids, *Acta Oto-Laryngol.,* 85, 282, 1978.
450. **Temesi, A., Bertók, L., and Pellet, S.,** Stimulation of human peripheral lymphocytes with endotoxin and radiodetoxified endotoxin, *Acta Microbiol. Hung.,* 30, 13, 1983.
451. **Thomas, D. P.,** Effects of catecholamines on platelet aggregation caused by thrombin, *Nature (London),* 215, 298, 1967.
452. **Thompson, J. and Van Furth, R.,** The effect of glucocorticosteroids on the kinetics of mononuclear phagocytes, *J. Exp. Med.,* 131, 429, 1970.
453. **Till, G. O.,** Cellular and humoral defense systems and inflammatory mechanisms in thermal injury, *Clin. Lab. Med.,* 3, 801, 1983.
454. **Tomonaga, A., Hirota, M., and Snyderman, R.,** Effect of membrane fluidizers on the number and affinity of chemotactic factor receptors on human polymorphonuclear leukocytes, *Microbiol. Immunol.,* 27, 961, 1983.
455. **Torres, C. R. and Hart, G. W.,** Topography and polypeptide distribution of terminal N-acetylglucosamine residues on the surfaces of intact lymphocytes; evidence for O-linked GLCNAC, *J. Biol. Chem.,* 259, 3308, 1984.
456. **Travis, J., Bowen, J., and Baugh, R.,** Human α-1-antichymotrypsin: interaction with chymotrypsin-like proteinases, *Biochemistry,* 17, 5651, 1978.
457. **Trump, B. F., Croker, B. P., Jr., and Mergner, W. J.,** The role of energy metabolism, ion, and water shifts in the pathogenesis of cell injury, in *Cell Membranes: Biological and Pathological Aspects,* Richter, G. W., Ed., Williams & Wilkins, Baltimore, MD, 1971, 84.
458. **Trump, B. F., Duttera, S. M., Byrne, W. L., and Arstila, A. V.,** Membrane structure: lipid protein interactions in microsomal membranes, *Proc. Natl. Acad. Sci. U.S.A.,* 66, 433, 1970.
459. **Trump, B. F. and Ginn, F. L.,** The pathogenesis of subcellular reaction to lethal injury, in *Methods Achiev. Exp. Pathol.,* Vol. 4, Bajusz, E. and Jasmin, G., Eds., S. Karger, Basel, 1969, 1.
460. **Trump, B. F. and Mergner, W. J.,** Cell injury, in *The Inflammatory Process,* Vol. 1, 2nd ed., Zweifach, B. W., Grant, L., and Mc Cluskey, R. T., Eds., Academic Press, New York, 1974, 115.
461. **Tsiganos, C. P. and Muir, H.,** The natural heterogeneity of proteoglycan of porcine and human cartilage, in *Chemistry and Molecular Biology of the Intercellular Matrix,* Vol. 2, Balazs, E. A., Ed., Academic Press, New York, 1970, 859.
462. **Turner, S. R., Tainer, J. A., and Lynn, W. S.,** Biogenesis of chemotactic molecules by the arachidonate lipoxygenase system of platelets, *Nature (London),* 257, 680, 1975.
463. **Unanue, E. R., Beller, D. I., Lu, C. Y., and Allen, P. M.,** Antigen presentation: comments on its regulation and mechanism, *J. Immunol.,* 132, 1, 1984.
464. **Unkeless, J. C., Tobia, A., Ossowski, L., Quigley, J. P., Rifkin, D. B., and Reich, E.,** An enzymatic function associated with transformation of fibroblasts by oncogenic viruses. I. Chick embryo fibroblast cultures transformed by avian RNA tumor viruses, *J. Exp. Med.,* 137, 85, 1973.
465. **Uvnäs, B.,** Modes of action of antigen-antibody reaction and compound 48/80 in histamine release, in *Molecular and Biological Aspects of the Acute Allergic Reaction,* Johansson, S. G. D., Strandberg, K., and Uvnas, B., Eds., Plenum Press, New York, 1976, 217.
466. **Valdorf-Hansen, J. F. and Zucker, M. B.,** Effect of temperature and inhibitors on serotonin-14C release from human platelets, *Am. J. Physiol.,* 220, 105, 1971.
467. **Van Asbeck, B. S., Marx, J. J. M., Struyvenberg, A., van Kats, J. H., and Verhoef, J.,** Effect of iron (III) in the presence of various ligands on the phagocytic and metabolic activity of human polymorphonuclear leukocytes, *J. Immunol.,* 132, 851, 1984.
468. **Vane, J. R.,** Prostacyclin: a hormone with a therapeutic potential, *J. Endocrinol.,* 95, 3P, 1982.
469. **Van Furth, R.,** The formation of immunoglobulins by circulating lymphocytes, *Semin. Hematol.,* 6, 84, 1969.
470. **Van Furth, R. and Cohn, Z. A.,** The origin and kinetics of mononuclear phagocytes, *J. Exp. Med.,* 128, 415, 1968.
471. **Van Furth, R., van der Meer, J. W., Toivonen, H., and Rytömaa, T.,** Kinetic analysis of the growth of bone marrow mononuclear phagocytes in long-term cultures, *J. Reticuloendothel. Soc.,* 34, 227, 1983.
472. **Velky, T. S., Greenburg, A. G., Yang, J. C., and Forbes, S.,** Modulators of plasma fibronectin response during sepsis, *Surgery,* 96, 190, 1984.
473. **Vergani, C. G., Plancher, A. C., Zuin, M., Cattaneo, M., Tramaloni, C., Maccari, S., Roma, P., and Catapano, A. L.,** Bile lipid composition and hemostatic variables in a case of high density lipoprotein deficiency (Tangier disease), *Eur. J. Clin. Invest.,* 14, 49, 1984.
474. **Violand, B. N. and Castellino, F. J.,** Mechanism of the urokinase-catalyzed activation of human plasminogen, *J. Biol. Chem.,* 251, 3906, 1976.
475. **Vischer, T. L., Bretz, U., and Baggiolini, M.,** In vitro stimulation of lymphocytes by neutral proteinases from human polymorphonuclear leukocyte granules, *J. Exp. Med.,* 144, 863, 1976.
476. **Vogt, W., Lufft, E., and Schmidt, G.,** Studies on the relation between the fifth component of complement and anaphylatoxinogen, *Eur. J. Immunol.,* 1, 141, 1971.

477. **Volkman, A. and Gowans, J. L.,** The production of macrophages in the rat, *Br. J. Exp. Pathol.*, 46, 50, 1965.

478. **Volpi, M., Naccache, P. H., and Sha'afi, R. I.,** Arachidonate metabolite(s) increase the permeability of the plasma membrane of the neutrophils to calcium, *Biochem. Biophys. Res. Commun.*, 92, 1231, 1980.

479. **Von Eyben, F. E. and Arends, J.,** Suppression of the mitogen response of normal lymphocytes by serum from patients with testicular germ cell tumors, *Am. J. Reprod. Immunol.*, 4, 5, 1983.

480. **Vroman, L.,** Possible relationships and interactions among events in clotting, platelet adhesion, immune surface reactions and granulocyte adhesion, *J. Theor. Biol.*, 105, 541, 1983.

481. **Vroon, D. H., Schultz, D. R., and Zarco, R. M.,** Separation of nine components and two inactivators of components of complement in human serum, *Immunochemistry*, 7, 43, 1970.

482. **Walker, I. D., Davidson, J. F., Young, P., and Conkie, J. A.,** Plasma fibrinolytic activity following oral anabolic steroid therapy, *Thromb. Diath. Haemorrh.*, 34, 236, 1975.

483. **Walsh, P. N. and Biggs, R.,** The role of platelets in intrinsic factor-Xa formation, *Br. J. Haematol.*, 22, 743, 1972.

484. **Ward, P. A.,** The chemosuppression of chemotaxis, *J. Exp. Med.*, 124, 209, 1966.

485. **Ward, P. A.,** A plasmin-split fragment of C 3 as a new chemotactic factor, *J. Exp. Med.*, 126, 189, 1967.

486. **Ward, P. A.,** Complement-derived leukotactic factors in pathological fluids, *J. Exp. Med.*, 134(Suppl.), 109s, 1971.

487. **Ward, P. A., Chapitis, J., Conroy, M. C., and Lepow, I. H.,** Generation by bacterial proteinases of leukotactic factors from human serum, and human C3 and C5, *J. Immunol.*, 110, 1003, 1973.

488. **Ward, P. A. and Hill, J. H.,** C5 Chemotactic fragments produced by an enzyme in lysosomal granules of neutrophils, *J. Immunol.*, 104, 535, 1970.

489. **Ward, P. A. and Schlegel, R. J.,** Impaired leukotactic responsiveness in a child with recurrent infections, *Lancet*, 2, 344, 1969.

490. **Ward, P. A. and Kunkel, S. L.,** Bacterial virulence and the inflammatory system, *Rev. Infect. Dis.*, (Suppl.)45, 793, 1983.

491. **Ward, P. A. and Zvaifler, N. J.,** Complement-derived leukotactic factors in inflammatory synovial fluids of humans, *J. Clin. Invest.*, 50, 606, 1971.

492. **Warren, L., Fuhrer, J. P., and Buck, C. A.,** Surface glycoproteins of cells before and after transformation by oncogenic viruses, *Fed. Proc.*, 32, 80, 1973.

493. **Wasserman, S. I., Goetzl, E. J., and Austen, K. F.,** Inactivation of slow reacting substance of anaphylaxis by human eosinophil arylsulfatase, *J. Immunol.*, 114, 645, 1975.

494. **Webster, M. E.,** The physiological and pathological role of the kallikrein-kallidin system, in *Hypotensive Peptides*, Erdös, E. G., Back, N., and Sicuteri, F., Eds., Springer-Verlag, New York, 1966, 263.

495. **Webster, M. E., Maling, H. M., Zweig, M. H., Williams, M. A., and Anderson, W., Jr.,** Evidence for kinins, histamine and complement as mediators of the inflammatory response, in *Protides of the Biological Fluids*, Peeters, H., Ed., Proc. 20th Colloquium, 1973, 371.

496. **Webster, M. E. and Ratnoff, O. D.,** Role of Hageman factor in the activation of vasodilator activity in human plasma, *Nature (London)*, 192, 180, 1961.

497. **Weigensberg, M., Morecki, S., Weiss, L., Fuks Z., and Slavin, S.,** Suppression of cell-mediated immune responses after total lymphoid irradiation (TLI). I. Characterization of suppressor cells of the mixed lymphocyte reaction, *J. Immunol.*, 132, 971, 1984.

498. **Weir, D. M., Blackwell, C. C., Stewart, J., Glass, E. J., and Oliver, A. M.,** Macrophage "receptors" for bacterial cell-wall sugars and immune response genes: possible determinants of susceptibility to infection, *Br. J. Rheumatol.*, 22(Suppl. 2), 161, 1983.

499. **Weiss, A. S., Gallin, J. I., and Kaplan, A. P.,** Fletcher factor deficiency: a diminished rate of Hageman factor activation caused by absence of prekallikrein with abnormalities of coagulation, fibrinolysis, chemotactic activity and kinin generation, *J. Clin. Invest.*, 53, 622, 1974.

500. **Weiss, S. J. and Putney, J. W., Jr.,** The relationship of phosphatidylinositol turnover to receptors and calcium-ion channels in rat parotid acinar cells, *Biochem. J.*, 194, 463, 1981.

501. **Weissmann, G., Smolen, J. E., and Korchak, H. M.,** Release of inflammatory mediators from stimulated neutrophils, *N. Engl. J. Med.*, 303, 27, 1980.

502. **Weissmann, G., Zurier, R. B., Spieler, P. J., and Goldstein, I. M.,** Mechanisms of lysosomal enzyme release from leukocytes exposed to immune complexes and other particles, *J. Exp. Med.*, 134, 149, 1971.

503. **Weissmann, G., Zurier, R. B., and Hoffstein, S.,** Leukocytic proteases and the immunologic release of lysosomal enzymes, *Am. J. Pathol.*, 68, 539, 1972.

504. **Weksler, B. B.,** Platelets and the inflammatory response, *Clin. Lab. Med.*, 3, 667, 1983.

505. **Werb, Z., Burleigh, M. C., Barrett, A. J., and Starkey, P. M.,** The interaction of alpha 2-macroglobulin with proteinases. Binding and inhibition of mammalian collagenases and other metal proteinases, *Biochem. J.*, 139, 359, 1974.

506. **Werb, Z. and Gordon, S.,** Elastase secretion by stimulated macrophages; characterization and regulation, *J. Exp. Med.*, 142, 361, 1975.

507. **West, G. B.**, Adrenaline and noradrenaline, *J. Pharm. Pharmacol.*, 7, 81, 1955.

508. **Westmoreland, N.**, Connective tissue alterations in zinc deficiency, *Fed. Proc.*, 30, 1001, 1971.

509. **Weston, W. L.**, Disorders of phagocyte function, *Arch. Dermatol.*, 112, 1589, 1976.

510. **White, R. R., Norby, D., Janoff, A., and Dearing, R.**, Partial purification and characterization of mouse peritoneal exudative macrophage elastase, *Biochim. Biophys. Acta*, 612, 233, 1980.

511. **Whitehouse, M. W. and Skidmore, I. F.**, Concerning the regulation of some diverse biochemical reactions, underlying the inflammatory response, by salicylic acid, phenylbutazone and other acidic antirheumatic drugs, *J. Pharm. Pharmacol.*, 17, 668, 1965.

512. **Wilhelm, D. L.**, Kinins in human disease, *Annu. Rev. Med.*, 22, 63, 1971.

513. **Williamson, D. H., Krebs, H. A., Stubbs, O., Page, M. A., Morris, H. P., and Weber, G.**, Metabolism of renal tumors in situ and during ischemia, *Cancer Res.*, 3p, 204y, 1970.

514. **Willis, A. L.**, Isolation of a chemical trigger for thrombosis, *Prostaglandins*, 5, 1, 1974.

515. **Willoughby, D. A., Coote, E., and Turk, J. L.**, Complement in acute inflammation, *J. Pathol.*, 97, 295, 1969.

516. **Wohlrab, H. and Jacobs, E. E.**, Copper-deficient mitochondria. Electron transport and oxidative phosphorylation, *Biochem. Biophys. Res. Commun.*, 28, 998, 1967.

517. **Wolf, G. and Johnson, B. C.**, Vitamin A and mucopolysaccharide biosynthesis, *Vitam. Horm. (N.Y.)*, 18, 439, 1960.

518. **Wolff, S. M., Dale, D. C., Clark, R. A., Root, R. K., and Kimball, H. R.**, The Chediak-Higashi syndrome: studies of host defense, *Ann. Intern. Med.*, 76, 293, 1972.

519. **Wolff, S. M., Kimball, H. R., Perry, S., Root, R., and Kappas, A.**, The biological properties of etiocholanolone, *Ann. Intern. Med.*, 67, 1268, 1967.

520. **Work, E.**, Production, chemistry and properties of bacterial pyrogens and endotoxins, in *Pyrogens and Fevers*, Ciba Found. Symp. Wolstenholm, G. E. W. and Birch, J., Eds., Churchill Livingstone, Edinburgh, 1971, 23.

521. **Wu, B. C., Valle, R. T., White, L. A. G., Sohal, R. S., Arcos, J. C., Argus, M. F., and Burch, G. E.**, Mitochondrial ultrastructure and energy transduction in rat heart during progressive thiamine deficiency, *Virchows Arch. B.*, 9, 97, 1971.

522. **Zeiger, R. S. and Colten, H. R.**, Histamine release from human eosinophils, *J. Immunol.*, 118, 540, 1977.

523. **Zeiger, R. S., Yurdin, D. L., and Colten, H. R.**, Histamine metabolism. II. Cellular and subcellular localization of the catabolic enzymes histaminase and histamine methyl transferase, in human leukocytes, *J. Allergy Clin. Immunol.*, 58, 172, 1976.

524. **Zigmond, S. H.**, Chemotaxis by polymorphonuclear leukocytes, *J. Cell Biol.*, 77, 269, 1978.

525. **Zigmond, S. H. and Hirsch, J. G.**, Leucocyte locomotion and chemotaxis. New method for evaluation, and demonstration of a cell-derived chemotactic factor, *J. Exp. Med.*, 137, 387, 1973.

526. **Zimmerman, A. N. E., Daems, W., Hülsmann, W. C., Snyder, J., Wisse, E., and Durrer, D.**, Morphological changes of heart muscle caused by successive perfusion with calcium-free and calcium-containing solutions (calcium paradox), *Cardiovasc. Res.*, 1, 201, 1967.

527. **Zoschke, D. C. and Bach, F. H.**, Specificity of antigen recognition by human lymphocytes in vitro, *Science*, 179, 1404, 1970.

528. **Zoumbos, N., Gascon, P., and Young, N.**, The function of lymphocytes in normal and suppressed hematopoiesis, *Blut*, 48, 1, 1984.

529. **Zucker, M. B., Pert, J. H., and Hilgartner, M. W.**, Platelet function in a patient with thrombasthenia, *Blood*, 28, 524, 1966.

530. **Zucker, M. B. and Peterson, J.**, Effect of acetylsalicylic acid, other nonsteroidal anti-inflammatory agents, and dipyridamole on human blood platelets, *J. Lab. Clin. Med.*, 76, 66, 1970.

531. **Zvaifler, N. J.**, Breakdown products of C'3 in human synovial fluids, *J. Clin. Invest.*, 48, 1532, 1969.

532. **Yecies, L. D. and Kaplan, A. P.**, The activation of plasminogen by the Hageman factor dependent plasminogen activator, *Fed. Proc.*, 35, 731, 1976.

533. **Yee, J. B. and Hutson, J. C.**, Testicular macrophages; isolation characterization and hormonal responsiveness, *Biol. Reprod.*, 29, 1319, 1983.

534. **Blackwell, G. J., Radomski, M., and Moncada, S.**, Inhibition of human platelet aggregation by vitamin K, *Thromb. Res.*, 37, 103, 1985.

535. **Dodds, R. A., Catterall, A., Bitensky, L., and Chayen, J.**, Effect on fracture healing of an antagonist of the vitamin K cycle, *Calcif. Tissue. Res.*, 36, 233, 1984.

FURTHER READINGS

Back, N. and Sicuteri, F., Eds., Vasopeptides, *Chemistry, Pharmacology and Pathophysiology,* Plenum Press, New York, 1972.

De Reuck, A. V. S., and Knight, J., Eds., *Cellular Injury,* Little, Brown, Boston, 1964.

Erdös, E. G., Ed., *Handbook of Experimental Pathology. Vol. 25 Supplement: Bradykinin, Kallidin, and Kallikreins,* Springer-Verlag, Berlin, 1979.

Hook, J. B., Ed., *Toxicology of the Kidney. Target Organ Toxicology Series,* Raven Press, New York, 1981.

Houck, J. C., *Chemical Messengers and the Inflammatory Process,* North Holland Biomedical Press, New York, 1979.

Houck, J. C., Ed., *Handbook of Inflammation,* Vols. 1 to 5, Elsevier/North Holland, Amsterdam, 1979 to 1982.

Kovach, A. G. B., Stoner, H. B., and Spitzer, J. J., Eds., *Neurohumoral and Metabolic Aspects of Injury,* Plenum Press, New York, 1973.

Lewis, G. P., Ed., *The Role of Prostaglandins in Inflammation,* Hans Huber, Berlin, 1976.

Mims, C. A., *The Pathogenesis of Infectious Disease,* 2nd ed., Academic Press, New York, 1982.

Ramwell, P. W. and Pharriss, B. B., Eds., *Prostaglandins in Cellular Biology,* Plenum Press, New York, 1972.

Silvestrini, B. and Spector, W. G., Eds., *Inflammation: Aetiopathogenetic, Clinical and Therapeutic Problems,* Excerpta Medica, Amsterdam, 1968.

Spector, W. G. and Willoughby, D. A., *The Pharmacology of Inflammation,* The English University Press, London, 1968.

Weissmann, G., Ed., *Mediators of Inflammation,* Plenum Press, New York, 1974.

Weissmann, G., Samuelsson, B., and Paoletti, R., *Advances in Inflammation Research,* Vols. 1 to 4, Raven Press, New York, 1979 to 1983.

Willoughby, D. A. and Giroud, J. P., Eds., *Inflammation: Mechanisms and Treatment,* MTP Press, Lancaster, England, 1980.

Willoughby, D. A., Giroud, J. P., and Vello, G. P., *Perspectives in Inflammation, Future Trends and Developments,* MTP Press, Lancaster, England, 1977.

Zweifach, B. W., Grant, L., and McCluskey, R. T., *The Inflammatory Process,* Vols. 1 to 3, Academic Press, London, 1974 to 1976.

Chapter 2

ATHEROSCLEROSIS

I. INTRODUCTION

The success in the prevention and treatment of acute conditions due to infectious diseases, hormone insufficiency disorders, and hypertension has increased the average life expectancy in developed countries during the last 50 years. This represents 20 years or more at birth, but less than 2 years at the age of 65. The reason for the hardly increased lifespan at old age is mainly due to atherosclerosis.[371] Our habits have been altered remarkably during these decades, but many new habits became associated with the high incidence of premature death from heart attack. Substantial progress has been make in studying the pathogenesis of atherosclerosis, but many aspects of the evolution of atherosclerosis still remain obscure.[69,114,141,278,395,668,698] The difficulties in the study of the disease are derived from several factors: (1) due to the accumulation of many earlier insults to the body, mainly chronic conditions manifest after 60 to 65 years of age; (2) these conditions progress slowly and they are silent, without symptoms, for a long time; (3) chronic disease conditions are extremely difficult to reproduce experimentally in animals, more than any other disease; and (4) the initiation of the disease usually cannot be determined and usually is not connected with the action of pathogenic organisms, chemicals, or other injurious agents.

Based on investigations from animal models, modern pathology and epidemiology studies and biochemical techniques revealed major factors contributing to the development of the early lesions of atherosclerosis.[610,632] These early stages are even found in childhood, but apparently it takes at least a decade or more until more severe stages become manifest. The clinical symptoms of the disease are precipitated by the influence of the risk factors. These risk factors appear to be intimately related to the inception of the atherosclerotic lesions, but their causal association is still uncertain.

II. PATHOGENESIS

There are three major theories for the development and interrelationship of the various phases of the atherosclerotic process: (1) *inflammatory theory:* the atherosclerotic changes start with an injury to the endothelium of the vessel wall, associated with local metabolic changes and deposition of lipids. These lipids act as foreign bodies and initiate the inflammatory response,[438,470] (2) *thrombogenic theory:* the primary phase commences with thrombosis, and the microthrombus changes into a plaque which is subsequently followed by lipid deposition;[217,439] and (3) *perfusion theory:* according to this theory, blood elements cause an injury on the endothelium or subendothelial connective tissue.[449,450] Consequently, a local inflammation focus develops on the intima, manifest by the action of the inflammatory exudate originating from the blood. This local inflammation is followed by the degenerative process and the production of atheroma.

Recently, it has been reported that the pathologic features of the human atherosclerotic plaque show monoclonal origin.[54-56,493,575] Thus, the initiation of the cellular alteration may be associated with an inflammatory response. Increased formation of collagen in the blood vessels due to hypertension provides some support of this theory,[204,537,538] although polyclonal origin and proliferative heterogeneity of atherosclerotic lesions have also been found experimentally.[189,368]

The relationship of the various pathogenic factors to the different atherosclerotic lesions and clinical presentations of the disease is summarized in Figure 1. The early lesions are

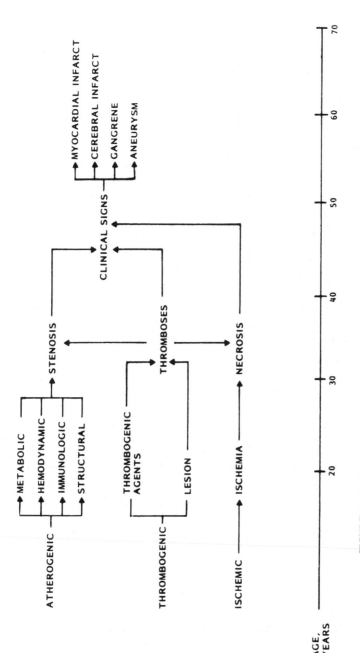

FIGURE 1.   Pathogenic factors and interactions leading to atherosclerosis and its complications.

observed in three forms: fatty dots and streaks, microthrombi, and gelatinous elevations.[346] These changes may be initiated by any minor injury to the endothelium or the intima as a result of mechanical, physical, chemical, or metabolic trauma. In response to these diverse injuries, the starting phase of atherosclerosis may develop according to different patterns. Mechanical trauma is associated with hypertension or with the collision of various blood cells with the vessel wall and subsequent release of permeability factors.[326] Chemical or metabolic changes are connected with hypoxia, due to disturbed metabolism, or toxemia representing the production of abnormal components or increased amounts of normal components. Local injury causes increased permeability of the arterial wall at the site and consequently, insudation of blood components into the intima with production microthrombi. The metabolism of lipids in the smooth muscle cell at a particular site is altered resulting in the appearance of fatty streaks. Stagnation and local hypoxia also brings about lipid accumulation. Under these circumstances, inhibition of protein metabolism causes gelatinous elevation.[76,85,232,539,540]

A. FATTY STREAKS

Fatty dots and streaks are found throughout the large vessels of the systemic arterial tree from early childhood to advanced age. Fatty streaking is prevalent even in infants between the ages of 1 and 12 months.[424] In these cases, the lesions are found near the aortic valve ring and, as the child grows, the aortic arch and the posterior wall of the thoracic aortic become more severely affected.[310] Fatty dots appear initially as minute round or oval yellow patches and elevated above the surface of the intima.[191,495] In these lesions, the number of fat-laden cells is usually small and may be concentrated immediately under the endothelium or more deeply within the intima. When these tiny lesions are raised, the intercellular ground substance is increased, probably due to edema.[276]

It has been suggested recently that blood monocytes can remove lipids from intimal lesions.[214] These cells penetrate into the intima of lesion-prone areas and accumulate during the development of the lesion. At the fatty streak stage, monocytes are the predominant cell elements. This invasion of the intima by monocytes may represent a clearance process. Once within the intima, the invading cells phagocytoze lipids and become the foam cells seen in experimental fatty streaking. This phenomenon is brought about by diets high in both fat and cholesterol.[432,663,664] When fibromuscular lesions develop in the arterial wall, modified smooth-muscle cells form the majority of foam cells.[601] The development of fatty streaks, other lesions, and further complications is depicted in Figure 2.

B. GELATINOUS ELEVATIONS

Gelatinous lesions are oval or elongated and translucent, found in all segments of the aorta. Biochemical analysis revealed that all constituents are probably derived from plasma. Portions of the intima with gelatinous lesions contain twice as much albumin and about four times as much fibrinogen and lipoprotein as in the normal intima. Thus, these lesions represent a form of focal intimal edema. In small lesions, the edema is limited, and in larger ones, the insudative process may involve the entire thickness of the intima. This is accompanied by separation of connective tissue elements, swelling of ground substance, and decrease of mucopolysaccharides.[595]

These lesions enter the advanced phase when the episodes of local injury occur repeatedly. Repeated hemorrhages, mural thrombosis or insudation, or the combination of these three conditions lead to the formation of atherosclerotic plaques.[661] There are white fibrous plaques without atheroma or more frequently, plaques with atheroma. The local effect is related to increased focal permeability and consequent insudation of blood into the intima as well as the production of microthrombi. The progress of plaque formation is dependent on the elevated lipid content of the insudation. The growth of the lesion is also accelerated by the

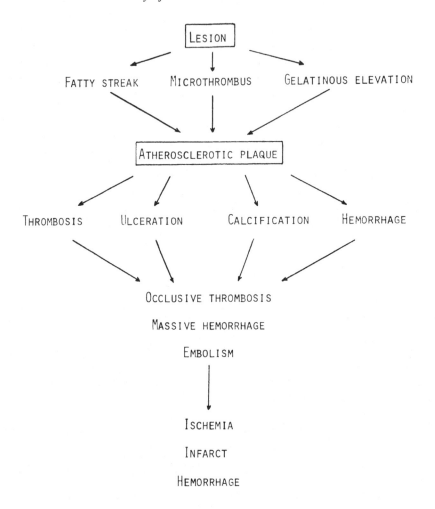

FIGURE 2.   Development of atherosclerotic lesions and clinical manifestations.

increased amount of lipid which promotes platelet sedimentation of thrombosis. Further local or general factors contribute to the conversion of early lesions to the advanced stage.[202] These factors include local degeneration of the connective tissue promoting mural thrombosis and calcification. Due to softening the capillary framework the atheroma becomes enlarged, massive hemorrhage or ulceration occurs, and subsequently, the emboli are discharged into the blood stream. Among general factors, hypertension plays an important role.

C. FIBROLIPID PLAQUES

Fibrolipid plaques or raised lesions are substantially elevated above the surface of the surrounding noninvolved intima. Often the underlying media shows no thinning, and the raised lesion may even exceed the total thickness of the intima and media.[3,214,476] The plaques consist of lipid-rich pools covered with connective tissue. In some of these lesions the connective tissue is the predominant element. In other lesions, lipids and other plasma-derived constituents and cell debris are accumulated and separated from the vessel lumen only by a thin sheet of fibrous or fibromuscular tissue. Complicating features such as ulceration and consequent thrombosis, hemorrhage, and calcification often superimpose the basic fibroid plaque pattern.

Raised lesions are further associated with changes in adventitial tissues such as increased fibrous tissue, increased vascularity, and high prevalence of cellular aggregates, mainly

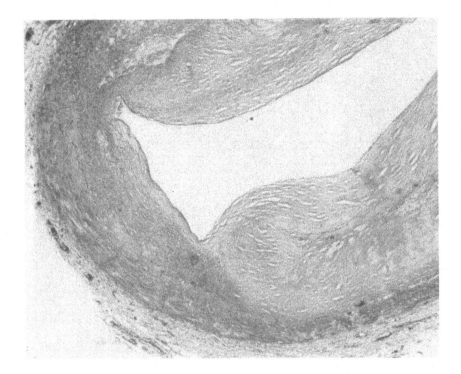

PLATE 1. Coronary sclerosis. Atherosclerotic intimal changes narrow the lumen of the vessel.

lymphocytes.[431] Atherosclerotic plaques often become calcified. Many forms of arterial calcification can occur in humans although three types appear with greater frequency and include focal calcification in severe atherosclerotic plaques, deposition of dense and extensive amounts of calcium in the media representing Mönckeberg's sclerosis, and diffuse deposition of calcium salts within the elastic fibres of the aorta.

Generally, as humans grow older the concentration of calcium increases in aortic elastic tissue. Between the ages of 20 and 50, the calcium content of the media is increased by about fivefold. This age-dependent calcification is diffuse and shows no relationship to the presence and severity of the atherosclerotic condition. In diabetic patients, the calcium content of the aorta is significantly higher than in age-matched nondiabetics,[38,639] possibly reflecting the vascular complications in diabetics. Moreover, calcified plaques are most numerous in the region of the coronary osteum and usually are accompanied by clinically significant disease. Calcified lesions are also greater both in the aorta and coronary artery branches in patients with history of ischemic heart disease. A case of calcified plaque is shown in Plate 1.

D. THROMBUS

In severely affected coronary arteries, the atherosclerotic plaques are associated with mural or occlusive thrombi.[472] In some cases the stenosis of the lumen is centrally situated, but more commonly found is the formation of eccentric thickening of the affected arterial segment.[688] This is seen in a case of coronary sclerosis (Plate 2). The complex plaque consists of alternating layers of connective tissue, lipid-rich atheromatous zones with cholesterol crystals, fibrin, and residual hemorrhage. This aspect of the plaque suggests that the growth of the lesion occurs in an alternating fashion connected with successive episodes of thrombosis. Fresh thrombi contain high amounts of fibrin and sometimes completely occlude a segmental length of artery, although sometimes the thrombi consist of aggregated platelets and virtually no fibrin.[348]

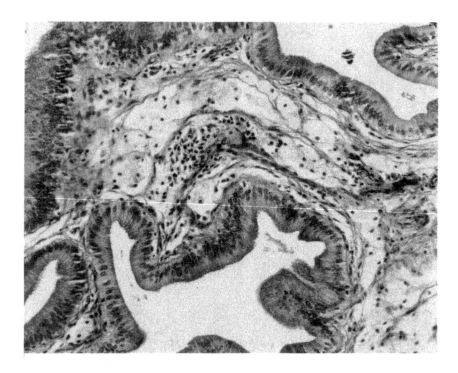

PLATE 2.   Cholesterolosis of gall bladder. Large vacuolated macrophages with centrally placed nuclei are deposited in the mucosa of the gall bladder.

The evolution of the primary lesions into more advanced or complicated phases is also connected with local and systemic factors. Local factors include decreased oxygen supply and low nutrients with reduction of enzymatic activity related to advancing age and increasing intimal thickness.[2,3] The resulting relative hypoxia, however, stimulates the ingrowth of capillaries and the thickened intima may become richly vascularized. If the intimal thickening is very rapid, the development of new vascular channels may not be fast enough to maintain adequate oxygenation and nutrition in the potentially hypoxic region of the arterial wall. In this event, ischemic necrosis of cellular elements can occur. Local and systemic factors facilitate the progress of the atherosclerotic process into thrombosis, ulcerations, calcifications, or hemorrhage. Hypertension is one of the major general factors in the precipitation of clinical manifestations.[137,151,323,571] In addition, hyperlipidemia, physical exertion, or cigarette smoking are contributing factors to the development of this phase. Terminal manifestations include occlusive thrombosis, massive hemorrhage within the atheroma, and distant embolism from ulcerated atheroma. Occlusive thrombosis is the most frequent cause of the downhill progress in atherosclerosis, presenting ischemia, infarct, and hemorrhage as cardinal clinical manifestations.[404]

III. CONTRIBUTING FACTORS

Atherosclerosis, a complex disease, represents a continuum of interrelated processes leading to irreparable vessel damage. The major contributing factors are hemodynamic forces, arterial tissue changes, and metabolic changes from blood components.[200] The development of this disease is presented as a complex phenomenon which reflects interactions between the blood components and structural and functional properties of the arterial wall, potentiated by processes which in turn regulate the circulation of blood elements.

A. HEMODYNAMIC FACTORS

Since atherosclerotic plaques are basically focal lesions of a systemic disease, the localization of the lesion and its severity seems to depend on the interaction between variations in the fluid mechanics of blood and changes in arterial tissue reactivity.[119,202,338,408,422,460,552] Blood flow and pressure exercise mechanical stresses on the arterial wall and influence its structure and composition.[112,209] Changes in blood pressure are important factors in the development of aneurysms.[513,530,603] The infiltration of the blood into the vessel wall depends on pressure and composition of the fluid phase on one hand,[202] and on the thickness, stability, and flexibility of the vascular media layer on the other.[525,526] Increased elocity causes changes constantly in the circulating blood cells which impinge on the endothelial surface thus leading to injury.[326] These hemodynamic factors influence the location, severity, and progression of the primary injury foci to secondary lesions.[338] More plaques are found in arteries where focal mechanical stresses are greater due to higher blood flow and pressure.[113,400,458] Usually, the arterial wall can adapt to these mechanical stresses, but narrowings, bends, and branchings may restrict the flexibility, thus limiting adaptability, making certain areas more susceptible to atherosclerotic changes.[221,554,587] Primary atherosclerotic lesions occur close to points of branching, where wall shear rates are low and the development of such lesions is inhibited where wall shear rates are high.[112,551]

Fatty streaks are more frequent in the thoracic than in the abdominal aorta.[119] This may be related to the concentration of cholesterol in the arterial wall. The regional distribution of fibroid plaques is markedly different from that of fatty streaks. These lesions are found more frequently in the abdominal aorta. Raised lesions also occur in the lateral and anterior aspects of the wall of the thoracic aorta. These differences are predominantly due to hemodynamic conditions in the various portions of the arterial bed. The medial tension per unit of laminar flow in the human abdominal aorta is greater than in the thoracic aorta.

The incidence of atherosclerosis is relatively low in renal, pulmonary, and mesenteric arteries. When lesions occur in these sites, alterations in blood flow dynamics are causally related to the lesions.[222] Experimental renal vein ligation in hypercholesterolemic rabbits is associated with the appearance of plaques in renal arteries. Similarly, bronchial ligation followed by collapse of the lung and increased resistance to pulmonary blood flow leads to plaque production in the pulmonary artery.

Increased shearing stress also shows effects on the vessel wall, including endothelial cytoplasmic swelling, deformation of nuclei, granulation and disintegration, repair attempts by migratory cells from subendothelial connective tissue, destruction of endothelial cells, erosion of the remaining cellular structures, and finally, formed blood elements from deposits on the damaged raw surface. Shearing stress and increased turbulence at certain local points of the vessel, such as at branches and bends predispose to endothelial damage.[340,363] In vessels where the demand for blood flow is greater, high wall shearing stress can occur, as is the case in coronary or renal arteries.[553]

The potential for adaptability of the wall to stress is related to other atherogenic factors.[209,322] The arrangement and composition of the medial layers, the depth of the degree of permeation of vasa vasorum into these layers, and the occurrence and organization of subendothelial thickenings modulate the normal differentiation of the vessel walls and the response to tension or pressure. The nature and magnitude of these responses largely depend on the effective diameter of the vessels and coexisting blood pressure conditions. The association of collagen and elastin components of the medial layers prevents the disruption of the media by mechanical stresses whenever pressure exceeds normal limits. However, hypertension produces a widening of the lamellar units of various vessels and facilitate the progress of atherosclerotic lesions.

The blood flow rate varies from the center to the inner wall surface of the vessels. Thus, there is decreased velocity and turbulence at the surface of the wall boundary altering the number of circulating blood cells causing endothelial injury.[112,218,362] These changes are obviously more prone to occur at narrowings, curves, and branches. The accretion of fibrin or circulation cellular elements on the intimal surface is also related to the properties of the boundary layers. To some extent, shearing and drag forces determine the rate of proliferation of intimal cells and the extent of accumulation of fibrous material within the subendothelial compartment.[699]

Some arteries or arterial segments are more severely involved in the injury process than others. The increased susceptibility is attributed to inherent metabolic differences among vessels and to special mechanical or structural conditions which prevail at the level of the individual arteries.[76] The alteration of the coagulation process also influences the effects of hemodynamic forces, the location of injury, and the severity of lesions, notwithstanding that increased coagulability is directly related to high blood lipid levels.

1. Thrombosis and Atherogenesis

Thrombosis superimposed on preexisting vascular lesions and subsequent arterial occlusion is the most important event in the development of complications resulting from thromboembolism and leading to clinical manifestations.[14,66,158,241,259,274,554] The formation of thrombi is a response of blood to various stimuli, such as elevated blood pressure, lipid content, or stasis. The mural thrombus can become organized and cause thickening of the wall, an important step in the development of subsequent stages.[261] Platelets are involved in the initial stages of the thrombus formation.[185,287,291,342,608] When the epithelial layer is damaged, the collagen from the vessel wall is exposed to the circulating blood and platelets aggregate onto the surface of the intima, interacting with collagen by means of the arginine ε-amino groups. Abnormal plasma lipoprotein composition in hypercholesterolemic patients induces platelet activation.[651]

Most aortic thrombi are composed of fibrin, which initially is exposed to the bloodstream, but soon a layer of endothelium covers its surface, and followed by the production of fibrous tissue layers on the subendothelial zone.[140,396] Two different changes follow this process which eventually favor the development of the mural thrombus: (1) condensation of fibrin forming fibrous tissue network and (2) organization of the thrombus. Condensation of fibrin occurs frequently, and in recurring thromboses, deposits are overlayered.[382] Newly formed fibrin deposits are reticular and flocculated, although older deposits are compact. In the aorta, thrombosis tends to recur with the formation of multiple deposits.

Mechanical stimulation caused by hemodynamic changes triggers the development of intimal lesions following the cohesion of platelets on the surface.[263,440,448,544] The aggregation of platelets on the endothelium brings about the release of permeability factors, causing intensified infiltration and deposition of lipoproteins in the vessel wall[18] (Figure 3). Intravascular stimulation derived from bacteria, viruses, or antigen-antibody complexes can also bring about intimal lesions and initiate the adhesion of platelets to the intimal surface. When platelets stick to collagen, their constituents or mediators are released into the general circulation, such as the discharge of amine storage granules.[554] Some of these components exert inhibitory activity on atherosclerosis.[405] This process is similar to the release that takes place in other cells, such as leukocytes or mast cells.[562] Platelet granules contain serotonin, ATP, ADP, and divalent ions, and these substances affect endothelial and smooth muscle cells from the vessel wall.[604] Lysosomes become unstable, and lysosomal enzymes are discharged initiating cell injury reactions.[136,582,652] Platelets also release elastases, these proteolytic enzymes digest certain connective tissue constituents. Proteins and other coagulation factors present in plasma are altered by the components released from platelets, leading ultimately to the conversion of soluble fibrinogen into fibrin and thus to the formation of insoluble deposits.[375,599]

A characteristic feature of early changes in the arterial wall is the focal disposition of

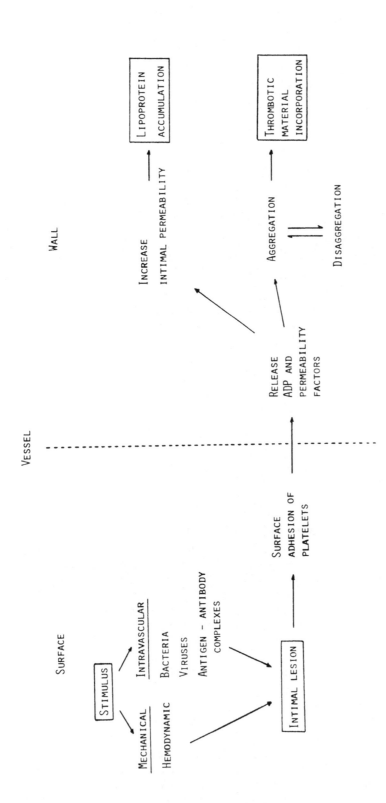

FIGURE 3. Mechanism of platelet aggregation. The adhesion of platelets on the surface of the endothelium leads to increased infiltration and deposition of plasma lipoproteins in the wall.

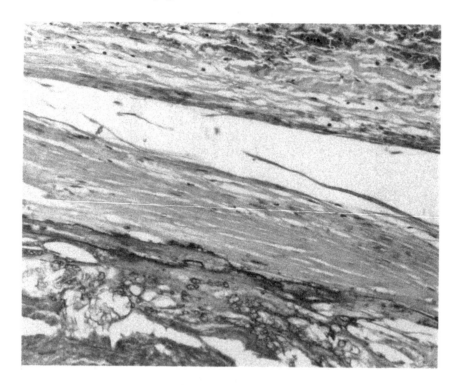

PLATE 3.   Atherosclerotic changes in aorta. Calcified intimal plaque is seen in the middle of the photo micrograph.

the lipid accumulation and intimal thickening.[358,598,599] This is seen in a case showing sub-intimal proliferation and calcification (Plate 3). Early alterations of the wall cause local adhesion of platelets and polymorphonuclear leukocytes, including some erythrocytes.[644,654] Mediators released by these cells increase the permeability of the tissue to plasma proteins and edema results. When the wall of the vessel is damaged, more platelets adhere to the area of injury, bringing about more adhesions, with build up of platelet aggregates and development of a platelet mass.

The primary damage caused by platelet aggregation and release of contents may be slight and reversible.[306,394] However, the combination of hyperlipidemia and hypertension predisposes to lipid deposition in the arterial intima resulting in fatty spots and streaks.[233] Slight impairment of the endothelial lining is sufficient to alter the intimal surface thereby causing recurrent platelet aggregation.

Blood platelets contain high amounts of ADP and ATP. The concentration of ADP in platelets decreases during the clotting of the platelet-rich plasma. When the thrombus is first formed, platelets, red, and white cells are disrupted and release ADP into the plasma (Figure 4). This released ADP triggers the adhesion of platelets, probably initiating the first step in the production of hemostatic plugs and thrombi. The size of platelet aggregates is related to the amount of ADP released and to the pattern of blood flow. Large platelet aggregates form in areas where there is disturbed blood flow. The platelet mass formed by the action of ADP is unstable and will fragment and not adhere unless fresh platelets arrive at the site. The platelet aggregation phenomenon is independent of the clotting mechanism and does not necessarily promote fibrin formation. When platelets aggregate under the influence of ADP, proteins and a specific phospholipid are released. This phospholipid seems to be essential for the normal clotting mechanism. Certain saturated fatty acids also elicit aggregation of platelets and activate blood clotting. The rapid infusion of saturated fatty acids

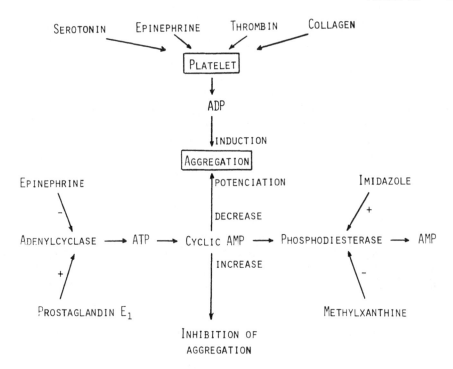

FIGURE 4. Regulation of platelet aggregation by cyclic AMP and pharmacological control.

produces thrombosis in experimental animals; subsequently, the formation of fibrin stabilizes the platelet mass.

Generation of prostacyclin (PGI$_2$) by arterial wall cells protects the vessel wall from the deposition of platelet aggregates.[79,187,248,272,319,459] This process explains why the contact of platelets with healthy endothelial cells does not provide a stimulus for platelet aggregation.[435] The endothelium from arterial wall can synthesize PGI$_2$ from intracellular precursors and also from arachidonic acid within platelets.[50,436,645] There is a homeostatic mechanism which maintains the balance between the powerful proaggregating substance thromboxane A$_2$ (derived from platelet endoperoxides, see Figure 16, Chapter 1) and the antiaggregating and vasodilating substance PGI$_2$. Impairment of this balance could lead to either a bleeding tendency, such as in uremia, or cause a tendency to produce emboli and thrombi, as in thrombotic thrombocytopenic purpura.[382]

In animal experiments, the high capacity to synthesize thromboxane A$_2$ by platelets and reduced ability of the arterial wall to produce PGI$_2$ leads to the formation of microthrombi at points where hemodynamic stress is apparent. This mechanism is responsible in part for the progression of atherosclerotic lesions since human atherosclerotic plaques do not possess sources to generate PGI$_2$.[138,678] Inhibition of prostacyclin production by impairment of prostacyclin synthetase and related to lipid peroxidation can trigger off some or all reactions in the neighboring arterial wall. Lipid peroxidation, resulting from free radical formation in a wide variety of pathologic conditions, thus accentuates atherosclerotic lesions.

Epidemiological studies among Eskimos from Greenland support the evidence that alterations of lipid metabolism can modify the prostacyclin system. The incidence of ischemic heart disease is very low among these people. These low rates of morbidity due to heart disease are attributed to low levels of cholesterol, triglycerides, LDL and VLDL, and high levels of HDL.[28] These plasma lipid patterns are regulated by the diet.[27] Dietary habits have influencing effects on platelet function and platelet-vessel wall interactions.[158] Moreover, Eskimos significantly have lower bleeding time due to decreased platelet aggregation.

High intake of eicosapentaenoic acid (C20:5) is one of the important features of the Eskimo diet. Eskimos also have high plasma levels of this fatty acid and low arachidonic acid concentration.[27] In contrast to arachidonic acid, eicosapentaenoic acid does not cause platelet aggregation and is the precursor of thromboxane A_3. In contrast to thromboxane A_2 derived from arachidonic acid, thromboxane A_3 does not have platelet aggregation functions. Cyclooxygenase in the vessel wall can generate an antiaggregating substance, probably PGI_3, and the impairment of the balance between pro- and antiaggregating substances is responsible for the low incidence of intra-arterial thrombosis in this population.

Evidence for the role of lipid factors in thrombosis and atherosclerosis exists in Type IIa hyperlipidemic patients. These patients are highly sensitive to aggregating agents such as ADP, collagen, or epinephrine.[369] The lipid composition of platelets is not different from normals, however, Type IIa subjects produce more thromboxane A_2 from arachidonic acid than normals. Type IIa patients also exhibit increased kallikrein activation and have high levels of circulatory soluble fibrin complexes. This finding is consistent with platelet-mediated activation of the intrinsic coagulation system. Treatment of these patients with clofibrate or other lipid regulating agents returns the ADP-sensitivity of platelets to normal, while modifying the plasma lipid profile.

In humans, homocystinemia is connected with progressive atherogenesis. Long-term infusion of homocystine in primates leads to the loss of the aortic endothelium.[262] Platelet consumption is increased threefold in these animals indicating an enhanced adhesion and aggregation to the areas of damaged endothelium. After 3 months of homocystinemia, experimental animals show typical atherosclerotic plaques with connective tissue matrix and modified intra- and extracellular lipid.

2. Mechanisms of Platelet Aggregation

The aggregation of platelets is stimulated by a variety of compounds, including some physiological substances: serotonin, epinephrine, thrombin, and collagen.[20,365,546] Such compounds cause the release of ADP from platelets, initiating aggregation. The involvement of ADP in this process prompted investigations to search for release inhibitors. This led to the finding that adenosine and derivatives elicit potent but transient inhibitory properties. Several adenosine-like compounds have been studied as potential drugs for the control of platelet adhesion and aggregation and substances structurally unrelated to adenosine nucleotides have also been tested. Prostaglandin E_1, and 8-isoprostaglandin E_1 in very low concentrations inhibit aggregation, pointing to a regulatory mechanism involved in this process.[79] Experiments on the hemostatic processes in rats *in vivo* have shown that prostaglandin E_1 is the most active inhibitor of ADP-induced platelet aggregation.[357]

Calcium ions and cyclic nucleotides are also involved as intracellular secondary messengers in the response of blood platelets to extracellular stimuli. Cyclic AMP or its dibutyryl derivative reduce platelet aggregation and the effect of prostaglandins is mediated through cyclic AMP, associated with an alteration of adenyl cyclase activity. Adenyl cyclase is an enzyme localized in the platelet membrane and not detectable in the cytoplasmic fraction. Prostaglandin increases the synthesis of cyclic AMP, which is subsequently metabolized by phosphodiesterases, with no effects on platelet phosphodiesterase. Other substances elicit different responses: imidazole stimulates, caffeine inhibits thus affecting the cyclic AMP levels in a different fashion, whereas caffeine and prostaglandin act synergistically.

The inhibition of platelet aggregation by prostaglandin E_1 is not dependent on the nature of the stimulating substance, suggesting a common mechanism.[630] Cyclic AMP blocks the aggregation induced by ADP, epinephrine, and collagen, and it is likely that this molecule occupies a central role in the inhibitory mechanism. Substances which alter the level of cyclic AMP also alter platelet responses. Increased cyclic AMP levels by either stimulation of adenyl cyclase or inhibition of phosphodiesterase, inhibit platelet aggregation and induce disaggregation. In contrast, reduction of cyclic AMP by either decreasing adenyl cyclase activity or simulating phosphodiesterase induces or potentiates aggregation. Some other prostaglandins also increase cyclic AMP levels, but to a considerably lesser degree. The relative activities of prostaglandin E_1, prostaglandin A_1, and prostaglandin F_1, in the stimulation of cyclic AMP synthesis, run parallel with their relative abilities to inhibit ADP-induced platelet aggregation.

Besides these natural substances, a variety of pharmacological agents bring about the inhibition of platelet adhesion and aggregation or release of contents.[213,263,467,480] Nonsteroidal anti-inflammatory drugs cause reduction of platelet release and of secondary ADP- or epinephrine-induced aggregation. Pyrimido-pyrimidine derivatives block both primary and secondary ADP- or epinephrine-induced aggregation and the aggregation caused by thrombin or collagen. These drugs also decrease platelet retention, they affect cyclic AMP by enhancing adenyl cyclase and inhibiting phosphodiesterase activity to a certain extent. Platelet aggregation is decreased in primary biliary cirrhosis.[30]

In the homocystinemia model,[262,264] experimental animals were treated with a phosphodiesterase inhibitor drug, dipyridamole. This drug did not alter the endothelial loss induced by homocystine, but inhibited both the formation of a thick thrombus in the areas of endothelial cell loss and the increase of platelet consumption. Dipyridamole probably interferes with certain platelet functions, connected with primary and secondary ADP-induced platelet aggregation and platelet release reactions.[480]

B. ARTERIAL WALL

The arterial wall consists of three layers: inner or intima, intermediate or media, and external or adventitia. These layers are composed by three principal tissues: endothelium, elastic and collagen fibres, and smooth muscle cells or fibroblasts. The intima starts at the lumen of the vessel and consists of the endothelium, the subendothelial layer, and the internal elastic lamina. The media consists essentially of smooth muscle cells and elastic fibers extending up to the adventitia, which represents a loose network of collagen and elastic fibres containing blood vessels, lymphatics, and nerve fibres.

In the newborn, the arterial intima consists of a single layer of endothelial cells. Age-associated changes start as early as the 34th week of gestation and there is a steady increase in intimal thickness until the end of the 4th decade. Such diffuse intimal thickening constitutes part of normal arterial growth and modeling. Diffuse intimal thickening, however, does not occur to the same extent and degree in all arteries. Thus, the distribution of arterial wall thickness follows the distribution of atherosclerotic lesions.[570] The intima of the aorta is not uniform and tends to be thicker at those sites which are especially prone to develop lesions.[45,62] During the atherosclerotic process changes are present in the composition of the arterial wall (Figure 5).

1. Endothelium and Endothelial Transport

The arterial endothelium performs a wide range of metabolic and secretory functions.[255,580,669,670] Some of these functions have relevance in atherogenesis. The arterial endothelial lining represents the interphase between the arterial wall and blood. The surface of the normal endothelium is nonthrombogenic, but it is altered when the normal hemostatic mechanism is disturbed. The endothelium is not a passive barrier for diffusion, but a dynamic structure with various properties and functions.[217,708] These functions include the ability to regenerate,[220,374,569] control of endothelial transport and permeability,[53,580,588,589] release and conversion of angiotensin,[523,545,604] uptake of serotonin,[306,579] and phagocytosis.[679] Many important components of hemostasis and inflammatory reactions are produced by endothelial cells such as thromboplastins,[706] plasminogen activator and fibrinolysin,[506] certain prostaglandins,[219] histamine,[293] heparin,[104] Von Willebrand factor, and Factor VIII[314,315] (Table

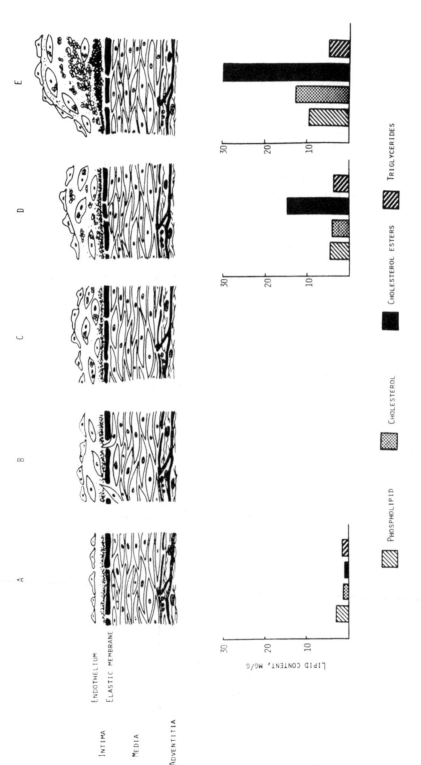

FIGURE 5.   Factors and stages in the development of atherosclerosis.   The normal artery and its layers: intima bounded by the endothelium toward the lumen and elastic membrane, media, and adventitia (A). The intima increases slowly with age in thickness and cell content. Increased serum cholesterol and triglyceride level associated with increased quantity of β- and pre-β-lipoproteins, increased tendency of platelet stickiness and clotting and increased permeability to plasma proteins due to hypertension, vasoactive amines from platelets. Toxins and anoxia cause decreased metabolism and proliferation of medial cells and the initial phase of a developing lesion (B). Subsequent or parallel to the proliferation of smooth muscle cells local lipoprotein metabolism becomes poor and intercellular lipid accumulates in medial cells (C). Extracellular lipid also occurs resulting in the formation of a fatty streak (D).

TABLE 1
Substances Synthesized by the Endothelial Cell[a]

Function	Substance
Blood coagulation	Fibrinolysin (plasminogen activator)
	Thromboplastin
	Factor VIII (antihaemophilic factor)
	Factor X (Von Willebrand factor)
Platelet aggregation	Prostaglandin E
	Prostacyclin (PGI$_2$)
	Platelet inhibitor
Other	Serotonin uptake
	Angiotensin I convertase
	Collagen

[a]   References 116,301,306,314—316,523,545, and 604.

1). Cytoplasmic contractile proteins, collagen, and basement membrane material are essential constituents of the endothelium.[407,301,316]

Other important properties are the existence of surface receptors for lipoproteins, hormones and drugs, and the specific immunological receptors. Lipoprotein lipase is an enzyme attached to endothelial membrane which exerts regulatory control in the metabolism of the smooth muscle cells of the media of the artery.[446] Lipoprotein lipase activity participates in the conversion of VLDL to LDL and in the degradation of chylomicrons to cholesterol-rich residues.[602] During the degradation process of lipoproteins, free fatty acids are released exerting an injurious action on the endothelium, relevant to atherogenesis.[546]

The vascular endothelium is permeable to a wide range of molecules. The permeability of the endothelium involves the presence of a pore system and the vesicular transport. Physiological studies on capillary transport revealed the existence of a two-pore system, one with small pores of approximately 9 μm in diameter and the other with large pores about 50 μm in diameter. Molecules up to 500,000 Da cross the endothelium by vesicular transport. The vesicular transport is bidirectional or emits invaginations on the luminal plasma membrane. LDL of about 22 μm in diameter can move across the normal endothelium in pinocytotic vesicles. This type of transport is unlikely for the larger chylomicrons and intact VLDL molecules.[568] Albumin and fibrinogen cross the arterial endothelium, and there are focal and regional differences in the permeability to these macromolecules.

There are active and inactive vesicles in endothelial cells, and the vesicular uptake of macromolecules is regulated, determining the rate of endothelial transport. Therefore, factors regulating permeability are important since this process represents a key step in atherogenesis. The modulation of the influx of components produced by the endothelium, platelet components, and lipoproteins influence the metabolism and proliferation of cells in the underlying media of the vessel wall.[158,406] The various sequences in the progress of atherosclerosis is given in Figure 6.

Under normal circumstances, the arterial endothelium also functions as a nonthrombogenic surface. This property derives from surface glycoproteins which prevent the adhesion of platelets and the activation of coagulation processes. Endothelial cells bind and inactivate substances which initiate or enhance platelet aggregation. These include the inactivation of serotonin[579] and thrombin.[20] The endothelial-platelet interaction determines whether the adhesion and aggregation of platelets to the arterial wall leads to thrombus formation. Once platelet aggregates are in contact with collagen or for other reasons, activated phospholipase A$_2$ acts upon the phospholipids in the platelet membrane with consequent release of arachidonic acid and formation of endoperoxides by the membrane bound cyclooxygenase system.

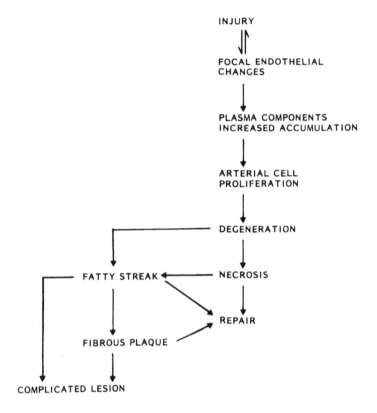

FIGURE 6.   Pathological sequences in the progress of human atherosclerosis.

Another enzyme system in platelets, thromboxane synthetase produces thromboxane A_2 which causes further platelet aggregation and release of adenosine diphosphate and serotonin.[434,435,436] The action of thromboxane A_2 is connected with changes in the intracellular Ca^{2+} and rise in cyclic GMP. Cyclic AMP concentrations usually remain unaltered. Some prostaglandins and prostacyclins which inhibit platelet aggregation, increase adenyl cyclase activity, and the production of cyclic AMP.

2. Metabolic Processes

The selective susceptibility of various segments of the arterial vasculature to develop atherosclerotic lesions indicates that the metabolism in arteries plays an active role in the pathogenesis of the disease.[82,143,168,199,269,274,275,381,383,614,621,624,707] The arterial wall is an active tissue and has its own metabolism. To fulfill essentially mechanical functions, it requires circulating metabolites to meet energy requirements and to permit adaptation of its structure and composition to long-term mechanical demands. Normal metabolic adaptations which are associated with the usual range of mechanical stresses may be insufficient to cope with abnormal blood components or even normal blood constituents if they are present in excessive quantities. On the other hand, abnormal mechanical stresses may result in inappropriate reactions of the arterial wall even when the concentrations of blood constituents are normal.

The vascular smooth muscle cells of the arterial wall derive their major fraction of energy from reactions linked to metabolic respiration. The tissue contains only a single layer of endothelial cells, but these cells are active in respiratory processes. Subsequently, anoxia and acute irreversible injury may develop in the endothelium. The oxygen consumption of the normal artery is quite low relative to that of other organs such as kidney or liver. Oxygen consumption is increased in the artery in the areas where fatty streaks develop. This rise is apparent before gross lesions are observed. The synthesis of ATP in these arteries, however,

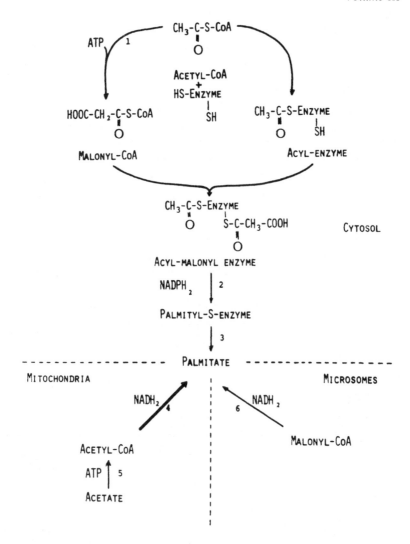

FIGURE 7. Synthesis of fatty acids in arterial tissue. Three major pathways function simultaneously. The cytoplasmic route regulated by acetyl-CoA carboxylase (1), fatty acid synthetase (2), and acyl-S-enzyme deacylase (3). The mitochondrial system synthetizes fatty acids from acetyl-CoA by chain elongation through the sequential addition of two carbon atom units involving some modification of the ω-oxidation system (4) or directly from acetate by acetyl thiokinase (5). The *de novo* synthesis of fatty acids occurs in the endoplasmic reticulum by alternating chain elongation and desaturation (6) using malonyl-CoA as substrate. The heavy arrow indicates the pathway which is increased in the atherosclerotic artery.

is lower than what is predicted from the oxygen consumption, suggesting a defect in oxidative phosphorylation.[266] The limited availability of oxygen aggravates the accumulation of lipids and lipoproteins in the artery.[271,347]

3. Lipid Synthesis in the Arterial Tissue

Among the various metabolic functions of the arterial wall, the local synthesis of lipids is essential[689] (Figure 7). The production of most fatty acids takes place in the cytosol and occurs in two major steps. The first reaction is the carboxylation of acetyl-CoA to form malonyl-CoA, catalyzed by acetyl-CoA carboxylase. This is the rate limiting step, and the enzyme has two active sulfhydryl groups. The peripheral sulfhydryl binds acetate, producing the acyl enzyme, which is then attached to the malonyl radical by the central sulfhydryl. The second step is catalyzed by the multienzyme complex fatty acid synthetase which requires NADPH and forms palmitic acid after cycling seven times through the first steps. Fatty acids are also synthetized by chain elongation in mitochondria using NADH as cofactor.[302,303] The extension of the carbon chain takes place by the addition of two carbon units to the existing acyl-CoA resulting in a variety of saturated and unsaturated fatty acids of various lengths, primarily C:18 and C:20 containing two, four, or more double bonds.[393] Acetate is also an efficient precursor of fatty acids in arterial tissue mitochondria. Acetyl-CoA is synthetized by an acetate thiokinase enzyme. The mitochondrial system depends on the availability of all fatty acyl receptors present in the tissue, which is influenced by the diet. The endoplasmic reticulum is also involved in fatty acid synthesis where chain elongation and desaturation occur as alternating processes. Malonyl-CoA is a major precursor for the microsomal action, but acetyl-CoA can also be utilized to a smaller extent.[121,123,201,611,612,613,614]

In atherosclerotic arterial tissue, fatty acid synthesis is considerably enhanced particularly when there is a rise in oleic acid.[686] Cholesteryl oleate is the only lipid that increases significantly in the atherosclerotic artery due to augmented esterification of the newly synthetized oleic acid to cholesterol. A marked increase also occurs in the production of C20:2 and C22:5 involved mainly in mitochondrial chain elongation. This action may be related to an impairment of NADH oxidation. Conditions that increase the NADH/NAD ratio, such as hypoxia or inhibitors of cytochrome oxidation, stimulate fatty acid synthesis.[352,665] Furthermore, cholesterol administration to experimental animals also enhances fatty acid formation. It is not clear, however, whether the change in fatty acid production occurs only when the disease has progressed to a relatively advanced phase or if the derangement itself initiates the progression of atherosclerosis.

The arterial wall can synthetize a great variety of phospholipids (Figure 8). Phospholipid synthesis is increased in the atherosclerotic vessel and this is stimulated by the elevation of cholesterol.[122] Newly synthetized fatty acids are incorporated into phospholipids *in situ*. Two major pathways are connected with the production of lecithin. The Kennedy pathway involves the *de novo* synthesis from α-glycerophosphate.[330] Using this substrate, fatty acids are esterified to position 1 of lecithin by this pathway. In atherosclerosis, the synthesis and content of lecithin are increased according to the extent of proliferation of the endoplasmic reticulum.[170,413,484,498-500] However, when lysolecithin is applied as a precursor, considerable amounts of fatty acids are bound to position 2, suggesting a direct esterification of fatty acids.[361,501,502] Increased levels of lysolecithin stimulate the Lands pathway. The enzyme catalyzing this process, fatty acyl CoA:lysophosphatidylcholine fatty acyl transferase, is located on the plasma membrane. The activity of this enzyme is enhanced in the atherosclerotic tissue probably due to the increased amount of lysolecithin coming from the plasma. Some lecithin is formed by methylation of ethanolamine utilizing *S*-adenosylmethionine as methyl donor. The Bremer-Greenberg pathway is attached to the endoplasmic reticulum in the liver;[52] it is probably localized on the same cellular organelle within the muscle cell.[84,441,442]

The synthesis of phospholipids is also enhanced in arteries with lesions as compared to normal arteries.[421] The composition of phospholipids changes as atherosclerotic lesions evolve. The relative roles of deposition and synthesis of phospholipids in the accumulation are uncertain, but there is evidence that local synthesis of phospholipids plays a greater role than the deposition from the plasma.[709] The rate of arterial wall phospholipid synthesis is greater in cholesterol-fed animals.[685] Among individual phospholipids, the greatest absolute rise occurs in lecithin, but in relative terms sphingomyelin accumulation in the arterial lesions also increases significantly. Whenever lysolecithin concentration is raised several fold, phosphatidylethanolamine content shows no change.[498] Furthermore, the sphingomyelin level is enhanced during the early stages of development although lecithin concentrations are elevated

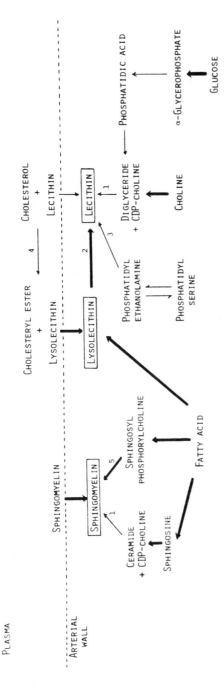

FIGURE 8.   Synthesis of phospholipids in arterial tissue. Phospholipids are incorporated into the muscle cell from the plasma and also produced in large quantities in the arterial wall. Mainly two pathways participate in the elevated levels of lecithin due to atherosclerosis. Through the Kennedy pathway, it is produced from CDP-choline and α, β-diglyceride by the phosphoryl choline glyceride transferase (1) or through the Lands pathway from lysolecithin and fatty acyl-CoA by lysolecithin:fatty acyl-CoA acyl transferase (2). The Bremer-Greenberg pathway, stepwise methylation of phosphatidyl ethanolamine by S-adenosylmethionine, occupies only a minor role (3). The balance between lecithin and lysolecithin in the plasma is associated with the function of lecithin:cholesterol acyl transferase (4). Sphingomyelin is synthetized from sphingosine or sphingosyl phosphorylcholine by the Kennedy pathway (1) or by fatty acyl-CoA transfer (5). Heavy arrows indicate processes which are increased in the atherosclerotic artery.

CHOLESTEROL + FATTY ACID $\overset{1}{\rightleftharpoons}$ CHOLESTERYL ESTER + H$_2$O

CHOLESTEROL + ACYL-CoA $\overset{2}{\rightleftharpoons}$ CHOLESTERYL ESTER + CoASH

CHOLESTEROL + LECITHIN $\overset{3}{\rightleftharpoons}$ CHOLESTERYL ESTER + LYSOLECITHIN

FIGURE 9.   Pathways of cholesteryl ester biosynthesis. Enzymes catalyzed these reactions are cholesterol esterase or cholesteryl ester hydrolase (1), acyl-CoA:cholesterol acyl transferase (2), and lecithin:cholesterol acyl transferase (LCAT)(3).

only after the lesions have reached an advanced phase. The sphingomyelin content of the arteries rises with age, and this accumulation of sphingomyelin is probably due to slow degradation of β-lipoproteins which are rich in this component. Removal of phospholipids from the arteries is also reduced. This may be connected with changes in the activity of various phospholipid hydrolases, particularly sphingomyelin phosphocholine hydrolase, which decreases with age.

The rate of cholesterol synthesis is quite slow in the normal arterial wall. The sterol portion of cholesteryl ester comes from the blood, and the esterification takes place in the wall.[1,251,269,270,443,505,613] Three enzyme systems participate in the production of these esters (Figure 9). Fatty acyl-CoA:cholesterol acyl transferase, a microsomal enzyme, plays a major role in the accumulation of cholesteryl ester. Cholesteryl ester synthetase, a cytoplasmic enzyme, is active at acid pH. This enzyme may be derived from lysosomes and functions as cholesteryl ester hydrolase. The activity of lecithin:cholesterol acyl transferase in arterial tissue is very low.[681] In the normal artery, the esterification of cholesterol is minimal *in situ* as compared to that of phospholipids and glycerol. In atherosclerotic tissue, however, there is a shift in the esterification process, and the majority of newly synthetized fatty acids are found to be esterified to cholesterol. This increase is stimulated during the early phases of the development of atherosclerotic lesion and is mainly due to the enhanced action of fatty acyl-CoA:cholesterol acyl transferase.

4. Lipid Composition of the Arterial Wall

Tissues of the arterial wall contain significant amounts of lipids and average 4.3 mg/100 mg dry tissue in patients between 6 months and 20 years of age. With normal growth and aging there is a steady increase in total lipid content.[596] The increase includes free cholesterol, triglyceride, and phospholipid about 0.2 mg/100 mg dry tissue for every 10 years of life. Cholesterol to total phospholipid ratio is constant at 1:1 molar ratios over the age range between 1 and 60 years.[600,601] Esterified cholesterol is very low below 20 years, 0.72 μg/100 mg, and rises very rapidly in the age range between 40 to 60 so that cholesterol ester constitutes 42% of total lipid in the arterial intima.

In the atherosclerotic artery, a number of tissue parameters are altered. The total lipid content is raised according to the severity of the lesions; it is less in fatty streaks than in plaques and in more advanced lesions. Parallel with the increased total lipid, the proportion of various lipid classes is altered including increased free:ester cholesterol ratio and decreased phospholipid, while triglycerides remain essentially unchanged.

Cholesterol and cholesteryl esters accumulate in greatest amount at all stages of the evolution of atherosclerotic lesions.[73,107,595,596] Accumulation of cholesterol can cause occlusion of the lumen of the affected blood vessels (Plate 4). The principal source of cholesterol

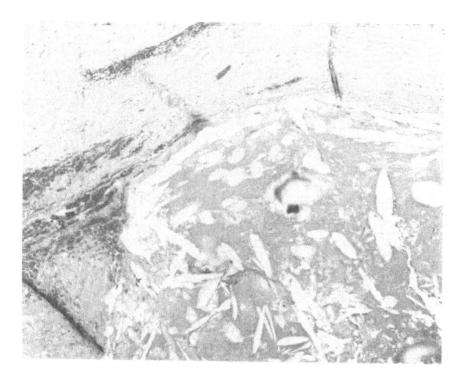

PLATE 4.   Coronary sclerosis. Atheromatous plaque containing spaces of dissolved cholesterol crystals causes near complete occlusion of the lumen.

is the blood plasma and the presence of the protein portion from plasma lipoproteins in the arterial lesions suggests that the cholesterol crosses the endothelial barrier in the form of lipoproteins. Lipoproteins can go from the vessel lumen into the lining endothelial cells by a passive transport process and are transported through the endothelial cell into the intima by either passive or active mechanisms. Lipids go through or are exchanged independently of the protein moiety. However, feeding experiments with labeled cholesterol have shown that it is incorporated into plasma lipoproteins and that it also appears in the aorta.

In addition to overall lipid changes in the arterial wall, the pattern of fatty acid composition also shows alterations. In lesion-free intima from young subjects, palmitic (C16:10) and palmitoleic (C16:1) acids constitute about 33% and linoleic acid (C18:2) 18% of the total fatty acid fraction. In this early age range, plasma low density lipoproteins (LDL) contain 48% of 18:2 acids, similar to the composition of adult-type plasma LDL. In contrast, in the aorta of 40- to 60-year-old patients, C18:2 acids are increased to 39%. This indicates that the accumulating cholesterol esters in the lesion-free intima associated with aging are derived from plasma LDL.[350]

a. Role of Lysosomes

The accumulation of lipids in the arteries is associated with lysosomal activity.[695-697] Esterified cholesterol is incorporated into the vessel wall attached to low density lipoproteins. Experiments with human fibroblasts show the possible mechanism of this incorporation (Figure 10). The initial event is the binding of the LDL molecule to the receptor on the cell surface. When LDL is bound to the LDL receptor, it enters the cell and is incorporated into endocytic vesicles. Fusion of this complex takes place with lysosomes followed by digestive action. Lysosomal proteolytic enzymes hydrolyze the protein part to free amino acids, while the cholesteryl ester is cleaved by acid lipase. The resulting free cholesterol is transferred to the endoplasmic reticulum where it modulates two enzymes: first, it suppresses 3-hydroxy-

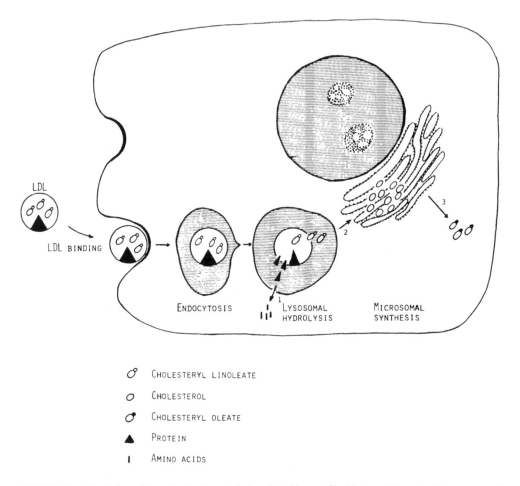

LDL

LDL BINDING

ENDOCYTOSIS

LYSOSOMAL
HYDROLYSIS

MICROSOMAL
SYNTHESIS

σ CHOLESTERYL LINOLEATE

o CHOLESTEROL

σ CHOLESTERYL OLEATE

▲   PROTEIN

| AMINO ACIDS

FIGURE 10. Metabolism of low density lipoprotein in cultured human fibroblast, and the role of lysosomes and the endoplasmic reticulum in cholesterol accumulation. LDL binds on the cell surface by LDL receptors then the complex molecule enters the cell where it becomes incorporated into endocytotic vesicles which combines with lysosomes. Lysosomal proteolytic enzymes (1) hydrolyze proteins and amino acids are released. Cholesteryl ester is degraded by lysosomal acid cholesteryl ester hydrolase (2). Free cholesterol is transferred to the endoplasmic reticulum where it is converted back to cholesteryl ester by acyl-CoA:cholesterol acyl transferase (3). The original cholesteryl ester contains more polyunsaturated fatty acids then the final ester.[100]

3-methylglutaryl coenzyme A reductase and therefore decreases endogenous cholesterol synthesis; and second, it is also reesterified by the enzyme acyl-CoA:cholesterol acyl transferase, thus accumulating in the cell. In contrast to the cholesteryl esters of plasma LDL which are rich in polyunsaturated fatty acids, the endogenously reesterified cholesterol is preferentially combined with monounsaturated or saturated fatty acids. As a consequence of this pathway, a 10-fold increase in cholesterol and 50-fold increase in cholesteryl ester content is found in severely diseased arteries. This changeover to a different fatty acid pattern is associated with the low activity of lecithin:cholesterol acyl transferase in the arterial tissue. This enzyme catalyzes the transfer of polyunsaturated fatty acids from position 2 of lecithin.[82]

In hypertension, the influx into the arterial wall of many plasma components increases; thus, evoking enhanced lysosome formation. Accordingly, increased numbers of lysosomes may deal adequately with the increased load, but degeneration and damage of the vascular wall may ensue. In atherosclerosis, higher levels of circulating cholesteryl ester-rich LDL gain access to the wall, binding to receptors. In cases of hypertension and hyperlipidemia, the endothelial cell is presented with increasing amounts of cholesteryl esters, thus over

TABLE 2
Activity of the Endoplasmic Reticulum Bound Enzymes in the Development of Atherosclerosis[483]

Liver: Cholesterol 7a-hydroxylase: cytochrome P-450 dependent-regulation of cholesterol metabolism
Vitamin D_2: decreases mixed function oxidase by binding cytochrome P-450 — vascular calcification
Ascorbic acid deficiency — reduced mixed function oxidase — hypercholesterolemia
Carbon monoxide: inhibition of cytochrome P-450 — enhanced development of advanced lesions
Fatty acid desaturase: unsaturated fatty acids reduce the risk of cardiovascular disease
Aorta: Wall contains mixed function oxidases — activation of promutagens leading to primary lesions
Blood: Platelets contain monooxygenases involved in the synthesis of prostaglandins and thromboxanes

whelming the lysosomal hydrolytic capacity. Consequent accumulation of cholesteryl esters causes cell overloading and death despite attempts of the cell to increase lysosomal activity.[93,98,99,100,230]

The protein part of the lipoprotein unit has also been identified in the wall of vessels. The proportion of free to esterified cholesterol is 1:3 in the plasma and 1:1 in the aorta, indicating that the lipid transport may be selective. Low density lipoproteins, synthetized in the liver, having a 1:1 free:esterified cholesterol ratio may penetrate into the wall at faster rates than other lipoproteins. In this regard, the accumulation of cholesterol alters the permeability of the endothelium.

b. Role of the Endoplasmic Reticulum

This unique cell organelle is fundamentally involved in the etiology of cardiovascular disease, primarily through its function in oxidative reactions. Atherosclerotic plaques have monoclonal origin, and focal proliferation of smooth muscle cells in the intima is required for the development of atherosclerosis.[54,55] Environmental mutagens can be activated by enzymes bound to the endoplasmic reticulum of cells in the arterial wall, and consequently, trigger local somatic mutations which lead to subsequent atherosclerotic lesions,[212] similar to the action of environmental chemicals on the function of the hepatic endoplasmic reticulum.[180-182] This mechanism may represent an initiating event which is advanced by other factors involved in this disease, producing the complete clinical symptoms of atherosclerosis.

The walls of the human aorta possess microsomal mixed function oxidase activity, and this enzyme system has been demonstrated in various animals.[321] This enzyme system has a wide spectrum of substrates and is similar to hepatic mixed function oxidases; it can be induced by polychlorinated biphenyls or polycyclic aromatic hydrocarbons.[72] Treatment of animals with benzo(a)pyrene or 7,12-dimethylbenz(a)anthracene increases the rate and number of atherosclerotic plaques without changes in serum cholesterol.[9]

Another aspect of the endoplasmic reticulum involvement is its role in lipid metabolism. Serum cholesterol levels are dependent on the action of microsomal hydroxylases including cholesterol 7α-hydroxylation, representing the first step in the conversion of cholesterol to bile acids.[77] Impaired enzyme function can lead to progressive accumulation of cholesterol in the liver and other tissues (Table 2). Excessive amounts of lipids accumulate in the endoplasmic reticulum membranes and disturb their normal fluidic structure. This may result in impaired mixed function oxidase system with accompanying increased nonspecific hydroxylation and peroxidation. Generation of lipid peroxides can damage endothelial prostacyclin synthetase, leading to suppression of PGI_2 in the heart, aorta, and mesenteric arteries.[248,322] Under the same conditions, the production of thromboxane A_2 by platelets is enhanced contributing to the progression of atherosclerotic lesions.

5. Lipid Association with Lesions

The presence of lipid is a distinguishing feature of atherosclerotic lesions.[477] It is an established fact that local injury and reaction predispose to lipid accumulation. Some ob-

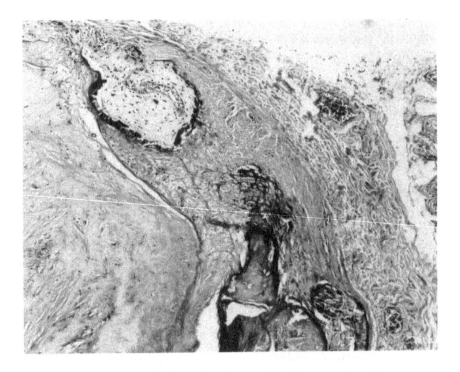

PLATE 5.   Severe coronary sclerosis with subintimal proliferation and calcification.

servations indicate the biochemical nature of these primary changes, and they relate to the effects of saccharides or amino acids. Localized alterations of mucopolysaccharides or collagen in the artery have been suggested as sites of initial injury. Cholesterol can be accumulated in various places of the body (Plate 5). Homocystinemia is also associated with lipid accumulation.[262,264] This metabolic disorder causes formation of abnormal mucopolysaccharides in the intima.

As the atherosclerotic process advances, cholesterol accumulates in the arterial wall.[365] In the age range of 40 to 60 years, 65 to 80% of total lipid is cholesterol, with a high ratio of esterified to free in most lesions. The rate of cholesterol influx is greater in an artery with fatty streaks than in normal; coupled with lower efflux, the resulting effect is net accumulation. In plaques, the influx of cholesterol is higher than in fatty streaks, and the influx of cholesterol ester exceeds the free cholesterol rate. The fatty acid pattern of cholesterol esters differs in fibrous plaques from plasma of atherosclerotic patients and from that of juvenile fatty streaks. The principal fatty acid in fibrous plaques is linoleic acid (C18:2), whereas in juvenile fatty streaks, oleic acid (C18:1) is predominant.

The lipid pattern of raised lesions is not homogenous. There is an overall increase of total lipids and increased proportion of cholesterol. The proportion of oleic acid is decreased and linoleic acid increased. There is a massive accumulation of cholesterol in the basal pool, up to 94.8 mg/100 mg dry tissue.[596,597] Triglycerides do not constitute a major component of either fatty streaks or raised lesions. Phospholipid content enhances significantly, but does not increase during atherosclerosis to the same extent as free or esterified cholesterol. Phosphatidylcholine is produced in significant amounts while sphingomyelin is not. However, the greatest increase is seen in the sphingomyelin fraction which is synthesized *in situ*.[4,462]

6. Connective Tissue in the Plaque
a. Collagen
Extracellular connective tissue elements make up the greatest part of the plaque in many

instances. Morphologically, these elements are collagen fibres, elastic tissue elements, ground substance, basement membrane, and extracellular microfilaments. Connective tissue components are four major classes of macromolecules: collagens, elastins, structural glycoproteins, and proteoglycans.[279,415,417,454]

Collagen constitutes the major component of atherosclerotic plaques and in diffuse intimal thickening. The soluble precursor of collagen, procollagen, contains specific *a* chains which exist in four genetically determined forms. These eventually produce four different types of collagen.[427,673] Collagen Types I and III predominate in the normal arterial wall; 30% is Type I and 70% is Type III. Type I is associated with fibroblasts and Type III with medial smooth muscle.[416] Small amounts of Type IV collagen are found in the vessel wall in basal laminae.

In atherosclerosis, connective tissue is increased in the intima in association with endothelial changes,[108] proliferation of arterial smooth muscle cells,[617] and retention of lipid and lipoproteins.[594,595] The explosive proliferation of endothelial cells enhances cell turnover and is responsible for the increased biosynthesis of connective tissue containing collagen and elastin, enhancing the formation of the intimal lesion. Atherosclerotic lesions synthesize collagen at a rate between 5 and 20 times higher than that found in lesion-free areas of the same arteries.[203] The degree of stimulation of collagen synthesis is related to the severity of the atherosclerotic process. In plaques, however, the distribution of various types of collagens is reversed; 65% is Type I, and 35% is Type III.[416,517] During regression there is a conversion to Type III. Experimentally, the process of collagen production can be reversed by reduction or complete removal of the atherogenic agent, i.e., cholesterol,[23] or surgically modifying its concentration by ileal bypass,[334] or by treatment with tyramine,[60] or generally by inhibiting protein synthesis.[655]

The role of catecholamines in collagen biosynthesis and its relation to experimental atherosclerosis has been recognized.[658] Collagen synthesis precedes the formation of fibrinous plaques on the wall. Nerve factors also play a role in atherogenesis, perhaps through the induction of hyperlipidemia and endothelial injury.

b. Elastin

Elastic fibres constitute important components of the extracellular connective tissues of the arterial wall. In the thoracic aorta, 40% of the total protein is elastic fiber, falling to about 20% in the abdominal portion. Elastin is produced in specialized mesenchymal cells, particularly in smooth muscle cells. Its immediate precursor is tropoelastin which is formed from a larger precursor, proelastin.[549] Tropoelastin aggregates on microfibrils and lysine oxidase catalyzes the formation of covalent bonds between amino acids producing desmosine and isodesmosine.[487]

In the early stages of atherosclerosis, changes occur in structural elastic tissue.[277] This is related to changes in elastase activity, which have been detected in atherosclerosis and in chronic obstructive lung disease.[295] Although aging is connected with loss of elastic tissue and increased distensibility of arteries, atherogenesis is accompanied by an increase in elastin in absolute terms.[348,349] In contrast with the fairly uniform increase in collagen, elastin levels are more variable. Elastins form protein-lipid complexes both in normal tissue and in atherosclerotic plaques. The amount of lipid is small in lesion-free segments, but there is a marked increase with the development of lesions. Most of the lipid is cholesterol ester and probable prerequisite of this binding is the amino acid transformation mentioned above.[348,349] This binding involves a transfer of the esterified cholesterol from LDL and VLDL. No association exists between elastin-lipid complexes and HDL.[350] Moreover, the complex binding is strong and it is difficult to remove lipids bound to plaque elastin. Elevated calcium, found in the lesions, is also bound to the elastin-lipid macromolecule.[517]

TABLE 3
Chemical Composition of Human Serum Lipoproteins[8,577]

Component	Lipoprotein class				
	Chylomicron	VLDL	LDL	HDL₂	HDL₃
Protein	2[a]	8	21	41	55
Triglycerides	84	50	11	4.5	4.1
Cholesterol					
Free	2	7	8	5.4	2.9
Ester	5	12	37	16	12
Phospholipids	7	18	22	30	23

[a]   Data are expressed in weight percent per particle.

c. Proteoglycans

Proteoglycans or glycosoaminoglycans represent the third major component of the extracellular matrix of the arterial wall.[454,511] This group of macromolecules contains complex carbohydrates in the form of heteropolysaccharides. These heteropolysaccharides can be divided into two classes: (1) nonsulfated, such as hyaluronic acid and chondroitin, and (2) sulfated, such as heparin, heparin sulfate, dermatan sulfate, keratan sulfate, chondroitin-4-sulfate, and chondroitin-6-sulfate.[116,535,682] They are attached to proteins to form proteoglycans.

The arterial collagen-elastin framework is embedded into a glycoprotein containing medium as an interfibrous matrix. Adjacent small elastic fibres are joined by proteoglycan molecules suggesting that one function of the arterial proteoglycans is to hold elastic fibres together.

During atherosclerosis, glycoproteins are increased,[279] and with this rise, the glycoprotein matrix of the lesion increases. If the cholesterol level is high the intimal connective tissue progresses toward plaque formation with increasing concentration of extracellular lipid. Moreover, the endothelial basement membrane becomes thickened containing the complex connective tissue product. The thickening represents a nonspecific response to injury.

C. COMPOSITION OF THE BLOOD

Lipids in the blood are associated with proteins to form lipoprotein water-soluble complexes.[595] Carbohydrates are present in lipids as glycosphingolipids in relatively small amounts, and their role in lipoproteins is still unknown. The binding between lipids and proteins is nonconvalent. These interactions are strong and the macromolecules withstand dissociation during normal fractionation procedures.

A common characteristic of all serum lipoproteins is that they contain polar and nonpolar lipids in various proportions[8] (Tables 3 and 4). Lipids occupy either the core of the surface of the lipoprotein particles, which may be essential in the organization and stability of these macromolecules. The basic lipid components of the plasma are cholesterol either in free and esterified form, triglycerides, or free fatty acids and phospholipids.[30,457,463]

Among fatty acids, the C16:1, C18:1, and C18:2 species are the most abundant, but minor saturated and unsaturated components are also present (Table 5). The heterogeneity of fatty acids may be important in maintaining appropriate fluidity. Lipid concentration varies with age, sex, and diet. However, the determination of various lipid fractions is especially important for the diagnosis of coronary atherosclerosis.[201,205,250-252,378]

Normal fasting blood plasma shows the lipid components distributed in four main lipoprotein groups: chylomicra, pre-β-lipoproteins or very low density lipoproteins (VLDL), low density lipoproteins (LDL), and α-lipoproteins or high density lipoproteins (HDL).

Chylomicrons are spherical lipid particles and consist mainly of triglycerides, normally

TABLE 4
Molecular Composition of Human Serum Lipoproteins[8,577]

Component	Chylomicron	VLDL	LDL	HDL$_2$	HDL$_3$
			Lipoprotein class		
Protein	102.000[a]	15.656	4.830	1.476	963
Triglycerides	507.000	11.500	298	19	10
Cholesterol					
Free	25.840	3.539	475	50	13
Ester	27.700	3.600	1.310	90	32
Phospholipids	45.160	4.545	653	137	51

[a]　Data represent molecules per particle and are expressed in terms of amino acids.

TABLE 5
Fatty Acid Composition of Human Serum Lipoproteins[593]

Fatty Acid	VLDL TG[a]	VLDL PL[a]	VLDL CE[a]	LDL TG	LDL PL	LDL CE	HDL TG	HDL PL	HDL CE
16:0	24.7[b]	36.4	22.8	24.9	32.1	10.8	24.5	30.2	10.7
16:1	4.1	1.3	2.9	4.2	1.6	3.3	4.0	1.4	3.2
18:0	3.9	18.7	6.1	4.8	15.9	1.3	4.6	16.1	1.2
18:1	35.2	13.2	34.6	35.6	12.0	19.3	35.9	12.4	18.9
18:2	22.5	16.1	26.0	17.2	20.0	51.9	17.1	20.8	52.2
20:4	1.1	4.3	1.9	1.4	6.7	5.6	1.3	8.5	6.3

[a]　TG, triglycerides; PL, phospholipids; CE, cholesteryl esters.
[b]　Data are expressed in weight percent per particle.

representing a small fraction of total plasma lipids.[519] Most plasma lipids are present in the circulation associated with α- or β-globulins thus terming them α- or β-lipoproteins. All these macromolecular protein-phospholipid complexes contain cholesterol, cholesterol esters, triglycerides, phospholipids, and other lipids in varying amounts where the lipids are bound to the protein moiety by secondary bonds.[504] There are major differences in the cholesterol and triglyceride contents of the lipoprotein fractions. An association has been described between cholesterol, cholelithiasis, and coronary heart disease.[75]

1. Cholesterol
a. Biosynthesis and Metabolism

The predominant lipid in atherosclerotic lesions is cholesterol.[97,152,505,509] This molecule is synthetized from acetate through various steps primarily in the liver (Figure 11) and it is then released into the blood, providing part of the plasma pool.[16,34,37,48] Cholesterol synthesis takes place to a smaller extent in the arterial wall, skin, adrenal cortex, gonads, and intestinal mucosa. The plasma concentration of cholesterol is dependent on two opposite processes, namely, its rate of synthesis and removal or degradation.[101,103] Metabolic studies revealed significant variations in plasma cholesterol levels in normal men.[647] The excess cholesterol synthetized in the liver is released into the bile canaliculi together with bile salts. The biliary cholesterol and bile salts mix with dietary cholesterol and other endogenous lipids facilitating the absorption and reabsorption of all lipids from the small intestine. Both endogenous and exogenous cholesterol are equilibrated in the serum. The contribution of dietary cholesterol to the total cholesterol pool is about half of the endogenous production. In the intracellular regulation of cholesterol biosynthesis, several enzymes play an important role. Although

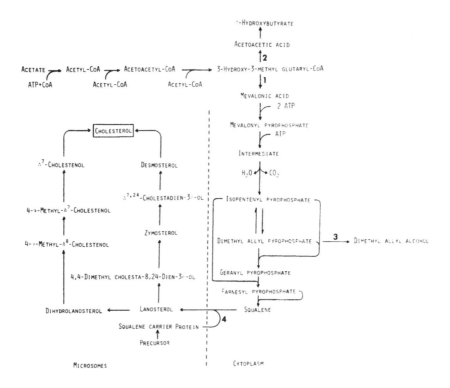

FIGURE 11.   Biosynthesis of cholesterol in the liver. Microsomes and supernatant fractions are required for the conversion of acetate to cholesterol. The conversion of 3-hydroxy-3-methylglutaryl-CoA to mevalonic acid by HMG-CoA reductase (1) is also microsome bound. This is a rate-limiting irreversible step and the formation of ketone bodies (2) and 3,3-dimethyl allylalcohol (3) provide a shunt as regulating side reactions. All subsequent processes are almost specific to sterol synthesis. Squalene is converted to lanosterol by cyclization and through two independent pathways cholesterol is produced. In the specific enzyme reactions, squalene and sterol carrier protein plays an important role (4) by the formation of a precursor-microsomal enzyme complex. Sterol carrier protein also participates in the formation of HDL lipoproproteins and in the initial stages of cholesterol metabolism.

some findings are still controversial, several abnormalities in enzyme activities have been found to be associated with the impairment of cholesterol synthesis and increased risk of cardiovascular disease. The condensation of acetyl-CoA with acetoacetyl-CoA produces 3-hydroxy-3-methylglutaryl-CoA, which can be cleaved to acetyl-CoA and acetoacetate yielding further ketone bodies or may be reduced to mevalonate. The mevalonate reaction is catalyzed by 3-hydroxy-3-methylglutaryl-CoA reductase, a microsomal enzyme. This enzyme elicits the principal control in the synthesis of isoprenoid compounds and cholesterol. The synthesis of this enzyme is very rapid with a half-life of 3 to 4 h,[24,163,290] and increased dietary cholesterol decreases the incorporation of acetate into endogenous cholesterol by inhibiting enzyme formation.[162,289] Another important control mechanism lies in the dehydrogenation of 3,3-dimethylallyl alcohol derived from mevalonate via dimethylallyl pyrophosphate to 3,3-dimethylacrylic acid.[124] This shunt utilizes a significant portion of intermediates which otherwise lead to the production of cholesterol. The significance of this regulation has been demonstrated in hypercholesterolemic patients;[190] a decrease in the enzyme activity results in a great excess of cholesterol being accumulated.

b. Balance

In addition to synthesis, dietary cholesterol intake also contributes to the input of this molecule. The role of plant sterols is relatively small since they are poorly absorbed by the intestine. Even the absorption of dietary cholesterol from the gut is incomplete, with only 20 to 40% taken up in man. This also reflects variations depending upon amounts present in the different body pools, including plasma, liver, and intestines. Many processes participate in the disposition of cholesterol (Figure 12).

The elimination of cholesterol metabolites takes place entirely through the stool, either as unchanged cholesterol, or bile acids produced in the liver, or coprostanol formed from cholesterol by bacterial action (Figure 13). Small amounts of cholesterol are converted to steroid hormones. The excreted cholesterol mixes with dietary cholesterol and probably limited amounts reenter the pool. Bile acids are reabsorbed efficiently via the enterohepatic circulation into the liver, and only small quantities leave the body (Figure 14). A fraction of cholesterol is excreted through the skin and in the milk during lactation. In the production of bile acids, the conversion of cholesterol to 7α-hydroxycholesterol is the rate-limiting step. The enzyme is located in the microsomal fraction of the hepatocyte and has a short half-life of 2.5 to 3.0 h. Bile salts returning to the liver via the portal circulation exercise a feedback control on 7α-hydroxylase.[521,576]

The sterol balance is a useful concept because the sterol nucleus does not undergo metabolic biotransformation in the body.[149,247,509,605] Oxidation, reduction, and hydroxylation processes occur on the steroid nucleus or side chains, but the basic ring system is indefinitely preserved. If the input into the organism exceeds the output which compensates for the matabolic inertness, cholesterol is accumulated in various tissues of the body. Atherosclerosis represents in part a positive sterol balance in the arterial wall. The influx of cholesterol into the intima is greater than the amount leaving, and the gradual storage in the artery ultimately leads to progressively severe lesions.

c. Association with Lesion

Evidence for a limited causal relationship between elevated cholesterol level and atherosclerosis has been provided by animal experiments. Arterial lesions resembling those of human atherosclerosis can be produced in a variety of animal species by procedures that lead to the elevation of serum cholesterol levels. Success in the production of lesions depends on the degree to which lipid levels can be raised and the length of time these levels can be maintained. In the dog and rat, for example, feeding cholesterol is sufficient to produce marked hypercholesterolemia, but ineffective in producing lesions. Appropriate procedures devised for achieving high serum cholesterol levels in these species include: (1) stress by the administration of adrenocorticotropin or by regulating the feedback mechanism by corticosteroids; (2) antithyroid treatment, by which reduction of thyroxine and triiodothyronine bring about decreased tissue metabolism; (3) toxic chemicals, such as carbon tetrachloride, causing impaired microsomal hydroxylation and altered transport; and (4) estrogens, which labilize lysosomes, triggering off cell injury.

Procedures for producing experimental atherosclerosis always included cholesterol feeding as the means to assess the role of serum cholesterol levels in the pathogenesis of the disease.[636,638] It has now been shown both in animals and in man that changes in the intake of neutral fat, independent of cholesterol intake, can also induce hypercholesterolemia. Severe atherosclerosis has been produced in rabbits by feeding high levels of saturated fats. It seems quite clear that serum cholesterol levels in humans are more responsive to the amount and nature of neutral fat in the diet than to the cholesterol level, although this dietary component may also play a role under some circumstances. The precise mechanism whereby dietary neutral fats influence serum lipoprotein levels has not been clarified, but considerable evidence indicates that the end result is an increased rate of conversion of cholesterol to bile acids. Cellular lipoprotein receptors also influence cholesterol homeostasis.[392] Atherogenic diets generally lead to elevation of all classes of serum lipids. For example, there can be a fivefold rise in triglyceride levels, and a sevenfold rise in phospholipid levels in rabbits fed cholesterol, although the rise in cholesterol levels is proportionately the greatest.

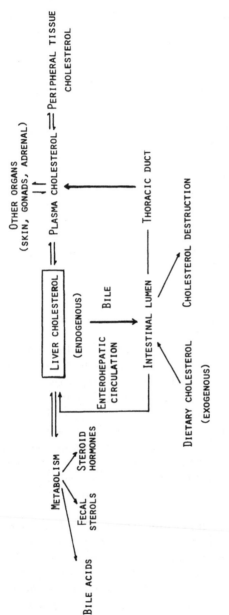

FIGURE 12.   Disposition of cholesterol.

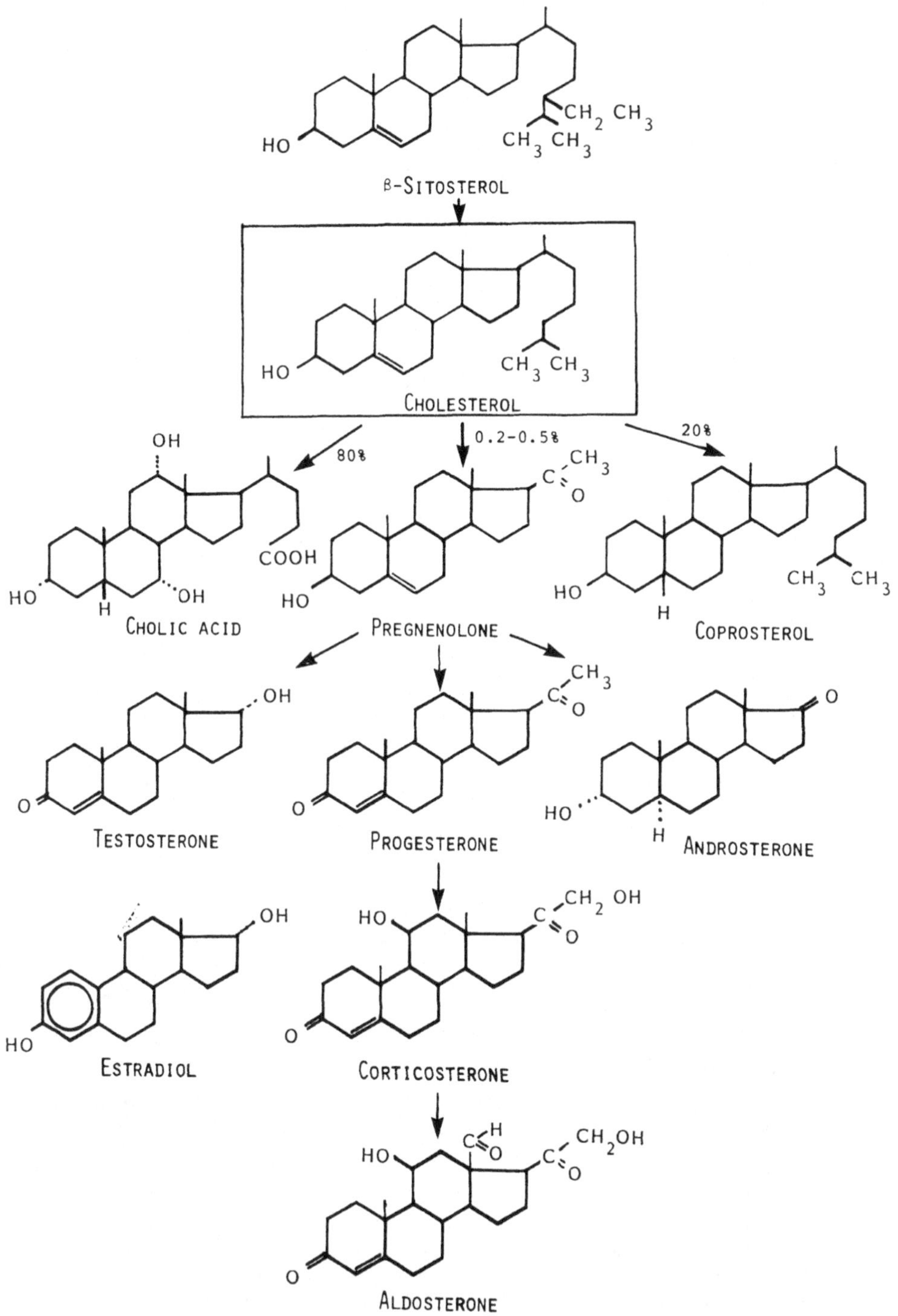

FIGURE 13.   Pathways of cholesterol metabolism influencing physiological balance.

In familial hypercholesterolemia or xanthomatosis, a marked elevation of plasma cholesterol is present, and in these individuals clinical symptoms of coronary artery disease are
evident at an early age as compared to normolipemic patients. The nature of the lesions in
humans is similar to those in rabbits fed high cholesterol-containing diets.

A study of coronary heart disease over a period of 12 years in Framingham, MA

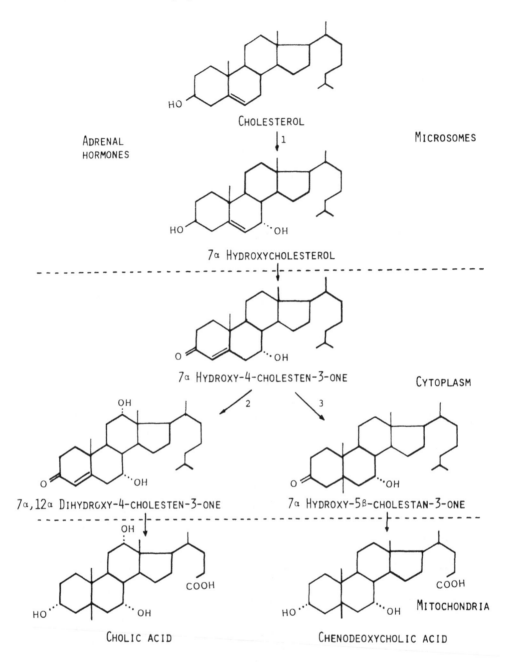

FIGURE 14.   Conversion mechanism of cholesterol to bile acids. In the breakdown of cholesterol microsomes, cytoplasm and mitochondria participate sequentially. 7α-Hydroxylation (1) is the rate-limiting step and involves the participation of the mixed function oxidase which also catalyzes the metabolism of drugs. The activity of this enzyme is dependent on adrenal hormones. 12α-Hydroxylase (2) is also microsome bound, but it is not inducible, Δ$_4$-5β-reductase (3) is a soluble enzyme.[77,240]

demonstrated that elevated cholesterol levels were associated with clinical signs of coronary artery disease.[74] The Framingham study also showed that in healthy individuals the increased susceptibility to ischemic heart disease runs parallel with increasing plasma cholesterol concentrations. Individuals with cholesterol levels lower than 200 mg/dl had about 50% less morbidity as a group, whereas cholesterol levels exceeding 260 mg/dl were associated with nearly twice the average death rate of control subjects.

The fat content of the human diet also affects cholesterol metabolism either by the actual amount or by the fatty acid composition. Increased dietary intake of saturated fatty acids causes elevated cholesterol levels and coronary heart disease.[196] The mechanism of this relationship is not yet clearly understood. Cholesterol absorption is especially reduced when dietary fat is absent or very low. Within the usual range of fat intake, however, it is unlikely that fat has a great effect on cholesterol absorption. When larger amounts of dietary fat are absorbed, the formation of chylomicrons is promoted in the mucosal cells of the intestine, and thus more cholesterol is absorbed from the gut. Dietary fat has no direct effect on hepatic cholesterol synthesis *de novo* other than providing acetate as precursor. In this respect, the action of dietary fat does not differ from that of dietary carbohydrates or proteins, but the importance of this precursor's role should not be underrated in the causation of hyperlipidemia.[419]

Endocrine factors such as thyroid hormones and estrogens[33,78,207,354,355] also influence serum cholesterol levels. Hypothyroid patients have elevated cholesterol, whereas in the serum of hyperthyroid individuals, cholesterol levels are low. This effect is connected with the direct action of thyroid hormones on the breakdown of cholesterol by increasing its metabolism. Estrogens have a decreasing effect in this respect and bilateral ovariectomy, may cause a rise. Similar increases may be observed in postmenopausal women. The lower incidence of atherosclerotic lesions and coronary heart diseases in females may reflect the modulating effect of estrogens on cholesterol metabolism.

2. Triglycerides

Dietary triglycerides are the major constituents of lipid fractions.[352,354,361,418] These neutral lipids are transported in the plasma as lipoprotein complexes, mainly in the form of chylomicrons or as VLDL, derived primarily from the liver. Triglycerides are also found to a lesser extent in the intestine and thoracic lymph. Part of the endogenous lipid from nondietary sources is also absorbed from the intestinal lumen.[573] Lipids are transferred from the lumen into the absorptive cells in very fine aqueous dispersions or in the form of mixed bile salt micelles. Triglyceride particles are transported almost entirely by the lymph, and fat absorption is accompanied by increased lymph flow. Chylomicrons are partially degraded in the intestinal mucosa by lipoprotein lipase to monoglycerides and fatty acids. Part of the free acids is transported into the circulation.[345,460,463,648] After absorption, triglycerides are reconstituted within the absorptive cells by reesterification of the mono- and diglycerides. Fatty acids containing less than ten carbon atoms enter the portal blood directly. These medium chain fatty acids are neither reesterified nor incorporated into triglycerides, but from the blood stream. The precursor pool of fatty acids includes dietary and endogenous components. The resynthetized di- and triglycerides are stored in the depot fat where later they are broken down largely into glycerol and free fatty acids.

The release of triglycerides from the cells is under hormonal and pharmacological control. The metabolic control of hepatic triglycerides is related to the control of VLDL triglyceride production.[331] Apart from chylomicrons, glucose is the major source of adipose tissue triglycerides, providing both the glycerol moiety via glycerophosphate and the fatty acid fraction by way of acetyl-CoA (Figure 15). Amino acids can also contribute to depot fat since after deamination to keto acids, they give rise to glucose.

3. Lipoproteins

a. Structure

Plasma lipoproteins are very heterogenous molecules with a lipid:protein ratio varying from 99:1 in chylomicrons to 1:99 in the albumin-free fatty acid complex. Whereas the protein fraction is mainly globulin, the lipid fraction is different. Hence, variations in lipid composition between lipoprotein classes are quantitative rather than qualitative (Table 6).

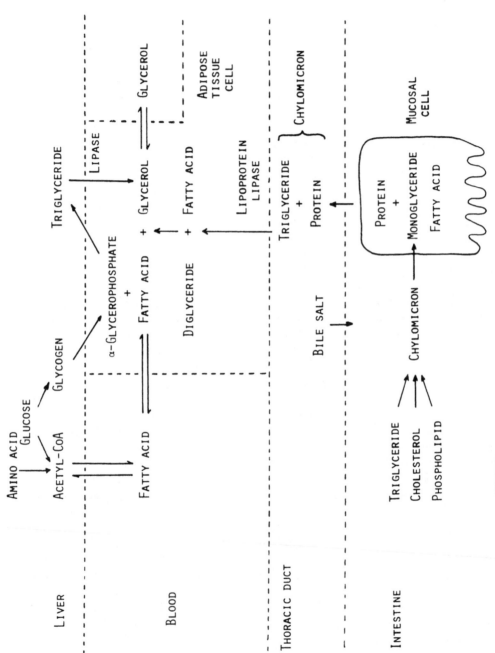

FIGURE 15.   Major pathways of triglyceride deposition and mobilization.

TABLE 6
Characteristics of Human Lipoprotein Classes

Lipoprotein	Density (g/ml)	Molecular weight (Da)	Diameter (nm)	Protein, mobility	Lipid: protein ratio
Chylomicrons	<0.97	0.4—30×10^9	75 — 1000		99: 1-98: 2
VLDL	0.97—1.006	5—10×10^6	30 — 80	Pre-β-globulin	92: 8
iDL	1.006—1.063	2.2—3.5×10^6		β-Globulin	79: 21
LDL$_1$	1.003	2.7—3.5×10^6	20.2 — 30		
LDL$_2$	1.034	2.2—2.7×10^6	20 — 20.2		
HDL	1.063—1.125	1.0—3.9×10^5	7 — 12	α-Globulin	59: 41-44: 56
HDL$_2$	1.094	1.75—2.6×10^5	8.5 — 10		
HDL$_3$	1.145	1.5—1.75×10^5	7.0 — 8.5		
Albumin-FFA Complex	1.125—1.210	69×10^3		Albumin	1: 99
Lipoprotein A	1.050—1.120	5×10^6		Pre-β-globulin	

Note: The classification and nomenclature of lipoproteins are based on density and charge as determined by electrophoretic mobility and ultracentrifugal flotation rate.[312,556,557,592,593]

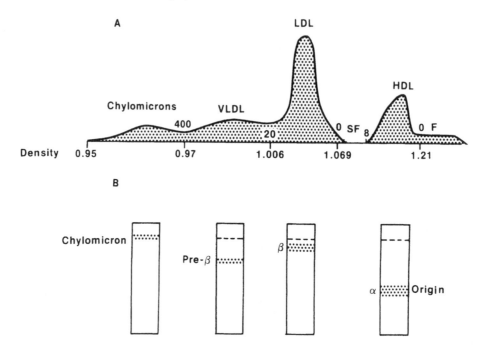

FIGURE 16.   The serum lipoprotein spectrum. Separation by ultracentrifugation (A) or agarose-gel electrophoresis (B). Flotation rates (S_f) are inversely related to density. Electrophoretic mobility at pH 8.6
shows that the increasing negative charge is different from density and molecular size.

The lipid moieties are linked to proteins with weak forces so that they can be separated.
Only small amounts of lipid are bound covalently due to important structural organization
requirements. The lipid:protein ratio determines the density of lipoproteins. This property
is applied for separating them into different classes by ultracentrifugation. However, the
separation is also dependent upon differences in the protein moiety. Although this classification of lipoproteins is arbitrary, most lipoprotein classes have different structural organization and stability and play distinctly characteristic roles in lipid transport and in
atherosclerosis. On the basis of different density and electrophoretic mobility, they are
divided into low and high density lipoproteins (HDL).[273,312,445,555,559] Low density lipoproteins
are separated into low density lipoproteins (LDH) and very low density lipoproteins (VLDL)
(Figure 16). Each class represents a family of closely related moieties with a different lipid
protein ratio which can be further divided into subgroups characterized by molecular size
and ultracentrifugal floatation rates.

The chemical composition of human lipoproteins shows significant differences[592,593]
(Table 7). Low density lipoproteins or β-lipoproteins contain large amounts of cholesterol
in both free and ester form.[32,159,184,258,366,380,568] They are constituted by 20 to 25% protein
and 75 to 80% lipid. The lipids distribution is cholesterol 40%, triglycerides 10%, and
phospholipids 30%. Sphingomyelin comprises about 26% of total phospholipid, with a
lecithin content that is also higher than in any other lipoprotein. LDL molecules exhibit a
spherical structure upon electronmicroscopy examination, with granular substructure. The
apoprotein portion contains approximately 12 polypeptide subunits joined together by lipid
bridges stabilizing the complex molecule.

VLDL or pre-β-lipoproteins contain a large amount of triglycerides;[35,367,401,508,552] with
a protein content of 8 to 10% and 90 to 92% lipids. The total lipid in VLDL is divided into
total cholesterol 20%, triglycerides 50% and phospholipids 18%. In VLDL the free choles-
terol:cholesterol ester ratio is higher than in any other lipoproteins. The main phospholipid

TABLE 7
Chemical Composition of Human Lipoproteins[a]

Component	Chylomicrons	VLDL	LDL	HDL	HDL$_2$	HDL$_3$
Proteins	2 — 3[b]	5 — 12	17 — 25	33 — 59	41	55
Lipids						
Total	97 — 98	88 — 95	75 — 83	45 — 66	4.5	4.1
Triglycerides	81 — 88	54 — 68	9 — 16	12 — 19	4.5	4.1
Cholesterol						
Total	2 — 7	15 — 18	36 — 59	24 — 30	22	15
Free	1 — 3	4 — 7	10 — 12	6 — 10	5	3
Ester	3 — 8	15 — 23	30 — 50	24 — 35	16	12
Free Fatty Acids	Trace	1 — 2	None			
Phospholipids						
Total	6 — 9	13 — 21	21 — 32	44 — 50	30	23
PE	5 — 6	2 — 10	2 — 10	5 — 10		
PC	75 — 81	60 — 74	50 — 68	70 — 75		
LPC	2 — 5	2 — 15	5 — 15	3 — 11		
SM	9 — 14	15 — 23	25 — 35	5 — 13		

[a] Most lipoproteins are heterogeneous in size and composition. Data show the generally accepted ranges.[457,559,592,593]

[b] Data are expressed in weight percent per particle.

is lecithin. Variations have been found in the amount of phospholipids, probably related to sex differences.

HDL constitute the smallest lipoprotein molecules. These lipoproteins exist in several isomeric forms in human plasma; HDL$_1$ is a minor component, and the HDL$_2$:HDL$_3$ ratio is influenced by various physiological and pathological parameters.[8,174,344,431,492,633]

HDL$_2$ may be related to estrogens, since its amount in premenopausal women is about three times greater than in men. This lipid:protein ratio is about 1:1, and it contains 32% cholesterol, 10% triglycerides and 51% phospholipids. In the HDL$_2$ component, lecithin constitutes 70 to 80% of the total sphingomyelin (12 to 14%). The predominant fatty acid in cholesteryl esters is linoleic acid. The concentration of HDL lecithin is influenced by risk factors, including coronary heart disease.[567]

Apart from those mentioned above, minor lipoproteins have also been identified and these are lipoprotein *a* and lipoprotein *x*.[524,666,675]

The lipid composition of lipoprotein *a* is similar to LDL, but it contains different proteins. The distribution of apolipoproteins in normal humans is given in Table 8. Although the presence of this lipoprotein has been confirmed in 75 to 78% of the population, it does not show any correlation with the occurence of coronary heart disease. Lipoprotein *x* was found in the serum of patients with lecithin: cholesterol acyl transferase deficiency and with biliary obstruction. It has been suggested that an altered apoA is the protein constituent which does not bind lipid. From the serum of cholestatic patients with significantly reduced hepatic lipase activity, a new lipoprotein was isolated which may mediate the disposition of chylomicrons.[451] An abnormally low density lipoprotein has been isolated in obstructive jaundice,[572] and the structure of a very high density lipoprotein in human serum has been elucidated.[7]

Since the protein moiety of these lipoproteins is essential in lipid transport, many studies dealt with the character and composition of apoproteins and the amino acid sequence of the peptide chains in most major constituents (Table 9).[6,25,26,102,313,344,414,556-558,584,585] The number of amino acids varies between 57 and 245. Some structures have not yet been established, mainly due to the methodologic problems to separate lipid free and soluble proteins. ApoA-I is most abundant and consists of a linear chain of 245 amino acids with a molecular weight

TABLE 8
Distribution of Apolipoproteins in the Plasma of Normal Fasting Subjects[557,558]

Apoprotein[a]	Plasma Concentration[b]		Lipoprotein class			
	μm	Mole %[c]	VLDL	LDL	IDL	HDL
ApoA-I	46	38				100
ApoA-II	23	20				100
ApoB	5	4	2	82	8	
ApoC-I	18	16	2		1	97
ApoC-II	3	3	30		10	60
ApoC-III	13	12	20	10	10	60
ApoD	5	4				100
ApoEII, III, IV	2	2	20	10	20	50

[a] The nomenclature for apoproteins represents lipoprotein families; however, trivial names indicating major amino acid component or appearance have also been adopted in the early literature, such as glycine-rich, arginine-rich, and highly polar apoproteins.
[b] Data are based on total plasma apolipoprotein concentration.
[c] The distribution of apoproteins in various lipoprotein classes represents mole percent for each apoprotein.

TABLE 9
Apoprotein Composition of Human Plasma Lipoproteins[557,558]

Aproprotein	Lipoprotein class				
	MW Da × 10³	VLDL[a]	LDL[a]	IDL[a]	HDL[a]
ApoA-I	28.4				45
ApoA-II	17.4				22
ApoB	255.0	2	13	75	
ApoC-I	6.6	8	26		17
ApoC-II	8.7	20	9		2
ApoC-III	8.7	60	41	22	7
ApoD	22.0				5
ApoE-II, III, IV	35.0	9	13	3	1

[a] Mole percent of total protein.

of 28,331 Da (Figure 17).[26] ApoA-I and ApoA-II are the major constituents of HDL.[86,87] ApoA-I is structurally similar in various species, probably representing a common physiological role.[385] It is an activator of lecithin:cholesterol acyl transferase. ApoA-I also regulates membrane lipid content and membrane cholesteryl esters during the disposition of VLDL. ApoA-II occurs in monomer or dimer form and contains two identical polypeptide chains linked together by cysteine disulfide bonds (Figure 18), each polypeptide chain is built from 77 amino acids, with a molecular weight of 8707 Da.[87] The characterization of apoB has not yet been achieved because it is difficult to separate from the lipid residue,[146,478] although apoB-48 is found as a constant constituent in VLDL of human.[117] In contrast, ApoC-1 contains a single polypeptide chain, (Figure 19) and it can be isolated from both VLDL and HDL.[378] ApoC-1 consists of 57 amino acid residues, aggregates in solutions not containing desaturating agents, and is an activator of plasma lecithin:cholesterol acyl transferase and lipoprotein lipase. ApoC-II is also a potent activator of lipoprotein lipase containing 78 amino acids with an estimated molecular weight of 8837 Da (Figure 20).[311,609] ApoC-III is the most abundant of the C-apoproteins in VLDL and HDL[88] and contains a polysaccharide made up by one molecule of galactose and galactosamine without or with one or two molecules of *N*-acetyl-neuraminic acid (Figure 21). ApoC-III is also an inhibitor of lipoprotein lipase as the substrate concentration exceeds 2%.

Asp-Glu-Pro-Pro-Gln-Ser-Pro-Trp-Asp-Arg-Val-Lys-Asp-Leu-Ala-Thr-Val-Tyr-Val-Asp-
Val-Leu-Lys-Asp-Ser-Gly-Arg-Asp-Tyr-Val-Ser-Gln-Phe-Gln-Gly-Ser-Ala-Leu-Gly-Lys-
Gln-Leu-Asn-Leu-Lys-Leu-Leu-Trp-Asp-Asp-Val-Thr-Ser-Thr-Phe-Ser-Lys-Leu-Arg-Gln-
Glu-Leu-Gly-Pro-Val-Thr-Glu-Glu-Trp-Phe-Asn-Asp-Leu-Gln-Gln-Lys-Leu-Asn-Leu-Glu-
Lys-Glu-Thr-Gly-Glu-Leu-Arg-Gln-Glu-Met-Ser-Lys-Asp-Leu-Glu-Glu-Val-Lys-Ala-Lys-
Val-Gln-Pro-Tyr-Leu-Asp-Asp-Phe-Gln-Lys-Lys-Trp-Glu-Glu-Met-Glu-Leu-Tyr-Arg-Glu-
Lys-Val-Glu-Pro-Leu-Arg-Ala-Glu-Leu-Gln-Glu-Gly-Ala-Arg-Gln-Lys-Leu-His-Glu-Leu-
Gln-Glu-Lys-Leu-Ser-Pro-Leu-Gly-Glu-Glu-Met-Arg-Asp-Arg-Ala-Arg-Ala-His-Val-Asp-
Ala-Leu-Arg-Thr-His-Leu-Ala-Pro-Tyr-Ser-Asp-Glu-Leu-Arg-Gln-Arg-Leu-Ala-Ala-Arg-
Leu-Glu-Ala-Leu-Lys-Glu-Asn-Gly-Ala-Gly-Arg-Leu-Ala-Glu-Tyr-His-Ala-Lys-Ala-Thr-
Glu-His-Leu-Ser-Thr-Leu-Ser-Glu-Lys-Ala-Lys-Pro-Ala-Leu-Glu-Asp-Leu-Arg-Gln-Gly-
Leu-Leu-Pro-Val-Leu-Glu-Ser-Phe-Lys-Val-Ser-Phe-Leu-Ser-Ala-Leu-Glu-Glu-Tyr-Thr-
Lys-Leu-Asn-Thr-Gln

FIGURE 17. Amino acid sequence of human very low density apolipoprotein, apoA-I[25,26]

Val-AspNH₂-Phe-Leu-Ser-Tyr-Phe-Val-Glu-Leu-Gly-Thr-GluNH₂-Pro-Ala-Thr-GluNH₂
|
Leu-Glu-Thr-Gly-Ala-Lys-Lys-Ileu-Leu-Pro-Thr-Leu-GluNH₂-Glu-Lys-Ser-Glu-Phe-Tyr-Ser
                                                                                    \
Asp-Tyr-Gly-Lys-Asp-Leu-Met-Glu-Lys-Val-Lys-Ser-Pro-Glu-Leu-GluNH₂-Ala-GluNH₂-Ala-Lys
|
Thr-Val-Thr-GluNH₂-Ser-Val-Leu-Ser-Glu-Val-Cys-Pro-Glu-Lys-Ala-PCA
                                           |
Thr-Val-Thr-GluNH₂-Ser-Val-Leu-Ser-Glu-Val-Cys-Pro-Glu-Lys-Ala-PCA
|
Asp-Tyr-Gly-Lys-Asp-Leu-Met-Glu-Lys-Val-Lys-Ser-Pro-Glu-Leu-GluNH₂-Ala-GluNH₂-Ala-Lys
                                                                                    /
Leu-Glu-Thr-Gly-Ala-Lys-Lys-Ileu-Leu-Pro-Thr-Leu-GluNH₂-Glu-Lys-Ser-Glu-Phe-Tyr-Ser
|
Val-AspNH₂-Phe-Leu-Ser-Tyr-Phe-Val-Glu-Leu-Gly-Thr-GluNH₂-Pro-Ala-Thr-GluNH₂

FIGURE 18. Amino acid sequence of human high density-apolipoprotein apoA-II (Apo-LP-GluNH₂-II). The apoprotein contains two identical polypeptide chains linked together by a disulfide bond between cysteine moieties. The amino terminals are unusual pyrrolidone carboxylic acid residues (PCA).[86,87]

H₂N-Thr-Pro-Asp-Val-Ser-Ala-Leu-Asp-Lys-Leu-Lys-Glu-Phe-Gly-

Asn-Thr-Leu-Glu-Asp-Lys-Ala-Arg-Glu-Leu-Ile-Ser-Arg-Ile-Lys-

Gln-Ser-Glu-Leu-Ser-Ala-Lys-Met-Arg-Glu-Trp-Phe-Ser-Glu-Thr-

Phe-Gln-Lys-Val-Lys-Glu-Lys-Leu-Lys-Ile-Asp-Ser-COOH

FIGURE 19. The amino acid sequence of human plasma very low density apolipoprotein, apoC-I (apoLP-Ser). Peptide residues in the boxes represent regions that contain amphiphatic helical structures.[313,585]

H₂N-Thr-Glu-Gln-Pro-Gln-Gln-Asp-Glu-Met-Pro-Ser-Pro-Thr-Phe-Leu-

Thr-Glu-Val-Lys-Glu-Trp-Leu-Ser-Ser-Tyr-Gln-Ser-Ala-Lys-Thr-

Ala-Ala-Gln-Asn-Leu-Tyr-Glu-Lys-Thr-Tyr-Leu-Pro-Ala-Val-Asp-

Glu-Lys-Leu-Arg-Asp-Leu-Tyr-Ser-Lys-Ser-Thr-Ala-Ala-Met-Ser-

Thr-Tyr-Thr-Gly-Ile-Phe-Thr-Asp-Gln-Val-Leu-Ser-Val-Leu-Lys-

Gly-Glu-Glu-COOH

FIGURE 20.   The amino acid sequence of human plasma very low density apolipoprotein, apo C-II.[311]

Two more apoliproteins have been isolated from human HDL: ApoD or thinline protein, and arginine-rich protein.[512] The name thinline refers to a characteristic thin precipitation produced with anti-HDL. This apoprotein function has not been established, but it contains glucosamine and is present in LDL, VLDL, and HDL₃. Arginine-rich apoprotein occurs in greater amounts in VLDL and it is increased in Type III hyperlipoproteinemia and hypothyroidism. New mutants of apoE have been described, associated with atherosclerosis, but not Type III hyperlipoproteinemia[705] (Figure 22).

b. Biosynthesis

The major sites of lipoprotein synthesis are liver and intestine.[37,152,167,256,309,312,373,519,531,532,619] The protein component is synthetized by ribosomes bound to the rough endoplasmic reticulum, while lipids are produced by both rough and smooth endoplasmic reticulum membranes. A high percentage of fatty acids originates from dietary fats. Fat absorption occurs in the upper part of the small intestine, and in man the jejunal mucosa is the major site of chylomicron assembly. Following intraluminal digestion, triglycerides are produced and released as chylomicrons into the lymph. Partial hydrolysis takes place in various tissues, including adipocytes. Within hepatocytes, apolipoproteins pass into the channels of the endoplasmic reticulum where carbohydrates are attached to proteins. The coupling of protein and lipid moieties occurs in the endoplasmic reticulum and in the Golgi apparatus. The newly synthetized lipoproteins are secreted into the space of Disse and, subsequently, into the sinusoids. The esterification of glycerol with fatty acyl-CoA derivatives is catalyzed by microsomal enzymes. Many factors, such as enzyme actions and exchange of lipids during circulation modify the lipid portion of new lipoproteins. A high fat diet inhibits hepatic fatty acid synthesis, and high carbohydrate regimens diet bring about a rise by conversion into fatty acids. Key enzymes which regulate fatty acid synthesis are acetyl-CoA carboxylase, fatty acid synthetase, and acyl-CoA:carnitine transferase (Figure 23). Phospholipid synthesis also occurs predominantly in the endoplasmic reticulum.[52,330] Cholesterol metabolism is influenced by dietary intake and by tissue metabolic activity, mainly the rate of hepatic synthesis. The regulation of this process is associated with lipoprotein metabolism through the squalene carrier protein and the activity of 3-hydroxy-3-methyl-glutaryl-CoA reductase. It has been suggested that the carrier protein not only mediates the absorption of precursors of cholesterol synthesis, but itself is probably the precursor protein of low density lipoproteins. The conversion of 3-hydroxy-3-methylglutaryl-CoA to mevalonic acid is the rate-

H₂N-SER-GLY-GLU-ALA-GLU-ASP-ALA-SER-LEU-SER-PHE-MET-GLUNH₂-GLY-TYR-MET-LYS-HIS-ALA-THR-

LYS-THR-ALA-LYS-ASP-ALA-LEU-SER-SER-VAL-GLUNH₂-SER-GLUNH₂-GLUNH₂-VAL-ALA-ALA-GLUNH₂-GLUNH₂-ARG-

GLY-TRP-VAL-THR-ASP-GLY-PHE-SER-SER-LEU-LYS-ASP-TYR-TRP-SER-THR-VAL-LYS-ASP-LYS-

PHE-SER-GLU-PHE-TRP-ASP-LEU-ASP-PRO-GLU-VAL-ARG-PRO-THR-SER-ALA-VAL-ALA-ALA-COOH
                                                                    |
                                                             (GAL,GAL)-(NAN)
                                                                    |
                                                                   NH₂

FIGURE 21. The amino acid sequence of human plasma very low density apolipoprotein, apoC-III (ApoLP-Ala).[88] In this protein, a disaccharide galactosyl-galactosamine is attached to the protein chain which may be extended with one or two residues of *N*-acetylneuraminic acid.

H₂N-Lys-Val-Glu-Gln-Ala-Val-Glu-Thr-Glu-Pro-
Glu-Pro-Glu-Leu-Arg-Gln-Gln-Thr-Glu-Trp-Gln-
Ser-Gly-Gln-Arg-Trp-Glu-Leu-Ala-Leu-Gly-Arg-
Phe-Trp-Asp-Tyr-Leu-Arg-Trp-Val-Gln-Thr-Leu-
Ser-Glu-Gln-Val-Gln-Glu-Glu-Leu-Leu-Ser-Ser-Gln-
Val-Thr-Gln-Glu-Leu-Arg-Ala-Leu-Met-Asp-Glu-
Thr-Met-Lys-Glu-Leu-Lys-Ala-Tyr-Lys-Ser-Glu-
Leu-Glu-Glu-Gln-Leu-Thr-Pro-Val-Ala-Glu-Glu-
Thr-Arg-Ala-Arg-Leu-Ser-Lys-Glu-Leu-Gln-Ala-
Ala-Gln-Ala-Arg-Leu-Gly-Ala-Asp-Met-Glu-Asp-
Val-Cys-Gly-Arg-Leu-Val-Gln-Tyr-Arg-Gly-Glu-
Val-Gln-Ala-Met-Leu-Gly-Gln-Ser-Thr-Glu-Glu-
Leu-Arg-Val-Arg-Leu-Ala-Ser-His-Leu-Arg-Lys-
Leu-Arg-Lys-Arg-Leu-Leu-Arg-Asp-Ala-Asp-Asp-
Leu-Gln-Lys-*Cys*-Leu-Ala-Val-Tyr-Gln-Ala-Gly-Ala-
Arg-Glu-Gly-Ala-Glu-Arg-Gly-Leu-Ser-Ala-Ile-Arg-
Glu-Arg-Leu-Gly-Pro-Leu-Val-Glu-Gln-Gly-Arg-
Val-Arg-Ala-Ala-Thr-Val-Gly-Ser-Leu-Ala-Gly-Gln-
Pro-Leu-Gln-Glu-Arg-Ala-Gln-Ala-Trp-Gly-Glu-
Arg-Leu-Arg-Ala-Arg-Met-Glu-Glu-Met-Gly-Ser-
Arg-Thr-Arg-Asp-Arg-Leu-Asp-Glu-Val-Lys-Glu-
Gln-Val-Ala-Glu-Val-Arg-Ala-Lys-Leu-Glu-Glu-Gln-
Ala-Gln-Gln-Ile-Arg-Leu-Gln-Ala-Glu-Ala-Phe-Gln-
Ala-Arg-Leu-Lys-Ser-Trp-Phe-Glu-Pro-Leu-Val-
Glu-Asp-Met-Gln-Arg-Gln-Trp-Ala-Gly-Leu-Val-
Glu-Lys-Val-Gln-Ala-Ala-Val-Gly-Thr-Ser-Ala-Ala-
Pro-Val-Pro-Ser-Asp-Asn-His-COOH

FIGURE 22.   The amino acid sequence of human B-very low density apolipoprotein, apo E.[88,102,675]

limiting step in cholesterol synthesis (Figure 11). Dietary cholesterol has biphasic influences on this enzyme; it can cause an immediate cholesterol synthesis inhibition and, subsequently, can inhibit protein synthesis. The regulation of synthesis is also connected with the presence of lipoproteins. Studies have shown that low density lipoproteins suppress 3-hydroxy-3-methylglutaryl-CoA reductase, while very low density lipoproteins are less effective and high density lipoproteins are inactive.

The synthesis of various apoproteins also occurs in the liver and intestines.[320,429,692,693,704] Apoproteins to VLDL and HDL are produced also in both organs, but apoC proteins are synthetized in liver and carried into the lymph.[295] The apoC fraction of intestinal VLDL is probably formed by transfer from other lipoproteins.[690] ApoC is exchanged reversibly between VLDL and HDL, whereas LDL does not participate in this transfer. The distribution of apoC between VLDL and HDL is related to the plasma triglyceride concentration. In man, during alimentary lipemia apoC is transferred from HDL to chylomicrons and probably to VLDL.

The smooth endoplasmic reticulum and Golgi apparatus play important roles in the formation of apoB.[318] Abetalipoproteinemia is a rare autosomal recessive disease characterized by fat malabsorption, acanthocytosis, and retinitis pigmentosa. Hepatocytes from patients with this disease contain large fat droplets and are deficient in smooth endoplasmic reticulum membranes with very low number of Golgi vacuoles.[519] In these patients, apoB is completely absent, and consequently, chylomicrons, VLDL, and LDL are not synthetized properly. In contrast, apoB levels in the serum have shown a correlation with the extent of coronary occlusion.[650] The metabolism of apoB in large triglyceride rich VLDL particles shows differences between normal and hypertriglyceridemic subjects.[478,479]

LDL originates from the degradation of VLDL. This process is reversible and dependent on the degree of triglyceride hydrolysis by lipoprotein lipase and on the rate of removal of cholesterol and phospholipids. A decreased rate of LDL production and lower plasma cholesterol levels have been found in patients with hypobetalipoproteinemia, a rare autosomal dominant disorder.[336] LDL may exert cytotoxic actions.[651]

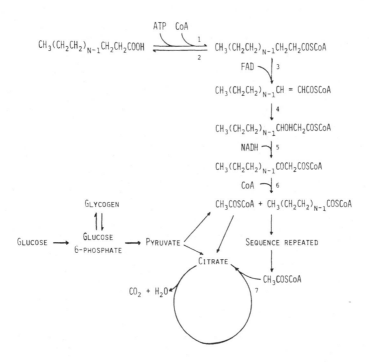

FIGURE 23. Fatty acid metabolism in the muscle and interrelations with glucose metabolism. Fatty acid degradation follows the β-oxidation pathway, starting with activation by thiokinase (1) which requires ATP and CoA. The reversible process is catalyzed by thiophorase (2). Through subsequent steps, desaturation is catalyzed by acyl dehydrogenase (3), uptake of water by enoyl hydratase (4), NAD-dependent β-hydroxy acyl dehydrogenase (5), and cleavage to form acetyl-CoA. Fatty acid derivatives short of two carbon atoms are produced by β-ketothiolase (6). The reaction sequence is repeated until the fatty acid chain is completely degraded to acetyl-CoA. A competition exists between fatty acid and glucose metabolism, both enter the acetyl-CoA pool which is completely oxidized through the citric acid cycle (7). Glucose and fatty acids regulate each other's release into the blood stream and subsequent metabolism. Fatty acids exert a feedback on glycolysis. High levels of fatty acids reduce the amount of glucose utilized in the muscle. This is particularly important in the metabolism of the heart.[516,565]

HDL is synthesized in the liver with both apoA and apoC; intestinal HDL contains only apoA. The production of HDL is reduced markedly in patients suffering from Tangier disease. In these patients, plasma triglycerides are elevated and total cholesterol is very low. However, abnormal amounts of cholesteryl esters are deposited in the reticuloendothelial system, causing liver and spleen enlargement. This defect is probably related to the deficiency of apoA-I synthesis resulting in the reduction of HDL and cholesteryl ester accumulation.

HDL fractions represent heterogeneous particles with two major subclasses, HDL_2 and HDL_3, which can be demonstrated by zonal ultracentrifugation.[578] These fractions can be further separated into subfractions by chromatography, electrophoresis, or ultracentrifugation. Levels of HDL_2 and HDL_3 fractions show sex-related differences. After puberty, HDL concentrations are higher in females than in males. The relative amounts of HDL_2 and HDL_3 are also influenced by diet, exercise, cigarette smoking, alcohol, and drugs.[133] HDL_3 can be converted to HDL_2 through the transfer of VLDL surface components during its degradation by hepatic lipoprotein lipase. This process is involved in the transfer of cholesterol and phospholipid from HDL to hepatocytes.[464]

The preferential synthesis of various lipoproteins indicates that through the formation of apoproteins, and depending upon the amount of various lipids present, there is an inter-conversion among these complex molecules. This represents a dynamic state, a continuous equilibrium between production and degradation, modulation of the synthesis and catabolism of lipids and proteins, and to exchange processes catalyzed by essential enzymes.[296] The summation of these processes determines eventually the half-life of the individual proteins.[409,410] Chylomicrons are rapidly cleared from the blood, hence their half-life is less than 1 h. During this process, nascent chylomicrons are produced in the intestine with the addition of apoA and apoB. In the circulation apoC is transferred from HDL to chylomicrons. These are then partially degraded, and triglycerides are hydrolyzed by triglyceride lipase. This lipase is activated by apoC-II, present in the capillary endothelium of extra hepatic tissues which produce diglycerides and fatty acids. Free fatty acids are released into the blood, and diglycerides are incorporated into vacuoles and endothelial microvesicles. In subsequent steps, the chylomicron triglyceride-poor particles are removed by the liver and degraded to glycerol and fatty acids, while apoC proteins are transferred back to HDL (Figure 24).

c. Metabolism

The metabolism of lipoproteins is connected with the lipids and the specific polypeptides forming the apoprotein part of these complexes.[245,246,377] Chylomicrons are not present in the blood of fasting subjects. LDL and HDL are responsible for the majority of cholesterol transport. LDL carries cholesterol throughout the body and HDL mediates its transport into the liver.[425] VLDL are triglyceride-rich particles. The metabolic relationship between the different lipoproteins is shown in Figure 25.[561,605] The normal daily intake of fat is about 120 grams containing 0.5 to 1.0 g of cholesterol.[247] Exogenous fat is transferred to chylomicrons in the mucosal cells of the gut. Apoprotein exchange occurs between chylomicrons and other circulating lipoproteins; apoC and apoE are transferred as essential steps for subsequent catabolism.

In the presence of apoC, especially apoC-II, chylomicrons interact with lipoprotein lipase located on the endothelical surfaces of the capillaries of skeletal muscle and adipose tissue cells. This enzyme breaks down the triglyceride core of the particle, producing a remnant rich in cholesterol and protein. The chylomicron remnant is taken up by the liver by binding to the high affinity apoE receptor located on the surface of the hepatocyte. The end result of this process is that dietary cholesterol is transferred to the liver, and triglycerides are transported to peripheral storage and utilization sites.

After the absorption phase, the liver maintains the availability of lipids in circulation.[128] This function regulates the production and discharge of triglyceride-rich VLDL particles. The metabolic pathway of VLDL is similar to that of chylomicrons (Figure 26), and lipoprotein lipase converts VLDL to intermediate density lipoprotein (IDL). During this process, cholesteryl esters are removed from the particles and apoB remains as the sole protein component in the lipoprotein complexes. IDL is further converted to LDL in the liver by a lipase by break down of triglycerides to fatty acids (Figure 27). Nascent HDL is rich in protein, phospholipid, and cholesterol, but deficient in cholesteryl ester. The reduction of HDL production is associated with the retention of cholesteryl ester in tissues. These findings suggest that HDL is pivotal for the removal of cholesteryl esters from peripheral tissues, including blood vessels, to the liver where they are metabolized.[24,63,150,224,406,466,471,532,577,619,620,622]

LDL is the major vehicle for the transport of plasma cholesterol. It is metabolized along two pathways: (1) through LDL receptors and (2) scavenger catabolism. In the high-affinity LDL receptor pathway, cell membrane receptors bind the lipoprotein and transfer it to lysosomes which catabolize it into further metabolites.[582] This process is regulated by a substrate feedback mechanism. In the scavenger pathway, the reticuloendothelial system is responsible for the daily metabolism of certain amounts of LDL.

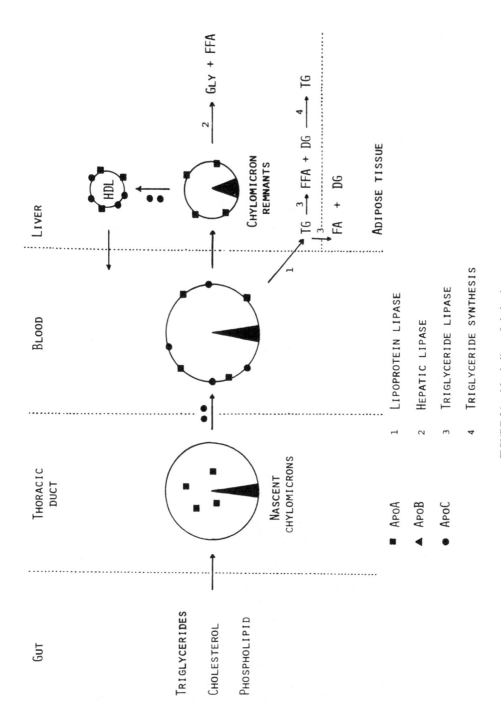

FIGURE 24. Metabolism of chylomicrons.

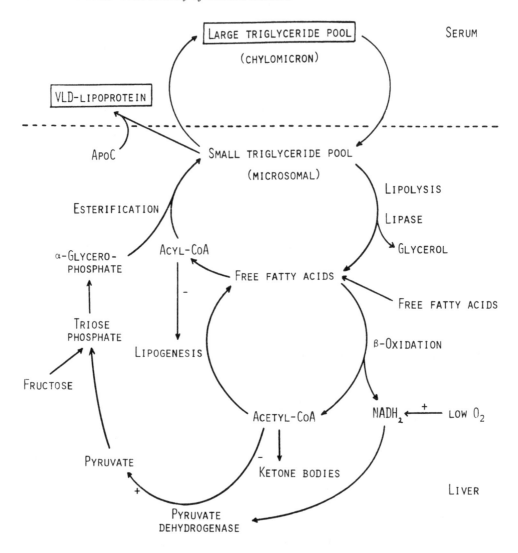

FIGURE 25.   Metabolism of lipoproteins in man.

HDL exchanges all components with every lipoprotein present in blood. This includes cholesteryl ester, phospholipid, and apoprotein. Both the liver and the gastrointestinal tract are responsible for HDL synthesis.[234,671] Nascent HDL is a complex of free cholesterol, phospholipid, and apoprotein. Plasma lecithin:cholesterol acyl transferase adds to this complex more cholesterol from other lipoproteins and tissue membranes, and through esterification, the process results in the circulating form of HDL.[681] This process is very dynamic, where HDL transfers cholesteryl ester to other lipoproteins and accepts cholesterol from various tissues.[225,297,503,524,574,607,680]

4. Antiatherogenicity of High Density Lipoproteins

Cholesterol-rich lipoproteins such as LDL and chylomicron remnants are considered to be atherogenic when in contact with cells in the atherosclerotic lesion, such as smooth muscle cells and macrophages. In contrast, HDL or one of its subfractions shows potential antiatherogenic activity,[109,333,428] with the removal of cholesteryl ester from tissues.[623]

Studies have indicated a strong reverse correlation between the prevalence of ischemic heart disease and HDL cholesterol levels[115,284] where these levels are abnormally low in

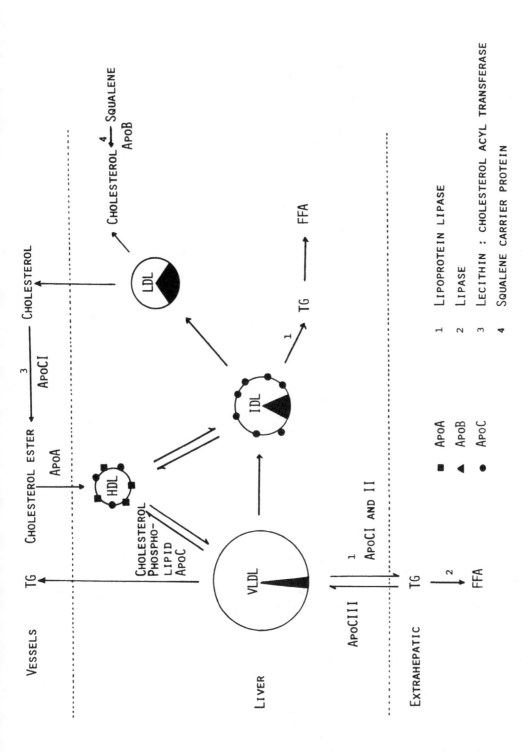

FIGURE 26. Regulation of very low density lipoprotein synthesis, and its association with triglyceride metabolism.

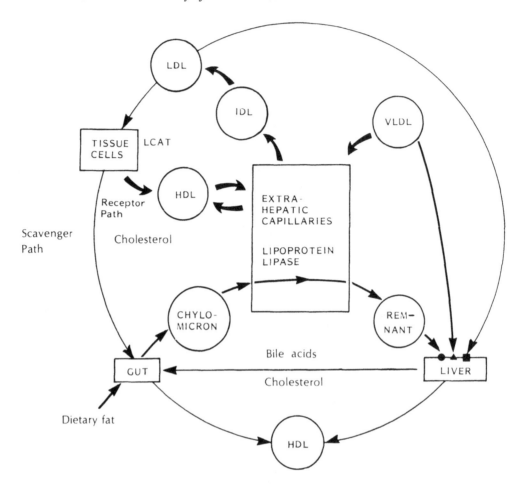

LDL

IDL

VLDL

TISSUE CELLS   LCAT

HDL   EXTRA-HEPATIC CAPILLARIES

Receptor Path

Scavenger Path   Cholesterol   LIPOPROTEIN LIPASE

CHYLO-MICRON   REM-NANT

Bile acids   LIVER

GUT   Cholesterol

Dietary fat   HDL

■ LDL RECEPTOR: ApoB,E RECEPTOR
● REMNANT RECEPTOR: ApoE RECEPTOR
▲ β-VLDL RECEPTOR

FIGURE 27.   Regulation of very low density lipoprotein catabolism, and its association with cholesterol metabolism.

relation to the development of progressive atherosclerosis.[280,281,389] Similarly, in heart attack survivors, HDL levels were lower than in healthy individuals, and among the various subfractions HDL_2 showed the most striking difference.[429]

In Tangier disease, the spleen enlargement is connected with the accumulation of cholesteryl esters within reticuloendothelial cells.[193] The disease is characterized by extremely low plasma HDL cholesterol and HDL apoproteins. In this disease, the primary defect is the abnormality in apoA-I structure, leading to a binding failure with HDL lipids and increased clearance.[12,193,194,560] The susceptibility to atherosclerosis is increased in Tangier disease, but not to the extent shown by the epidemiological relationship between ischemic heart disease and HDL cholesterol in the general population.[561] There are other genetic conditions where low HDL concentrations are connected with enhanced atherogenesis. Genetically determined familial hyperalphalipoproteinemia with high plasma HDL levels is rarely accompanied with clinical complications of atherosclerosis.[226] Abnormalities have

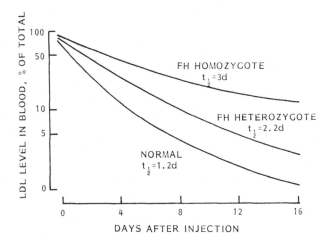

FIGURE 28. Assessment of the number of low density lipoprotein (LDL) receptors. Labeled LDL injected to various groups of patients and the loss of radioactivity from the blood was measured. This reflects the cellular uptake of LDL, which is dependent on the number of LDL receptors in the cell membrane. Normal subjects show a relatively fast LDL uptake. The removal of LDL from the bloodstream is slower in patients with homozygous and heterozygous form of familial hypercholesterolemia (FH).

been reported recently in HDL in homozygous familial hypercholesterolemia.[227] Also, high HDL cholesterol levels have been associated with increased mortality from carcinoma,[333,701] but this possibility was not supported by a comprehensive study.[96,280,284,286]

5. Lipoprotein Receptors

Recent findings showed that a receptor, bound to the surface of cells, mediates the uptake of LDL and extended the role of lipoprotein receptors into the degradation of other lipoproteins.[563,564] These receptors regulate plasma lipoprotein concentrations, serve as a target for cholesterol delivery into cells, and play part in the homeostasis of cholesterol.[231,387,388] Three receptors have been identified: (1) the apoB-E receptor, that binds LDL and apoE containing HDL and occurs in hepatocytes and certain peripheral tissues,[308,551] (2) the apoE receptor, which does not bind normal LDL, but interacts with chylomicron remnants and HDL containing apoE;[305,307] and (3) the β-VLDL receptor of macrophages, which plays a role in tissue levels of cholesterol, connected with the early stages of atherosclerosis and with xanthoma formation.[253]

a. ApoB-E Receptor

The important role of the LDL receptor in atherosclerosis was established when its absence in familial hypercholesterolemia was discovered (Figure 28).[307,640] These receptors are localized on the surface of cells and can bind LDL particles, thus removing them from the bloodstream. The number of receptors on the surface of cells varies with the demands for cholesterol. When demand is low, excess cholesterol accumulates in the cell which subsequently produces fewer receptors and takes up LDL at a decreased rate. This represents a protective mechanism for the cell against increased cholesterol content, but at the same time, LDL levels in the blood are increased. The LDL receptor is found in cultured fibroblasts, blood cells, and on membranes of cells in many different tissues.[308] Liver cells contain the highest concentration and these cells are responsible for about 75%, the receptor-mediated removal of LDL.[390] The ovaries and the adrenal glands are also rich in LDL receptors. These organs have particularly large requirements for cholesterol.

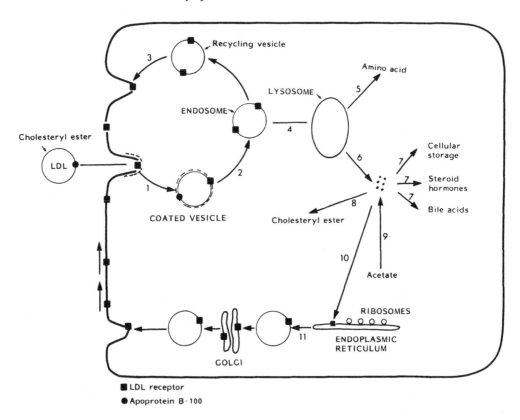

FIGURE 29. Regulation of low density lipoprotein (LDL) metabolism. Circulating LDL is incorporated into the cell by receptor-mediated endocytosis (1) and LDL is bound to receptor which invaginates and form a coated vesicle and endosome (2). In the acidic environment, LDL dissociates from the receptor which is recycled (3). Lysosomes engulf LDL where enzymes break up the lipoprotein (4). Apo B-100 is hydrolyzed into amino acids (5). Cholesteryl ester is hydrolyzed to free cholesterol (6), which is used for the synthesis of steroid hormones, bile acids, and new membranes (7), or stored as cholesteryl ester produced by acyl-CoA:cholesterol acyl transferase (8), which is activated by cholesterol. The cellular level of cholesterol is regulated by a feedback mechanism. Excess cholesterol inhibits endogenous synthesis of cholesterol by blocking the activity of the rate limiting enzyme, the hydroxymethylglutanyl CoA reductase (9), and inhibits the synthesis of LDL receptors by the endoplasmic reticulum (10) by suppressing the receptor gene into messenger RNA. In the presence of a low level of cholesterol, LDL receptor is produced and transported to the cell membrane (11).

LDL contains a large apoprotein molecule, apoB-100. The LDL receptor is a glycoprotein which protrudes from the cell surface. These glycoprotein receptors bind the apoB-100 part of the LDL. The binding is highly specific and sensitive with concentrations of less than 10^{-9} molar LDL bound to receptors. LDL bound to the receptor is carried into the cell by endocytosis. Inside, the cell LDL particle is separated from the receptors and becomes fused with lysosomes. The mechanism of LDL uptake into the cell and cellular metabolism includes the hydrolytic breakdown of the LDL particle, and unesterified cholesterol leaves the lysosome and becomes incorporated into newly synthesized membranes (Figure 29).

The amount of cholesterol released from LDL regulates the metabolism of the cell. The accumulation of exogenous cholesterol controls the reduction of the synthesis of endogenous cholesterol by inhibition of the synthesis of the CoA reductase, a key enzyme in cholesterol biosynthesis.[384] Subsequently, the cell becomes dependent on exogenous cholesterol. The LDL-derived cholesterol increases the storage of cholesterol within the cell by activating acyl-CoA:cholesterol acyltransferase. This enzyme converts free cholesterol and triggers a feedback mechanism that affects the cell to stop producing new LDL receptors.

LDL originates from VLDL particles which contain apoB-100 and apoE proteins, both of which can be bound by the LDL receptor. When VLDL circulates into adipose tissue or muscle, the triglyceride fraction is removed, and an intermediate density lipoprotein relatively rich in cholesteryl ester (IDL) is formed. IDL particles are quickly removed from the bloodstream because they bind very highly to liver cells. This tight binding is due to the presence of apoE with affinity for LDL receptors on the liver cell greater than that of apoB-100. In time, apoE disassociate from the receptor binding site and are converted to LDL.

The function of the LDL receptor in atherosclerosis is supported by morbidity data. High intake of cholesterol causes cholesterol accumulation in the liver cell which suppresses the synthesis of LDL receptor. This leads to increased serum LDL levels connected with advanced atherosclerosis. Animal experiments support this concept, and high-fat diets cause reduction of LDL receptors in the liver. High cholesterol-containing diets can decrease the synthesis of hepatic LDL receptors as much as 90% and consequently, the serum levels of both LDL and IDL is increased. In animals maintained on low fat diets, the number of LDL receptors is high, and they rapidly metabolize LDL with the resulting reduction in LDL levels.

b. Hepatic ApoE Receptor

In familial hypercholesterolemic patients, the absence of apoB-E receptor causes increased concentrations of apoE-enriched HDL and β-VLDL. These lipoproteins, however, are not elevated indicating the presence of another receptor, known as apoE receptor.[59,80] Experiments with young dogs established the receptor-mediated binding of apoE HDL$_c$ to hepatocyte membranes.[305,308] The existence of apoE receptors has also been confirmed in the liver of baboons, swine, and humans.[307] Chemical modification of the lysyl or arginyl residues in apoE abolishes the binding of apoE HDL$_c$ to the apoE receptor, this is similar to the failure of chemically modified LDL to bind to apoB-E receptors.[305] Patients with Type III hyperlipoproteinemia have abnormalities in apoE structure.[703] ApoE exists at least in three major isomer forms (E2, E3, and E4).[515,705] Patients with Type III hyperlipoproteinemia are homozygous for apoE2, which is structurally abnormal. The abnormality is probably due to the substitution of the cystine for arginine at site 158 of the peptide chain.[173,676] In hypothyroidism, the LDL catabolism may indicate the role of apoE receptors.[308] During the conversion of hypertriglyceridemic VLDL to LDL, the receptor binding determinants switch from apolipoprotein E to apolipoprotein B.[80]

c. Macrophage β-VLDL Receptor

Employing mouse peritoneal macrophages, it was found that β-VLDL can stimulate macrophage cholesteryl ester synthesis.[231,387] β-VLDL from Type III hypercholesterolemic patients and cholesterol-fed animals can induce the accumulation of lipoprotein cholesterol by mouse peritoneal macrophages, indicating the similarity (or genesis) of foam cells.[176] β-VLDL is rich in apoB and apoE, but its uptake by macrophage β-VLDL receptors is not mediated by the presence of either apoprotein because neither apoE-enriched HDL$_c$ nor apoB-enriched LDL are able to stimulate cholesteryl ester accumulation in macrophages.[391] It seems that the macrophage contains the specific receptor, since chemical modification of the arginyl residues of β-VLDL blocks its binding and uptake by macrophages.[309]

6. Enzymatic Regulation

There is a continuous exchange of lipid and protein components between the various lipoproteins and between lipoproteins and cell constituents. The transfer of apoC is reversible between VLDL and HDL and LDL does not take part in this process. Lipids are freely transferable between each lipoprotein. Two major enzymes involved in lipoprotein metabolism are lipoprotein lipase and lecithin:cholesterol acyl transferase. These enzymes are associated with the production of the lipoprotein structure.[164,265,280,328,332,343,361,398,455,507,702]

TABLE 10
Distribution of Cholesterol Between LDL and HDL
Fractions

	Age (Year)	Total (mg %)	Cholesterol	
			HDL	LDL
Newborn	—	65	43	57
Women	18—35	187	34	66
	45—65	250	24	76
Men	18—35	197	25	75
	45—65	240	22	78
Myocardial infarct		260	14	86
Nephrosis		577	6	94
Diabetes		254	20	80
Familial xanthomatosis		423	7	93

Note: Figures represent average values.[33,90]

Lipoprotein lipase is present in many tissues; adipose tissue and skeletal muscle constitute major sites. This lipase is primarily responsible for the hydrolysis of plasma lipoprotein triglyceride.[351] Lipoprotein lipase differs from other lipases in that it needs apoC-II as a cofactor and is activated by low concentrations of heparin.[629] Lipoprotein lipase activity can show wide fluctuations representing an adaptive mechanism whereby plasma triglyceride fatty acids are removed from circulation according to need.[465] During postprandial triglyceride storage, the adipose tissue lipase activity is high. When triglycerides are mobilized as in starvation, lipase activity is low. This decrease in enzyme activity on the endothelial surface can result in an increased accumulation of VLDL and chylomicrons in the circulation. There are two pathological conditions connected with reduced lipoprotein lipase activity in adipose tissue: (1) uncontrolled diabetes mellitus[317,332,507] and (2) familial hyperchylomicronemia (Type I hyperlipoproteinemia).[566] In diabetes mellitus, lipase deficiency of adipose tissue is due to reduced levels of circulating insulin. Following treatment with this hormone, the enzyme activity returns to normal.[329,360] There is an interaction between lipoprotein lipase and heparin-like polysaccharides.[57]

Triglyceride lipase catalyzes the initial step in the catabolism of chylomicron and VLDL, producing diglycerides and fatty acids from triglycerides. In normal individuals, the enzyme activity is low, and heparin causes a release of triglyceride lipase from tissues, mainly from the liver. The postheparin lipolytic enzyme is activated by apoC-I, and this governs the breakdown of di- and monoglycerides. The total clearing of chylomicrons is therefore dependent on the function of the postheparin lipoprotein lipase.

Transfer of triglycerides occurs from VLDL to LDL and HDL.[464] Phospholipids also show a rapid exchange between LDL and HDL, that is independent from lecithin:cholesterol acyl transferase activity. These lipoproteins play an important role in the transfer of phosphatidylcholine into many cell structures, such as microsomes, mitochondria, and erythrocytes. The exchange is continuous and a phospholipid exchange protein participates in the process.[142,169,183,607] Free cholesterol is also readily transferred between the different lipoprotein classes. The cholesteryl ester exchange proceeds only very slowly, related to the fact that these components are deep inside the protein skeleton. Most cholesteryl esters are formed by the transfer of the fatty acids in position 2 from phosphatidylcholine to cholesterol catalyzed by lecithin: cholesterol acyl transferase (Figure 9). This enzyme elicits greater affinity to unsaturated than to saturated fatty acids. HDL and LDL are the major sources of cholesterol and phosphatidylcholine (Table 10). Large amounts of lecithin:cholesterol acyl transferase occur in the liver, with higher levels in males than in females and activity dependent on the presence of apoA-I. Lecithin:cholesterol acyl transferase deficiency, a rare hereditary disorder, causes increased plasma cholesterol and lecithin and decreased lysole-cithin and cholesteryl esters. Lipid composition of erythrocytes is abnormal, and their lifespan is reduced. LDL and HDL are very heterogenous and contain greater amounts of free cholesterol and more phosphatidylcholine than normal lipoproteins.

Lecithin:cholesterol acyl transferase (LCAT) is an extracellular enzyme produced in the liver which circulates in plasma and acts on HDL. LCAT converts lecithin and unesterified cholesterol to HDL cholesteryl ester and indirectly affects the composition of other plasma lipoproteins and plasma membranes. LCAT promotes the nonenzymatic transfer of lecithin and free cholesterol chylomicron residues and plasma membranes to HDL and the transfer of cholesterol ester from HDL to VLDL and LDL. These reactions control the levels of lecithin and free cholesterol in plasma lipoproteins and facilitate the removal of cholesterol from plasma. LCAT also plays a role in cholesterol transport within the arterial wall, removing cholesterol from arteries and other tissues.[177] Furthermore, the reaction catalyzed by LCAT represents the major source of LDL cholesteryl esters and therefore probably takes part in the deposition of extracellular lipids in fibrous plaques.[225]

LCAT has clear specificity for acyl groups bound by ester linkage to phospholipids,[225] also exerting specificity for fatty acids. The plasma enzyme transfers fatty acids in the following rates: linoleic acid > oleic acid > arachidonic acid > palmitic acid.[574] These relative rates account for the typical fatty acid composition of plasma cholesteryl esters and probably for the high proportion of cholesteryl linoleate found in atherosclerotic plaques.[225] HDL is the substrate of this enzyme, and it is activated by apoA-I, the principal apoprotein of HDL. ApoA-II partially blocks this activation, whereas apoC-I also shows some activation.

In patients with familial LCAT deficiency, high plasma concentrations of free cholesterol and relatively high amounts of free cholesterol and lecithin are found in all major lipoprotein fractions.[680] VLDL is frequently elevated, and LDL fractions are very heterogenous containing mainly free cholesterol and lecithin. HDL is even more heterogenous than LDL and also contains mainly free cholesterol and lecithin. Patients with familial LCAT deficiency generally have atherosclerosis of the abdominal aorta and the renal arteries.[297] Most cholesterol in atheromatous lesions is unesterified, and cholesteryl esters contain less linoleic acid than that found in spontaneous atheroma patients. This finding indicates that LCAT normally contributes cholesteryl esters to atherosclerotic plaques, and the reaction can influence the removal of extracellualar unesterified cholesterol and cholesterol esters from fibrous plaques.[242] The absence of LCAT does not prevent atherosclerosis, however, the incidence and severity may, however, show variations.

Enzymes for cholesteryl ester synthesis and degradation and phospholipases also are found in the arterial wall.[548] The development of the atherosclerotic plaque is characterized by the accumulation of free and esterified cholesterol. Oleate esters largely accumulate in smooth muscle cells forming inclusions. As the severity of the lesion is enhanced, the cholesteryl esters show similarity to those of LDL.[600] Although smooth muscle produces cholesterol *de novo*, the major part comes from LDL. Inside the cell, lipids and apoproteins are metabolized also by monolysosomal acid hydrolases. Free cholesterol enters the cell and becomes esterified by microsomal enzymes predominantly to oleate and synthesized *de novo*. The synthesis of cholesterol esters follows three pathways (Figure 9). Of these pathways, acyl CoA:cholesterol acyl transferase is the most active and responsible for most cholesteryl ester synthesis in atherogenesis. The esters are insoluble in water and they aggregate to form a separate phase. This process continues with continuing influx of cholesterol until cell death. During regression cholesteryl esters are hydrolyzed, and the free cholesterol leaves the cell by direct exchange with serum lipoproteins. The exchange with HDL represent the principal mechanism for the elimination of cholesterol from foam cells.[623]

Phospholipases are found in small amounts in membranes and they are relevant to atherosclerosis. Phospholipases can degrade lipoproteins in the blood or in the cell.[168,169,519]

These enzymes play a role in thrombosis through control of the synthesis of prostaglandins and thromboxanes. The action of phospholipase A_2 on phospholipid substrates leads to free fatty acids and lysophosphatidic acid. In most naturally occurring phospholipids, unsaturated fatty acids occupy position 2 of the glycerol skeleton which is cleared by phospholipase A_2. This enzyme, therefore is able to release arachidonic acid which is the immediate precursor of potent substances such as prostaglandins and thromboxanes. The other product of hydrolysis, lysophosphatide, exerts a detergent action and promotes lysis of membranes.

7. Hormonal and Pharmacologic Regulation

Triglycerides in adipose tissue are continually hydrolyzed by lipolysis and resynthetized by esterification; these processes are related to different enzymatic reactions. Nutritional, metabolic, hormonal, and pharmacologic interventions influence the regulation of these processes by acting on hydrolysis or reesterification.[106,144,179,207,210,283,402,452,454,499,625] The balance of these opposing reactions determines the amount of free fatty acid pool in adipose tissue, which is the source of plasma fatty acids, also associated with the metabolism of other tissues, such as muscle and liver. The regulation of fatty acid release, therefore, has profound effects on blood lipoprotein levels. Free fatty acids in blood may increase rapidly in response to many endogenous or environmental factors. High levels may represent the pathogenic link between risk and disease; such conditions occur in metabolic disorders such as diabetes, carbohydrate intolerance, and obesity.

Hormonal stimulation or inhibition of free fatty acid mobilization acting on different steps in the mechanism influence fatty acid plasma levels (Figure 30). The most important hormones are insulin and prostaglandins. The rate of fatty acid release from adipose tissue into the plasma is reduced by insulin, while it enhances lipogenesis (Figure 31). Insulin inhibits the activity of adipolytic lipase and thus decreases the discharge of glycerol into the circulation. The action of insulin probably depends on the amount of glucose, and glucose uptake into adipose tissue is increased.[516,565] Other hormones increase the rate of lipolysis and accelerate the release of fatty acids,[161] these include many peptide hormones such as glucagon, epinephrine, norepinephrine, vasopressin, adrenocorticotropic hormone, growth hormone, thyroid-hormone, and melanocyte-stimulating hormone. These substances activate the hormone-sensitive lipase and increase the utilization of glucose. The optimal activity of the lipolytic processes is also associated with thyroid hormones and glucocorticoids, affecting lipolysis by influencing the activity of a hormone-sensitive triglyceride lipase. There are di- and monoglyceride lipases in adipose tissue not dependent on hormones, but it is the hormone-sensitive lipase that is considered the rate-limiting enzyme in lipolysis.[332] Lipase exists in an inactive form, and cyclic AMP converts it to an active form. Glucagon, adrenocorticotrophic hormone, thyrotropic hormone, epinephrine, and norepinephrine stimulate adenyl cyclase, and lipolysis is largely dependent on the amount of cyclic AMP present in tissues. Insulin depresses the level of cyclic AMP by inhibiting adenyl cyclase activity.[360] Nicotinic acid and prostaglandin E probably act at the same site. The prominent role of insulin in the regulation of triglyceride metabolism is also related to its controlling action in diabetes mellitus.[659] Growth hormone acts in the presence of corticosteroids, and its effect is probably related to the synthesis of adipolytic triglyceride lipase. Thyroid hormones inhibit phosphodiesterase activity and raise the cyclic AMP levels which can be inhibited also by caffeine and theophylline. Therefore, they cause increased cyclic AMP levels and, consequently, a prolonged elevation of plasma free fatty acids.

8. Dietary Regulation

Plasma lipoproteins and cholesterol are largely synthesized in the liver. Thus, plasma and liver cholesterol content can be considered as a single metabolic pool. There are contradictory reports on the effects of dietary cholesterol on serum cholesterol lev-

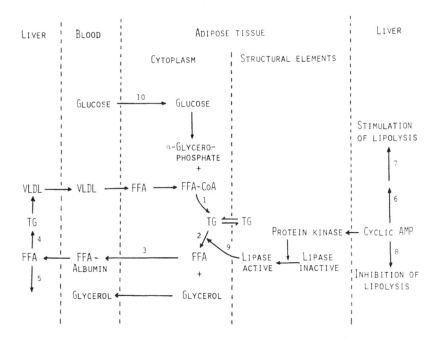

FIGURE 30. Hormonal and pharmacological regulation of fatty acid release and triglyceride metabolism. Free fatty acid concentration in the plasma is determined by the balance between esterification (1) and lipolysis (2). The mobilization of free fatty acids is dependent on the activation of hormone sensitive lipase. Activation is carried out by a protein kinase which is catalyzed by cyclic AMP. The liberated free fatty acids become bound to albumin (3), and a large fraction is taken up by the liver where it may be incorporated into triglycerides of VLDL (4) or oxidized (5). Hormonal stimulation of lipolysis can be fast (ACTH and other peptide hormones), catecholamines; (6) or delayed (glucocorticoids, thyroid hormones); (7), by increasing cyclic AMP system or decreasing fatty acid reesterification (glucocorticoids). Hormonal inhibition of lipolysis (insulin, prolactin, vasopressin, oxytocin, prostaglandins); (8), is also related to cyclic AMP. Insulin reduces fat mobilization by decreasing the activity of the hormone-sensitive lipase (9) and by promoting glucose transport (10) and triglyceride synthesis. There are many pharmacological agents with direct effect on adipose tissues (adrenergic blocking agents, nicotinic acid, salicylates, pyrazoles). Their action is probably associated with the inhibition of adenyl cyclase activity (8). The inhibitory effect of several pharmacological inhibitors is indirect, related to their action on the central nervous system, on sympathetic nerve terminals, or in blocking sympathetic ganglions.

els.[91,103,134,149,710] Some studies suggest that dietary uptake can reduce hepatic cholesterol synthesis by a feedback mechanism, leading to an overall decrease in plasma cholesterol levels. Other experiments with dietary cholesterol show variations within usual limits, indicating that the amount of cholesterol in the diet exerts little influence on the plasma cholesterol concentration. This discrepancy may be related to the fact that the equilibration of dietary cholesterol with plasma cholesterol takes several days, and several weeks with tissue cholesterol. Moreover, the catabolism of cholesterol in the liver is rapid with a half-life of several days; the total body turnover takes several weeks.

The concentration of triglycerides in the diet has also been implicated in the etiology of atherosclerosis for many years.[298,299] When dietary triglyceride content is increased, the serum cholesterol concentration is also enhanced. Saturated fatty acids and monounsaturated fatty acids elevate cholesterol levels, whereas polyunsaturated acids bring about a reduction. When the dietary intake of linoleic acid is raised above normal levels, plasma free cholesterol decreases and the proportion of cholesterol linoleate increases. The ratio of long-chain saturated acids plus the monoenoic acids contrasted with the dietary polyunsaturated fatty

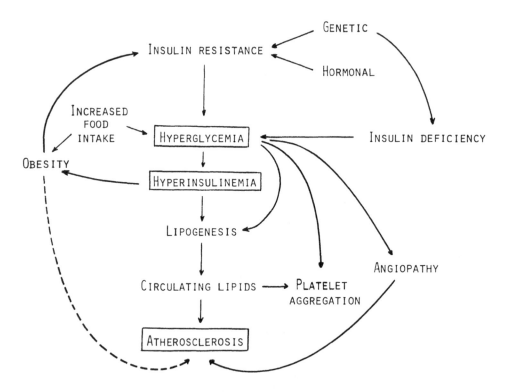

FIGURE 31.   Interrelationship between altered glucose metabolism and atherosclerosis. The association between metabolic components and hormonal regulation of carbohydrate tolerance and incidence of vascular disease reflects a form of vicious circle. Raised glucose level increases the prevalence of atherogenesis, the link being probably changes in circulating insulin level. Hyperinsulinemia favors local accumulation of triglycerides and inhibits lipogenesis. Elevated insulin level is also associated with obesity which itself may be related to atherosclerosis. Obesity causes insulin resistance which in turn raises blood glucose level. Insulin resistance also develops by the effect of hormonal and genetic factors. This may elicit insulin deficiency associated with hyperglycemia and the circle starts again.

acids determines the plasma cholesterol concentration. The mechanism by which polyunsaturated fatty acids influence the cholesterol content has not yet been elucidated. In certain animals, the increase of dietary linoleate content brings about an increased rate of cholesterol synthesis; and the rate of catabolism and removal is also accelerated to an even greater degree. The net result is that the turnover rate of plasma cholesterol is increased following a linoleate-rich diet. However, it is not known whether linoleic acid enhances excretion of cholesterol or its breakdown to bile acids.

There are some suggestions that the role of polyunsaturated fatty acids may be connected with the synthesis of prostaglandins. These compounds decrease blood pressure and also reduce platelet aggregation, among other pharmacological properties. Essential fatty acids are precursors of these compounds and their participation in prostaglandin synthesis could explain the antiatherogenic effect of unsaturated fatty acids. It is possible, that the lowering of cholesterol concentration is secondary or unrelated to the prostaglandin effect, rather than directly associated with the formation of cholesteryl esters.

Miscellaneous dietary components have been shown to be associated with the development of atherosclerosis, such as vitamin D supplementation or zinc deficiency.[179,188] Oral administration of zinc sulfate had a beneficial effect in the treatment of severe symptomatic atherosclerotic patients. Copper is antagonistic to zinc in many respects, since it enhances atherosclerosis.[653] Chromium deficiency is a causal factor in atherosclerosis, and manganese may also be involved in this disease. Cadmium has been shown to cause hypertension.

Imbalances of these trace metals may influence directly the course of cardiovascular diseases or may have a secondary role.[335,497,662]

D. ABNORMALITIES OF LIPOPROTEIN SYNTHESIS AND SECRETION
1. Genetic

Hereditary factors involving either structural or regulating genes can affect lipoprotein synthesis and degradation.[282] In Tangier's disease, HDL is significantly decreased and the reduced HDL found is mainly composed of apoA-II.[193,312] ApoA-I is reduced with slightly decreased LDL, but VLDL and fasting chylomicrons are increased. In abetalipoproteinemia, apoB is absent in the circulation. In this disease, normal VLDL and LDL are absent in the plasma, LCAT activity and cholesterol esterification are reduced, the polypeptide composition of HDL is modified. In heterozygous patients with familial hypobetalipoproteinemia there is no obvious defect of lipid transport although serum cholesterol, LDL cholesterol, and apoB concentrations are about 20 to 25% of normal. This may be caused by reduced LDL synthesis. In familial hypercholesterolemia the rate-limiting enzyme of sterol synthesis, β-hydoxy-β-methylglutaryl-CoA reductase, is suppressed.[92,95,229]

2. Fatty Liver

Acute or chronic consumption of alcohol causes the accumulation of triglycerides in the liver and increased VLDL in plasma.[29,372,376] Neutral fat accumulation reduces VLDL catabolism, and there is an increased availability of fatty acids for the synthesis of triglycerides and lipoproteins. Fatty acids may derive from the diet, from adipose tissue, or from increased hepatic fatty acid synthesis and decreased fatty acid oxidation. In patients with alcoholic hepatitis, VLDL contains apoB almost exclusively. LDL is deficient in cholesteryl esters and LCAT deficiency is severe.[451] All these changes are reversed to normal following recovery.

VLDL is mostly originated from the liver.[125,165,619] The endoplasmic reticulum plays a role in synthesis of both components, where the apoprotein originates from the rough membranes and the triglyceride from the smooth reticulum. The secretion of the VLDL particles is influenced by osmiophylic particles in the Golgi vesicles. This action is modified by perfusion of the liver with free fatty acids,[320] partial hepatectomy, administration of alcohol,[550] or corticosterone.[518] In contrast, the Golgi vesicles are essentially empty when protein synthesis is inhibited by cycloheximide,[655] or when the synthesis of apoprotein B is blocked,[486] or when the production of VLDL precursors and their transfer to the endoplasmic reticulum is inhibited by orotic acid.[468,483] In these cases, fat accumulates in the cell with the exception of cycloheximide treatment. Thus, the induction of fatty liver is the consequence of an impairment of the balance between transport of triglyceride precursors and the metabolism or transport of triglycerides as VLDL into plasma. This impairment can be caused by acute ethanol intoxication, cortisone or cathecholamines. These agents increase VLDL production and release into the blood. However, fat accumulates in the liver due to defects in transport.[36]

Many fatty livers are associated with the reduction of protein synthesis, and due to the depression of apolipoprotein synthesis, the liver is unable to export triglycerides. These conditions include the effects of most hepatotoxins. In fatty liver produced by orotic acid feeding in rats, the bulk of the stored lipid is found in the cisternae of the endoplasmic reticulum.[468] Lipid inclusions, also called liposomes, contain many of the apolipoproteins found in VLDL. Consequently, both VLDL and LDL in plasma are reduced to negligible level.[469] HDL is present, but also reduced.

In Menkes' disease the synthesis of lipids, lipoproteins, and apolipoproteins is modified.[68] In hepatocellular failure serum apoB levels are considerably altered.[637,646]

IV. RISK FACTORS

A number of variables, some related to the patient and some to his environment, have been implicated as risk factors that might promote the development of atherosclerosis.[10,105,294,324] Risk factors represent various abnormalities. Habits,[403] physical activities,[364,385,496,514,481] traits, stress factors,[153,236] and other conditions[235,237,482,520] cause a significant increase in the susceptibility of an individual to atherosclerotic disease, usually associated with the premature development of lesions and early onset of clinical symptoms.[154,235,237,631] The genetic epidemiology of coronary heart disease has also been investigated.[114] Identification of the potentially reversible risk factors is important since significant progress in controlling clinical arterial disease can only be made if severe atherosclerosis can be prevented.[616]

A. AGE

Complicated atherosclerotic lesions and clinical manifestations increase with advancing age.[235,495,672,502] This factor has the strongest and most consistent association with vascular lesions. It is probable that continuous exposure to various etiological factors and not to an intrinsic aging process of the arteries is the cause. Lesions appear in the aorta during the first decade of life, in the coronary arteries in the second, and in central arteries in the third.[67] The effect of increasing age on the wall of the artery may be linked with increases of blood glucose levels which are more or less inevitable consequences of aging.[2,529]

B. SEX

Atherosclerotic lesions are far more common and usually more extensive in men than in women.[15,285,397] Males also have more lesions in the coronary arteries and more frequent clinical coronary heart disease during the middle decades of life. Premenopausal women are likely to be relatively free of severe coronary disease compared with men until late into middle age. Estrogens seem to be the prime reason for this difference, since sex differences gradually diminish and in the sixties, heart attacks strike women almost as frequently as men. Controversies about age relationships have also been reported.[615] Serum cholesterol levels are not essentially different between young men and women. Large differences exist, however, in the distribution of cholesterol between the various lipoprotein fractions (Table 10). Estrogens do not lower serum cholesterol content, but increase the concentration in α-lipoproteins with a shift of cholesterol from LDL to the HDL fraction and reduction of cholesterol:phospholipid ratio as well.[402]

C. RACE

Striking geographical variations in the prevalence of clinical coronary artery disease correspond roughly to the distribution of various ethnic groups.[28,58,160,397,412,528,641] Detailed comparisons among various race goups in New Orleans, LA show that atherosclerosis is more prevalent in the white population than in blacks.[394] Blacks also have less extensive lesions than whites. Sex differences in blacks are not as marked as in whites. In Durban, South Africa, Bantus have less atherosclerosis than Asian Indians.[456] The genetic or racial effect may be biased to a certain extent by the socioeconomic differences or cultural factors which exist between the race groups evaluated in these studies. Moreover, large intragroup variations suggest that racial background alone does not confer immunity or increased susceptibility to atherosclerosis. Studies on migrant populations show greater influences due to environmental factors. Japanese living in California have a higher frequency of ischemic heart disease.[334] Similarly, recently emigrated Yemenite Jews showed lower prevalence of ischemic heart disease than those who lived in Israel for more than 15 years.[641] Variations were found in cholesterol autooxidation, health status, and arteriosclerosis in developed countries.[494]

D. DIET

Several investigations indicate some contradiction on dietary influences.[133,166,171,292,356,536,656,667] Among various populations, atherosclerotic lesions show a correlation between the fat content of the diet and the levels of serum cholesterol. No positive association was found between lesions and dietary lipids within a population.[467,514,522] Other studies suggest no parallelism between dietary triglyceride levels and atherosclerotic lesions. Recent studies in Oslo, Norway reveal that although individual variations are wide, mean values for raised lesions increases with increasing cholesterol levels.[606] In Puerto Rico, similar data were obtained between serum cholesterol levels and atherosclerosis.[210] The presence of polyunsaturated fat in diet influences plasma lipids and lipoproteins.[70]

E. OBESITY

Excess weight is considered as a secondary risk factor in coronary heart disease.[254,426,547] The effects of obesity may become manifest through concommitant hyperlipidemia, hypertension, or diabetes. More recent studies, however, did not support a strong direct association between the extent and severity of atherosclerosis and obesity.[490]

F. SMOKING

Smoking alone does not appear to lead to the development of coronary heart disease, but in heavy smokers the habit contributes to the severity of atherosclerotic conditions.[151,257,292,338,353,490] Lesions are usually more extensive than in nonsmokers.[212,420] Males between 40 and 50 years of age and who smoke more than 15 cigarettes a day, triple the risk of dying from ischemic heart disease; those who smoke more than 40 cigarettes per day have a risk five times greater.[151,257] The mechanism of how smoking mediates the increased risk to atherosclerosis is not clear. In those who stop smoking, the risk of coronary heart disease decreases quickly and within a few years such risk is not greater than in the matched nonsmoking population.[237,510] As a result of smoking, fatty streaks progress to raised lesions.[642]

Constituents of the cigarette smoke are considered to play a pathogenic role, and carbon monoxide has been suggested as a mediator of intimal injury.[13,488] Possible hypersensitivity to tobacco antigens was also proposed.[260] When volunteers were inoculated with a glycoprotein of 1800 Da molecular weight, an immediate cutaneous hypersensitivity developed. The glycoprotein contains rutin, closely related to quercetin, a compound which activates Hageman factor.[46] The tobacco glycoprotein acting through the Hageman factor shortens partial thromboplastin, and in time, it activates plasminogen and generates bradykinin. Rutin or similar constituents in cigarette smoke cause an inflammatory reaction which injures the arterial intima thus resulting in an enhanced growth of atherosclerotic plaques or initiation of thrombus formation.[46,151]

G. DIABETES MELLITUS

Diabetes constitutes a potent risk factor. This disease has additive effects on the severity of atherosclerosis (Table 11).[156,178,211,529,543,683] Particularly, in the most common form, mild maturity-onset diabetes provides significantly enhanced risk. Diabetics have atherosclerotic disease more frequently, more prematurely, and more advanced than nondiabetics.[129] The effective control of diabetes results in delaying of atherosclerotic complications. Conversely, men with manifestations of atherosclerosis exhibit more frequent glucose tolerance abnormalities.[206,437] Plasma insulin response to intravenous glucose injections is different between normal and hypertriglyceridemic subjects. Macrovascular complications of diabetes show an association with differing dietary, metabolic, and clinical risk factors of atherosclerosis.[482]

The mechanism of action of diabetes may be correlated with: (1) increase of the extent of atherosclerosis within the arterial bed, (2) acceleration of the rate of plaque growth and

TABLE 11
Relation between Diabetes or Gout and Death Associated with Arteriovascular Events

Diagnosis and test		Mortality rate			
		Vascular renal disease	Coronary heart disease	Sudden death	Stroke
Normal		75	52	26	19
Suspect or definite diabetes		149	108	22	41
1 H Glucose	< 205 mg/dl	24	15	9	6
	≥ 205	42	42	20	0
Uric acid	< 5.0 mg/dl	54	38	12	15
	5.0 — 6.9	58	35	19	17
	≥ 7.0	112	72	32	23

Note: Subjects were men aged 40 to 59, free of definite coronary heart disease in 1958. Diagnosis and primary tests were carried out in 1958 and followed long-term without systematic intervention. The data represent age adjusted death rate/1000. Further tests were carried out: diabetes, between 1958 to 1970; glucose tolerance test, between 1965 to 1970; uric acid test, between 1962 to 1970.[616]

greater tendency for necrosis and thrombosis, (3) microangiopathic changes, (4) changes in platelet function or in fibrinolytic action, and (5) changes in susceptibility of underperfused tissues. Increased incidence of fatty streaks was found on the intimal surface of vessels indiabetics,[529] and raised lesions within the aorta and the coronary arteries are significantly increased in diabetics. Animal experiments have shown that ^{14}C-glucose or ^{14}C-acetate are incorporated into aortic lipids of diabetic rats in greater amounts when insulin was not administered.[386]

In uncontrolled juvenile diabetes, plasma concentrations of triglycerides are high and can be reduced to normal levels by insulin treatment. Oral antidiabetic agents are not effective in restoring lipid levels to normal. Obesity, associated with insulin-controlled diabetes, causes hypertriglyceridemia. In adult-onset diabetes the relationship with increased plasma triglycerides is not conclusive. More recently, it was found that HDL concentrations are significantly lower in maturity-onset diabetics.[329] Diabetes modifies thromboxane B2 formation in clotting whole blood.[49]

The effect of diabetes on atherosclerosis may represent a metabolic association, where the relationship between hyperglycemia and atherosclerosis is largely due to a link between glucose levels as a consequence of hormonal and metabolic deregulation,[178,437] causing increased incidence of atherosclerotic arterial disease.[161,332,547] The blood glucose level-arterial disease relationship is associated with changes in circulating insulin levels and lipid metabolism in the blood and/or in various tissues including the arterial wall (Figure 31).

In contrast to the effect of elevated serum glucose levels on lipid metabolism, fatty acids in blood interfere with intracellular glucose metabolism (Figure 32). There are three lipid fractions which readily enter tissue metabolism: chylomicrons, VLDL binding amounts of triglycerides, and the free fatty acid-albumin complex. Fatty acids are released from these lipids and the increased fatty acids compete with glucose because they are preferentially utilized with respect to glucose. Subsequently, the action of insulin on glucose metabolism is inhibited. In insulin deficient diabetics, glucose utilization is reduced despite hyperglycemia, while plasma fatty acid utilization is increased and due to accelerated turnover rates, high levels of lipids accumulate, constituting an additional risk to the atherosclerotic patient.

H. HYPERTENSION

Atherosclerosis is usually associated with arterial hypertension, although race and age differences obscure the comparisons between hypertensive and normotensive pa-

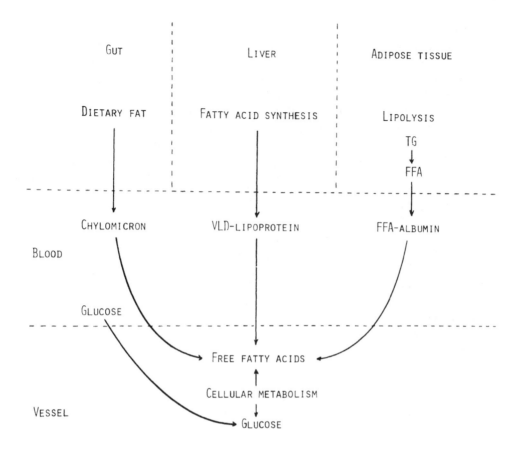

FIGURE 32.   Interference between blood lipids and the metabolism of cellular glucose.

tients.[135,160,212,327,335,379,529] Elevated systemic blood pressure is an important risk factor for premature coronary and cerebrovascular disease. Hypertension is arbitrarily defined as systolic arterial blood pressure greater than 140 mmHg together with diastolic pressure over 90 mmHg. When both systolic and diastolic blood pressures are considered together, men with hypertension are at greater risk of heart disease than normotensive men of the same age.[325,473] The diastolic measurement seems to be more important, since the elevation of diastolic pressure without the elevation of systolic pressure is associated with more extensive lesions. Atherosclerosis occurs only in parts of the vascular system which is perfused at high pressure. Lesions are not found in the pulmonary arterial tree except in cases of long-standing hypertension. Hypertension is additive to other major risk factors such as hypercholesterolemia and cigarette smoking.[456,649]

The effect of hypertension on vascular complications may include disturbances in flow pattern, causing endothelial injury.[425] High levels of catecholamines and other vasoactive substances increase endothelial permeability and mediate the entry of lipids and other plasma constituents into the arterial wall. The production of prostaglandins is associated with hypertension.[671] Moreover, the induction of high blood pressure in rats and rhesus monkeys causes significant increase of arterial smooth muscle lysosomal hydrolases, which reverted to normal when the blood pressure was restored to normal. The lysosomal changes are probably secondary to the mechanical actions of hypertension. Significant rise in pressure and rheologic and metabolic consequences in the arterial tree constitute the dominant factors in hypertension-related atherosclerotic lesions.

I. ARTERIOSCLEROSIS

Arteriosclerosis is usually associated with arterial hypertension.[222,294] The causes of hypertension can be: (1) nonspecific renal failure, (2) renal neoplasm and ischemia, (3) hyperactive tumor of the adrenal cortex or medulla, (4) complicated pregnancy, and (5) obesity. Arteriosclerosis affects the kidney more than any other organ, but the most important complications of hypertension involve the heart. Hypertension promotes the development of coronary atherosclerosis and subsequent myocardial infarction by increased workload to the heart and increased peripheral resistance. In response to this increased output demand the heart undergoes hypertrophy, and it dilates when a critical level is reached. Eventually heart failure ensues, the most common cause of death in hypertensive patients. Reduced heart function decreases the renal blood flow and filtration potentiating the vicious circle. Patients with hypertension can be controlled by means of medication, and most complications of hypertensive cardiovascular disease are thus avoided. However, some of the drugs used can be toxic and cause severe side effects. Antihypertensive agents can be phenyl piperazine derivatives, or β-adrenoceptor blockers, among others. Cardiotonic agents are commonly used in heart failure to increase the contractile force of the myocardium. It is not unusual to add agents to control the rhythm since electric disturbances are usually present.

J. HYPERURICEMIA AND GOUT

Persons suffering from hyperuricemia or gout are found to have also an increased risk of premature coronary heart disease or stroke (Table 11).[81] Nutritional and pharmacologic therapy can correct hyperuricemia, thus retarding the development of sclerotic lesions.

Other diseases which are accompanied by prolonged elevation of LDL and VLDL in the blood or with a shift of cholesterol between LDL and HDL proteins, such as hypothyroidism, lipid nephrosis, and hyperlipemia, are frequently associated with premature or more severe atherosclerosis.[154,239]

V. PHENOTYPING

Phenotyping is the most accepted method for diagnosing various types of hyperlipidemia.[43,195,197] Noninvasive techniques for the assessment of atherosclerosis have been recently suggested.[69]

High speed centrifugation, or electrophoresis in certain conditions, has been applied for the separation of various lipoproteins. Ultracentrifugation separates lipoprotein fractions according to their density. During electrophoresis lipoprotein particles move according to their electric charge, and the migration provides a characteristic separation.

These semiquantitative screening methods demonstrate the presence of chylomicrons in a fasting sample if it is due to any abnormalities, and the appearance of α- and β-lipoproteins whether or not they are present in excessive amounts. The various methods have been simplified[195,196,273] and accordingly, five different phenotypes may be distinguished (Figure 33). The more common hyperlipoproteinemic phenotypes II, III, and IV predispose to the development of premature and severe atherosclerotic disease.

Chylomicrons are present in the plasma in excessive amounts but the lipoprotein bands are normal in Type I hyperlipoproteinemia or familial lipoprotein lipase deficiency, due to molecular defects of lipoprotein lipase activity.[464] This disorder is associated with removal of exogenous or dietary fat from the plasma. The elevated triglyceride levels are probably due to the inability to clear chylomicrons resulting from low plasma postheparin lipoprotein lipase activity (Figure 34). The activity of other lipases is apparently normal. This condition may be corrected therefore by reducing the dietary intake of fat. High carbohydrate diets can also increase VLDL due to conversion of carbohydrate to lipids in the liver.

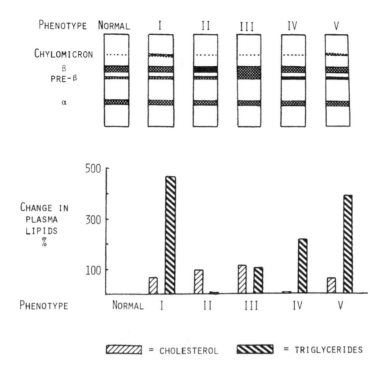

FIGURE 33.   Electrophoretic patterns of lipoproteins and cholesterol and triglyceride levels of plasma. These parameters are applied for the diagnosis of different types of atherosclerosis in patients.[43,195]

In Type II familial hypercholesterolemia, due to the deficiency or absence of LDL membrane receptor function, the plasma cholesterol concentrations are raised;[94] fasting triglyceride levels are normal or only slightly elevated, and the plasma is therefore clear. The β-lipoprotein band and α-lipoproteins and LDL receptors are normal, but as a result of LDL overproduction β-lipoprotein levels are increased. Postheparin lipoprotein lipase activity is also normal. Lipid deposition is common in tissues, leading to xanthoma or atheroma. Type II pattern may be secondary as a result of hypothyroidism. Reduction of dietary cholesterol and triglyceride is used for treatment. This phenotype can be subdivided into two categories. Type IIa is characterized by high plasma cholesterol levels, with triglyceride mostly within normal limits. The increased cholesterol synthesis is associated with reduced receptor binding leading to practically unlimited cholesterol synthesis. Milder forms are due to dietary causes, and severe forms are associated with genetic abnormalities manifested by xanthomas of the skin or tendons.[253] In Type IIb phenotype the β-lipoproteins and cholesterol are elevated, while triglyceride varies from normal to increased levels. In some cases this hyperlipidemia shows a familial origin, as in patients exhibiting the same pattern but with moderate elevation of β-lipoproteins. This type probably represents several different disorders, some of which are also due to genetic abnormalities. The Type IIb disorder is sensitive to caloric intake restriction and balanced composition of the diet.

In familial dysbetalipoproteinemia or Type III lipoprotein disorder, remnant lipoproteins accumulate in plasma. This is due to substitution of cysteine for arginine in apoE.[479] Plasma concentration of cholesterol and triglycerides are increased; the plasma appears turbid. The electrophoretogram shows an elevated β-lipoprotein band extended diffusely into the pre-β-lipoprotein zone. Since apoE is essential for the efficient clearance of chylomicrons and VLDL remnants from the plasma,[172] affected individuals have highly elevated levels of these lipoproteins in their bloodstream. The abnormality of the β-lipoprotein band is related to an abnormal triglyceride content many time greater than that found in normal β-lipoproteins.

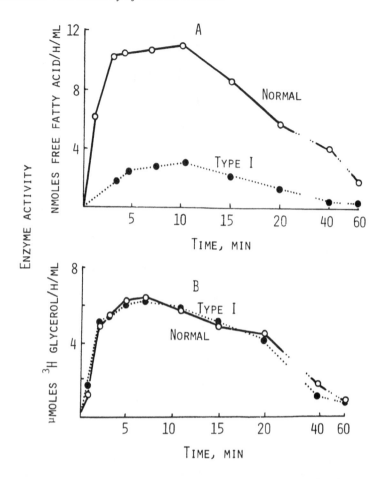

FIGURE 34.   Lipase activities of a normal and type I hyperlipoproteinemic patient. Enzyme activity is measured in plasma using adequate substrates (A) glyceryl
[1-^{14}C] trioleate:triglyceride lipase or (B) [^{3}H] glyceryl-monooleate:monoglyceride
hydrolase, after intravenous injection of heparin, 100 units/kg body weight.[282,566]

Postheparin lipoprotein lipase activity is low. Xanthomas and other clinical signs of atherosclerosis are present.[253] Low cholesterol and unsaturated fatty acid diets are usually advised.

In Type IV hyperlipidemia or familial hypertriglyceridemia there is a lipoprotein overproduction or reduced catabolism.[478,586] Due to this molecular defect, plasma VLDL are
increased. Triglyceride concentrations are also greatly elevated due to increased endogenous
production.[453] Plasma cholesterol is sometimes raised in proportion to the hypertriglyceridemia, and hence, the plasma may be turbid. Marked increase of the pre-β-lipoprotein band
is the characteristic change in the electrophoretogram. In the congenital form of this type
inadequate amounts of VLDL are available. In secondary form it is also found in connection
with obesity, maturity onset diabetes, alcoholism, or as a side effect of oral contraceptive
intake.

Type V hyperlipemia or familial apoC-II deficiency shows various molecular defects.
Two specific forms have been estabished: (1) ApoC-II deficiency is connected with the
defective clearance of triglyceride-containing particles from plasma[83] and (2) sequence abnormality in apoA-I producing gross hypertriglyceridemia.[59] It is classified as a mixed
lipoprotein abnormality showing a complex lipoprotein pattern. VLDL and chylomicrons
are the major lipoproteins accumulating in plasma.[583] Plasma cholesterol and triglyceride
levels are raised, and triglycerides exceed cholesterol concentrations. The plasma is invar-

iably turbid, and an elevated pre-β band and the presence of chylomicrons on the electrophoretogram characterize the disorder. Xanthomas occur frequently, usually the glucose tolerance test is abnormal due to obesity or preexisting diabetes. The association with pancreatitis has also been reported.

VI. IMMUNOLOGICAL ASPECTS OF ATHEROSCLEROSIS

A relationship was established between circulating immune complexes, immunoglobulins, complement, antibodies to dietary antigens and cholesterol, and lipoprotein levels in patients with occlusive coronary lesions.[42] Recently, some correlation was found between the death rate due to ischemic heart disease and the frequency of HLA_8 and haptotype 1-8.[412] HLA_8 frequency and serum cholesterol levels are correlated, and the high mortality rate from ischemic heart disease and high serum cholesterol levels in Finland may be connected with the combination of HLA_8 and W_{15} antigens. These various histocompatibility genes determine the pattern of immune response and HLA_8. It is linked to genes that predispose several autoimmune diseases such as chronic active hepatitis, juvenile-onset diabetes mellitus, Graeves' disease, and Addison's disease.

In some instances, immunization can induce arteriopathies.[337,370] Injury to the arterial tissue results from repeated injections of antigens, and fresh histological lesions are formed in the arterial wall due to trapping of the soluble antigen-antibody complexes.[126,215]

The subsequent accumulation of these complexes in arteries is widespread, mainly involving small capillaries. Immune complexes, however, also deposit in the coronary arteries and aorta, at sites where hydrodynamic conditions are favorable.[339]

In experimental conditions, the early lesions are destructive, showing severe changes inthe elastic structure of the wall of the vessels containing little or no lipid. It is possible to induce atherosclerotic plaques in rabbits by the combination of cholesterol containing diet and immunization.[45,628,635]

This may indicate that the immunization process induces an injury to the artery, and subsequent abnormal metabolic conditions lead to the secondary development of atherosclerosis. The production of the lesions is attributed to the penetration of the immune complex into the arterial wall. In some cases the sensitization process may incude antiartery or antielastin antibodies or hyperlipidemia and autoimmune hyperlipidemia.[39-41,44,45,139,618]

Autoimmune hyperlipidemia is a metabolic disease in which the lipolysis of lipoproteins is inhibited by circulating autoantibodies.[39] This disorder is the result of disturbed immunoglobulin synthesis and may coexist with rheumatoid arthritis, systemic lupus erythematosus, myeloma, lymphoma, and nephrotic syndrome.[216] Often, ischemic diseases are associated with autoimmune hyperlipidemia, but genuine atherosclerosis is the most frequent complication of this disorder. The hyperlipidemia represents the major factor in the development of atherosclerosis, where circulating lipoprotein-immunoglobulin complexes potentiate the severity of the sclerotic changes.

Different types of autoantibodies can cause autoimmune hyperlipidemia. The type of hyperlipidemia induced at the site of action in the lipolytic process shows variations.[40,42] The two major types include autoimmune hyperlipidemia induced with (1) antilipoprotein antibodies or (2) antilipoprotein lipase antibodies. In the antilipoprotein type, lipolysis is inhibited by antibodies blocking the surface of lipoproteins. The hyperlipoproteinemia can be Type IIa, III, or V. The metabolism of ingested lipids is reduced in these conditions as indicated by fat tolerance tests. Postheparin lipase activity is usually normal but spontaneous agglutination of serum particles often occurs.[433]

In the antienzyme type of autoimmune hyperlipidemia, the inhibition of lipolysis is due to antibodies that interfere with (1) lipase activation, (2) lipase function, or (3) lipase synthesis. The hypolipoproteinemia may be type I, IV, or V. There is no agglutination, fat tolerance tests are abnormal, and postheparin lipase activity is decreased.

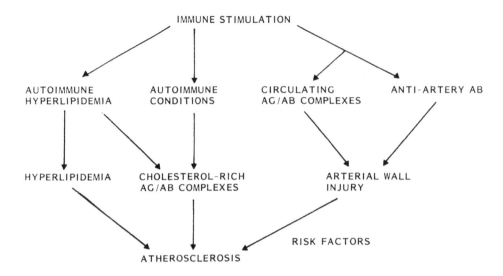

FIGURE 35.   Mechanisms of immunological production of atherosclerosis. Hyperlipidemia by anti-immune
reactions alone can be atherogenic by transporting excess amounts of lipid-rich macromolecules through the
artery. (1) Cholesterol-rich antigen-antibody complexes can cause direct damage on arteries and the overflow
of lipid containing macromolecules occurs secondarily. (2) Immune inductions produce circulating antigen-
antibody complexes or anti-artery antibody which cause an arterial wall damage, and associated risk factors
potentiate the development of atherosclerosis (3).

Several pathogenic sequences can be traced leading to arterial wall disease by immunogenic mechanisms. Immune reactions cause specific molecular interactions with high
affinity, and the disturbed flow of macromolecules through the arterial wall finally results
in the atherogenic lesion. Arterial lesions may be secondary to the increase of circulating
lipoproteins induced by the antienzyme type autoimmune hyperlipidemia. In this case,
atherosclerosis is the result of the increase lipid level, and there is no immune reaction in
the vessel walls. On the other hand, the arterial lesion may be secondary to the infiltration
of cholesterol-rich antigen-antibody complexes. In this case, atherosclerosis is the consequence of a variety or a sequence of autoimmune reactions, where antigen-antibody complexes are of different composition, some containing antielastin or antiartery antibodies. In
this case, the antigen-antibody complexes cause immunological injury to the arterial wall
preceding atherosclerosis (Figure 35).[139]

VII. ACTION OF ANTIATHEROSCLEROTIC DRUGS

Atherosclerosis, being a multifunctional disease requires several approaches to treatment.[174] Prevention with balanced diet, weight reduction, and cessation of smoking are
important in reducing mortality trends with severe manifestations. Drugs play a role in the
profilaxis and treatment. Drugs given attention in the therapy of atherosclerosis are (1)
hypolipidemic agents, (2) drugs affecting coagulation, in particular antiaggregating agents,
and (3) other agents which influence certain phases of the atherogenesis process, such as
heparin and other mucopolysaccharides, heparinoids, phthalasines, pyridinol-carbonate, and
other drugs. Recent studies have evolved from finding drugs affecting plasma lipid levels
to the modulation of lipoprotein profiles or to the prevention of ischemic heart disease.

A. HYPOLIPIDEMIC DRUGS

Since primarily cholesterol elevation has been implicated in atherosclerosis, attempts to
control this disease have been concentrated mainly on cholesterol-reducing drugs (Figure
36).[90,341,527] The endogenous production of cholesterol is the major contributor to the body

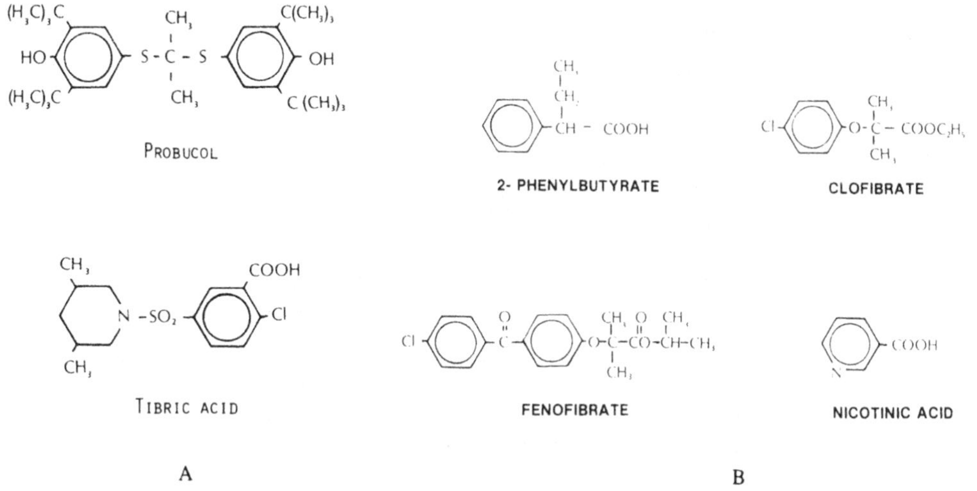

FIGURE 36.   Structure of some hypolipidemic drugs.

cholesterol pool. Thus, the possibility of controlling cholesterol synthesis by pharmacological means can be effective, and some types of hyperlipoproteinemia can be influenced. Cholesterol-lowering agents act by interference with one or more steps in the metabolic pathway of cholesterol. Accordingly, the application of drugs is based on (1) inhibition of cholesterol biosynthesis, (2) interference with cholesterol and bile acid absoption from the bile, (3) agents with predominant action on plasma lipid transport, (4) indirect hormone action on cholesterol synthesis, and (5) indirect metabolic action on plasma lipids.

Elevated triglycerides also represent a characteristic symptom of coronary heart disease parallel to elevated cholesterol. Therefore, the reduction of abnormal serum triglyceride levels has become another aim of drug therapy.[111,411] In most cases, it is difficult to envisage any structural relationship between the antiatherosclerotic drugs and intermediates of cholesterol biosynthesis (Figure 37). Their mechanism of action is therefore related to inhibition of enzymes by blocking active sites or to competition with cofactors.

Many drugs inhibit cholesterol synthesis, such as 2-phenylbutyric acid and derivatives.[19,64,132,198,461,541,542,626,700] Application of this drug in clinical trials has resulted in toxic manifestations. Derivatives of this compound reduce acetyl-CoA formation. The currently employed clofibrate has some effect on cholesterol biosynthesis at the level of 3-hydroxy-3-methylglutaryl-CoA reductase.[21] There are some other drugs blocking cholesterol synthesis at other steps. Benzmalacene (*N*-[1-methyl-2,3-*bis*(*p*-chlorophenyl)propyl]maleamic acid or 4-[[2,3-*bis*⟨4-chlorophenyl⟩-1-methylpropyl]amino]-4-oxo-2-butenoic acid) inhibits the incorporation of mevalonic acid into cholesterol in rat liver homogenates. However, benzamalacene given to animals has a toxic effect and results in liver damage.[207,304] This drug has been among the first compounds used clinically. It is structurally related to a series of nonsteroidal estrogens and estogen antagonists.

One of the most widely studied compounds is triparanol (4-chloro-α-[4-[2-⟨diethylamino⟩ethoxy]phenyl]-⟨4-methylphenyl⟩benzeneethanol, MER-29).[17,71,192] Triparanol lowers blood cholesterol by inhibiting 75% or more of the endogenous synthesis. It blocks the reduction of the 24, 25 double bond in the steroid side chain, leading to the accumulation of 25-dehydrocholesterol, as it is commonly known, desmosterol.[627] Desmosterol replaces cholesterol in lipoproteins, and therefore, triparanol therapy leads to the accumulation of the precursor compound in the blood in place of cholesterol. The lipoprotein pattern returns to normal in Type II patients but not in Type IV. Probucol has no consistent action on lipogenesis in experiments, but apparently decreases endogenous cholesterol synthesis and intestinal reabsorption.

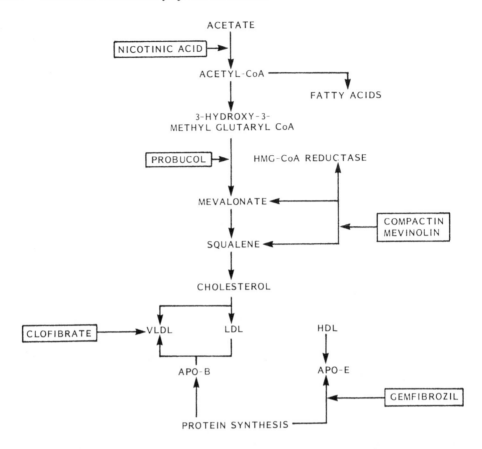

FIGURE 37.   Effect of hypolipidemic drugs on cholesterol biosynthesis and lipoprotein assembly. The boxes indicate the most recently established mechanism of action of each compound.

Tibric acid reduces triglycerides in Type IV patients, it causes marginal decrease in Type IIb, but has no effect on cholesterol level.[65,591] This drug stimulates mitochondrial α-glycerophosphate dehydrogenase in the liver. α-Glycerophosphate as a fatty acid acceptor is oxidized by this enzyme, and therefore, the rate of triglyceride synthesis is lowered. Tibric acid is not in use due to adverse reactions observed in clinical trials.

Fenofibrate (1-methylethyl 2[4-⟨4-chlorobenzoyl⟩phenoxy]-2-methyl propanoate, Procetofen) has been recently applied in human therapy in Europe. This drug lowers both serum cholesterol and triglycerides. Animal experiments demonstrated that the drug may enhance cholesterol transfer from the tissues by activating HDL.[89]

B. PREVENTION OF CHOLESTEROL ABSORPTION

The effect of dietary cholesterol on serum cholesterol has not been unequivocally established. Some reports indicated that dietary cholesterol contributes to elevated serum levels. Inhibition of cholesterol absorption is, therefore, an important route for control. Experiments have shown that various sterols of plant origin, such as β-sitosterol, stigmasterol, and ergosterol, can prevent hypercholesterolemia and atherosclerosis.[288,634] β-Sitosterol has been the most frequently applied steroid; administration of large daily amounts reduce cholesterol and LCAT activity; a fall in β-lipoprotein level is also observed.[677] Side effects are minimal, but the drug has an unpleasant taste and is no longer commonly prescribed. β-Sitosterol competes with cholesterol for the site of esterification.

Absorption of cholesterol only occurs in the presence of bile acids. If bile acid uptake is blocked, this effect will result in reduced cholesterol absorption.[238,240,268,300,447,485,673,691]

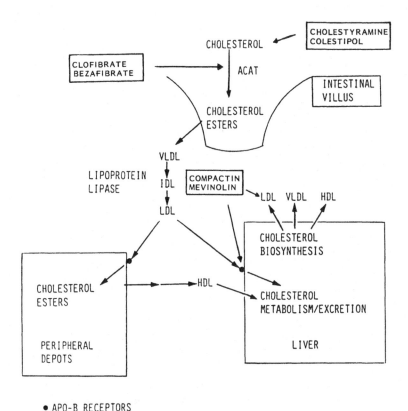

FIGURE 38.   Site of action of hypolipidemic drugs in cholesterol metabolism and binding to carrier proteins. Effects on target organs, including liver, peripheral depots, and intestines, are indicated.

Various anion exchange resins have been used to decrease cholesterol intake from the intestine. Cholestyramine or DDAE Sephadex exert hypocholesterolemic action by removing bile acids in the form of insoluble complexes which are then excreted in the stool.[638] Cholestyramine increases the turnover of bile acids at the expense of cholesterol (Figure 38). The major disadvantage of this therapy is not only the bulk, but resins are not specific absorbents for bile acids preventing at the same time other compounds from being taken up. Observed side effects with resins mainly include constipation. Linoleamides are also inhibitors of cholesterol absorption. One of the most potent representatives of these drugs, moctamide, inhibits dietary induced hypercholesterolemia.[636]

Clinical manifestations of atherosclerosis are rare in women before menopause. In view of this observation, estrogens have been used with some success in males. Long term studies showed sustained depression of lipids, but the beneficial effect on myocardial infarction in males was slight to nonexistent. Feminizing side effects obviously limited the use of this substance on a wide basis.

Related nonsteroid estrogens have been tested which exert hypolipemic action without estrogenic side effects. One successful compound was Colargil (hexestrol bis (β-diethyl aminoethyl ether) which had excellent coronary vasodilator properties. Prolonged administration of this drug reduced cholesterol levels, but induced severe phospholipidosis, including the liver.[147,148] Hence its application has been banned after epidemic proportions. Side effects were seen in Japan. The relation between hexestrol diethylaminoethyl ether and estradiol is seen in Figure 39. A detailed study using conjugated equine estrogen resulted in a significant increase of ischemic and thrombotic episodes.[130]

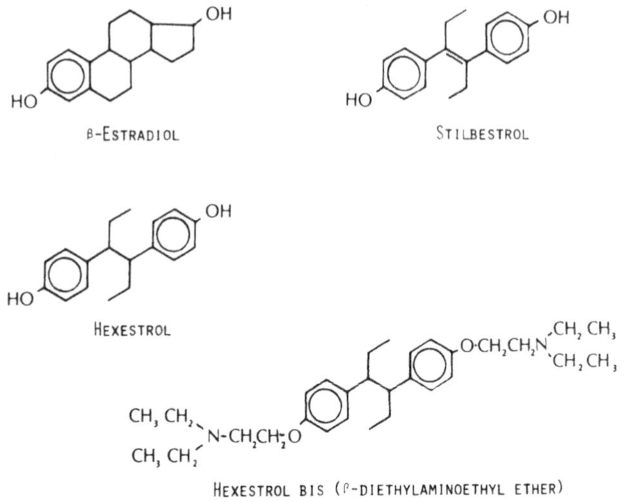

β-ESTRADIOL

STILBESTROL

HEXESTROL

HEXESTROL BIS (β-DIETHYLAMINOETHYL ETHER)

FIGURE 39. Structural relationship betwen estradiol and hexestrol bis(β-diethylaminoethyl ether).

The action of thyroid hormones on serum cholesterol levels has been known for many years. Hyperthyroidism is associated with hypocholesterolemia, whereas hypothyroidism increased cholesterol levels. The application of thyroid hormones as drugs has been of limited value since they increase basal metabolism and the rate of oxygen consumption of the myocardium, aggravating the symptoms of coronary or myocardial insufficiency. Structurally related compounds have been developed and D-thyroxine and choloxine are available.[131,452]

In the case of D-thyroxine, plasma cholesterol and LDL protein level can be lowered. The action on basal metabolic rate, however, is only slight. The mechanism of action of thyroid therapy may be associated with effects on cholesterol degradation to bile acids. Occasionally, however, some patients exhibited severe anginal attacks indicating an elevated metabolic requirement of the myocardium and suggesting caution in the administration of this drug. Moreover, treatment with D-thyroxine may lead to enhanced incidence of ischemic and thrombotic complications.[131]

Many other drugs have also been tested in the management of hyperlipidemias.[22,243,423,674] Nicotinic acid has been used successfully by a large number of investigators. There are several suggestions for its mechanism.[11,175,228,430,447,489] Cholesterol synthesis requires CoA and nicotinic acid may reduce the amount of the available coenzyme for cholesterol production. Nicotinic acid dilates blood vessels and increases circulation; its competition with nicotinamide nucleotides and participation in cholesterol biosynthesis, or its effects on cyclic AMP production provide some explanation for its actions. Considering the results of many attempts to synthesize a potent antiatherosclerotic drug which blocks cholesterol synthesis, transport, and deposition into the vessels, as well as the results of many trials, successes, and failures of atherosclerosis therapy, it may be that combination treatments may provide a better way of controlling the disease (Figure 40).

C. MODIFICATION OF LIPOPROTEIN DISTRIBUTION

A reciprocal change has been observed between VLDL- and LDL-cholesterol following carbohydrate restriction or drug treatment or in combination with or without the addition of nicotinic acid.[111] Among these circumstances, patients develop increased LDL cholesterolemia if their starting cholesterol level is lower than 150 mg/dl and HDL in the normal range; if the starting cholesterol level is higher than 150 mg/dl, the opposite may occur.

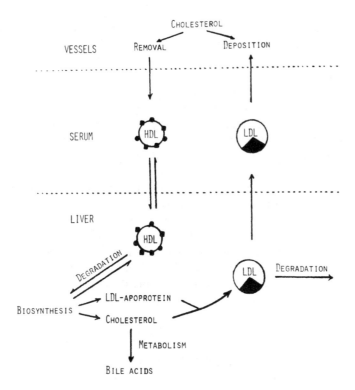

FIGURE 40.   Scheme for possible drug interactions in the mechanism of
lipoprotein metabolism. Several drugs bring about a reduction in the biosynthesis of cholesterol and apoproteins of low density lipoproteins and an increase
in the biosynthesis of high density lipoproteins in the liver. Consequently, this
results in an enhanced mobilization of cholesterol from the periphery by a
transport action associated with the high density lipoproteins. When the breakdown of low density lipoproteins is increased; this also raises the metabolism
of cholesterol to bile acids. On the other hand, some drugs enhance the
degradation of low density lipoproteins and the metabolism of cholesterol to
bile acids. These drugs may, however, elicit no effect on the elimination of
the depot cholesterol from the vessels by high density lipoproteins-mediated
transport processes. These actions show an essential difference between the
various antihypercholesterolemic drugs, thus indicating that in the manifestation of atherosclerosis, different mechanisms may coincide and that multiple
drug therapy may lead to a greater success.

This shows that VLDL may be replaced partly by LDL which enhances atherogenesis. It
has been suggested that the addition of an exchange resin to clofibrate may counteract the
increased LDL.[534] Some new hypolipidemic drugs may reduce plasma lipid levels without
affecting LDL. Gemfibrozil, a clofibrate analog, may cause some increase of LDL cholesterol, but to a smaller degree than clofibrate.[186] Recent studies have shown that gemfibrozil
may even raise HDL levels, thus the modulating effect manifests on the lipoprotein profile.
    During the development of atheroma sulfated mucopolysaccharides and glycoproteins
are increased.[687] These substances interact with plasma lipoproteins and extract lipoproteins
from the arterial wall, especially sulfate-rich mucopolysaccharides which react with LDL.
Based on these observations heparin, chondroitin sulfate, and different heparinoids were
suggested for *in vivo* studies. These substances may saturate LDL binding sites that lipoproteins cannot bind and become incorporated into smooth muscle cells. Sulfated mucopolysaccharides may enhance the release of lipoprotein lipase from the arterial endothelium and
increase LDL release and degradation. The major problem of application of heparin and

heparinoids in therapy is due to their great expense, requirement of prolonged parenteral administration which may cause long-term side effects.

D. ANTIPLATELET DRUGS

Since platelet functions are correlated with coronary heart disease, drugs modifying platelet aggregation have also been considered for atherosclerosis therapy.[155,581,630] Following treatment with nonsteroidal anti-inflammatory drugs platelet aggregation is decreased. Current antiplatelet therapy in coronary prevention include the study of the effects of aspirin, sulfinpyrazone, dipyridamole, and oral anticoagulant drugs.[97] Aspirin inhibits the conversion of arachidonic acid to prostaglandins.

Considering the contesting actions of various prostaglandins on platelet aggregation, this raises the possibility of the treatment of cardiovascular diseases with anticoagulants[118,127] and perhaps certain prostaglandins.[5,51,61,120,244,474,357] Prostaglandin E_1 is the most potent vasodilator and also a powerful inhibitor of ADP-induced platelet aggregation.[137,590] Prostacyclin is also a very potent antiaggregation agent, and it is responsible for maintaining the endothelium free from aggregated platelets.[110,145,249] These substances may have a potential role in therapy of atherosclerosis especially in conditions involving thrombotic complications.

REFERENCES

1. **Abdulla, Y.H., Orton, C. C., and Adams, C. W. M.,** Cholesterol esterification by transacylation in humans and experimental atheromatous lesions, *J. Atheroscler. Res.,* 8, 967, 1968.
2. **Adams, C. W. M.,** *Vascular Histochemistry in Relation to the Chemical and Structural Pathology of Cardiovascular Disease,* Lloyd-Luke, London, 1967, 139-140.
3. **Adams, C. W. M. and Bayliss, O. B.,** The relationship between diffuse intimal thickness, medial enzyme failure and intimial lipid deposit in various human arteries, *J. Atheroscler. Res.,* 10, 327, 1969.
4. **Adams, C. W. M. and Bayliss, O. B.,** Histochemical observations on the localization of sphingomyelin, cerebroside and cholesterol in the normal and atherosclerotic human artery, *J. Pathol. Bacteriol.,* 85, 113, 1963.
5. **Adelman, B., Stemerman, M. B., Mendell, D., and Handin, R. I.,** The interaction of platelets with aortic subendothelium: inhibition of adhesion and secretion by prostaglandin I2, *Blood,* 58, 198, 1981.
6. **Alaupovic, P.,** Apolipoproteins and lipoproteins, *Atherosclerosis,* 13, 141, 1971.
7. **Alaupovic, P., Sanbar, S. S., Furman, R. H., Sullivan, M. L., and Walraven, S. L.,** Studies of the composition and structure of serum lipoproteins. Isolation and characterization of very high density lipoproteins of human serum, *Biochemistry,* 5, 4044, 1966.
8. **Albers, J. J., Chen, C. H., and Aladjem, F.,** Human serum lipoproteins. Evidence for three classes of lipoproteins in Sf0-2, *Biochemistry,* 11, 57, 1972.
9. **Albert, R. E., Vanderlaan, M., Burns, F. S., and Nishizumi, M.,** Effects of carcinogens on chicken atherosclerosis, *Cancer Res.,* 37, 2232, 1977.
10. **Alfred, C. A.,** An educational and behavioral approach for the primary prevention of premature cardiovascular disease, *J. Am. Diet. Assoc.,* 84, 1042, 1984.
11. **Altschul, R., Hoffer, A., and Stephen, J. D.,** Influence of nicotinuric acid on serum cholesterol in man, *Arch. Biochem.,* 54, 558, 1955.
12. **Assman, G., Capurso, A., Smootz, E., and Wellner, U.,** Apoprotein A metabolism in Tangier disease, *Atherosclerosis,* 30, 321, 1978.
13. **Astrup, P.,** Carbon monoxide in tobacco smoke and its influence on the development of vascular diseases, *Rehabilitation,* 25, 11, 1972.
14. **Astrup, T.,** Role of blood coagulation and fibrinolysis in the pathogenesis of arteriosclerosis, in *Connective Tissue, Thrombosis, and Atherosclerosis,* Page, I. H., Ed., Academic Press, New York, 1959, 223.
15. **Austin, G. E. and Moss, T. J.,** Gender and pre-atherosclerotic lesions. Effect on prevalence in human abdominal aortas, *Arch. Pathol. Lab. Med.,* 108, 811, 1984.
16. **Avigan, J., Bhathena, S. J., and Schreiner, M. E.,** Control of sterol synthesis and of hydroxymethylglutaryl CoA reductase in skin fibroblasts grown from patients with homozygous type II hyperlipoproteinemia, *J. Lipid Res.,* 16, 151, 1975.

17. **Avigan, J., Steinberg, D., Thompson, M. J., and Mosettig, E.,** The mechanism of action of MER-29, *Prog. Cardiovasc. Dis.,* 2, 525, 1960.
18. **Aviram, M. and Brook, J. G.,** Selective release from platelet granules induced by plasma lipoproteins, *Biochem. Med.,* 32, 30, 1984.
19. **Avoy, D. R., Swyryd, E. A., and Gould, R. G.,** Effects of alpha-p-chlorophenyloxyisobutyryl ethyl ester (CPIB) with and without androsterone on cholesterol biosynthesis in rat liver, *J. Lipid Res.,* 6, 369, 1965.
20. **Awlrey, B. J., Owen, W. G., Fry, G. L., Cheng, F. H., and Hoak, J. C.,** Binding of human thrombin to human endothelial cells and platelets, *Blood,* 46, 1046, 1975.
21. **Azarnoff, D. L., Tucker, D. R., and Barr, G. A.,** Studies with ethyl chlorophenoxyisobutyrate (clofibrate), *Metabolism,* 14, 959, 1965.
22. **Bagdon, R. E., Engstrom, R. G., Kelly, L. A., Hartman, H. A., Robison, R. L., and Visscher, G. E.,** Hyperlipidemic activity and toxicity studies of a styryl-hexahydroindolinol, 34-250, *Toxicol. Appl. Pharmacol.,* 69, 12, 1983.
23. **Bailey, A. J.,** The nature of collagen, in *Comprehensive Biochemistry,* Part B, Vol. 26, Florkin, M. and Stotz, E. H., Eds., Elsevier, Amsterdam, 1968, 297-424.
24. **Bailey, J. M. and Butler, J.,** Cholesterol uptake from doubly-labeled alpha-lipoproteins by cells in tissue culture, *Arch. Biochem. Biophys.,* 159, 580, 1973.
25. **Baker, A. N., Delahunty, T., Gotto, A. M., and Jackson, R. L.,** The primary structure of human plasma high density apolipoproteinglutamine-I, *Proc. Natl. Acad. Sci. U.S.A.,* 71, 3631, 1974.
26. **Baker, A. N., Gotto, A. M., and Jackson, R. L.,** The primary structure of human plasma high density apolipoprotein-glutamine-I (ApoA-I). II. The amino acid sequence and alignment of cyanogen bromide fragments IV, III, and I, *J. Biol. Chem.,* 250, 2725, 1975.
27. **Bang, H. O., Dyerberg, J., and Hjorne, N.,** The composition of food consumed by Greenland Eskimos, *Acta Med. Scand.,* 200, 69, 1976.
28. **Bang, H. O., and Dyerberg, J.,** Plasma lipids and lipoproteins in Greenlandic West Coast Eskimos, *Acta Med. Scan.,* 192, 85, 1972.
29. **Baraona, E., Savolainen, M., Karsenty, C. Leo, M. A., and Lieber, C. S.,** Pathogenesis of alcoholic hypertriglyceridemia and hypercholesterolemia, *Trans. Am. Assoc. Physicians,* 26, 306, 1983.
30. **Barclay, M.,** Lipoprotein class distribution in normal and diseased states, in *Blood Lipids and Lipoproteins: Quantitation, Composition and Metabolism,* Nelson, G. J., Ed., Wiley-Interscience, New York, 1972, 585-704.
31. **Barnhart, J. W., Sefranka, J. A., and McIntosh, D. D.,** Hypocholesterolemic effect of 4,4'(isopropylidenedithio)-bis(2,6-di-t-butylphenol) (probucol), *Am. J. Clin. Nutr.,* 23, 1229, 1970.
32. **Bar-on, H., Roheim, P. S., and Eder, H. A.,** Serum lipoprotein and apolipoprotein in rats with streptozotocin-induced diabetes, *J. Clin. Invest.,* 57, 714, 1976.
33. **Barr, D. P.,** Influences of sex and sex hormones upon development of atherosclerosis and upon lipoprotein of plasma, *J. Chronic Dis.,* 1, 63, 1955.
34. **Barter, P. J.,** Production of plasma esterified cholesterol in lean, normotriglyceridemic humans, *J. Lipid Res.,* 15, 234, 1974.
35. **Barter, P. J. and Nestel, P. J.,** The distribution of triglyceride in subclasses of very low density plasma lipoproteins, *J. Lab. Clin. Med.,* 76, 925, 1970.
36. **Baruch, Y., Brook, J. G., Eidelman, S., and Aviram, M.,** Increased concentration of high density lipoprotein in plasma and decreased platelet aggregation in primary biliary cirrhosis, *Atherosclerosis,* 53, 151, 1984.
37. **Bates, S. R. and Rothblat, G. H.,** Regulation of cellular sterol flux and synthesis by human serum lipoproteins, *Biochim. Biophys. Acta.,* 360, 38, 1974.
38. **Beach, K. W., and Strandness, D. E.,** Atherosclerosis obliterans and associated risk factors in insulin-dependent and non-insulin dependent diabetes, *Diabetes,* 29, 822, 1980.
39. **Beaumont, J. L.,** L'hyperlipidemie par auto-anticorps anti-beta-lipoproteines. Une nouvelle entite pathologique, *C. R. Acad. Sci. (Paris),* 261, 4563, 1965.
40. **Beaumont, J. L., Antonucci, M., Lagrue, G., Guedon, J., and Perol, R.,** Nephrotic syndrome, monoclonal gammapathy and autoimmune hyperlipidemia, *Clin. Exp. Immunol.,* 18, 25, 1974.
41. **Beaumont, J. L., Antonucci, M., and Berard, M.,** Autoimmune hyperlipidemia in the nephrotic syndrome, in *Proc. Int. Workshop-Conference on Atherosclerosis,* G. W. Manning and M. D. Haust, Eds., Plenum Press, New York, 1977, 53.
42. **Beaumont, J. L. and Beaumont, V.,** Immunological factors of atherosclerosis, in *Atherosclerosis III,* G. Schettler and A. Weizel, Eds., Springer-Verlag, Berlin, 1974, 579.
43. **Beaumont, J. L., Carlson, L. A., Cooper, G. R., Fejfar A., Fredrickson, D. S., and Strasser, T.,** Classification of hyperlipidaemias and hyperlipoproteinaemias, *WHO,* 43, 891, 1970.
44. **Beaumont, J. L. and Lorenzelli, L.,** Le phenomene d'agglutination des particules lipidiques. Son interet en sero-immunologie, *Pathol. Biol.,* 20, 357, 1972.

45. **Beaumont, V. and Beaumont, J. L.,** L'hyperlipidemie experimentale par immunisation chez le lapin, *Pathol. Biol.,* 16, 869, 1968.
46. **Becker, C. G. and Dubin, T.,** Activation of Factor XII by tobacco glycoprotein, *J. Exp. Med.,* 146, 457, 1977.
47. **Becker, C. G. and Murphy, G. E.,** Demonstration of contractile protein in endothelium and cells of the heart valves, endocardium, intima, arteriosclerotic plaques, and Aschoff bodies of rheumatic heart disease, *Am. J. Pathol.,* 55, 1, 1969.
48. **Beg, Z. H., Allmann, D. W., and Gibson, D. M.,** Modulation of 3-hydroxy-3-methylglutaryl coenzyme A reductase activity with AMP and with protein fractions of rat liver cytosol, *Biochem. Biophys. Res. Comm.,* 54, 1369, 1973.
49. **Beitz, A., Schimke, E., Honigmann, G., Beitz, J., Block, H. W., and Schliack, V.,** Thromboxane B2 formation in clotting whole blood of healthy and diabetic humans in vitro, *Biomed. Biochim. Acta,* 43, S455, 1984.
50. **Beitz, J. and Foster, W.,** Influence of human low-density and high-density lipoprotein cholesterol on the in vivo prostaglandin I_2 synthetase activity, *Biochim. Biophys. Acta,* 620, 353, 1980.
51. **Belch, J. J. F., McKay, A. J., McArdle, B., Leiberman, D. P. Pollock, J. G., Lowe, G. D. O., and Prentice, C. R. M.,** Epoprostenol (prostacyclin) and severe arterial disease, *Lancet,* 1, 315, 1983.
52. **Belina, H., Cooper, S. D., Farkas, R., and Feuer, G.,** Sex difference in the phospholipid composition of rat liver microsomes, *Biochem. Pharmacol.,* 24, 301, 1975.
53. **Bell, F. P., Gallus, A. S., and Schwartz, C. J.,** Focal, and regional patterns of uptake and the transmural distribution of 131₁-fibrinogen in the pig aorta in vivo, *Exp. Mol. Pathol.,* 20, 281, 1974.
54. **Benditt, E. P.,** Implications of the monoclonal character of human atherosclerotic plaques, *Ann. N.Y. Acad. Sci.,* 275, 96, 1976.
55. **Benditt, E. P. and Benditt, J. M.,** Evidence for a monoclonal origin of human atherosclerotic plaques, *Proc. Natl. Acad. Sci. U.S.A.,* 70, 1753, 1973.
56. **Benditt, E. P. and Schwartz, S. M.,** Atherosclerosis: what can we learn from studies on human tissues, *Lab. Invest.,* 50, 3, 1984.
57. **Bengtsson, G., Olivecrona, T., Hook, M., Riesenfeld, J., and Lindahl, U.,** Interaction of lipoprotein lipase with native and modified heparin-like polysaccharides, *Biochem. J.,* 189, 625, 1980.
58. **Berenson, G. S., Webber, L. S., Srinivasan, S. R., Cresanta, J. L., Frank, G. C., and Farris, R. P.,** Black-white contrasts as determinants of cardiovascular risk in childhood: precursors of coronary artery and primary hypertensive diseases, *Am. Heart J.,* 108, 672, 1984.
59. **Berensztajn, J. and Kotlar, T. J.,** Liver uptake of chylomicron remnants with high and low apoprotein E:C ratios, *Proc. Natl. Acad. Sci. U.S.A.,* 81, 5863, 1984.
60. **Bergen, S. S., Van Italie, T. B., Tennent, D. M., and Sebrell, W. H.,** Effect of an anion exchange resin on serum cholesterol in man, *Proc. Soc. Exp. Biol. Med.,* 102, 676, 1959.
61. **Bergman, G., Daly, R., Atkinson, L., Rothman, M., Richardson, P. J., Jackson, G., and Jewitt, D. E.,** Prostacyclin: haemodynamic and metabolic effects in patients with coronary artery disease, *Lancet,* 1, 569, 1981.
62. **Bertelson, S.,** Chemical studies on the arterial wall in relation to atherosclerosis, *Ann. N.Y. Acad. Sci.,* 149, 643, 1968.
63. **Bell, F. P.,** Transfer of cholesterol between serum lipoproteins, isolated membranes, and intact tissue, *Exp. Mol. Pathol.,* 19, 273, 1973.
64. **Best, M. M. and Duncan, C. H.,** Hypolipemia and hepatomegaly from ethyl chlorophenoxyisobutyrate (CPIB) in the rat, *J. Lab. Clin. Med.,* 64, 634, 1964.
65. **Bielmann, P., Brun, D., Moorjani, S., Gagne, C., Lupien, P., and Tetreault, L.,** Dose-response to tibric acid: a new hypolipidemic drug in type IV hyperlipoproteinemia, *Clin. Pharmacol. Ther.,* 17, 606, 1975.
66. **Bick, R. L.,** Clinical implications of molecular markers in hemostasis and thrombosis, *Semin. Thromb. Hemost.,* 10, 290, 1984.
67. **Bierman, E. L. and Ross, R.,** Ageing and atherosclerosis, in *Atherosclerosis Reviews,* Vol. 2, Paoletti, R. and Gott, A. M., Eds., Raven Press, New York, 1977, 79-81.
68. **Blackett, P. R., Lee, D. M., Donaldson, D. L., Fesmire, J. D., Chan, W. Y., Holcombe, J. H., and Rennert, O. M.,** Studies of lipids, lipoproteins, and apolipoproteins in (Menkes) disease, *Pediatr. Res.,* 18, 864, 1984.
69. **Blankenhorn, D. H., Rooney, J. A., and Curry, P. J.,** Noninvasive assessment of atherosclerosis, *Prog. Cardiovasc. Dis.,* 26, 295, 1984.
70. **Blaton, V., DeBuyzere, M., Declercq, B., Pracetyo, A., Vanderkelen, G., Delaughe, J., and Spin-cemaille, J.,** Effect of polyunsaturated isocaloric fat diets on plasma lipids, apolipoproteins and fatty acids, *Atherosclerosis,* 53, 9, 1984.
71. **Blohm, T. R., Kariya, T., and Laughlin, M. W.,** Effects of MER-29, a cholesterol synthesis inhibitor, on mammalian tissue lipids, *Arch. Biochem.,* 85, 250, 1959.

72. **Bond, J. A., Omiecinski, C. J., and Juchau, M. R.,** Kinetics, activation, and induction of aortic mono-oxygenase. Biotransformation of benzo[a]pyrene, *Biochem. Pharmacol.*, 28, 305, 1979.

73. **Bondjers, G. and Björkernd, F. J.,** Arterial repair and atherosclerosis after mechanical injury. 3. Cholesterol accumulation and removal in morphologically defined regions of aortic atherosclerotic lesions in the rabbit, *Atherosclerosis*, 17, 85, 1973.

74. **Borhain, N. O., Ed.,** *The Framingham Study,* Am. Heart Assoc., Council on Epidemiol., New York, 1971.

75. **Bortnichak, E. A., Freeman, D. H., Ostfeld, A. M., Castelli, W. P., Kannel, W. B., McNamara, P. M.,** The association between cholesterol cholelithiasis and coronary eart disease in Framingham, Massachusetts, *Am. J. Epidemiol.*, 12, 19, 1985.

76. **Bottcher, C. J. F.,** Phospholipids of atherosclerotic lesions in the human aorta, in *Evolution of the Atherosclerotic Plaque,* Jones, R. J., Ed., University of Chicago Press, IL, 109, 1963.

77. **Boyd, G. S. and Lawson, M. E.,** Studies on the catabolism of cholesterol to bile acids in the liver: cholesterol-7-alpha-hydroxylase, in *Atherosclerosis,* Jones, R. J., Ed., Springer-Verlag, New York, 1970, 286.

78. **Boyd, G. S. and Oliver, F. M.,** Thyroid hormones and plasma lipids, *Br. Med. Bull.*, 16, 138, 1960.

79. **Boxer, L. A., Allen, J. M., Schmidt, M., Yoder, M., and Baehner, R. L.,** Inhibition of polymorpho-nuclear adherence by prostacyclin, *J. Lab. Clin. Med.*, 95, 672, 1980.

80. **Bradley, W. A., Hwang, S. I., Karlin, J. B., Lin, A. H., Prasad, S. C., Gotto, A. M., and Gianturco, S. H.,** Low-density lipoprotein receptor binding determinants switch from apolipoprotein E to apolipoprotein B during conversion of hypertriglyceridemic: very-low-density lipoprotein to low-density lipoproteins, *J. Biol. Chem.*, 259, 14728, 1984.

81. **Brand, F. N., McGee, D. L., Kannel, W. B., Stokes, J., and Castelli, W. P.,** Hyperuricemia as a risk factor of coronary heart disease: the Framingham study, *Am. J. Epidemiol.*, 121, 11, 1985.

82. **Brecher, P. I. and Chobanian, A. V.,** Cholesterol ester synthesis in normal and atherosclerotic aortas of rabbits and rhesus monkeys, *Circ. Res.*, 35, 692, 1974.

83. **Breckenridge, W. C., Jr., Little, J. A., Steiner, G., and Poapst, J.,** Hypertiglyceridemia associated with deficiency of apolipoprotein C-II, *N. Engl. J. Med.*, 298, 1265, 1978.

84. **Bremer, J. and Greenberg, D. M.,** Enzymic methylation of foreign sulfhydryl compounds, *Biochim. Biophys. Acta,* 46, 205, 1961.

85. **Brest, A. N. and Moyer, J. H., Ed.,** *Atherosclerotic Vascular Disease,* Appleton-Century-Crofts Inc., New York, 1971.

86. **Brewer, H. B., Lux, S. E., Ronan, R., and John, K. M.,** Amino acid sequence of human apo-Lp-Gln-II (apoA-II), an apolipoprotein isolated from the high-density lipoprotein complex, *J. Biol. Chem.*, 247, 7519, 1972.

87. **Brewer, H. B., Lux, S. E., Ronan, R., and John, K. M.,** Amino acid sequence of human apo-Lp-Gln-II (apoA-II), an apolipoprotein isolated from the high-density lipoprotein complex, *Proc. Nat. Acad. Sci. U.S.A.,* 69, 1034, 1972.

88. **Brewer, H. B., Schulman, R., Herbert, P., Ronan, R., and Wehrly, K.,** The complete amino acid sequence of alanine apolipoprotein (apoC-3) and apolipoprotein from human plasma very low-density lipoproteins, *J. Biol. Chem.*, 249, 4969, 1974.

89. **Brodie, R. R., Chasseaud, L. F., and Elsom, F. F.,** Antilipidemic drugs. Part 4: the metabolic fate of the hypolipidemic agent. isopropyl-[4'-(p-chlorbenzoyl)-2-phenoxy-2-methyl]-pr(LF 178) in rats, dogs, and man, *Arzneim. Forsch.,* 26, 896, 1976.

90. **Bronte-Stewart, B.,** The relationship between the serum lipids and the development of ischaemic heart disease, *Postgrad. Med. J.,* 35, 198, 1959.

91. **Brown, J.,** Nutritional and epidemiologic factors related to heart disease, *World Rev. Nutr. Diet.,* 12, 1, 1970.

92. **Brown, M. S., Dana, S. E., and Goldstein, J. L.,** Regulation of 3-hydroxy-3-methylglutaryl coenzyme A reductase activity in cultured human fibroblasts. Comparison of cells from a normal subject and from a patient with homozygous familial hypercholesterolemia, *J. Biol. Chem.,* 249, 789, 1974.

93. **Brown, M. S. and Goldstein, J. L.,** Analysis of a mutant strain of human fibroblasts with a defect in the internalization of receptor-bound low density lipoproteins, *Cell,* 9, 663, 1974.

94. **Brown, M. S., and Goldstein, J. L.,** Familial hypercholesterolemia: a genetic defect in the low density lipoprotein receptor, *N. Engl. J. Med.,* 294, 1386, 1976.

95. **Brown, M. S. and Goldstein, J. L.,** Familial hypercholesterolemia: defective binding of lipoproteins to cultured fibroblasts associated with impaired regulation of 3-hydroxy-3-methyl-glutaryl coenzyme A reductase activity, *Proc. Natl. Acad. Sci. U.S.A.,* 71, 788, 1974.

96. **Brown, M. S. and Goldstein, J. L.,** How LDL receptors influence cholesterol and atherosclerosis, *Sci. Am.,* 251, 58, 1984.

97. **Brown, M. S., and Goldstein, J. L.,** General scheme for regulation of cholesterol metabolism in mammalian cells, in *Disturbances in Lipid and Lipoprotein Metabolism,* Dietschy, J. M., Gotto, A. M., and Ontko, J. A., Eds., American Physiological Society, Bethesda, MD, 1980, 173-180.

98. **Brown, M. S. and Goldstein, J. L.,** Receptor-mediated control of cholesterol metabolism, *Science,* 191, 150, 1976.

99. **Brown, M. S., Faust, J. R., and Goldstein, J. L.,** Role of the low-density lipoprotein receptor in regulating the content of free and esterified cholesterol in human fibroblasts, *J. Clin. Invest.,* 55, 783, 1975.

100. **Brown, M. S., Ho, Y. K., and Goldstein, J. L.,** The low-density lipoprotein pathway in human fibroblasts: relation between cell surface receptor binding and endocytosis of low-density lipoprotein, *Ann. N.Y. Acad. Sci.,* 275, 244, 1976.

101. **Brown, M. S., Kovanen, P. T., and Goldstein, J. L.,** Regulation of plasma cholesterol by lipoprotein receptors, *Science,* 212, 628, 1981.

102. **Brown, M. S., Levy, R. I., and Fredrickson, D. S.** Further characterization of apolipoproteins from the human plasma very low density lipoproteins, *J. Biol. Chem.,* 245, 6588, 1970.

103. **Bullock, B. C., Bond, M. G., Lehner, N. D. M., and Clarkson, T. B.,** Effect of plasma cholesterol concentration (200 vs. 300 mg/dl) in preexisting coronary atherosclerosis in rhesus monkeys, *Circulation,* 54, 11, 1976.

104. **Buonassisi, V. and Root, M.,** Enzymatic degradation of heparin-related mucopolysaccharides from the surface of endothelial cell cultures, *Biochim. Biophys. Acta,* 383, 1, 1975.

105. **Burch, P. R. J.,** Ischaemic heart disease: epidemiology, risk factors and cause, *Cardiovasc. Res.,* 14, 307, 1980.

106. **Butcher, R. W., Baird, C. E., and Sutherland, E. W.,** Effects of lipolytic and antilipolytic substances on adenosine 3', 5'-monophosphate levels in isolated fat cells, *J. Biol. Chem.,* 243, 1705, 1968.

107. **Camejo, G., Lopez, A., Vegas, H., and Paoli, H.,** The participation of aortic proteins in the formation of complexes between low density lipoproteins and intima-media extracts, *Atherosclerosis,* 21, 77, 1975.

108. **Caplan, B. A. and Schwartz, C.,** Increased endothelial cell turnover in areas of in vivo Evans blue uptake in the pig aorta, *Atherosclerosis,* 17, 401, 1973.

109. **Carew, T. E., Koschinsky, T., Hayes, S. B., and Steinberg, D.,** A mechanism by which high-density lipoproteins may slow the atherogenic process, *Lancet,* 1, 1315, 1976.

110. **Carlson, L. A., Irion, E., and Orö, L.,** Effect of infusion of prostaglandin E$_1$ on the aggregation of blood platelets in man, *Life Sci.,* 7, 85, 1968.

111. **Carlson, L. A., Olsson, A. G., Orö, L., Rössner, S., and Walldius, G.,** Effect of hypolipidemic regimens on serum lipoproteins, *Proc. Third Int. Symp. Atherosclerosis,* Springer-Verlag, Berlin, 1974, 768-781.

112. **Caro, C. G.,** Mechanical factors in atherogenesis, in *Cardiovascular Flow Dynamics and Measurements,* Hwang, W. H. C., and Norman, W. A., Eds., University Park Press, Baltimore, MD, 1977, 473-487.

113. **Caro, C. G. and Lever, M. J.,** The mass transport of the arterial wall: effects of mechanical stresses and vasoactive agents, including nitrates, *Z. Kardiol,* 72(Suppl.3), 178, 1983.

114. **Carter, C., Havlik, K., Feinleib, M., Kuller, L. H., Elston, R., and Rao, D. C.,** Genetic epidemiology of coronary heart disease. Past, present and future, *Arteriosclerosis,* 4, 510, 1984.

115. **Castelli, W. P., Doyle, J. T., Gordon, T., Hames, C. G., Hjortland, M. C., Hulley, S. B., Kagan, A., and Zukel, W. J.,** HDL cholesterol and other lipids in coronary heart disease. The cooperative lipoprotein phenotyping study, *Circulation,* 55, 767, 1977.

116. **Castellot, J. J., Addonizio, M. L., Rosenberg, R., and Karnovsky, M. J.,** Cultured endothelial cells produce a heparin like inhibitor of smooth muscle cell growth, *J. Cell Biol.,* 90, 372, 1981.

117. **Cazzolato, G., Bittolo, N. A., Bon, G., and Avogaro, P.,** Apoprotein B-48 is a constant finding in very low density lipoproteins of humans, *Arteriosclerosis,* 5, 88, 1985.

118. **Chalmers, T. C., Matt, R. J., Smith, H., and Kunsler, A. M.,** Evidence favoring the use of anticoagulants in the hospital phase of acute myocardial infarction, *N. Engl. J. Med.,* 297, 1091, 1977.

119. **Chien, S.,** Significance of macrorheology and microrheology in atherogenesis, *Ann. N.Y. Acad. Sci.,* 270, 10, 1976.

120. **Chierchia, S., Patrono, C., Crea, F., Ciabattoni, G. De Caterine, R., Cinotti, G. A., Distante, A., and Maseri, A.,** Effects of intravenous prostacyclin in variant angina, *Circulation,* 65, 470, 1982.

121. **Chin, D. J., Luskey, K. L., Anderson, R. G. W., Faust, J. R., Goldstein, J. L., and Brown, M. S.,** Appearance of crystalloid endoplasmic reticulum in compactin-resistant Chinese hamster cells with 500-fold increase in 3-hydroxy-3-methylglutaryl-coenzyme A reductase, *Proc. Natl. Acad. Sci. U.S.A.,* 79, 1185, 1982.

122. **Chobanian, A. V. and Hollander, W.,** Phospholipid synthesis in the human arterial intima, *J. Clin. Invest.,* 45, 932, 1966.

123. **Chobanian, A. V. and Manzur, F.,** Metabolism of lipid in the human fatty streak lesion, *J. Lipid Res.,* 13, 201, 1972.

124. **Christopher, J. and Popjak, G.**, Studies on the biosynthesis of cholesterol: XIV the origin of prenoic acids from allyl pyrophosphates in liver enzyme systems, *J. Lipid Res.*, 2, 244, 1961.

125. **Claude, A.**, Growth and differentiation of cytoplasmic membranes in the course of lipoprotein granule synthesis in the hepatic cell. I. Elaboration of elements of the Golgi complex, *J. Cell Biol.*, 47, 745, 1970.

126. **Cochrane, C. G.**, The role of immune complexes and complement in tissue injury, *J. Allergy*, 42, 113, 1968.

127. **Conard, J., Castel, M., and Samama, M.**, Antithrombin III and atherosclerosis, *Adv. Exp. Med. Biol.*, 164, 59, 1984.

128. **Cooper, A. D.**, Role of the liver in the degradation of lipoproteins, *Gastroenterology*, 88, 192, 1985.

129. **Cooper, R., Lin, K., Stamler, J., Schoenberger, J. A., Shekelle, R. B., Collette, P., and Shekelle, S.**, Prevalence of diabetes/hyperglycemia and associated risk factors in blacks and whites, *Am. Heart J.*, 108, 827, 1984.

130. The coronary drug project: initial findings leading to modifications of its research protocol, *JAMA*, 214, 1313, 1970.

131. The coronary drug project: findings leading to further modifications of its protocol with respect to dex-trothyroxine, *JAMA*, 220, 996, 1972.

132. **Cottet, J., Mathivat, A., and Redel, J.**, Etude thérapeutique d'un hypocholestérol émiant de synthèse: l'acide-ethyl-acétique, *J. Presse Med.*, 62, 939, 1954.

133. **Couzigon, P., Flenarg, P., Crockett, R., Rautou, J. J., Blanchard, P., Lemoine, F., Richard-Molard, B., Amouretti, M., and Bérau, C.**, High density lipoprotein cholesterol and apoprotein Al in healthy volunteers during long-term moderate alcohol intake, *Ann. Nutr. Metab.*, 28, 377, 1984.

134. **Crawford, T.**, *The Pathology of Ischaemic Heart Disease*, Butterworths, London, 1977, 32.

135. **Curb, J. D. and Taylor, A. A.**, Mild hypertension and atherosclerosis, in *Atherosclerosis Reviews*, Vol. 9, Gotto, A. M., and Paoletti, R., Eds., Raven Press, New York, 1982, 53—84.

136. **Curreri, P. W., Kothari, H. V., Bonner, M. J., and Miller, B. F.**, Increased activity of lysosomal enzymes in experimental atherosclerosis, and the effect of cortisone, *Proc. Soc. Exp. Biol. Med.*, 130, 1253, 1969.

137. **Curwen, K. D., Gimbrone, M. A., and Handin, R. J.**, In vitro studies in thromboresistance, the role of prostacyclin (PGI_2) in platelet adhesion to cultured normal and orally transformed human vascular endothelial cells, *Lab. Invest*, 42, 366, 1980.

138. **D'Angelo, V., Villa, S., and Mysliewic, M.**, Defective fibrinolytic and prostacyclin-like activity in human atheromatous plaques, *Thomb. Hemostasis*, 39, 535, 1978.

139. **Dallochio, M. Crokett, R., Razaka, G., Gandji, F. A., Bricuad, H., Pautrizel, R., and Broustet, P.**, Anticorps anti-aorte et lésions aortiques par injections répétées de broyats aortiques (etude chez le lapin), *Arch. Mal. Coeur.*, 3, 44, 1968.

140. **Davies, M. J. and Thomas, T.**, The pathological basis and microanatomy of occlusive thrombus formation in human coronary arteries, in *Interaction Between Platelets and Vessel Walls*, Born, G. V. R. and Vane, J. R., Eds., Royal Society, London, 1981, 9-12.

141. **Dairgnon, J.**, The lipid hypothesis. Pathophysiological basis, *Arch. Surg.*, 113, 28, 1979.

142. **Day, A. J., Newman, H. A. I., and Zilversmit, D. B.**, Synthesis of phospholipid by foam cells isolated from rabbit atherosclerotic lesions, *Circ. Res.*, 19, 122, 1966.

143. **Day, A. J. and Wilkinson, G. K.**, Incorporation of 14C-labeled acetate into lipid by isolated foam cells and by atherosclerotic arterial intima, *Circ. Res.*, 21, 593, 1967.

144. **Dayton, S., Dayton, J., Drimmer, F., and Kendall, F. E.**, Rates of acetate turnover and lipid synthesis in normal, hypothyroid and hyperthyroid rats, *Am. J. Physiol.*, 199, 71, 1960.

145. **De Gaetano, G., Remuzzi, C. T., Mysliwec, M., and Dawati, M. S.**, Vascular prostacyclin and plas-minogen activator activity in experimental and clinical conditions of disturbed haemostasis or thrombosis, *Haemostasis*, 8, 300, 1979.

146. **De Graeve, J., Bouissou, H., Thiers, J. C., Fouet, J., and Valdiguie', P.**, Is cutaneous apoprotein B a better discriminator than serum lipoproteins for atherosclerosis?, *Atherosclerosis*, 52, 301, 1984.

147. **de la Iglesia, F. A., Feuer, G., McGuire, E. J., and Takada, A.**, Morphological and biochemical changes in the liver of various species in experimental phospholipidosis after dimethylamino-ethoxyhexestrol treat-ment, *Toxicol. Appl. Pharmacol.*, 34, 28, 1975.

148. **de la Iglesia, F. A., Feuer, G., Takada, A. D., and Matsuda, Y.**, Morphologic studies on secondary phospholipidosis in human liver, *Lab. Invest.*, 30, 539, 1974.

149. **Dietschy, J. M. and Wilson, J. D.**, Regulation of cholesterol metabolism I, *N. Engl. J. Med.*, 282, 1128, 1970.

150. **Dole, V. P.**, Effect of nucleic acid metabolites on lipolysis in adipose tissue, *J. Biol. Chem.*, 236, 3121, 1961.

151. **Doll, R. and Hill, A. B.**, Mortality in relation to smoking. Ten years' observation of a British doctor, *Br. Med. J.*, 1, 1399, 1964.

152. **Dole, V. P. and Hamlin, J. T.,** Particulate fat in lymph and blood, *Physiol. Rev.,* 42, 674, 1962.
153. **Dorian, B. and Taylor, C. B.,** Stress factors in the development of coronary artery disease, *J. Occup. Med.,* 26, 747, 1984.
154. **Dormandy, J. A.,** The red cell as a risk factor in circulatory diseases, *Adv. Exp. Med. Biol.,* 164, 395, 1984.
155. **Douglas, A. S.,** Trials of antiplatelet drugs in coronary prevention, in *Atherosclerosis: Mechanisms and Approaches to Therapy,* Miller, N. E., Ed., Raven Press, New York, 1984, 77-90.
156. **Dunn, F. L., Raskin, P., Bilheimer, D. W., and Grundy, S. M.,** The effect of metabolic control on very low-density lipoprotein-triglyceride metabolism in patients with type II diabetes mellitus and marked hypertriglyceridemia, *Metabolism,* 33, 117, 1984.
157. **Dustan, H. P.,** Vascular diseases of hypertension: mechanism, recognition and control, in *Atherosclerosis Reviews,* Vol. 2, Paoletti, R. and Gotto, A. M., Eds., 1977, 1-25.
158. **Dyerberg, J. and Bang, H. O.,** Haemostatic function and platelet poly-unsaturated fatty acids in Eskimos, *Lancet,* 2, 433, 1979.
159. **Eder, H. A. and Roheim, P. S.,** Plasma lipoproteins and apolipoproteins, *Ann. N.Y. Acad. Sci.,* 275, 169, 1976.
160. Editorial, Hypertension in blacks and whites, *Lancet,* 2, 73, 1980.
161. **Edwards, J. C., Howell, S. L., and Taylor, K. W.,** Fatty acids as regulators of glucagon secretion, *Nature,* 224, 808, 1969.
162. **Edwards, P. A.,** Effect of plasma lipoprotein and lecithin-cholesterol dispersion on the activity of 3-hydroxy-3-methylglutaryl-coenzyme A reductase of isolated rat hepatocytes, *Biochim. Biophys. Acta,* 409, 30, 1975.
163. **Edwards, P. A. and Gould, R. G.,** Turnover rate of hepatic 3-hydroxy-3-methylglutaryl coenzyme A reductase as determined by use of cycloheximide, *J. Biol. Chem.,* 247, 1520, 1972.
164. **Edwards, P. A., Fogelman, A. M., and Popjak, G.,** Direct relationship between the amount of sterol lost from rat hepatocytes and the increase in activity of HMG-CoA reductase, *Biochem. Biophys. Res. Commun.,* 68, 64, 1976.
165. **Ehrenreich, J. H., Bergeron, J. J. M., Siekevitz, P., and Palade, G. E.,** Golgi fractions prepared from rat liver homogenates. I. Isolation procedure and morphological characterization, *J. Cell Biol.,* 59, 45, 1973.
166. **Eichner, E. R.,** Platelets, carotids and coronaries. Critique on antithrombotic role of antiplatelet agents, exercise and certain diets, *Am. J. Med.,* 77, 513, 1984.
167. **Eisenberg, S. and Levy, R. I.,** Lipoprotein metabolism, *Adv. Lipid Res.,* 13, 1, 1975.
168. **Eisenberg, S., Stein, Y., and Stein, O.,** Phospholipidases in arterial tissue. II. Phosphatide acyl-hydrolase and lysophosphatide acyl-hydrolase activity in human and rat arteries, *Biochim. Biophys. Acta,* 164, 205, 1968.
169. **Eisenberg, S. and Schurr, D.,** Phospholipid removal during degradation of rat plasma very low density lipoprotein in vitro, *J. Lipid Res.,* 17, 578, 1976.
170. **Eisenberg, S., Stein, Y., and Stein, O.,** Phospholipidases in arterial tissue. 3. Phosphatide acyl-hydrolase and sphingomyelin choline phosphohydrolase in rat and rabbit aorta in different age groups, *Biochim. Biophys. Acta,* 176, 557, 1969.
171. **Ellis, N. I., Lloyd, B., Lloyd, B. S., and Clayton, B. E.,** Selenium and vitamin E in relation to risk factors for coronary heart disease, *J. Clin. Pathol.,* 37, 200, 1984.
172. **Elmholm, C.,** Role of apolipoprotein E in the lipolytic conversion of beta-very low-density lipoproteins to low-density lipoproteins in type III hyperlipoproteinemia, *Proc. Natl. Acad. Sci. U.S.A.,* 81, 5566, 1984.
173. **Epstein, S. E. and Palmeri, S. T.,** Mechanisms contributing to precipitation of unstable angina and acute myocardial infarction: implications regarding therapy, *Am. J. Cardiol.,* 54, 1245, 1984.
174. **Ewing, A. M., Freeman, N. K., and Lingren, F. T.,** The analysis of human serum lipoprotein distributions, *Adv. Lipid Res.,* 3, 25, 1965.
175. **Failey, R. B., Jr., Brown, E., and Hodes, M. E.,** Effect of nicotinic acid on conjugation pattern of bile acids in man, *Circulation,* 20, 984, 1959.
176. **Fainaru, M., Mahley, R. W., Hamilton, R. L., and Innerarity, T. L.,** Structural and metabolic heterogeneity of β-very low density lipoproteins from cholesterol-fed dogs and humans with Type III hyperlipoproteinemia, *J. Lipid Res.,* 23, 702, 1982.
177. **Falcone, D. J., Hajjar, D. P., and Mimick, C. R.,** Enhancement of cholesterol ester accumulation in re-endothelialized aorta, *Am. J. Pathol.,* 99, 81, 1980.
178. **Fedele, D., Lapolla, A., Cardone, G., Baldo, G., and Crepaldi, G.,** Glycosylated hemoglobin in endogenous hypertriglyceridemia, *Acta Diabetol. Lat.,* 20, 303, 1983.
179. **Feenstra, D. L. and Wilkens, J. N.,** Cholesterol en vitamine D, *Ned. T. Geneesk.,* 109, 615, 1965.
180. **Feuer, G., Cooper, S. D., de la Iglesia, F. A., and Lumb, G.,** Microsomal phospholipids and drug action. Quantitative biochemical and electron microscope studies, *Int. J. Clin. Pharmacol. Therap. Toxicol.,* 5, 389, 1972.

181. **Feuer, G., Miller, D. R., Cooper, S. D., de la Iglesia, F. A., and Lumb, G.,** The influence of methyl groups on toxicity and drug metabolism, *Int. J. Clin. Pharmacol. Therap. Toxicol.,* 7, 13, 1973.

182. **Feuer, G., da la Iglesia, F. A., and Cooper, S.,** Role of hepatic endoplasmic reticulum enzyme markers in the preliminary safety evaluation of drugs and other foreign compounds, *Proc. Eur. Soc. Study Drug Toxicity,* 15, 142, 1973.

183. **Fielding, C. J.,** Phospholipid substrate specificity of purified human plasma lecithin: cholesterol acyltransferase, *Scand. J. Clin. Lab. Invest.,* 33(Suppl. 137), 15, 1974.

184. **Fisher, W. R.,** The structure of the lower-density lipoproteins of human plasma: newer concepts derived from studies with the analytical ultracentrifuge, *Ann. Clin. Lab. Sci.,* 2,198, 1972.

185. **Fitscha, P., Kaliman, J., Sinsinger, H., and Peskar, B. A.,** Follow-up of in vivo platelet function in patients with coronary heart disease, *Cor. Vasa,* 13, 338, 1984.

186. **Fitzgerald, J. E., Sanyer, J. L., Schardein, J. L., Lake, R. S., McGuire, E. J., and de la Iglesia, F. A.,** Carcinogen bioassay and mutagenicity studies with the hypolipidemic agent gemfibrozil, *J. Natl. Cancer Inst.,* 67, 1105, 1981.

187. **Fleischer, L. N., Tall, A. R., Miller, R. W., Uritte, L. D., and Cannon, P. J.,** Stimulation of arterial endothelial cell prostacyclin synthesis by high-density lipoproteins, Proc. 5th Intern. Conf. Prostaglandins, Florence, Italy, 1982, 597.

188. **Fleischman, A. I., Hayton, T., Bierenbaum, M. L., and Wildrick, E.,** Effect of calcium and vitamin D3 upon the fecal excretion of some metals in the mature male rat fed a high fat cholesterol diet, *J. Nutr.,* 95, 19, 1968.

189. **Florentin, R. A., Nam, S. C., Lee, K. T., and Thomas, W. A.,** Increased mitotic activity in aortas of swine after three days of cholesterol feeding, *Arch. Pathol.,* 88, 463, 1969.

190. **Fogelman, A. M., Edmond, J., and Popjak, G.,** Metabolism of mevalonate in rats and man not leading to sterols, *J. Biol. Chem.,* 250, 1771, 1975.

191. **Fowler, S. and DeDuve, C.,** Nature, location and mode of formation of intracellular lipid deposits in atherosclerotic lesions. Rapport du 42e Congrès Français de Médicine, Liége, Masson, Paris, 1979, 51.

192. **Frantz, I. D., Jr., Mobberley, M. L., and Schroepfer, G. J., Jr.,** Effects of MER-29 on the intermediary metabolism of cholesterol, *Prog. Cardivasc. Dis.,* 2, 511, 1960.

193. **Fredrickson, D. S., Altrocchi, P. H., Avioli, L. V., Goodman, D. S., and Goodman, H. C.,** Tangier disease, *Ann. Intern. Med.,* 55, 1016, 1961.

194. **Fredrickson, D. S., Gooto, A. M., and Levy, R. I.,** Familial lipoprotein deficiency, *Metabolic Basis of Inherited Disease,* 3rd ed., Stanbury, J. B., Wyngaarden, J. B., and Fredrickson, D. S., Eds., McGraw-Hill, New York, 1972, 493.

195. **Fredrickson, D. S. and Lees, R. S.,** A system of phenotyping hyper-lipoproteinemia, *Circulation,* 31, 321, 1965.

196. **Fredrickson, D. S., Levy, R. I., and Lees, R. S.,** Fat transport in lipoproteins: an integrated approach to mechanisms and disorders, *N. Engl. J. Med.,* 276, 94, 1967.

197. **Fredrickson, D. S., Levy, R. I., and Lees, R. S.,** Fat transport in lipoproteins. An integrated approach to mechanisms and disorders, *N. Eng. J. Med.,* 276, 34, 1967.

198. **Fredrickson, D. S. and Steinberg, D.,** Failure of alpha-phenylbutyrate and beta-phenylvalerate in treatment of hypercholesterolemia, *Circulation,* 15, 391, 1957.

199. **French, J.,** Atherosclerosis in relation to the structure and function of the arterial intima, with special reference to the endothelium, *Int. Rev. Exp. Pathol.,* 5, 253, 1966.

200. **Friedman, M.,** *Pathogenesis of Coronary Artery Disease,* McGraw-Hill, New York, 1969.

201. **Friedman, M. and Byers, S. O.,** The pathogenesis of neurogenic hypercholesterolemia. V. Relationship to hepatic catabolism of cholesterol, *Proc. Soc. Exp. Biol. Med.,* 144, 917, 1973.

202. **Fuchs, J., Weinberger, I., Rotenberg, Z., Erdberg, A., Davidson, E., Joshna, H., and Agnon, J.,** Plasma viscosity in ischemic heart disease, *Am. Heart J.,* 108, 435, 1984.

203. **Fuller, G. C. and Langnor, R. O.,** Elevations of aortic proline hydroxylase: a biochemical defect in experimental arteriosclerosis, *Science,* 168, 987, 1970.

204. **Fuller, G. C., Miller, E., Farber, T., and Van Loon, E.,** Aortic connective tissue changes in miniature pigs fed a lipid-rich diet, *Connect. Tissue Res.,* 1, 217, 1972.

205. **Fuller, J. H. and McCartney, M. A.,** Lipoproteins and C.H.D. [letter], *Lancet,* 1, 1291, 1976.

206. **Fuller, J.H., Shipley, M. J., Rose, G., Jarrett, R. H., and Keen, H.,** Coronary heart disease risk and impaired glucose tolerance, *Lancet,* 1, 1373, 1980.

207. **Furman, R. H. and Howard, R. P.,** The influence of gonadal hormones on serum lipids and lipoproteins: studies in normal and hypogonadal subjects, *Ann. Intern. Med.,* 47, 969, 1957.

208. **Furman, R. H., Howard, R. P., Norcia, L. N., and Robinson, C. W., Jr.,** Effect of N-(1-methyl-2,3-di-p-chlorphenyl)-maleic acid (benzmalacene) on serum lipids and lipoproteins, *Proc. Soc. Exp. Biol. Med.,* 103, 302, 1960.

209. **Fry, D. I.,** Responses of the arterial wall to certain physical factors, in CIBA Foundation Symposium No. 12 (new series), *Atherogenesis: Initiating Factors,* Porter, R. and Knight, J., Eds., Excerpta Medica, Amsterdam, 1973, 93-120.

210. **Garcia-Palmieri, M. R., Tillotson, J., Cordero, E., Costar, R. J., Sorlis, P., Gordon, T., Kannel, W. B., and Colon, A. A.,** Nutrient intake and serum lipids in urban and rural Puerto Rican men, *Am. J. Clin. Nutr.,* 30, 2092, 1977.

211. **Garcia-Webb, C., Bonser, A. M., Whiting, D., and Masarei, J. R.,** Insulin resistance — a risk factor for coronary heart disease? *Scand. J. Clin. Lab. Invest.,* 43, 677, 1983.

212. **Garg, J. P., Gupta, R. S., Agrawal, M. P., and Bhandarl, V. M.,** Effect of smoking on serum lipids and lipoproteins in healthy subject, and patients of old myocardial infarction and hypertension, *Indian J. Med. Sci.,* 57, 63, 1983.

213. **Genton, E., Gent, M., Hirsh, J., and Harker, L. A.,** Platelet-inhibiting drugs in the prevention of clinical thrombotic disease, *N. Engl. J. Med.,* 293, 1174, 1975.

214. **Gerrity, R. G.,** The role of monocyte in atherogenesis. I. Transition of blood-borne monocytes into foam cells in fatty lesions, *Am. J. Pathol.,* 103, 181, 1981.

215. **Germuth, F. G., Senterfit, L. B., and Pollack, A. D.,** Immune complex disease. I. Experimental acute and chronic glomerulonephritis, *John Hopkins Med. J.,* 120, 225, 1967.

216. **Gersh, I. and Catchpole, H. R.,** The nature of ground substance of connective tissue, *Persp. Biol. Med.,* 3, 282, 1960.

217. **Gertz, S. D., Uretzky, G., Wajnberg, R., Narvot, N., and Gotsmans, M. S.,** Endothelial cell damage and thrombus formation after partial arterial constriction, *Circulation,* 63, 476, 1981.

218. **Gessner, F. B.,** Haemodynamic theories in atherogenesis, *Circulation Res.,* 33, 259, 1973.

219. **Gimbrone, M. A., Jr., and Alexander, R. W.,** Angiotension II. Stimulation of prostaglandin in cultured human vascular endothelium *Science,* 189, 219, 1975.

220. **Gimbrone, M. A., Cotran, R. S., and Folkman, J.,** Human vascular endothelial cells in culture, *J. Cell Biol.,* 60, 673, 1974.

221. **Glagov, S.,** Hemodynamic factor in localization of atherosclerosis, *Acta Cardiol. Suppl.,* 11, 311, 1965.

222. **Glagov, S. and Ozoa, A. K.,** Significance of the relatively low incidence of atherosclerosis in the pulmonary, renal and mesenteric arteries, *Ann. N.Y. Acad. Sci.,* 149, 940, 1968.

223. **Gleich, G. J., Welsh, P. W., Yunginger, J. W., Hyatt, R. E., and Catlett, J. B.,** Allergy to tobacco, an occupational hazard, *N. Engl J. Med.,* 302, 617, 1980.

224. **Glickman, R. M. and Kirsch, K.,** Lymph chylomicron formation during the inhition of protein synthesis. Studies of chylomicron apoproteins, *J. Clin. Invest.,* 52, 2910, 1973.

225. **Glomset, J. A. and Norum, K.,** The metabolic role of lecithin: cholesterol acyltransferase: perspectives from pathology, *Adv. Lipid Res.,* 11, 1, 1973.

226. **Glueck, G. J., Gartside, P., Fallat, R. W., Sielski, J., and Steiner, P. M.,** Longevity syndromes: familial hypobeta- and familial hyperalphalipoproteinemia, *J. Lab. Clin. Med.,* 88, 941, 1976.

227. **Goldberg, R. B., Fless, G. M., Bakes, S. G., Joffe, B. I., Getz, G. S., Scanu, A. M., and Seftel, H. C.,** Abnormalities of high-density lipoproteins in homozygous familial hypercholesterolemia, *Arteriosclerosis,* 4, 472, 1984.

228. **Goldstein, J. L., Basu, S. K., Brunschede, G. Y., and Brown, M. J.,** Release of low-density lipoprotein from its cell surface receptors by sulfated glycosaminoglycans, *Cell,* 7, 85, 1976.

229. **Goldstein, J. L. and Brown, M. S.,** Familial hypercholesterolemia. A genetic regulatory defect in cholesterol metabolism, *Am. J. Med.,* 58, 147, 1975.

230. **Goldstein, J. L., Dana, S. E., Faust, J. R., Beaudec, A. L., and Brown, M. S.,** Role of lyosomal acid lipase in the metabolism of plasma low density lipoprotein. Observations in cultural fibroblasts from a patient with cholesteryl ester storage disease, *J. Biol. Chem.,* 250, 8487, 1975.

231. **Goldstein, J. L., Ho, Y. K., Brown, M. S., Innerarity, T. L., and Mahley, R. W.,** Cholesteryl ester accumulation in macrophages resulting from receptor-mediated uptake and degradation of hypercholesterolemic canine β-very low density lipoproteins, *J. Biol. Chem.,* 255, 1839, 1980.

232. **Gofman, J. W. and Young, W.,** The filtration concept of atherosclerosis and serum lipids in the diagnosis of atherosclerosis, in *Atherosclerosis and Its Origin,* Sandler, M. and Bourne, G. H., Eds., Academic Press, New York, 1963, 197-227.

233. **Goodnight, S. H., Harris, W. S., and Connor, W. E.,** The effects of dietary w³ fatty acids on platelet composition and function in man: a prospective, controlled study, *Blood,* 58, 880, 1981.

234. **Gotto, A. M. and Rifkind, B. M.,** The current status of high density lipoproteins, in *Atherosclerosis Reviews,* Vol. 9, Gotto, A. M. and Paoletti, R., Eds, Raven Press, New York, 1982, 1—12.

235. **Gorev, N. N., Kozhura, I. M., Kozhura, I. P., Polinskaya, V. I., Chayalo, P. P., and Cherkasskii, L. P.,** Some pathogenic factors of age-related specificities in experimental atherosclerosis, *Cor. Vasa,* 25, 196, 1983.

236. **Gordon, D., Guyton, J. R., and Karnovsky, M. T.,** Intimal alterations in rat aorta induced by stressful stimuli, *Lab. Invest.,* 45, 14, 1981.

237. **Gordon, T., Kannel, W. B., McGee, D., and Daber, J. R.,** Death and coronary attacks in man after giving up cigarette smoking. A report from the Framingham study, *Lancet,* 2, 1345, 1974.

238. **Grande, F., Anderson, J. T., and Keys, A.,** Phenyl butyramide and the serum cholesterol concentration in man, *Metabolism,* 6, 154, 1957.
239. **Green, D., Stone, N. J., and Krumlovsky, P. A.,** Putative atherogenic factors in patients with chronic renal failure, *Prog. Cardiovasc. Dis.,* 26, 133, 1983.
240. **Greim, H., Trülzsch, D., Czygan, P., Hutterer, F., Schaffner, F., Popper, H., Cooper, D. Y., and Rosenthal, O.,** Bile acid formation by liver microsomal systems, *Ann. N.Y. Acad. Sci.,* 212, 139, 1973.
241. **Griffith, M. J., Breitkreutz, L., Trapp, H., Briet, E., Noyes, C. M., Lundblad, R. L., and Roberts, H. R.,** Characterization of the clotting activities of structurally different forms of activated factor IX, *J. Clin. Invest.,* 75, 4, 1985.
242. **Griggs, T. R., Reddick, R. L., Sultzer, D., and Brinkhous, K. M.,** Susceptibility to atherosclerosis in aortas and coronary arteries of swine with von Willebrand's disease, *Am. J. Pathol.,* 102, 137, 1981.
243. **Grimm, R. H., Leon, A. S., Hunninghake, D. B., Lenz, K., Hannan, P., and Blackburn, H.,** Effect of thiazide diuretics on plasma lipids and lipoproteins in mildly hypertensive males, *Circ. Res. (Suppl I),* 26, 149, 1981.
244. **Groves, H. M., Kinlough-Rathbone, R. L., Casenave, D. P., Dejane, E., Richardson, M., and Mustard, J. F.,** Effect of dipyridamole and PGI2 on rabbit platelet adherence in vitro and in vivo, *J. Lab. Clin. Med.,* 99, 548, 1982.
245. **Grundy, S. M.,** Hyperlipoproteinemia: metabolic basis and rationale for therapy, *Am. J. Cardiol.,* 54, 206, 1984.
246. **Grundy, S. M.,** Modern management of hyperlipidemia, *Compo. Thes.,* 10, 46, 1984.
247. **Grundy, S. M., Ahrens, E. H., and Davignon, J.,** The interaction of cholesterol absorption and cholesterol synthesis in man, *J. Lipid Res.,* 10, 304, 1969.
248. **Gryglewski, R. J., Dembinska-Klec, A., Zmuda, A., and Gryglewska, T.,** Prostacyclin and thromboxane A2 biosynthesis capacities of heart, arteries and platelets at various stages of experimental atherosclerosis in rabbits, *Atherosclerosis,* 31, 385, 1978.
249. **Gryglewski, R., Bunting, S., Moncada, S., and Flower, R. J.,** Arterial walls are protected against deposition of platelet thrombi by a substance (prostaglandin X) which they make from prostaglandin endoperoxides, *Prostaglandins,* 12, 685, 1976.
250. **Gustafson, A., Alaupovic, P., and Furman, R. H.,** Studies of the composition and structure of serum lipoproteins. Separation and characterization of phospholipid protein residues obtained by partial delipidization of very low density lipoproteins of human serum, *Biochemistry,* 5, 632, 1966.
251. **Gutstein, W. H. and Farrell, G.,** Serum cholesterol responses to hypothalamic stimulation and fatty acid administration in the rat, *Proc. Soc. Exp. Biol. Med.,* 141, 137, 1972.
252. **Gutstein, W. H., Schneck, D. J., and Appleton, H. D.,** Association of increased plasma lipid levels with brain stimulation, *Metabolism,* 17, 535, 1968.
253. **Haber, C. and Kwiterovich, P. O.,** Dyslipoproteinemia and xanthomatosis, *Pediatr. Dermatol.,* 1, 261, 1984.
254. **Habert, H. B.,** The nature of the relationship between obesity and cardiovascular disease, *Int. J. Cardiol.,* 6, 268, 1984.
255. **Hajjar, D. P., Falcone, D. J., Fowler, S., and Minick, C. R.,** Endothelium modifies the altered metabolism of the injured aortic wall, *Am. J. Pathol.,* 102, 28, 1981.
256. **Hamilton, R. L.,** Synthesis and secretion of plasma lipoproteins, *Adv. Exp. Med. Biol.,* 26, 7, 1972.
257. **Hammond, E. C.,** Smoking in relation to diseases other than cancer. Total death rates, in Proc. 2nd World Conf. Smoking and Health, Richards, R. G., Ed., 1972, 24-34.
258. **Hammond, M. G. and Fisher, W. R.,** The characterization of a discrete series of low density lipoproteins in the disease, hyper-pre-beta-lipoproteinemia. Implications relating to the structure of plasma lipoproteins, *J. Biol. Chem.,* 246, 5454, 1971.
259. **Hanger, K. H., Kilgore, J., and James, E.,** Essential thrombocythemia and coronary artery disease, *Chest,* 86, 933, 1984.
260. **Harkavy, J.,** Tobacco allergy in cardiovascular disease: a review, *Ann. Allergy,* 26, 447, 1968.
261. **Harker, L. A. and Slichter, S. J.,** Arterial and venous thromboembolism, kinetic characterization and evaluation of therapy, *Thromb. Diath. Haemorrh.,* 31, 188, 1974.
262. **Harker, L. A., Ross, R., Slichter, S., and Scott, C.** Homocystine induced atherosclerosis: the role of endothelial cell injury and platelet response in its genesis, *J. Clin. Invest.,* 58, 731, 1976.
263. **Harker, L., Ross, R., and Glomset, J.,** Role of the platelets in atherogenesis, *Ann. N.Y. Acad. Sci.,* 275, 321, 1976.
264. **Harker, L. A., Slichter, S. J., Scott, C. R., and Ross, R.,** Homocystinemia: vascular injury and arterial thrombosis, *N. Engl. J. Med.,* 291, 537, 1976.
265. **Harlan, W. R., Winesett, P. S., and Wasseman, A. J.,** Tissue lipoprotein lipase in normal individuals and in individuals with exogenous hyperglyceridemia and the relationship of this enzyme to assimilation of fat, *J. Clin. Invest.,* 46, 239, 1967.

266. **Harmsen, E., de Tombe, P. P., de Jong, J. W., and Achterberg, P. W.,** Enhanced ATP and GTP synthesis from hypoxanthine or inosine after myocardial ischemia, *Am. J. Physiol.*, 246, H37, 1984.

267. **Harris, R. S., Jr., Gilmore, H. R., Bricker, L. A., Keim, I. M., and Rubin, E.,** Long-term oral administration of probucol (4,4'-isopropylidenedithio) bis(2,6-di-t-butylphenol) (DH-581) in the management of hypercholesterolemia, *J. Am. Geriatr. Soc.*, 22, 167, 1974.

268. **Hashim, S. A. and Van Italie, T. B.,** Cholestyramine resin therapy for hypercholesterolemia: clinical and metabolic studies, *J. Am. Med. Assoc.*, 192, 289, 1965.

269. **Hashimoto, S., Dayton, S., and Alfin-Slater, R. B.,** Esterification of cholesterol by homogenates of atherosclerotic and normal aortas, *Life Sci.*, 12, 1, 1973.

270. **Hashimoto, S., Dayton, S., Alfin-Slater, R. B., Bui, P. T., Baker, N., and Wilson, L.,** Characteristics of the cholesterol-esterifying activity in normal and atherosclerotic rabbit aortas, *Circ. Res.*, 34, 176, 1974.

271. **Haskell, W. L.,** Exercise-induced changes in plasma lipids and lipoproteins, *Prev. Med.*, 13, 23, 1984.

272. **Haslam, R. J. and McClenaghan, M. D.,** Measurement of circulating prostacyclin, *Nature (London)*, 292, 364, 1981.

273. **Hatch, F. T. and Lees, R. S.,** Practical methods for plasma lipoproteins analysis, *Adv. Lipid Res.*, 6, 7, 1968.

274. **Hauss, W. H.,** Role of arterial wall cells in sclerogenesis, *Ann. N.Y. Acad. Sci.*, 275, 286, 1976.

275. **Haust, M. D.,** Reaction patterns of intimal mesenchyma to injury and repair in atherosclerosis, *Adv. Exp. Med. Biol.*, 43, 35, 1974.

276. **Haust, M. D.,** The morphogenesis and fate of potential and early atherosclerotic lesions in man, *Hum. Pathol.*, 2, 1, 1971.

277. **Haust, M. D.,** Proliferation and degeneration of elastic tissue in aortic explants from normo- and hypercholesterolaemic rabbits — an ultrastructural study, *Exp. Mol. Pathol.*, 31, 169, 1977.

278. **Haust, M. D.** Arteriosclerosis. I. Concepts of disease, in *Textbook of Pathology*, Brunson, J. G. and Gall, E. A., Eds., Macmillan, New York, 1971, 451.

279. **Haust, M. D.,** Connective tissue in atherosclerosis, in *Atherosclerosis*, Proc. 4th Int. Symp. (Japan), Goto, Y., Hata, Y., and Klose, G., Eds., Springer-Verlag, Berlin, 1977, 30-35.

280. **Havel, R. J.,** Lipoprotein biosynthesis and metabolism, in *Lipoprotein Structure*, Scanu, A. M. and Landsberger, F. R., Eds., N.Y. Acad. Sci., 348, 1980, 16—29.

281. **Havel, R. J., Goldstein, J. L., and Brown, M. S.,** Lipoproteins and lipid transport, in *Metabolic Control and Disease*, Bondy, P. K. and Rosenberg, L. E., Eds., W. B. Saunders, Philadelphia, 1980, 393-494.

282. **Havel, R. J. and Gordon, R. S.,** Idiopathic hyperlipemia: metabolic studies in an affected family, *J. Clin. Invest.*, 39, 1777, 1960.

283. **Havel, R. J. and Kane, J. P.,** Drugs and lipid metabolism, *Annu. Rev. Pharmacol.*, 13, 287, 1973.

284. **Havlick, R. J., Wilson, P. W., Garrison, R. J., and Feinleib, M.,** Epidemiology of lipoproteins and the decline in coronary heart disease mortality, in *Lipoproteins and Coronary Atherosclerosis*, Noseda, G., Fragiacomo, C., Fumagalli, R., and Paoletti, R., Eds., Elsevier, Amsterdam, 1982, 61-68.

285. **Hazzard, W. R.,** Atherogenesis: why women live longer than men, *Geriatrics*, 40, 42, 1985.

286. **Heller, R. F., Miller, N. E., Wheeler, M. J., and Kind, P. R.,** Coronary heart disease in 'low risk' men, *Atherosclerosis*, 49, 187, 1983.

287. **Heptinstall, S.,** Properties of blood platelets that may be relevant to atherogenesis, *Cor. Vasa*, 13, 343, 1984.

288. **Hernandez, H. H., Peterson, D. W., Chaikoff, I. L., and Dauben, W. G.,** Absorption of cholesterol-4-C^{14} in rats fed mixed soybean sterols and beta-sitosterols, *Proc. Soc. Exp. Biol. Med.*, 83, 498, 1953.

289. **Higgins, M. and Rudney, H.,** Regulation of rat liver beta-hydroxy-beta-methylglutaryl-CoA reductase activity by cholesterol, *Nature (London)*, 246, 60, 1973.

290. **Higgins, M. J. P., Kawachi, T., and Rodney, H.,** The mechanism of the diurnal variation of hepatic HMC-CoA reductase activity in the rat, *Biochem. Biophys. Res. Commun.*, 45, 138, 1971.

291. **Hillis, L. D., Hirsh, P. D., Campbell, W. B., and Firth, B. G.,** Interactions of the arterial wall, plaque and platelets in myocardial ischemia and infarction, *Cardiovasc. Clin.*, 14, 31, 1983.

292. **Hjermann, I., Byre, K. V., Holme, I., and Leren, P.,** Effect of diet and smoking intravention on the incidence of coronary heart disease, *Lancet*, 2, 1303, 1981.

293. **Hollis, T. M. and Rosen, L. A.,** Histidine decarboxylase activity of bovine aortic endothelium and intima-media, *Proc. Soc. Exp. Biol. Med.*, 141, 978, 1972.

294. **Holme, I., Enger, S. C., Helgeland, A., Hjermann, I., Leren, P., Lund-Larsen, P. G., Solberg, L. A., and Stong, J. P.,** Risk factors and raised atherosclerotic lesion in coronary and cerebral vessels. Statistical analysis from the Oslo study, *Arteriosclerosis*, 1, 250, 1981.

295. **Hoonebeck, W., Potazman, J. P., De Cremoux, H., Bellon, G., and Robert, L.,** Elastase-type activity of human serum. Its variation in chronic obstructive lung disease and atherosclerosis, *Clin. Physiol. Biochem.*, 1, 285, 1983.

296. **Hooper, P. L. and Scallen, T. J.,** Modulation of high-density lipoprotein: the importance of protein phosphorylation/dephosphorylation, *Am. Heart J.*, 108, 1393, 1984.

297. **Hovig, T. and Gjone, E.**, Familial lecithin: cholesterol acyltransferase deficiency. Ultrastructural studies on lipid deposition and tissue reaction, *Scand. J. Clin. Lab. Invest.*, 33(Suppl 137), 135, 1974.

298. **Howard, A. N. and Gresham, G.A.**, Dietary aspects of atherosclerosis and thrombosis, *Int. J. Vit. Res.*, 38, 546, 1968.

299. **Howard, A. N.**, Recent advances in nutrition and atherosclerosis, in *Atherosclerosis*, Jones, R. J., Ed., Springer-Verlag, Berlin, 1980, 408.

300. **Howard, A. N. and Hyams, D. E.**, Combined use of clofibrate and cholestyramine or DEAE sephadex in hypercholesterolemia, *Br. Med. J.*, 2, 25, 1971.

301. **Howard, B. V., Macarak, E. J., Gunson, D., and Kefalides, N. A.**, Characterization of the collagen synthesized by endothelial cells in culture, *Proc. Natl. Acad. Sci. U.S.A.*, 73, 2361, 1976.

302. **Howard, C. F., Jr.**, De novo synthesis and elongation of fatty acids by subcellar fractions of monkey aorta, *J. Lipid Res.*, 9, 254, 1968.

303. **Howard, C. F.**, Aortic lipogenesis during aerobic and hypoxic incubation, *Atherosclerosis*, 15, 359, 1972.

304. **Huff, J. W. and Gilfillian, J. L.**, Benzmalacene: inhibition of cholesterol biosynthesis and hypocholesteremic effect in rats, *Proc. Soc. Exp. Biol. Med.*, 103, 41, 1960.

305. **Hui, D. Y., Innerarity, T. L., and Mahley, R. W.**, Lipoprotein binding to canine hepatic membranes: metabolically distinct apo-E and apo-B,E receptors, *J. Biol. Chem.*, 256, 5646, 1981.

306. **Inagaki, M., Kawamoto, S., and Hidaka, H.**, Serotonin excretion from human platelets may be modified by Ca^{2+}-activated phospholipid-dependent myosin phosphorylation, *J. Biol. Chem.*, 759, 14321, 1984.

307. **Innerarity, T. L., Hui, D. Y., and Mahley, R. W.**, Hepatic apoprotein E (remnant) receptors, in *Proc. Int. Symp. Lipoproteins and Coronary Atherosclerosis*, Noseda, G., Fragiacomo, C., Fumagali, R., and Paoletti, R., Eds., Elsevier/North-Holland Press, Amsterdam, 1982, 173-181.

308. **Innerarity, T. L. and Mahley, R. W.**, Enhanced binding by cultured human fibroblasts of apo-E-containing lipoproteins as compared with low density lipoproteins, *Biochemistry*, 17, 1440, 1978.

309. **Innerarity, T. L. and Mahley, R. W.**, Lipoprotein metabolism mediated by cell surface receptors. In vivo and in vitro parallel, in *7th Int. Symp. Drugs Affecting Lipid Metabolism*, Fumagalli, R., Kritchevsky, D., and Paoletti, R., Eds., Elsevier/North Holland Press, Amsterdam, 1980, 53-60.

310. **Insull, W. and Bartsch, G. E.**, Cholestrol, triglyceride, and phospholipid content of intima, media, and atherosclerotic fatty streak in human thoracic aorta, *J. Clin. Invest.*, 45, 513, 1966.

311. **Jackson, R. L., Baker, H. N., Gilliam, J. M., and Gotto, A. M.**, Primary structure of very low density apolipoprotein C-II of human plasma, *Proc. Natl. Acad. Sci., U.S.A.*, 74, 1942, 1977.

312. **Jackson, R. L., Morrisett, J. D., and Gotto, A. M.**, Lipoprotein structure and metabolism, *Physiol. Rev.*, 56, 259, 1976.

313. **Jackson, R. L., Sparrow, J. T., Baker, H. N., Morrisett, J. D., Taunton, O. D., and Gotto, A. M.**, The primary structure of apoprotein-serine, *J. Biol. Chem.*, 249, 5308, 1974.

314. **Jaffe, E. A., Hoyer, L. W., and Nachman, R. L.**, Synthesis of von Willebrand factor by cultured endothelial cells, *Proc. Natl. Acad. Sci. U.S.A.*, 71, 1906, 1974.

315. **Jaffe, E. A., Hoyer, L. W., and Nachman, R. L.**, Synthesis of antihaemophilic factor antigen by cultured human endothelial cells, *J. Clin. Invest.*, 52, 2764, 1973.

316. **Jaffe, E. A., Minick, C. R., Adelman, B., Becker, C. G., and Nachman, R. L.**, Synthesis of basement collagen by cultured human endothelial cells, *J. Exp. Med.*, 144, 209, 1976.

317. **Jaillard, J., Sezille, G., Fruchart, J. P., and Romon, M.**, Etude de l'activité de la lipoproteine-lipase et de la cellularité au niveau du tissue lipideux humain: influence de l'obesité et du diabète, *Diabet. Mecab. (Paris)*, 2, 5, 1976.

318. **Janus, E. D., Nicoll, A. M., Turner, P. R., Magill, P., and Lewis, B.**, Kinetic bases of the primary hyperlipidaemias. Studies of apoprotein B turnover in genetically defined subjects, *Eur. J. Clin. Invest.*, 10, 161, 1980.

319. **Johnson, M., Carey, F., and McMillan, R. M.**, Alternative pathways of arachidonate metabolism: prostaglandins, thromboxane and leukotrienes, *Essays Biochem.*, 15, 40, 1983.

320. **Jones, A. L., Ruderman, N. B., and Herrera, M. G.**, Electronmicroscopic and biochemical study of lipoprotein synthesis in the isolated perfused rat liver, *J. Lipid Res.*, 8, 429, 1967.

321. **Juchau, M. R., Bond, J. A., and Benditt, E. P.**, Aryl 4-monoxygenase and cytochrome P-450 in the aorta: possible role in atherosclerosis, *Proc. Natl. Acad. Sci. U.S.A.*, 73, 3723, 1976.

322. **Kaijser, L., Eklund, B., and Joreteg, T.**, Hemodynamic effects of PGE, and PGI2 in man, in *Prostaglandins in Clinical Medicine. Cardiovascular and Thrombotic Disorders*, Wu, K. K. and Rossi, E. C., Eds., Year Book Medical, Chicago, IL, 1982, 123-132.

323. **Kannel, W. B., Dawber, T. R., and McGee, D. L.**, Perspective on systolic hypertension: the Framingham study, *Circulation*, 61, 1179, 1980.

324. **Kannel, W. B. and Schatzkin, A.**, Risk factor analysis, *Prog. Cardiovasc. Dis.*, 26, 309, 1984.

325. **Kaplan, N. M.**, Whom to treat, the dilemma of mild hypertension, *Am. Heart J.* 101, 867, 1981.

326. **Karino, T. and Goldsmith, H. L.**, Role of blood cell-wall interactions in thrombogenesis and atherogenesis: a microrheological study, *Biorheology*, 21, 587, 1984.

327. **Keil, J. E., Sandifer, S. H., Loadbolt, C. B., and Boyle, E.,** Skin color and education effect on blood pressure, *Am. J. Public Health,* 71, 532, 1981.

328. **Kekki, M.,** Lipoprotein lipase action determining plasma high density lipoprotein cholesterol levels in adult normolipaemics, *Atherosclerosis,* 37, 143, 1980.

329. **Kennedy, A. L., Lappin, T. R. J., Lavery, T. D., Hadden, D. R., Weawer, J. A., and Montgomery, D. A. D.,** Relation of high density lipoprotein cholesterol concentration on type of diabetes and its control, *Br. Med. J.,* 2, 1191, 1978.

330. **Kennedy, E. P. and Weiss, S. B.,** The function of cytidine coenzymes in the biosynthesis of phospholipides, *J. Biol. Chem.,* 222, 193, 1956.

331. **Kennerly, D. A.,** Lipid metabolism and the imitation and regulation of mediator release from the mast cells, *Surv. Immunol. Res.,* 3, 304, 1984.

332. **Kessler, J. I.,** Effect of diabetes and insulin on the activity of myocardial and adipose tissue lipoprotein lipase of rats, *J. Clin. Invest.,* 42, 362, 1963.

333. **Keys, A.,** Alpha lipoprotein (HDL) cholesterol in the serum and the risk of coronary heart disease and death, *Lancet,* 2, 603, 1980.

334. **Keys, A., Kimura, N., Kusukawa, A., Bronte-Stewart, B., Larsen, N., and Keys, M. A.,** Lessons in cholesterol studies in Japan, Hawaii, and Los Angeles, *Ann. Intern. Med.,* 48, 83094, 1958.

335. **Khan, S. N., Rahman, M. A., and Samad, A.,** Trace elements in serum from Pakistani patients with acute and chronic ischemic heart disease and hypertension, *Clin. Chem.,* 30, 644, 1984.

336. **Kisselbah, A. H., Alfarsi, S., and Evans, D. J.,** Low-density lipoprotein metabolism in familial combined hyperlipemia. Mechanism of the multiple lipoprotein phenotypic expression, *Arteriosclerosis,* 4, 14, 1984.

337. **Klarfeld, D. M.,** Interactions of immune function with lipids and atherosclerosis, *CRC Int. Rev. Toxicol.,* 11, 333, 1983.

338. **Klein, L. W. and Gorlin, R.,** The systemic and coronary hemodynamic response to cigarette smoking, *N.Y. State J. Med.,* 83, 1264, 1983.

339. **Kniker, W. I. and Cochrane, C. G.,** Pathogenic factors in vascular lesions of experimental serum sickness, *J. Exp. Med.,* 122, 83, 1965.

340. **Knox, P.,** The cell surface in health and disease, *Mol. Aspects Med.,* 7, 117, 1984.

341. **Kolata, G.,** Cholesterol-heart disease link illuminated, *Science,* 221, 1164, 1983.

342. **Kortenhaus, H., Schroen, H., and Born, G. V. R.,** Quantification of the adhesion of platelets in hamster venules in vivo, *Proc. R. Soc. London (Biol.),* 215, 135, 1982.

343. **Kostner, G.,** Studies on the cofactor requirements for lecithin: cholesterol acyltransferase, *Scand. J. Clin. Lab. Invest.,* 33(Suppl. 137), 19, 1974.

344. **Kostner, G. and Alaupovic, P.,** Studies of the composition and structure of plasma lipoproteins. Separation and quantification of the lipoprotein families occurring in the high density lipoproteins of human plasma, *Biochemistry,* 11, 3419, 1972.

345. **Kostner, G. and Holasek, A.,** Characterization and quantitation of the apolipoproteins from human chyle chylomicrons, *Biochemistry,* 11, 1217, 1972.

346. **Kottke, B. A., Unnik, K., Carlo, I. A., and Subbiah, M. T.,** Early chemical and structural changes during regression of spontaneous atherosclerotic lesions after intestinal bypass surgery, *Circulation,* 50, 93, 1974.

347. **Kramer, J. B. and Corr, P. B.,** Mechanisms contributing to arrhythmias during ischemia and infarction, *Eur. Heart J.,* 5(Suppl. B), 11, 1984.

348. **Kramsch, D. M.,** The role of connective tissue in atherosclerosis, in *Drugs, Lipid Metabolism and Atherosclerosis,* Kritchevsky, D., Paoletti, R., and Holmes, W. L., Eds., Plenum Press, New York, 1978, 155-194.

349. **Kramsch, D. M., Franzblau, C., and Hollander, W.,** The protein and lipid composition of arterial elastin and its relationship to lipid accumulation in the atherosclerotic plaque, *J. Clin. Invest.,* 46, 66, 1971.

350. **Kramsch, D. M. and Hollander, W.,** Interaction of serum and arterial lipoproteins with elastin of the arterial intima and its role in the lipid accumulation in atherosclerotic plaques, *J. Clin. Invest.,* 52, 236, 1973.

351. **Krauss, R. M., Levy, R. I., and Fredrickson, D. S.,** Selective measurement of two lipase activities in post heparin plasma from normal subjects and patients with hyperlipoproteinemia, *J. Clin. Invest.,* 54, 1107, 1974.

352. **Kresse, V. H., Filipovic, I., and Buddecke, E.,** Gesteigerte 14C-Inkorporation in die Triglycerine (Triglyceride) des Arteriengewebes bei Sauerstoffmangel, *Hoppe Seyler's Z. Physiol. Chem.,* 350, 1611, 1969.

353. **Kristein, M. M.,** 40 years of U.S. cigarette smoking and heart disease and cancer mortality rates, *J. Chronic Dis.,* 37, 317, 1984.

354. **Kritchevsky, D.,** Effect of thyroid hormones on lipid metabolism, in *Action of Hormones on Molecular Processes,* Litwack, G. and Kritchevsky D., Eds., John Wiley & Sons, New York, 1964, 162-171.

355. **Kritchevsky, D., Cottrell, M. C., and Tepper, S. A.,** Oxidation of cholesterol by rat liver mitochondria: effect of thyroactive compounds, *J. Cell. Comp. Physiol.,* 60, 105, 1962.

356. **Kromhout, D. and de Lezenne Coulander, C.**, Diet, prevalence and 10-year mortality from coronary heart disease in 871 middle-aged men, *Am. J. Epidemiol.*, 119, 733, 1984.

357. **Kudryashov, S. A., Tertov, V. V., Orchkhov, A. N., Geling, N. G., and Smirnov, V. N.**, Regression of atherosclerotic manifestations in primary culture of human aortic cells: effects of prostaglandins, *Biomed. Biochim. Acta*, 43, S284, 1984.

358. **Kunz, F., Zwierzina, W. D., and Hörtnagl, H.**, Clot lipids in ischaemic heart disease, *Atherosclerosis*, 49, 195, 1983.

359. **Kurtz, S. M., Fitzgerald, J. E., Fisken, R. A., Schardein, J. L., Reutner, T. H., and Lucas, J. A.**, Toxicology studies on gemfibrozil, *Proc. R. Soc. Med.*, 69(Suppl. 2), 15, 1976.

360. **Lakshmann, M. R., Nepokroeff, C. M., and Porter, J. W.**, Control of the synthesis of fatty-acid synthetase in rat liver by insulin, glucagon and adenosine $3':5'$ cyclic monophosphate, *Proc. Natl. Acad. Sci. U.S.A.*, 69, 3516, 1972.

361. **Lands, W. E.**, Metabolism of glycerolipids 2. The enzymatic acylation of lysolecithin, *J. Biol. Chem.*, 235, 2233, 1960.

362. **Langille, L. B.**, Integrity of arterial endothelium following acute exposure to high shear stress, *Biotheology*, 21, 333, 1984.

363. **Lanir, Y.**, The possible role of intimal convective transport in atherogenesis, *Biorheology*, 21, 643, 1984.

364. **LaPorte, R. E., Adams, L. L., Savage, D. D., Brenes, G., Dearwacer, S., and Cook, T.**, The spectrum of physical activity, cardiovascular disease and health: an epidemiologic perspective, *Am. J. Epidemiol.*, 120, 507, 1984.

365. **Lechi, C., Zatti, M., Corradini, P., Bonadonna, G., Arioso, E., Pedrolli, G., and Lechi, A.**, Increased leukocyte aggregation in patients with hypercholesterolemia, *Clin. Chim. Acta*, 144, 11, 1984.

366. **Lee, D. M. and Alaupovic, P.**, Physicochemical properties of low-density lipoproteins of normal human plasma. Evidence for the occurrence of lipoprotein B in associated and free forms, *Biochemistry*, 9, 249, 1970.

367. **Lee, D. M. and Alaupovic, P.**, Composition and concentration of apolipoproteins in very low and low density lipoproteins of the normal human plasma, *Atherosclerosis*, 19, 501, 1974.

368. **Lee, K. T., Thomas, W. A., Florentin, R. A., Reiner, J. M., and Lee, W. M.**, Evidence for a polyclonal origin and proliferative heterogeneity of atherosclerotic lesions induced by dietary cholesterol in young swine, *Ann. N.Y. Acad. Sci.*, 275, 336, 1976.

369. **Lees, R. S. and Carvalho, A. C. A.**, Hypercholesterolaemia and platelets, in *Thrombotic Process in Atherogenesis*, Chandler, A. B., Ed., 1978, 301-308.

370. **Levy, L.**, A form of immunological atherosclerosis, in *The Reticuloendothelial System and Atherosclerosis*, Di Luzio, N. R. and Paoletti, R., Eds., Plenum Press, New York, 1967, 431.

371. **Levy, R. I.**, Declining mortality in coronary heart disease, *Atherosclerosis*, 1, 312, 1981.

372. **Lewis, B.**, *The Hyperlipidemias: Clinical and Laboratory Practice*, Blackwell Scientific, Oxford, 1976.

373. **Lewis, B.**, Metabolism of the plasma lipoproteins, in *The Scientific Basis of Medicine Annual Review*, Gilliland, I. and Frances, J., Eds., Athlone Press, London, 1972, 118.

374. **Lewis, L. J., Hoak, J. C., Maca, R. D., and Fry, G. L.**, Replication of human endothelial cells in culture, *Science*, 181, 453, 1973.

375. **Lewis, R. A. and Austen, K. F.**, Mediation of local homeostasis and inflammation by leukotrienes and other mast-cell-dependent compounds, *Nature (London)*, 293, 103, 1981.

376. **Lieber, C. S., Teschke, R., Hasumura, Y., and DeCarli, L. M.**, Differences in hepatic and metabolic changes after acute and chronic alcohol consumption, *Fed. Proc.*, 34, 2060, 1975.

377. **Liedtke, A. J., Nellis, S. H., and Mjos, O. D.**, Effects of reducing fatty acid metabolism on mechanical function in regionally ischemic hearts, *Am. J. Physiol.*, 247, H387, 1984.

378. **Lim, C. T., Chung, H. J., Kayden, H. J., and Scanu, A. M.**, Lipoproteins of human serum high density lipoproteins, *Biochim. Biophys. Acta*, 420, 332, 1976.

379. **Limas, C., Westrum, B., and Limas, C. T.**, The evolution of vascular changes in the spontaneously hypertensive rat, *Am. J. Pathol.*, 98, 357, 1980.

380. **Lindgren, F. T., Jensen, L. C., Wills, R. D., and Stevens, G. R.**, Subfractionation of Sf4-105, Sf4-20 and high density lipoproteins, *Lipids*, 7, 194, 1972.

381. **Lindy, S., Turoto, H., Uitto, J., Helin, P., and Lorenzen, I.**, Injury and repair in arterial tissue in the rabbit. Analysis of DNA, RNA, hydroxyproline and lactate dehydrogenase in experimental arteriosclerosis, *Circ. Res.*, 30, 123, 1972.

382. **Ljungner, H., Manhem, P., and Bergqvist, D.**, Decreased fibrinolytic activity in human atherosclerotic vessels, *Atherosclerosis*, 50, 113, 1984.

383. **Lofland, H. B., Moury, D. M., Hoffman, C. W., and Clarkson, T. B.**, Lipid metabolism in pigeon aorta during atherogenesis, *J. Lipid Res.*, 6, 112, 1965.

384. **Mabuchi, H., Haba, T., Tatami, R., Miyamoto, S., Sakai, Y., Wakasugi, T., Watanabe, A., Koizumi, J., and Takeda, R.**, Effect of an inhibitor of 3-hydroxy-3-methylglutaryl coenzyme. A reductase on serum lipoproteins and ubiquinone-10 levels in patients with familial hypercholesterolemia, *N. Engl. J. Med.*, 305, 478, 1981.

385. **Magnus, P., Borresen, A. L., Opstad, P. K., Bugge, J. F., and Berg, K.,** Increase in the ratio of serum levels of apolipoproteins A-I and A-II during prolonged physical strain and caloric deficiency, *Eur. J. Appl. Physiol.,* 53, 21, 1984.

386. **Mahler, R.,** Diabetes and arterial lipids, *Quart. J. Med.,* 34, 484, 1965.

387. **Mahley, R. W.,** Cellular and molecular biology of lipoprotein metabolism in atherosclerosis, *Diabetes,* 30, 63, 1981.

388. **Mahley, R. W.,** Atherogenic hyperlipoproteinemia, the cellular and molecular biology of plasma lipoproteins altered by dietary fat and cholesterol, in *Medical Clinics of North America: Lipid Disorders,* Havel, R. J., Ed., W. B. Saunders, Philadelphia, 1982, 375-402.

389. **Mahley, R. W., Francheschini, G., Sirtori, C. R., Capurso, A., and Weisgraber, K. H.,** A-I Milano Apoprotein. Decreased high density lipoprotein levels with significant lipoprotein modifications and without clinical atherosclerosis in an Italian family, *J. Clin. Invest.,* 66, 892, 1980.

390. **Mahley, R. W., Hui, D. Y., Innerarity, T. L., and Weisgraber, K. H.,** Two independent lipoprotein receptors on hepatic membranes of the dog, swine, and man: the apo-E receptors, *J. Clin. Invest,* 68, 1197, 1981.

391. **Mahley, R. W., Innerarity, T. L., Brown, M. S., Ho, Y. K., and Goldstein, J. L.,** Cholesteryl ester synthesis in macrophages: stimulation by β-very low density lipoproteins from cholesterol-fed animals of several species, *J. Lipid Res.,* 21, 970, 1980.

392. **Mahley, R. W. and Innerarity, T. L.,** Lipoprotein receptors and cholesterol homeostasis, *Biochim. Biophys. Acta,* 737, 197, 1983.

393. **Majerus, P. W. and Vagelos, P. R.,** Fatty acid biosynthesis and the role of the acyl carrier protein, *Adv. Lipid Res.,* 5, 1, 1967.

394. **Malcolm, G. T., Strong, J. P., and Restrepo, C.,** Atherosclerosis and lipid composition of the abdominal aorta. Comparison of autopsied New Orleans and Guatemalan men, *Lab. Invest.,* 50, 79, 1984.

395. **Malinow, M. R.,** Atherosclerosis: progression, regression and resolution, *Am. Heart J.,* 108, 1523, 1984.

396. **Mann, K. G.,** The biochemistry of coagulation, *Clin. Lab. Med.,* 4, 207, 1984.

397. **Manton, K. G.,** Sex and race specific mortality differentials in multiple cause of death data, *Gerontologist,* 20, 480, 1980.

398. **Mantulin, W. W., Massey, J. B., Gotto, A. M., Jr., and Pownall, H. J.,** Reassembled model lipoproteins, *J. Biol. Chem.,* 256, 10815, 1981.

399. **Marcus, A. J., Weksler, B. B., Jaffe, E. A., Brockman, M. J., Ullman, H. L., and Tack-Goldman, K.,** Interaction between stimulated platelets and endothelial cells in vitro, *Philos. Trans. R. Soc. (Biol.),* 294, 343, 1981.

400. **Marcus, M. L., Koyanagi, S., Harrison, D. G., Doty, D. B., Hiracaka, L. F., and Eastham, C. L.,** Abnormalities in the coronary circulation that occur as a consequence of cardiac hypertrophy, *Am. J. Med.,* 75, 62, 1983.

401. **Margolis, S.,** Separation and size determination of human serum lipoproteins by agarose gel filtration, *J. Lipid Res.,* 8, 501, 1967.

402. **Marmorston, J., Moore, F. J., Hopkins, C. E., Kuzma, O. T., and Weiner, J.,** Clinical studies of long-term estrogen therapy in men with myocardial infarction, *Proc. Soc. Exp. Biol. Med.,* 110, 400, 1962.

403. **Marmot, M. G.,** Life style and national and international trends in coronary heart disease mortality, *Postgrad. Med. J.,* 60, 3, 1984.

404. **Maroko, P. R., Ribeiro, L. G., and Goldberg, S.,** Acute myocardial infarction — coronary thrombosis and salvage of the ischemic myocardium, *Cardiovasc. Clin.,* 14, 191, 1983.

405. **Marra, R., Pagano, I., De Stefano, V., and Bizzi, B.,** Antithrombin III and factor Xa inhibitive in atherosclerosis, *Haemostasis,* 13, 209, 1983.

406. **Marsh, J. B.,** Lipoproteins in a nonrecirculating perfusate of rat liver, *J. Lipid Res.,* 15, 544, 1974.

407. **Marshall, F. N.,** Pharmacology and toxicology of probucol, *Artery,* 10, 7, 1982.

408. **Martin, J. F.,** A review of the clinical significance of physical events in the circulation, *Life Support Syst.,* 2, 153, 1984.

409. **Massey, J. B., Gotto, A. M., Jr., and Pownall, H. J.,** Thermodynamics of lipid-protein interactions: interaction of apolipoprotein A-II from human plasma high density lipoproteins with dimyristoylphosphatidylcholine, *Biochemistry,* 20, 1575, 1981.

410. **Massey, J. B., Gotto, A. M., Jr., and Pownall, H. J.,** Human plasma high density apolipoprotein A-I: effect of protein-protein interactions on the spontaneous formation of a lipid-protein recombinant, *Biochem. Biophys. Res. Commun.,* 99, 466, 1981.

411. **Mastaglia, F. L.,** Adverse effects of drugs on muscle, *Drugs,* 24, 304, 1982.

412. **Matthews, J. D.,** Ischaemic heart disease: possible genetic markers, *Lancet,* 2, 682, 1975.

413. **McCandless, E. L. and Zilversmit, D. B.,** Failure of bone marrow to form plasma phosphatides, *Acta Physiol. Pharmacol. Neerl.,* 5, 98, 1956.

414. **McConathy, W. J. and Alaupovic, P.,** Studies on the isolation and partial characterization of apolipoprotein D and lipoprotein D of human plasma, *Biochemistry,* 15, 515, 1976.

415. **McCullagh, K. A. and Baliau, G.,** Collagen characterization and cell transformation in human athero-sclerosis, *Nature (London)*, 258, 73, 1975.

416. **McCullagh, K. A. and Ehrhart, L. A.,** Induction of type I and regression of type III collagen synthesis in experimental canine atherosclerosis, *Circulation*, 54, 85, 1976.

417. **McCullagh, K. A. and Ehrhart, L. A.,** Increased arterial collagen synthesis in experimental canine atherosclerosis, *Atherosclerosis*, 19, 43, 1974.

418. **McGarry, J. D. and Foster, D. W.,** Regulation of ketogenesis and clinical aspects of the ketonic state, *Metabolism*, 21, 471, 1972.

419. **McGarry, J. D., Meier, J. M., and Foster, D. W.,** The effects of starvation and refeeding on carbohydrate and lipid metabolism in vivo and in the perfused rat liver, *J. Biol. Chem.*, 248, 270, 1973.

420. **McGill, H. C., Jr.,** Atherosclerosis: problems in pathogenesis, in *Atherosclerosis Review II*, Paoletti, R. and Gotto, A. M., Eds., 1977, 27-65.

421. **McMurray, W. C. and Magee, W. L.,** Phospholipid metabolism, *Annu. Rev. Biochem.*, 41, 129, 1972.

422. **Meade, T. W.,** Haemostatic function and ischaemic heart disease, *Adv. Exp. Med. Biol.*, 164, 3, 1984.

423. **Meittinen, T. A.,** Mode of action of a new hypocholesterolaemic drug (DH-581) in familial hypercholes-terolaemia, *Atherosclerosis*, 15, 163, 1972.

424. **Meller, J., Conde, C. A., Deppisch, L. M., Donoso, E., and Dack, S.,** Myocardial infarction due to coronary atherosclerosis in three young adults with systemic lupus erythematosus, *Am. J. Cardiol.*, 35, 309, 1975.

425. **Merode, T.,** Serum HDL/total cholesterol ratio and blood pressure in asymptomatic atherosclerotic lesions of the cervical carotid arteries in men, *Stroke*, 16, 34, 1985.

426. **Messeoli, A. H.,** Obesity in hypertension: how innocent a bystander?, *Am. J. Med.*, 77, 1077, 1984.

427. **Miller, E. J. and Matukas, V. J.,** Biosynthesis of collagen. The biochemists view, *Fed. Proc.*, 33, 1197, 1974.

428. **Miller, N. E.** High-density lipoprotein, atherosclerosis and ischaemic heart disease, in *Atherosclerosis: Mechanisms and Approaches to Therapy*, Miller, N. E., Ed., Raven Press, New York, 1984, 153-168.

429. **Miller, N. E., Hammett, F., Saltissi, S., Rao, S., Van Zeller, H., Coltart, J., and Lewis, B.,** Relation of angiographically defined coronary artery disease to plasma lipoprotein subfractions and apolipoproteins, *Br. Med. J.*, 282, 1741, 1981.

430. **Miller, O. N., Hamilton, J. G., and Goldsmith, G. A.,** On the mechanism of action of nicotinic acid in lowering serum lipids, *Am. J. Clin. Nutr.*, 10, 285, 1962.

431. **Mitchell, J. R. A. and Schwartz, C. J.,** Study of cardiovascular disease at necropsy, in *Arterial Disease*, Blackwell Scientific, Oxford, 1965, 377.

432. **Minick, C. R. and Murphy, G. E.,** Experimental induction of atheroarteriosclerosis by the synergy of allergic injury to arteries and lipid-rich diet. II. Effect of repeatedly injected foreign protein in rabbits fed a lipid-rich, cholesterol-poor diet, *Am. J. Pathol.*, 73, 265, 1973.

433. **Moncada, S., Gryglewski, R. J., Bunting, S., and Vane, J. R.,** An enzyme isolated from arteries transforms prostaglandin endoperoxides to an unstable substance that inhibits platelet aggregation, *Nature (London)*, 261, 663, 1976.

434. **Moncada, S. and Vane, J. R.,** Prostacyclin in the cardiovascular system, *Adv. Prostagland. Thromb. Res.*, 6, 43, 1980.

435. **Moncada, S. and Vane, J. R.,** Arachidonic acid metabolites and the interactions between platelets and blood vessel walls, *N. Engl. J. Med.*, 300, 1143, 1979.

436. **Moncada, S. and Vane, J. R.,** Unstable metabolites of arachidonic acid and their role in hemostasis and thrombosis, *Br. Med. Bull.*, 34, 129, 1978.

437. **Mondola, P., Patti, L., Santangelo, F., and Coraggio, S.,** Changes in serum apolipoprotein B concen-tration oral glucose or intramuscular insulin, *Acta Diabetol. Lat.*, 21, 235, 1984.

438. **Moon, H. D.,** Connective tissue reactions in the development of arteriosclerosis, in *Connective Tissue, Thrombosis and Atherosclerosis*, Page, I. H., Ed., Academic Press, New York, 1959, 33.

439. **Moore, S.,** Injury mechanism in atherosclerosis, in *Vascular Injury and Atherosclerosis*, Moore S., Ed., Marcel Dekker, New York, 1981, 131-148.

440. **Moore, S., Friedman, R. J., Singal, D. P., Gauldie, J., and Blajchman, M.,** Inhibition of injury induced thromboatherosclerotic lesions by anti-platelet serum in rabbits, *Thromb. Diath. Haemorragh.*, 35, 70, 1976.

441. **Morin, R. J.,** Phospholipid composition and synthesis in male rabbit aortas, *Metabolism*, 17, 1051, 1968.

442. **Morin, R. J.,** Effects of estradiol on the in vitro incorporation of acetate-1-14C and choline-1,2,-14C into the phospholipids of human peripheral arteries, *Experientia*, 26, 1214, 1970.

443. **Morin, R. J., Edralin, G. G., and Woo, J. M.,** Esterification of cholesterol by subcellular fractions from swine arteries and inhibition by amphipathic and polyanionic compounds, *Atherosclerosis*, 20, 27, 1974.

444. **Morita, T. and Bing, R. J.,** Lipid metabolism in perfused human coronary arteries, *Proc. Soc. Exp. Biol. Med.*, 140, 617, 1972.

445. **Morrisett, J. D., Jackson, R. L., and Gotto, A. M.,** Lipoproteins: structure and function, *Annu. Rev. Biochem.,* 44, 183, 1975.

446. **Morrison, A. D., Berwick, L., Orci, L., and Winegrad, A. L.,** Morphology and metabolism of an aortic intima-media preparation in which an intact endothelium is preserved, *J. Clin. Invest.,* 57, 650, 1976.

447. **Moutafis, C. D., Myant, N. B., Mancini, M., and Oriente, P.,** Cholestyramine and nicotinic acid in the treatment of familial hyperbetalipoproteinaemia in the homozygous form, *Atherosclerosis,* 14, 247, 1971.

448. **Mustard, J. F. and Packham, M. A.,** Factors influencing platelet function: adhesion, release, and aggregation, *Pharmacol. Rev.,* 22, 97, 1970.

449. **Mustard, J. F., Packham, M. A., and Kinlough-Rathborne, R. L.,** Platelets and atherosclerosis, in *Atherosclerosis: Mechanisms and Approaches to Therapy,* Miller, N. E., Ed., Raven Press, New York, 1983, 29-43.

450. **Mustard, J. F., Packham, M. A., and Kinlough-Rathborne, R. L.,** Platelets, atherosclerosis and clinical complications, in *Vascular Injury and Atherosclerosis,* Moore, S., Ed., Marcel Dekker, New York, 1981, 79-110.

451. **Muller, P., Fellin, R., Lambrecht, J., Agostinin, B., Wieland, H., Rost, W., and Seidel, D.,** Hypertriglyceridaemia secondary to liver disease, *Eur. J. Clin. Invest.,* 4, 419, 1974.

452. **Myant, N. B.,** The thyroid and lipid metabolism, in *Lipid Pharmacology,* Paoletti, R., Ed., Academic Press, New York, 1964, 299-323.

453. **Myher, J. J., Kuksis, A., Breckenridge, W. C., and Little, J. A.,** Studies of triacylglycerol structure of very low-density lipoproteins of normolipemic subjects and patients with type III and type IV hyperlipoproteinemia, *Lipids,* 19, 683, 1984.

454. **Nakashima, Y., Di Ferrante, N., Jackson, R. L., and Pownall, H. J.,** The interaction of human glycosaminoglycans with plasma lipoproteins, *J. Biol. Chem.,* 250, 5386, 1975.

455. **Nakaya, Y., Schaefer, E. J., and Brewer, H. B.,** Activation of human post-heparin lipoprotein lipase by apolipoprotein H, *Biochem. Biophys. Res. Commun.,* 95, 168, 1980.

456. **Neaton, J. D., Kuller, L. H., Wentworth, D., and Borhani, N. O.,** Total and cardiovascular mortality in relation to cigarette smoking, serum cholesterol concentration, and diastolic blood pressure among black and white males followed up for five years, *Am. Heart J.,* 108, 759, 1984.

457. **Nelson, G. J., Ed.,** *Blood Lipids and Lipoproteins: Quantitation, Composition and Metabolism,* John Wiley & Sons, New York, 1972.

458. **Nerem, R. M.,** Atherogenesis: hemodynamics, vascular geometry and the endothelium, *Biorheology,* 21, 649, 1984.

459. **Neri Semeri, G. G., Gensini, G. F., Masotti, G., Abbate, R., Morettini, A., Poggesi, L., and Fortini, A.,** Role of prostacyclin and thromboxane A2 in ischaemic heart disease, *Adv. Exp. Med. Biol.,* 164, 175, 1984.

460. **Nestel, P. J.,** Relationship between plasma triglycerides and removal of chylomicrons, *J. Clin. Invest.,* 43, 943, 1964.

461. **Nestel, P. J., Hirsch, E. Z., and Couzens, E. A.,** The effects of chlorophenoxyisobutyric acid and ethinylestradiol on cholesterol turnover, *J. Clin. Invest.,* 44, 891, 1965.

462. **Newman, H. A. I., McCandless, E. L., and Zilversmit, D. B.,** The synthesis of C14 lipids in rabbit atheromatous lesions, *J. Biol. Chem.,* 236, 1264, 1961.

463. **Nichols, M.,** Functions and interrelationships of different classes of plasma lipoproteins, *Proc. Natl. Acad. Sci. U.S.A.,* 64, 1128, 1969.

464. **Nikkila, E. A., Kuusi, T., and Taskinen, M. R.,** Role of lipoprotein lipase and hepatic endothelial lipase in the metabolism of high density lipoproteins: a novel concept on cholesterol transport in HDL cycle, in *Metabolic Risk Factors in Ischemic Cardiovascular Disease,* Carlson, L. A. and Pernow, B., Eds., Raven Press, New York, 1982, 205-215.

465. **Nikkila, E. A. and Pykalisto, O.,** Regulation of adipose tissue lipoprotein lipase synthesis by intracellular free fatty acid, *Life Sci.,* 7, 1303, 1968.

466. **Noel, S. P. and Rubinstein, D.,** Secretion of apolipoproteins in very low density and high density lipoproteins by perfused rat liver, *J. Lipid Res.,* 15, 301, 1974.

467. **Nordoy, A., Lagarde, M., and Reneaud, S.,** Platelets during alimentary hyperlipemia induced by cream and cod liver oil, *Eur. J. Clin. Invest.,* 14, 339, 1984.

468. **Novikoff, P. M. and Edelstein, D.,** Reversal of orotic acid-induced fatty liver in rats by clofibrate, *Lab. Invest.,* 36, 215, 1977.

469. **Novikoff, P. M., Roheim, P. S., Novikoff, A. B., and Edelstein, D.,** Production and prevention of fatty liver in rats fed clofibrate and orotic acid containing sucrose, *Lab. Invest.,* 30, 732, 1974.

470. **O'Brien, J. R.,** Effect of anti-inflammatory agents on platelets, *Lancet,* 1, 894, 1968.

471. **Ockner, R. K., Hughes, F. B., and Isselbacher, K. J.,** Very low density lipoproteins in intestinal lymph: role in triglyceride and cholesterol transport during fat absorption, *J. Clin. Invest.,* 48, 2367, 1969.

472. **O'Connor, N. T., Cederholm-Williams, S., Copper, S., and Colter, L.,** Hypercoagulability and coronary artery disease, *Br. Heart J.,* 52, 614, 1984.
473. **O'Malley, K. and O'Brien, E.,** Management of hypertension in the elderly, *N. Engl. J. Med.,* 302, 1397, 1980.
474. **Olsson, A. G.,** Clinical uses of prostaglandins in cardiovascular disease, in *Atherosclerosis: Mechanisms and Approaches in Therapy,* Miller, N. E., Ed., Raven Press, New York, 1983, 91-103.
475. **Olsson, A. G., Rossner, S., Walldius, G., and Carlson, L. A.,** Effect of Gemfibrozil on lipoprotein concentrations in different types of hyperlipoproteinaemia, *Proc. R. Soc. Med.,* (Suppl. 2)69, 28, 1976.
476. **Orekhov, A. N., Andereeva, E. R., Shekhonin, B. V., Tertov, V. V., and Smirnov, V. N.,** Content and localization of fibronectin in normal intima, atherosclerotic plaque and underlying media of human aorta, *Atherosclerosis,* 53, 213, 1984.
477. **Owens, J. S. and Gillett, M. P.,** Plasma lipids, lipoproteins and cell membranes, *Biochem. Soc. Trans.,* 11, 336, 1983.
478. **Packard, C. J., Shepherd, J., Joerns, G., Gotto, A. M., and Taunton, J.,** Apolipoprotein B metabolism in normal, Type IV and Type V hyperlipoproteinemic subjects, *Metabolism,* 29, 213, 1980.
479. **Packard, C. J., Munro, A., Lorimer, A. R., Gotto, A. M., and Shepherd, J.,** Metabolism of apolipoprotein B in large triglyceride-rich very low-density lipoproteins of normal and hypertriglyceridemic subjects, *J. Clin. Invest.,* 74, 2178, 1984.
480. **Packham, M. A. and Mustard, J. F.,** Non-steroidal anti-inflammatory drugs, pyrimido-pyridine compounds: effect on platelet function, in *Platelets, Drugs and Thrombosis,* Hirsch, J., Cade, J. F., Gallus, A. S., and Schönbaum, E., Eds., S. Karger, Basel, 1975, 111-123.
481. **Paffenbarger, R. S. and Hyde, R. T.,** Exercise in the prevention of coronary heart disease, *Prev. Med.,* 13, 3, 1984.
482. **Paisey, R. B., Arredondo, G., Villalobos, A., Lozano, O., Guevara, I., and Kelly, S.,** Association with differing dietary, metabolic and clinical risk factors with macrovascular complications of diabetes, *Diabetes Care,* 7, 421, 1984.
483. **Parke, D. V.,** The endoplasmic reticulum: its role in physiological functions and pathological situations, in *Concepts of Drug Metabolism,* Part B, Jenner, P. and Testa, B., Eds., Marcel Dekker, New York, 1981, 1-52.
484. **Parker, F., Ormsby, J. W., Peterson, N. F., Odland, G. F., and Williams, R. H.,** In vitro studies of phospholipid synthesis in experimental atherosclerosis, *Circ. Res.,* 19, 700, 1966.
485. **Parkinson, T. M.,** Hypolipemic effects of orally administered dextran and cellulose anion exchangers in cockerels and dogs, *J. Lipid Res.,* 8, 24, 1967.
486. **Partin, J. S., Partin, J. C., Schubert, W. K., and McAdams, A. J.,** Liver ultrastructure in abetalipoproteinemia: evolution of micronodular cirrhosis, *Gastroenterology,* 67, 107, 1974.
487. **Partridge, S. M.,** Isolation and characterization of elastin, in *Chemistry and Molecular Biology of the Intercellular Matrix,* Balass, E. A., Ed., Academic Press, London, 1977, 593-616.
488. **Parsons, W. B., Jr.,** The effect of nicotinic acid on serum lipids, *Am. J. Clin. Nutr.,* 8, 471, 1960.
489. **Parsons, W. B., Jr.,** Treatment of hypercholesteremia by nicotinic acid. Progress reports with review of studies regarding mechanism of action, *Arch. Intern. Med.,* 107, 653, 1961.
490. **Patel, Y. C., Eggen, D. A., and Strong, J. P.,** Obesity, smoking and atherosclerosis. A study on interassociations, *Atherosclerosis,* 36, 481, 1980.
491. **Patsch, J. R., Prasad, S., Gotto, A. M., and Bengtsson-Olivecrona, G.,** Postprandial lipemia. A key for the conversion of high-density lipoprotein 2 into high-density lipoprotein 3 by hepatic lipase, *J. Clin. Invest.,* 74, 2017, 1984.
492. **Patsch, J. R., Sailer, S., Kostner, G., Sandhoper, F., Holasek, A., and Braunsteiner, H.,** Separation of the main lipoprotein density classes from human plasma by rate-zonal ultra-centrifugation, *J. Lipid Res.,* 15, 356, 1974.
493. **Pearson, T. A., Dillman, J. M., and Heptinstall, R. H.,** The clonal characteristics of human aortic intima. Comparison with fatty streaks and normal media, *Am. J. Pathol.,* 113, 33, 1983.
494. **Peng, S. K. and Taylor, C. B.,** Cholesterol autooxidation, health and arteriosclerosis. A review on situations in developed countries, *World Rev. Nutr. Diet,* 44, 117, 1984.
495. **Petermans, J.,** Prevalence of disease of the large arteries in an elderly Belgian population: relationship with some metabolic factors, *Acta Cardiol. (Brux),* 39, 365, 1984.
496. **Poole, G. W.,** Exercise, coronary heart disease and risk factors. A brief report, *Sports Med.,* 1, 311, 1984.
497. **Pories, W. J. and Strain, W. H.,** Zinc and wound healing, in *Zinc Metabolism,* Prasod, A. S. and Thomas, C. C., Eds., Charles C. Thomas, Springfield, IL, 1966, 378.
498. **Portman, O. W.,** Atherosclerosis in nonhuman primates: sequences and possible mechanisms of change in phospholipid composition and metabolism, *Ann. N.Y. Acad. Sci.,* 162, 120, 1969.
499. **Portman, O. W., Alexander, M., and Maniffo, C. X.,** Nutritional control of arterial lipid composition in squirrel monkeys: major ester classes and types of phospholipids, *J. Nutr.,* 91, 35, 1967.

500. **Portman, O. W., Alexander, M., and Osuga, T.,** Heterogeneity of lipid composition of microsome subfractions from aorta and liver, *Biochem. Biophys. Acta,* 187, 435, 1969.

501. **Portman, O. W. and Alexander, M.,** Lysophosphatidylcholine concentrations and metabolism in aortic intima plus inner media: effect of nutritionally induced atherosclerosis, *J. Lipid Res.,* 10, 158, 1969.

502. **Portman, O. W. and Alexander, M.,** Changes in arterial subfractions with aging and atherosclerosis, *Biochim. Biophys. Acta,* 260, 460, 1972.

503. **Pownall, H. J., Hu, A., Gotto, A. M., Jr., Albers, J. J., and Sparrow, J. T.,** Activation of lecithin: cholesterol acyltransferase by a synthetic model lipid-association peptide, *Proc. Natl. Acad. Sci. U.S.A.,* 77, 3154, 1980.

504. **Pownall, H. J., Hickson, D., and Gotto, A. M., Jr.,** Thermodynamics of lipid-protein association, *J. Biol. Chem.,* 256, 9849, 1981.

505. **Proudlock, J. W. and Day, A. J.,** Cholesterol esterifying enzymes of atherosclerotic rabbit intima, *Biochim. Biophys. Acta,* 260, 716, 1972.

506. **Pugatch, E. M. J., Foster, E. A., MacFarlane, D. E., and Poole, J. C. F.,** The extraction and separation of activators and inhibitors of fibrinolysis from bovine endothelium and mesothelium, *Br. J. Haematol.,* 18, 669, 1970.

507. **Pykalisto, O. J., Smith, P. H., and Burnsell, J. D.,** Determinants of human adipose tissue lipoprotein lipase. Effect of diabetes and obesity on basal and diet induced activity, *J. Clin. Invest.,* 56, 1108, 1975.

508. **Quarfordt, S. H., Nathans, A., Dowdee, M., and Hilderman, H. L.,** Heterogeneity of human very low density lipoproteins by gel filtration chromatography, *J. Lipid Res.,* 13, 435, 1972.

509. **Quintao, E., Grundy, S. M., and Ahrens, E. H.,** Effects of dietary cholesterol on the regulation of total body cholesterol in man, *J. Lipid Res.,* 12, 233, 1971.

510. **Rabkin, S. W.,** Effect of cigarette smoking cessation on risk factors for coronary atherosclerosis, *Atherosclerosis,* 53, 173, 1984.

511. **Radhakrishnamurthy, B., Ruiz, H., and Berenson, D. S.,** Isolation and characteristics of proteoglycans from bovine aorta, *J. Biol. Chem.,* 252, 4831, 1977.

512. **Ragland, J. B., Bertram, P. D., and Sabesin, S. M.,** Identification of nascent high density lipoproteins containing arginine-rich protein in human plasma, *Biochem. Biophys. Res. Commun.,* 80, 81, 1978.

513. **Rail, D. L.,** The role of atheromatous plaque rupture in the genesis of myocardial infarction, *Med. Hypotheses,* 14, 261, 1984.

514. **Rainville, S. and Vaccaro, P.,** Lipoprotein cholesterol levels, coronary artery disease and regular exercise: a review, *Am. Correct. Ther. J.,* 37, 161, 1983.

515. **Rall, S. C., Jr., Weisgraber, K. H., and Mahley, R. W.,** Human apolipoprotein E: the complete amino acid sequence, *J. Biol. Chem.,* 257, 4171, 1982.

516. **Randle, P. J., Garland, P. J., Hales, C. N., and Newsholm, E. A.,** The glucose fatty-acid cycle: its role in insulin sensitivity and the metabolic disturbances of diabetes relations, *Lancet,* 1, 785, 1963.

517. **Rauterberg, J. and Allan, S. S.,** Occurrence of type I and Type II collagen in normal and atherosclerotic human aortas, in *Atherosclerosis IV, Proc. 4th Int. Symp.,* Schettler, G., Goto, Y., Hata, Y., and Klose, G., Eds., Springer-Verlag, Berlin, 1977, 368.

518. **Reaven, E. P., Kolterman, O. G., and Reaven, G. M.,** Ultrastructural and physiological evidence for corticosteroid-induced alteration in hepatic production of very low density lipoprotein particles, *J. Lipid Res.,* 15, 74, 1974.

519. **Redgrave, T. G.,** The role in chylomicron formation of phospholipase activity of intestinal Golgi membranes, *Aust. J. Exp. Biol. Med. Sci.,* 51, 427, 1973.

520. **Renaud, S.,** Risk factors for coronary heart disease and platelet functions, *Adv. Exp. Med. Biol.,* 164, 129, 1984.

521. **Renson, J., Van Cantfort, J., Robaye, B., and Gielen, J.,** Mesures de la demi-vie de la cholesterol-7-alpha-hydroxylase, *Arch. Int. Physiol.,* 77, 972, 1969.

522. **Ribeiro, J. P., Hartley, L. H., Sherwood, J., and Herd, J. A.,** The effectiveness of a low lipid diet and exercise in the management of coronary artery disease, *Am. Heart J.,* 108, 1183, 1984.

523. **Richardson, J. B. and Beaulnes, A.,** The cellular site of action of angiotensin, *J. Cell Biol.,* 51, 419, 1971.

524. **Ritland, S., Blomhoff, J. P., and Gjone, E.,** Lecithin: cholesterol acyl-transferase and lipoprotein-X in liver disease, *Clin. Chem. Acta,* 49, 251, 1973.

525. **Robert, L.,** The elastic element in the arterial wall: biosynthesis and degradation, in *Atherosclerosis V, Proc. 5th Int. Symp.,* Gotto, A. M., Smith, L. C., and Allen B., Eds., Springer-Verlag, Berlin, 1980, 136-139.

526. **Robert, L., Robert, B., and Robert, A. M.,** Molecular biology of elastin as related to aging and atherosclerosis, *Exp. Gerontol.,* 5, 339, 1970.

527. **Roberts, W. C.,** Reducing the blood cholesterol level reduces the risk of heart attack, *Am. J. Cardiol.,* 53, 649, 1984.

528. **Robertson, W. B.,** Some factors influencing the development of atherosclerosis. A survey in Jamaica, West Indies, *J. Atherosclerosis Res.,* 2, 79, 1962.

529. **Robertson, W. B. and Strong, J. P.,** Atherosclerosis in persons with hypertension and diabetes mellitus, *Lab. Invest.,* 18, 538, 1968.

530. **Robinson, F. C.,** Aneurism of the coronary arteries, *Am. Heart J.,* 109, 1, 1985.

531. **Rogers, J. B. and Bochenek, W.,** Localization of lipid re-esterifying enzymes of the rat small intestine: effect of jejunal removal on ileal enzyme activities, *Biochim. Biophys. Acta,* 202, 426, 1970.

532. **Roheim, P. S., Gidez, L. I., and Eder, H. A.,** Extrahepatic synthesis of lipoproteins of plasma and chyle: role of the intestine, *J. Clin. Invest.,* 45, 297, 1966.

533. **Romano, E. L., Sotolongo-Pons, M., Camejo, G., and Soyano, A.,** Circulating immune complexes, immunoglobulins complement, antibodies to dietary antigens, cholesterol and lipoprotein levels in patients with occlusive coronary lesions, *Atherosclerosis,* 53, 119, 1984.

534. **Rose, H. G., Haft, G. K., and Juliano, J.,** Clofibrate-induced low density lipoprotein elevation: therapeutic implications and treatment by colestipol resin, *Atherosclerosis,* 23, 413, 1976.

535. **Rosenberg, R. D., Fritze, L. M., Castellot, J. J., and Karnovsky, M. J.,** Heparin-like molecules as regulations of atherogenesis, *Nouv. Rev. Fr. Hematol.,* 26, 255, 1984.

536. **Rosenthal, M. B., Barnard, R. J., Rose, D. P., Inkeles, S., Hall, J., and Pritikin, N.,** Effects of a high-complex-carbohydrate, low-fat, low-cholesterol diet on levels of serum lipids and estradiol, *Am. J. Med.,* 78, 23, 1985.

537. **Ross, R.,** Atherosclerosis: a problem of the biology of arterial wall cells and their interactions with blood components, *Artherosclerosis,* 1, 293, 1981.

538. **Ross, R. and Glomset, J. A.,** Atherosclerosis and the arterial smooth muscle cell: proliferation of smooth muscle is a key event in the genesis of the lesions of atherosclerosis, *Science,* 180, 1332, 1973.

539. **Ross, R. and Glomset, J. A.,** The pathogenesis of atherosclerosis, *N. Engl. J. Med.,* 295, 369, 1976.

540. **Ross, R. and Glomset, J. A.,** The pathogenesis of atherosclerosis, *N. Engl. J. Med.,* 295, 420, 1976.

541. **Rossi, B. and Rulli, V.,** The hypocholesterolemic effect of phenylethylacetic acid amide in hypercholesterolemia atherosclerotic patients, *Am. Heart J.,* 53, 277, 1957.

542. **Rouffy, J., Dreux, C., Goussault, Y., Dakkak, R., and Renson, F. J.,** Antilipidemia drugs. Part V. Evaluation of the hypolipidemic effect of LF 178 in 191 patients affected by the atherogenic form of endogenous hyperlipoproteinemia (Types IIa, IIb, and IV), *Arzneim. Forsch.,* 26, 901, 1976.

543. **Ruderman, N. B. and Haudenschild, C.,** Diabetes as an atherogenic factor, *Prog. Cardiovasc. Dis.,* 26, 373, 1984.

544. **Rutherford, R. B. and Ross, R. J.,** Platelet factors stimulate fibroblasts and smooth muscle cells quiescent in plasma serum to proliferate, *Cell Biol.,* 69, 196, 1976.

545. **Ryan, J. W., Ryan, U. S., and Schultz, D. R.,** Subcellular localization of pulmonary angiotensin-converting enzyme (kininase II), *Biochem. J.,* 145, 497, 1975.

546. **Saba, S. R. and Mason, R. G.,** Studies of an activity from endothelial cells that inhibit platelet aggregation, serotonin release and clot retraction, *Thromb. Res.,* 5, 747, 1974.

547. **Salans, L. B., Knittle, J. L., and Hirsch, J.,** The role of adipose cell size and adipose tissue insulin sensitivity in the carbohydrate intolerance of human obesity, *J. Clin. Invest.,* 47, 153, 1968.

548. **Sakurada, T., Orimo, H., Okale, H., Noma, A., and Murakami, M.,** Purification and properties of cholesterol ester hydrolase from human aortic intima and media, *Biochim. Biophys. Acta,* 424, 204, 1976.

549. **Sandberg, L. B., Gray, W. R., Foster, J. A., Torres, A. R., Alvarez, V. L., and Janata, J.,** Primary structure of porcine tropoelastin, in *Elastin and Elastic Tissue. Advances in Experimental Biology,* Vol. 79, Sandberg, L. B., Gray, W. R., and Franzblau, C., Eds., Plenum Press, New York, 1977, 277-284.

550. **Sane, T., Nikkilä, E. A., Taskinen, M. R., Välimäki, M., and Ylikahri, R.,** Accelerated turnover of very low-density lipoprotein triglyerides in chronic alcohol users. A possible mechanism for the up-regulation of high density lipoprotein by ethanol, *Atherosclerosis,* 53, 185, 1984.

551. **Sarno, A., Raineri, A., Assennato, P., and Caimi, G.,** Evaluation of the haemorheological determinants in coronary heart disease, *Adv. Exp. Mol. Biol.,* 164, 411, 1984.

552. **Sata, T., Havel, R. H., and Jones, A. L.,** Characterization of subfractions of triglyceride-rich lipoproteins separated by gel chromatography from blood plasma of normolipemic and hyperlipemic humans, *J. Lipid Res.,* 13, 757, 1972.

553. **Sawyer, P. N., Himmelfarb, E., Lustrin, I., and Zisking, H.,** Measurements of streaming potentials of mammalian blood vessels, aorta and vena cava, in vivo, *Biophys. J.,* 6, 641, 1966.

554. **Sawyer, P. N. and Srisivasan, S.,** The role of electrochemical surface properties in thrombosis at vascular interfaces: cumulative experience of studies in animals and man, *Bull. N.Y. Acad. Med.,* 48, 235, 1972.

555. **Scanu, A. M.,** Structure of human serum lipoproteins, *Ann. N.Y. Acad. Sci.,* 195, 390, 1972.

556. **Scanu, A. M.,** Plasma lipoproteins: an introduction., in *The Biochemistry of Atherosclerosis,* Scanu, A. M., Wissler, R. W., and Getz, G. S., Eds., Marcell Dekker, New York, 1979, 3-8.

557. **Scanu, A. M., Edelstein, C., and Gordon, J. I.,** Apolipoproteins of human plasma high-density lipoproteins. Biology, biochemistry and clinical significance, *Clin. Physiol. Biochem.,* 2, 111, 1984.

558. **Scanu, A. M. and Teng, T. L.,** Apolipoproteins of plasma lipoproteins: behavior in solution, in *Biochemistry of Atherosclerosis*, Scanu, A. M., Wissler, R. W., and Getz, G. S., Eds., Marcell Dekker, Basel, 1979, 107-122.

559. **Scanu, A. M. and Wisdom, C.,** Serum lipoprotein structure and functions, *Annu. Rev. Biochem.*, 41, 703, 1972.

560. **Schaefer, E. J., Zech, L. A., Schwartz, D. E., and Brewer, H. B.,** Coronary heart disease prevalence and clinical features in familial high density lipoprotein deficiency (Tangier Disease), *Ann. Intern. Med.*, 93, 261, 1980.

561. **Schaefer, E. J., Eisenberg, S., and Levy, R. I.,** Lipoprotein apoprotein metabolism, *J. Lipid Res.*, 19, 667, 1978.

562. **Schleimer, R. P., MacGlashan, D. W., Schulman, E. S., Peters, S. P., Adams, G. K., Adkinson, N. F., and Lichtenstein, L. M.,** Human mast cells and basophils-structure, function, pharmacology and biochemistry, *Clin. Rev. Allergy*, 1, 327, 1983.

563. **Schneider, W. J., Kovanen, P. T., Brown, M. S., Goldstein, J. L., Utermann, G., Weber, W., Havel, R. J., Kotie, L., Kane, J. P., Innerarity, T. L., and Mahley, R. W.,** Familial dysbetalipoproteinemia: an abnormal binding of mutant apoprotein E to low density lipoprotein receptors of human fibroblasts and membranes from liver and adrenal of rats, rabbits, and cows, *J. Clin. Invest.*, 68, 1075, 1981.

564. **Schonfeld, G.,** Disorders of lipid transport-update 1983, *Prog. Cardiovasc. Disc.*, 26, 89, 1983.

565. **Schonfeld, G. and Kipnis, D. M.,** Effects of fatty acids on carbohydrate and fatty acid metabolism of rat diaphragm, *Am. J. Physiol.* 215, 513, 1968.

566. **Schreibman, P. H., Arons, D. L., Saudak, C. D., and Arky, R. A.,** Abnormal lipoprotein lipase in familial exogenous hypertriglyceridemia, *J. Clin. Invest.*, 52, 2075, 1973.

567. **Schriewer, H., Schulte, H., and Assmann, G.,** HDL phosphatidyl choline and risk-factors of coronary heart disease, *J. Clin. Chem. Biochem.*, 22, 515, 1984.

568. **Schumaker, V. N.,** Hydrodynamic analysis of human low density lipoproteins, *Acc. Chem. Res.*, 6, 398, 1973.

569. **Schwartz, S. M., Gajdusek, C. M., and Selden, S. C.,** Vascular wall growth control: the role of the endothelium, *Atherosclerosis*, 1, 107, 1981.

570. **Schwartz, S. M., Stemerman, M. B., and Benditt, E. P.,** The aortic intima: II. Repair of the aortic lining after mechanical denudation, *A. J. Pathol.*, 81, 15, 1975.

571. **Schwartz, S. M. and Ross, R.,** Cellular proliferation in atherosclerosis and hypertension, *Prog. Cardiovasc. Dis.*, 26, 355, 1984.

572. **Seidel, D. and Alaupovic, P.,** Ein abnormales Low-density-lipoprotein bei Cholestase. I. Isolierung und Charakterisierung, *Med. Wchschr.*, 95, 1774, 1970.

573. **Senior, J. R.,** Intestinal absorption of fats, *J. Lipid Res.*, 5, 495, 1964.

574. **Sgoutas, D. S.,** Fatty acid specificity of plasma phosphatidylcholine: cholesterol acyltransferase, *Biochemistry*, 11, 293, 1972.

575. **Shadle, P. J. and Barondes, S. H.,** Platelet-collagen adhesion: inhibition by a monoclonal antibody that binds glycoprotein IIb, *J. Cell Biol.*, 99, 2056, 1984.

576. **Shefer, S., Hauser, S., Bekersky, I., and Mosbach, E. H.,** Feedback regulation of bile acid biosynthesis in the rat, *J. Lipid Res.*, 10, 645, 1969.

577. **Shen, B. W., Scanu, A. M., and Kezdy, F. J.,** Structure of human serum lipoproteins inferred from compositional analysis, *Proc. Natl. Acad. Sci. U.S.A.*, 74, 837, 1977.

578. **Shepherd, J., Caine, E. A., Bedford, D. K., and Packard, C. J.,** Ultracentrifugal subfractionation of high-density lipoprotein, *Analyst*, 109, 347, 1984.

579. **Shepro, D., Batbouta, J. C., Robbler, L. S., Carson, M. P., and Belamarich, F. A.,** Serotonin transport by cultured bovine aortic endothelium, *Circ. Res.*, 36, 799, 1975.

580. **Sheps, S. G. and Colville, D. S.,** Occlusive renovascular disease, *Cardiovasc. Clin.*, 13, 219, 1983.

581. **Sherry, S.,** Role of platelet-active drugs in coronary artery disease, *Cardiovasc. Clin.*, 14, 173, 1983.

582. **Shio, H. M., Farquar, G., and De Duve, C.,** Lysosomes of the arterial walll. IV. Cytochemical localization of acid phosphatase and catalase in smooth muscle cells and foam cells and foam cells from rabbit atheromatous aorta, *Am. J. Pathol.*, 76, 1, 1974.

583. **Shore, V. G. and Shore, B.,** Heterogeneity of human plasma very low density lipoproteins. Separation of species differing in protein components, *Biochemistry*, 12, 502, 1973.

584. **Shore, B. and Shore, V. G.,** Isolation and characterization of polypeptides of human serum lipoproteins, *Biochemistry*, 8, 4510, 1969.

585. **Shulman, R. S., Herbert, P. N., Wehrly, K., and Fredrickson, D. S.,** The complete amino acid sequence of C-I (apoLp-Ser), an apolipoprotein from human very low density lipoproteins, *J. Biol. Chem.*, 250, 182, 1975.

586. **Sigurdsson, G., Nicoll, A., and Lewis, B.,** Conversions of very low density lipoprotein to low density lipoprotein, *J. Clin. Invest.*, 56, 1481, 1975.

587. **Silberberg, A.,** Conditions of flow at interfaces with flexible walls, *Ann. N.Y. Acad. Sci.,* 275, 2, 1976.

588. **Simionescu, N., Simionescu, M., and Palade, G. E.,** Permeability of muscle capillaries to exogenous myoglobin, *J. Cell Biol.,* 57, 424, 1973.

589. **Simionescu, N., Simionescu, M., and Palade, G. E.,** Permeability of muscle capillaries to small heme-peptides. Evidence for the existence of patent transendothelial channels, *J. Cell Biol.,* 64, 586, 1975.

590. **Sinzinger, H., Schernthaner, G., and Kaliman, J.,** Sensitivity of platelets to prostaglandins in coronary heart disease and angina pectoris, *Prostaglandins,* 22, 773, 1981.

591. **Sirtori, C. R., Zoppi, S., Quarisa, B., and Agradi, E.,** Clinical evaluation of tibric acid (CP 18,524) a new hypolipidemic agent, *Pharmacol. Res. Commun.,* 6, 445, 1974.

592. **Skipski, V. P., Barclay, M., Barclay, R. K., Fitzes, V. A., Good, J. J., and Archibald, F. M.,** Lipid composition of human serum lipoproteins, *Biochem. J.,* 104, 340, 1967.

593. **Skipski, V. P.,** Lipid composition of lipoproteins in normal and diseased states, in *Blood Lipids and Lipoproteins: Quantitation, Composition and Metabolism,* Nelson, G. J., Ed., Wiley-Interscience, New York, 1972, 471-584.

594. **Smith, E. B.,** The relationship between plasma and tissue lipids in human atherosclerosis, in *Advances in Lipid Research,* Vol. 12, Paoletti, R. and Kritchevsky, D., Eds., Academic Press, New York, 1984, 1-49.

595. **Smith, E. B.,** Development of the atheromatous lesion, in *The Smooth Muscle of the Artery. Advances in Experimental Medicine and Biology,* Vol. 57, Wolf, S. and Werthessen, N. T., Eds., Plenum Press, New York, 1975, 254.

596. **Smith, E. B.,** The influence of age and atherosclerosis on the chemistry of aortic intima, Parts 1 and 2. The lipids, *J. Atheroscler. Res.,* 5, 224 and 248, 1965.

597. **Smith, E. B. and Ashall, C.,** Low density lipoprotein concentration in interstitial fluid from human atherosclerosis lesions. Relation to theories of endothelial damage and lipoprotein binding, *Biochim. Biophys. Acta,* 754, 249, 1983.

598. **Smith, E. B., Evans, P. H., and Downham, M. D.,** Lipid in the aortic intima. The correlation of morphological and chemical characteristics, *J. Atheroscler. Res.,* 7, 171, 1967.

599. **Smith, E. B., Slater, R. S., and Hunter, J. A.,** Quantitative studies on fibrinogen and low-density lipoprotein in human aortic intima, *Atherosclerosis,* 18, 479, 1973.

600. **Smith, E. B. and Smith, R. H.,** Early changes in aortic intima, in *Atherosclerosis Reviews,* Vol. 1, Paoletti, R. and Gotto, A. M., Ed., Raven Press, New York, 1976, 119-136.

601. **Smith, E. B.,** Development of the atheromatous lesion, in *The Smooth Muscle of the Artery. Advances in Experimental Medicine and Biology,* Vol. 57, Wolf. S. and Werthessen, N. T., Eds., Plenum Press, New York, 1975, 254.

602. **Smith, L. C., Voyta, J. C., Kinnunen, P. K. J., Gotto, A. M., Jr., and Sparrow, J. T.,** Lipoprotein lipase interaction with synthetic N-dansyl fragments of apolipoprotein C-11, *Biophys. J.,* 37, 174, 1982.

603. **Smith, M. D., Cowley, M. J., and Vetrovec, G. W.,** Aneurysms of the left main coronary artery: a report of three cases and review of the literature, *Cathet. Cardiovasc. Diagn.,* 10, 583, 1984.

604. **Smith, U. and Ryan, J. W.,** Pulmonary endothelial cells and the metabolism of adenine nucleotides, kinins and angiotensin 1, *Adv. Exper. Biol.,* 21, 267, 1972.

605. **Sodhi, H. S. and Kudchodkar, B. J.,** Correlating metabolism of plasma and tissue cholesterol with that of plasma-lipoproteins, *Lancet,* 1, 1973.

606. **Solberg, L. S., Hjorman, I., Helgeland, H., Holme, I., Lerne, P. A., and Strong, J. P.,** Association between risk factors and atherosclerotic lesions based on autopsy findings in the Olso study: a preliminary report, in *Atherosclerosis IV,* Schettler, G., Gotto, Y., Hata, Y., and Klose, G., Eds., 1977, 98-102.

607. **Soutar, A. K., Garner, C. W., Baker, H. N., Sparrow, J. T., Jackson, R. L., Gotto, A. M., and Smith, L. C.,** Effect of the human plasma apolipoproteins and phosphatidylcholine acyl donor on the activity of lecithin: cholesterol acyltransferase, *Biochemistry,* 14, 3057, 1975.

608. **Spaet, T. H.,** Platelets and atherogenesis, *Haematologia (Budap.),* 15, 355, 1982.

609. **Sparrow, J. T. and Gotto, A. M.,** Synthetic fragments of apolipoprotein CII: phospholipid binding studies, *Circulation,* 62, 77, 1980.

610. **St. Clair, R. W.,** Atherosclerosis: regression in animal models current concepts of cellular and biochemical mechanisms, *Prog. Cardiovasc. Dis.,* 26, 109, 1983.

611. **St. Clair, R. W., Lofland, H. B., Jr., and Clarkson, T. B.,** Fatty acid synthesis in cell-free system from rabbit aorta, *J. Lipid Res.,* 9, 739, 1968.

612. **St. Clair, R. W., Lofland, H. B., and Clarkson, T. B.,** Composition and synthesis of fatty acids in atherosclerotic aortas of the pigeon, *J. Lipid Res.,* 9, 739, 1969.

613. **St. Clair, R. W., Lofland, H. B., and Clarkson, T. B.,** Influence of duration of cholesterol feeding on esterification of fatty acids by cell-free preparation of pigeon aorta, *Circ. Res.,* 27, 213, 1970.

614. **St. Clair, R. W.,** Metabolism of the arterial wall and atherosclerosis, in *Atherosclerosis Reviews,* Vol. 1, Paoletti, R. and Gotto, A. M., Eds., Raven Press, New York, 1976, 61.

615. **Stamler, J., Pick, R., Katz, L. N., Pick, A., Kaplan, B. M., Berkson, D. M., and Century, D.,** Effectiveness of estrogens for therapy of myocardial infarction in middle-age men, *JAMA,* 183, 632, 1963.

616. **Stamler, J., Berkson, D. M., and Lindberg, H. A.,** Risk factors: their role in the etiology and pathogenesis of the atherosclerotic diseases, in *The Pathogenesis of Atherosclerosis,* Wissler, R. C. and Greer, J. C., Eds., Williams & Wilkins, Baltimore, 1972, 41.

617. **Stary, H. C.,** Proliferation of arterial cells in atherosclerosis, *Adv. Exp. Med. Biol.,* 43, 59, 1974.

618. **Stein, F., Pezess, M. P., Poullain, N., and Robert, L.,** Anti-elastin antibodies in normal and pathological human sera, *Nature (London),* 207, 312, 1965.

619. **Stein, O., Bar-on, H., and Stein, Y.,** Lipoproteins and the liver, *Prog. Liver Dis.,* 4, 45, 1972.

620. **Stein, O. and Stein, Y.,** The removal of cholesterol from Landschütz ascites cells by high-density apolipoprotein, *Biochim. Biophys. Acta,* 326, 232, 1973.

621. **Stein, O. and Stein, Y.,** Cholesterol content and sterol synthesis in human skin fibroblasts and rat aortic smooth muscle cells exposed to lipoprotein-depleted serum and high density apolipoprotein phospholipid mixtures, *Biochim. Biophys. Acta,* 431, 347, 1976.

622. **Stein, O., Weinstein, D. B., Stein, Y., and Steinberg, D.,** Binding, internalization, and degradation of low density lipoprotein by normal human fibroblasts and by fibroblasts from a case of homozygous familial hypercholesterolemia, *Proc. Natl. Acad. Sci. U.S.A.,* 73, 14, 1976.

623. **Stein, Y., Glangland, M. C., Fainam, M., and Stein, O.,** The removal of cholesterol from aortic ascites cells by fractions of human high-density apolipoprotein, *Biochim. Biophys. Acta,* 380, 106, 1975.

624. **Stein, Y., Stein, O., and Shapiro, B.,** Enzymic pathway of glyceride and phospholipid synthesis in aortic homogenates, *Biochim. Biophys. Acta,* 70, 33, 1963.

625. **Steinberg, D.,** Catecholamine stimulation of fat mobilization and its metabolic consequences, *Pharmacol. Rev.,* 18, 217, 1966.

626. **Steinberg, D. and Fredrickson, D. S.,** Inhibition of lipid synthesis by alpha-phenyl-N-butyrate and related compounds, *Proc. Soc. Exp. Biol. Med.,* 90, 232, 1955.

627. **Steinberg, D., Avigan, J., and Feigelson, E. B.,** Identification of 24-dehydrocholesterol in the serum of patients treated with MER-29, *Prog. Cardiovasc. Dis.,* 2, 586, 1960.

628. **Stemerman, M. B., Pitlick, F. A., and Dembitzer, H. M.,** Electron microscopic immunohistochemical identification of endothelial cells in the rabbit, *Circl. Res.,* 38, 146, 1976.

629. **Stocks, J. and Galton, D. J.,** Activation of phospholipase A, activity of lipoprotein lipase by apoprotein CII, *Lipids,* 15, 186, 1980.

630. **Strano, A. and Davi, G.,** Platelet function tests and coronary heart disease, *Adv. Exp. Mol. Biol.,* 164, 31, 1984.

631. **Strong, J. P. and McGill, H. C.,** The natural history of aortic atherosclerosis: relationship to race, sex and coronary lesions in New Orleans, *Exp. Mol. Pathol.,* 2(Suppl. 1), 15, 1963.

632. **Strong, J. P., Eggen, D. A., and Oalmann, M. C.,** The natural history, geographic pathology and epidemiology of atherosclerosis, in *The Pathogenesis of Atherosclerosis,* Wissler, R. W. and Greer, J. C., Eds., Williams & Wilkins, Baltimore, 1972, 20-40.

633. **Sundaram, G. S., Mackenzie, S. L., and Sodhi, H. S.,** Preparative isoelectric focusing of human serum high-density lipoprotein (HDL3) *Biochim. Biophys. Acta,* 337, 196, 1974.

634. **Swell, L., Trout, E. C., Jr., Field, H., Jr., Treadwell, C. R.,** Intestinal metabolism of C-14-phytosterols, *J. Biol. Chem.,* 234, 2286, 1959.

635. **Szigeti, I., Ormos, J., Jákó, J., and Tószegi, A.,** The atherogenic effect of immunization with homologous complex great vessel wall in rabbit, *Acta Allergol. (Suppl.),* 7, 374, 1960.

636. **Takeuchi, N. and Yamamura, Y.,** Effects of egg yolk and moctamide on serum lipids in man, *Clin. Pharmacol. Ther.,* 116, 368, 1974.

637. **Tarantino, G., Buda, G. R., Amato, M., and Infascelli, R. M.,** Serum Apo B levels in hepatocellular failure, *Boll. Chim. Farm.,* 122, 7S, 1983.

638. **Tennent, D. M., Siegel, H., Zanetti, M. E., Kuron, G. W., Ott, W. H., and Wolf, F. J.,** Plasma cholesterol lowering action of bile acid binding polymers in experimental animals, *J. Lipid Res.,* 1, 469, 1960.

639. **Terpstra, A. H., and Beynen, A. C.,** Density profile and cholesterol concentration of serum lipoproteins in experimental animals and human subjects on hypercholesterolaemic diets, *Comp. Biochem. Physiol. B,* 77, 523, 1984.

640. **Thompson, G. R., Soutar, A. K., Spengel, F. A., Jadhav, A., Gavigan, S. J. P., and Myant, N. B.,** Defects of receptor-mediated low density lipoprotein catabolism in homozygous familial hypercholesterolemia and hypothyroidism in vivo, *Proc. Natl. Acad. Sci. U.S.A.,* 78, 2591, 1981.

641. **Toor, M., Katchalsky, S., Agmon, J., and Allalouf, D.,** Serum lipids and atherosclerosis among Yemenite immigrants in Israel, *Lancet,* 1, 1270, 1957.

642. **Tracy, R. E., Toca, U. T., Strong, J. P., and Richards, M. L.,** Relationship of raised atherosclerotic lesions to fatty streaks in cigarette smokers, *Atherosclerosis,* 38, 347, 1981.

643. **Trelstad, R. L.,** Human aorta collagens: evidence for three distinct species, *Biochem. Biophys. Res. Commun.,* 57, 717, 1974.

644. **Tschopp, T. B. and Baumgarmer, H. R.,** Platelet adhesion and mural platelet thrombus formation on aortic subendothelium, *J. Lab. Clin. Med.,* 98, 402, 1981.

645. **Tremoli, E., Colli, S., Maderna, P., and Paoletti, R.,** Platelets and arachidonic acid metabolism in human and experimental hypercholesterolemia, *Cor. Vasa,* 13, 333, 1984.

646. **Tso, P. and Simmonds, W. J.,** The absorption of lipids and lipoprotein synthesis, *Lab. Res. Methods Biol. Med.,* 10, 191, 1984.

647. **Turner, P. R., Konarska, R., Revill, J., Masana, I., LaVille, A., Cortese, S., Swan, A. V., and Lewis, B.,** Metabolic study of variation in plasma cholesterol level in normal men, *Lancet,* 2, 663, 1984.

648. **Tytgat, G. N., Rubin, C., and Saunders, D. P.,** Synthesis and transport of lipoprotein particles in intestinal absorptive cells in man, *J. Clin. Invest.,* 50, 2065, 1971.

649. **Udenfriend, S., Ooshima, A., Cardinale, G., Fuller, G. C., and Spector, S.,** Increased formation of collagen in the blood vessels of hypertensive rats, *Ann. N.Y. Acad. Sci.,* 275, 101, 1976.

650. **Vander Heiden, G. L., Barbosiak, J. J., Sasse, E. A., and Yorde, D. E.,** Correlation of the extent of coronary occlusion with Apo B levels, *Atherosclerosis* 50, 29, 1984.

651. **Van Hingsbergh, V. W.,** LDL cytotoxicity. The state of art, *Atherosclerosis,* 53, 113, 1984.

652. **Van Hoof, F.,** *Lysosomes and Storage Diseases,* Herz, H. G. and Van Hoof, F., Eds., Academic Press, New York, 1973, 218-261.

653. **Van Reen, R.,** Effects of excessive dietary zinc in rat and interrelationship with copper, *Arch. Biochem.,* 46, 337, 1953.

654. **Vargaftig, B. B., Chignard, M., and Benveniste, J.,** Present concept on the mechanisms of platelet aggregation, *Biochem. Pharmacol.,* 30, 263, 1981.

655. **Verbin, R. S., Goldblatt, P. J., and Farber, E.,** The biochemical pathology of inhibition of protein synthesis in vivo. The effects of cycloheximide on hepatic parenchymal cell ultrastructure, *Lab. Invest.,* 20, 529, 1969.

656. **Vessby, B. and Lithell, M.,** Dietary effects on lipoprotein hyperlipoproteinemia. Delineation of two subgroups of hypertriglyceridemia, *Artery,* 1, 63, 1976.

657. **Viener, A., Brook, J. G., and Aviram, M.,** Abnormal plasma lipoprotein composition in hypercholesterolaemic patients induces platelet activiation, *Eur. J. Clin. Invest.,* 14, 207, 1984.

658. **Volicer, L. and Hynie, S.,** Effect of catecholamines and angiotensin on cyclic AMP in rat aorta and tail artery, *Eur. J. Immunol.,* 15, 214, 1971.

659. **Volpe, J. J. and Vagelos, P. R.,** Regulation of mammalian fatty-acid synthetase. The roles of carbohydrate and insulin, *Proc. Natl. Acad. Sci. U.S.A.,* 71, 889, 1974.

660. **Volpe, J. J. and Vagelos, P. R.,** Mechanism and regulation of biosynthesis of saturated fatty acids, *Physiol. Rev.,* 56, 339, 1976.

661. **Vracko, R. and Benditt, E. P.,** Capillary basal lamina thickening. Its relationship in endothelial cell death and replacement, *J. Cell Biol.,* 47, 281, 1970.

662. **Wacker, W. E., Ulmer, D. D., and Vallee, B. L.,** Metalloenzymes and myocardial infarction; malic and lactic dehydrogenase activities and zinc concentration in serum, *N. Eng. J. Med.,* 255, 449, 1956.

663. **Wahlqvist, M. L. and Day, A. J.,** Phospholipid synthesis by foam cells in human, *Exp. Mol. Pathol.,* 11, 275, 1969.

664. **Wahlquist, M. L., Day, A. J., and Tume, R. K.,** Incorporation of oleic acid into lipid by foam cells in human atherosclerotic lesions, *Circ. Res.,* 24, 123, 1969.

665. **Wakil, S. J., McLain, L. W., and Warshaw, J. B.,** Synthesis of fatty acids by mitochondria, *J. Biol. Chem.,* 235, 31, 1960.

666. **Walli, A. K., and Seidel, D.,** Role of lipoprotein-X in the pathogenesis of cholestatic hypercholesterolemia, *J. Clin. Invest.,* 74, 867, 1984.

667. **Walter, A. R. P.,** Sugar intake and coronary heart disease, *Atherosclerosis,* 14, 137, 1971.

668. **Walton, K. W.,** Pathogenetic mechanism in atherosclerosis, *Am. J. Cardiol.,* 35, 542, 1975.

669. **Warren, B. A. and Khan, S.,** The ultrastructure of the lysis of fibrin by endothelium in vitro, *Br. Exp. Pathol.,* 55, 138, 1974.

670. **Warren, B. A. and Khan, S.,** The scanning electron microscopy of the lysis of fibrin by endothelium, *Br. Exp. Pathol.,* 56, 340, 1975.

671. **Weber, P. C., Scherer, B., and Siess, W.,** Prostaglandins and hypertension, *Adv. Exp. Med. Biol.,* 164, 269, 1984.

672. **Webber, L. S., Cresanta, J. L., Voors, A. W., and Berenson, G. S.,** Tracking of cardiovascular disease risk factor variables in school-age children, *J. Chronic Dis.,* 36, 647, 1983.

673. **Webster, H. D. and Bollert, J. A.,** Toxicologic, reproductive and teratologic studies of colestipol hydrochloride, a new bile acid sequestrant, *Tox. Appl. Pharmacol.,* 28, 57, 1974.

674. **Weilly, H. S. and Genton, E.,** Altered platelet function in patients with prosthetic mitral valves. Effects of sulfinpyrazone therapy, *Circulation,* 42, 967, 1970.

675. **Weisgraber, K. H. and Mahley, R. W.,** Apoprotein (E-AII) complex of human plasma lipoproteins *J. Biol. Chem.,* 253, 6281, 1978.

676. **Weisgraber, K. H., Innerarity, T. L., and Mahley, R. W.,** Abnormal lipoprotein receptor binding activity of the human E apoprotein due to cysteine-arginine interchange at a single site, *J. Biol. Chem.,* 257, 2518, 1982.

677. **Weisweiler, P., Heinemann, V., and Schwandt, P.,** Serum lipoproteins and lecithin: cholesterol acyltransferase activity in hypercholesterolemic subjects given β-sitosterol, *Int. J. Clin. Pharmacol. Ther. Toxicol.,* 22, 204, 1984.

678. **Weksler, B. B., Marcus, A. J., and Jaffe, E. A.,** Synthesis of prostaglandin I₂ (prostacyclin) by cultured human and bovine endothelial cells, *Proc. Natl. Acad. Sci. U.S.A.,* 74, 3922, 1977.

679. **Welsh, M. J., Lewis, L. J., and Hoak, J. C.,** Phagocytosis by cultured human endothelial cells, *Fed. Proc.,* 33, 632, 1974.

680. **Wengeler, H., Greten, H., and Seidel, D.,** Serum cholesterol esterifications of lecithin: cholesterol acyltransferase and lipoprotein-X, *Eur. J. Clin. Invest.,* 2, 372, 1972.

681. **Wengeler, H. and Seidel, D.,** Does lipoprotein-X (LP-X) act as a substrate for the lecithin: cholesterol acyltransferase (LCAT), *Clin. Chim. Acta,* 45, 429, 1973.

682. **Wessler, S.,** Clinical implications of heparin, *Adv. Exp. Med. Biol.,* 52, 309, 1974.

683. **West, K. M., Ahuja, M. M., Bennett, P. H., Czyzyk, A., De Agosta, O. M., Fuller, G. H., Grab, B., Grabanskas, V., Jarrett, R. J., and Kosaka, K.,** The role of circulating glucose and triglyceride concentrations and their interactions with other risk factors' as determinants of arterial disease in nine diabetic population samples from the WHO multinational study, *Diabetes Care,* 6, 361, 1983.

684. **Whereat, A. F.,** Fatty acid synthesis in cell-free system from rabbit aorta, *J. Lipid. Res.,* 7, 671, 1966.

685. **Whereat, A. F.,** Recent advances in experimental and molecular pathology. Atherosclerosis and metabolic disorder in the arterial wall, *Exp. Mol. Pathol.,* 7, 233, 1967.

686. **Whereat, A. F.,** Is atherosclerosis a disorder of intramitochondrial respiration?, *Ann. Int. Med.,* 73, 125, 1970.

687. **Wight, T. N. and Ross, R.,** Proteoglycans in primate arteries. I ultrastructural localization and distribution in the intima, *J. Cell. Biol.,* 67, 660, 1975.

688. **Wilens, S. L.,** The nature of diffuse intimal thickening of arteries, *Am. J. Pathol.,* 27, 825, 1951.

689. **Williams, C. D. and Avigan, D. S.,** In vitro effects of serum proteins and lipids on lipid synthesis in human skin, fibroblasts and leukocytes grown in culture, *Biochim. Biophys. Acta,* 260, 423, 1972.

690. **Wilson, D. E. and Lees, R. S.,** Metabolic relationships among the plasma lipoproteins, *J. Clin. Invest.,* 51, 1051, 1972.

691. **Wilson, D. J.,** The role of bile acids in the overall regulation of steroid metabolism, *Arch. Intern. Med.,* 130, 493, 1972.

692. **Windmueller, H. G., Lindgren, F. T., Lossow, W. J., and Levy, R. I.,** On the nature of circulating lipoproteins of intestinal origin in the rat, *Biochim. Biophys. Acta,* 202, 507, 1970.

693. **Windmueller, H. G. and Spaeth, A. E.,** Fat transport and lymph and plasma lipoprotein biosynthesis by isolated intestine, *J. Lipid Res.,* 13, 92, 1972.

694. **Wissler, R. W., Vesselinovitch, D., Borensztajn, J., and Hughes, R.,** Regression of severe atherosclerosis in cholestyramine-treated rhesus monkeys with or without a low-fat, low-cholesterol diet, *Circulation,* 52, 11, 1975.

695. **Wolinsky, H.,** Role of lysosomes in vascular disease; a unifying theme, *Ann. N.Y. Acad. Sci.,* 275, 238, 1976.

696. **Wolinsky, H. and Fowler, S.,** Participation of lysosomes in atherosclerosis, *N. Engl. J. Med.,* 299, 1173, 1978.

697. **Wolinsky, H., Goldfischer, S., and Daly, M. M.,** Arterial lysosomes and corrective tissues in primate atherosclerosis and hypertension, *Circ. Res.,* 36, 553, 1975.

698. **Woolf, N.,** *Pathology of Atherosclerosis,* Butterworth Scientific, London, 1982, 62.

699. **Wright, H. P.,** Mitosis patterns in aortic endothelium, *Atherosclerosis,* 15, 93, 1971.

700. **Wulfert, B., Majoie, B., and de Ceaurriz, A.,** Antilipidemic drugs: Part 6, LE178, in man. A preliminary note on a multicenter investigation bearing on 393 subjects with pure or mixed form of hyperlipidemia, *Arzneim. Forsch.,* 26, 906, 1976.

701. **Yaari, S., Goldbourt, U., Even-Zohar, S., and Neufeld, H. N.,** Associations of serum high density lipoprotein and total cholesterol with total, cardiovascular and cancer mortality in a 7-year prospective study of 10,000 men, *Lancet,* 1, 1011, 1981.

702. **Yamada, N. and Murase, T.,** Modulation of lipoprotein lipase activity by apolipoprotein E. *Biochem. Biophys. Res. Commun.,* 94, 710, 1980.

703. **Yamamura, T., Yamamoto, A., Sumiyoshi, T., Hiramori, K., Nishioeda, Y., and Namu, S.,** New mutants of apolipoprotein E associated with atherosclerotic disease but not to type III hyperlipoproteinemia, *J. Clin. Invest.,* 74, 1229, 1984.

704. **Yousef, I. M. and Kuksis, K.**, Release of chylomicrons by isolated cells of rat intestinal mucosa, *Lipids,* 7, 380, 1972.
705. **Zannis, V. I., Just, P., and Breslow, J.**, Human apolipoprotein E isoprotein subclasses are genetically determined, *Am. J. Hum. Genetc.*, 33, 11, 1981.
706. **Zeldis, S. M., Nemerson, Y., Pitlich, F. A., and Lentz, T. L.**, Tissue factor (thromboplastin) localization to plasma membranes by peroxidase-conjugated antibodies, *Science,* 175, 766, 1972.
707. **Zemplenyi, T.**, *Enzyme Biochemistry of the Arterial Wall as Related to Atherosclerosis*, Lloyd-Luke Medical Books, London, 1968.
708. **Zilversmit, D. B.**, A proposal linking atherogenesis to the interaction of endothelial lipoprotein lipase with triglyceride-rich lipoproteins, *Circ. Res.*, 33, 633, 1973.
709. **Zilversmit, D. B.**, Exchange of phospholipid classes between liver microsomes and plasma: comparison of rat, rabbit, and guinea pig, *J. Lipid Res.*, 12, 36, 1971.
710. **Zilversmit, D. B.**, Atherogenesis: a post-prandial phenomenon, *Circulation,* 60, 473, 1979.
711. **Marks, J., Ed.**, *Dyslipoproteinaemia — Aspects of Gemfibrosil Therapy*, Vol. 4, Research and Clinical Forums, Kent, England, 1982.

FURTHER READINGS

Bristow, M. R., Ed., *Drug-Induced Heart Disease*, Elsevier/North-Holland, Amsterdam, 1980.
Chazov, E., Smirnov, V., and Dhalla, N. S., Eds., *Advances in Myocardiology*, Vol. 3, Plenum Medical Book Company, New York, 1982.
Chazov, E., Smirnov, V.,, and Rona, G., Eds., *Advances in Myocardiology,* Vol. 4, Plenum Medical Book Company, New York, 1983.
Dhalla, N. S. and Hearse, D. J., Eds., *Advances in Myocardiology,* Vol. 6, Plenum Medical Book Company, New York, 1985.
Donoso, E., Ed., *Drugs in Cardiology*, Medical Book Corp., New York, 1975.
Gotto, A. M., Jr. and Paoletti, R., Eds., *Atherosclerosis Reviews,* Vol. 7 to 12, Raven Press, New York, 1976 to 1984.
Harris, P. and Poole-Wilson, P. A., Eds., *Advances in Myocardiology,* Vol. 5, Plenum Medical Book Company, New York, 1984.
Havel, R. J. and Kane, J. P., Drugs and lipid metabolism, *Ann. Rev. Pharmac.*, 26, 1, 1972.
Kritchevsky, D., *Handbook of Experimental Pharmacology — Pharmacology of Hypolipidemic Agents*, Springer-Verlag, Berlin, 1975.
Miller, N. E., *Atherosclerosis: Mechanisms and Approaches to Therapy*, Raven Press, New York, 1984.
Myant, N. B., Effect of drugs on the metabolism of bile acids, *Adv. Exp. Biol. Med.*, 26, 137, 1972.
Porter, R. and Knight, J., Ed., *Atherogenesis: Inititating Factors*, Elsevier, Amsterdam, 1973.
Scanu, A. M., Wissler, R. W., and Getz, G. S., Ed., *The Biochemistry of Atherosclerosis*, Marcel Dekker, New York, 1979.
Schettler, G. and Weizel, A., Ed., *Atherosclerosis*, Springer-Verlag, Berlin, 1974.
Woolf, N., *Pathology of Atherosclerosis*, Butterworth Scientific, London, 1982.

Chapter 3

LIVER DISEASES

I. INTRODUCTION

The liver is one of our vital organs; it has several roles which include metabolic, synthetic, secretory, and excretory functions. In the fetus it is a hematopoietic organ, and a processing, storage, and defense organ throughout our lifespan. Whereas the liver is one of the largest and most complex functioning organs in the body, its architecture is relatively simple. The liver parenchymal cell structure and constituent subcellular organelles reflect the diverse and highly specialized functions of this organ (Figure 1). The liver operates like a complex chemical factory, producing many essential blood proteins and lipids (lipoproteins), metabolizing foodstuffs and foreign compounds, altering and synthesizing new substances, and regulating plasma concentrations of many molecules. It filters materials of various origins from the bloodstream, secretes and transports useful compounds into other organs,[375] eliminates byproducts, detoxifies drugs and other foreign substances,[27] and reduces hormone activity through inactivation. The various operations of the hepatic cell, such as processing, secretory, excretory, and phagocytic activities proceed largely independent of each other.

Diseases of the liver are related to one or more functions; changes in the biochemical bases of these functions, therefore, lead to hepatic ailments. The control of synthesis and metabolism represents the maintenance of homeostasis. If any failure occurs in the hepatic ability of regulating molecular interconversion, homeostatic diseases become readily apparent. In particular, the upset in metabolic balance causes metabolic disorders, whereas deficiencies in the regulation of bile secretion are associated with biliary diseases. Abnormal synthesis and altered function of the structural elements of the hepatocytes result in parenchymatous diseases. The liver affects other organs by its endocrine and exocrine behavior. Breakdown of regulation may cause neurological disorders, malfunction of endocrine glands, and many other interrelated diseases. The involvement of impaired hepatic metabolism is considered a factor in inflammation,[183] in thermal injury,[515] and in sudden infant death syndrome[75,244]

II. STRUCTURAL CHANGES ASSOCIATED WITH DISEASE

The integrity of the plasma membrane structure is essential for the maintenance of normal hepatic functions. Hepatocytes cannot perform properly the various biochemical processes when the membranes of their constituent subcellular organelles show any abnormalities or if the turnover of the individual components does not proceed correctly. The turnover rate of hepatocytic subcellular organelles is variable; the biological half-life of human hepatocytes and plasma membranes varies between 6 and 12 months. In contrast, protein and phospholipid synthesis and renewal takes from 1 to 20 d. Some particular processes proceed even faster. This constant replacement of constituent molecules in the membranes by rapid biochemical processes assures the maintenance of structural continuity and integrity of the bilayer, as well as the proper architecture of the membrane. Many reactions are very complex and are responsible not only for the proper topology of the membrane, but are also involved in catalytic functions. The level at which these processes operate is continually being controlled by the changing internal cell environment. Structural and functional relationships are closely enmeshed, and in disease processes, these undergo reciprocal changes (Figure 2). There are also processes which are dependent on the given structural unit and its development.

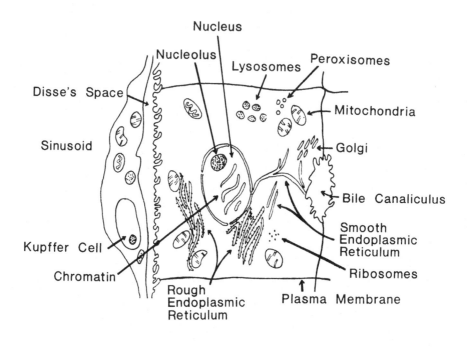

FIGURE 1.   Schematic representation of the liver cell. The various subcellular organelles elicit diverse biochemical functions associated with different enzyme activities.

The importance of membrane structure in relation to hepatobiliary disease is mostly concerned with the endoplasmic reticulum and the plasma membrane. The formation of smooth endoplasmic reticulum membranes is particularly complex; any process modification may affect the normal cellular processes. Pathologic changes in protein and phospholipid synthesis not only represent an error in the biogenesis of the endoplasmic reticulum, but also cause changes in the activity of detoxication enzymes which metabolize and eliminate foreign compounds, such as drugs and carcinogens from liver cells. Any interference with the biosynthesis of proteins and phospholipids in the smooth endoplasmic reticulum leads to functional and structural changes. The impairment of these processes thereby leads to cell injury with ensuing disease. The plasma membrane of the hepatocyte is linked with the secretion of a wide range of substances such as proteins, lipoproteins, smaller moieties, and mainly bile. The hepatocyte membrane can be separated into two components. One facing the sinusoids is concerned with the exchange of substances to and from the blood. The other membrane surface separates neighboring cells and is capable of bile secretion at the level of the bile canaliculus, exchanging ions and other substances between cells. Damage to the hepatocyte plasma membrane brings about disorders associated with abnormal transport processes.

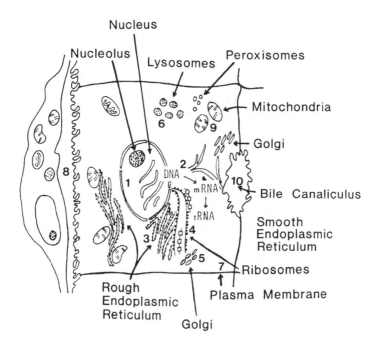

FIGURE 2.   Diseases and subcellular target organelles.

1 Mutation, Neoplasia	6 Storage
2 Inborn Error	7 Transport
3 Degranulation - Toxicity	8 Intake
4 Dilatation - Toxicity	9 Respiration
	- Swelling
5 Selection	10 Elimination

III. HEPATOCELLULAR DEGENERATION AND NECROSIS

Hepatic diseases reflect changes both in the function and in the microscopic appearance of the cell.[484] As a consequence of these changes, hepatocellular degeneration ranges functionally and clinically from minimal insufficiency to fatal hepatic failure. The common basis of most cell injury is the lack of oxygen. The reaction to this hypoxia is a relatively stereotyped cellular response. During this process, the first morphological sign is cloudy swelling, consisting of a granular appearance of the cytoplasm caused by swelling and disruption of mitochondria. This change is associated with reversible denaturation of cellular proteins, especially those which function as enzymes necessary for oxydative processes. Denaturation is often linked with calcium uptake from the interstitial fluid and, subsequently, the injured cells accumulate calcium fairly readily.

Mitochondria are the center of oxidation, and with oxygen deprivation, they become unable to metabolize various substrates and to produce adequate amounts of adenosine triphosphate and other high energy-containing phosphates.[308,482,485] Adenosine triphosphate is essential for the maintenance of membrane integrity in the mitochondria as well as in the cell membrane. Thus, with the loss of adenosine triphosphate, changes occur in the cell permeability. The membrane of the normal cell is semipermeable; it allows the free passage of some metabolites, but excludes others. In particular, it keeps out sodium via the mechanism of the sodium pump utilizing active metabolic processes. The cell efficiently maintains a high intracellular electrolyte level. In case of impairment, sodium enters the cell from the interstitial fluid. In further stages of cell injury, water accumulates to the extent that vesicles are formed in the cytoplasm. In this phase, the hydropic degeneration represents a further advance of the injury, but it is still reversible. Further structural changes occur in the liver parenchymal cells as well as in other organs associated with fat accumulation.[307,490] Fatty change develops following damage to the metabolic systems which normally carry out the processing and elimination of neutral lipids. Fat accumulation appears as a result of various toxic actions: in acute alcoholism and in malnutrition, there is a pathologic mobilization of excess fat from tissue depots. This excess of lipid exhausts the capacity of the hepatocyctic fat-utilization system and fat accumulates within the cell. Moreover, hypoxia suppresses the production of enzymes necessary for processing the mobilized fatty acids. Subsequently, the failure to synthesize adequate enzymes limits cellular activity of eliminating the large amounts of incoming lipid. Defective fat mobilization is recurring in diabetic patients often associated with incomplete fatty acid oxidation. The accumulating intermediates are responsible for the symptoms of acidosis. Hypoxic injury of tissues is frequently followed by hydropic degeneration, and further changes develop in the form of severe fatty change. This stage is always associated with the partial suppression of protein synthesis by the cell.

If the process of hypoxia is severe enough, the prolonged deterioration of cellular activity proceeds further to cellular necrosis. This occurs when cells are disrupted irreversibly; cell death follows irreversible injury. In severe hepatocellular degeneration signs of hepatic coma are apparent, usually associated with a characteristic encephalopathy.

A. CHOLESTASIS

Obstruction of the normal bile outflow from hepatocytes causes either abnormal retention of bile within the liver cell or the accumulation of abnormal amounts of biliary substances in the blood.[40,312,611] These are representative of the mechanisms of intrahepatic or extrahepatic cholestasis. Increased retention of bile in bile passages produces stagnation and mechanical dilatations of bile canaliculi and ductules. This stasis influences intrahepatic blood circulation and metabolism. Increased amounts of biliary substances in the blood may cause toxic injury to the hepatic cells.[445,447] Extrahepatic biliary obstruction produces different degrees of injury.

Centrilobular cholestasis is the most common form of hepatic disease in which several organelles are altered around the bile canaliculus as a result of the increased intracellular pressure and impaired bile transport processes. The alterations of the endoplasmic reticulum and mitochondria may be associated with the detergent action of bile acids. However, changes in the bile duct system are probably secondary to the parenchymal lesions. Many causes of cholestasis include primary hepatocellular damage resulting in a defect in bile acid oxidation and exerting qualitative changes in bile composition. Changes in intracellular structures coincide with the formation of bile thrombi which bring about a mechanical obstruction or induce a defect in the excretion of conjugated bilirubin regurgitating into the sinusoids. Cell membranes and extralobular ductules develop increased permeability to water and electrolytes and, consequently, lesion the sodium pump leading to changes in the concentration of canalicular bile. Obstructive or destructive phenomena occurring in the intralobular ductules and bile ducts are also considered in the pathogenesis of certain types of intrahepatic cholestasis, particularly in primary biliary cirrhosis.[279,445,518]

The morphological features of intrahepatic and extrahepatic cholestasis show typical characteristics, including hepatomegaly without significant changes in the lobular pattern. In later stages, bile stasis and inflammatory processes become manifest. Electron microscopic studies have revelaed the possible sites of lesions responsible for the development of cholestasis (Figure 3). These include dilatation of the bile canaliculi, alteration of microvilli, deposition of dense amorphous or fibrillar material throughout the cell cytoplasm, and variable changes in the smooth endoplasmic reticulum membranes and mitochondria.

Several mechanisms have been proposed to explain the biochemical changes underlying intrahepatic cholestasis. Bile secretion from the liver cell can be divided into two fractions:

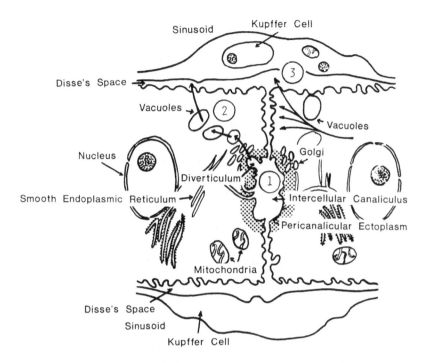

FIGURE 3. Schematic representation of changes in the liver cell in cholestasis. The intercellular canaliculus is dilated and the structure of microvilli is damaged showing a diverticulum and widened pericanalicular ectoplasm. The intercellular space is widened containing irregular microvilli. The Golgi apparatus and smooth endoplasmic reticulum are hypertrophied, mitochondrial cristae are curled, and intracytoplasmic vacuoles are present. The intercellular excretion of bile constituents from the canaliculus into the blood stream is reduced (1), transhepatocytic regurgitation of bile constituents through vacuoles is apparent (2), and overflow causes elimination into the blood stream. Reversed secretory polarity of the hepatocytes renders secretion of bile constituents into the intercellular space rather than secreting into the paralyzed canaliculus (3). Such reversed polarity and widened intercellular spaces provide the possibility for a more diffuse and widespread overflow of bile constituents toward the hepatocyte-blood stream barrier (modified from References 124 and 125).

one is bile acid-dependent and the other bile acid-independent. Both fractions are altered by sex steroid hormones or exogenous bile acids. The bile acid-independent fraction is modulated by the sodium pump using sodium/potassium-activated adenosine triphosphatase. This fraction contains mainly electrolytes, and the greater part of the excretion product is reabsorbed in the bile duct and gallbladder. The bile acid-dependent fraction contains bile acids and heterogeneous micelles which are composed of polyionic complexes formed from bile salts, cholesterol, and phospholipids. Hyperbilirubinemia is produced when the elimination of this fraction is disturbed.[59,149,262,310,311] Hydrophylic bile acids promote the formation of these aggregates which also carry other anions including bilirubin. In normal circumstances, the micelle and bile flow follow unidirectionally from the sinusoids toward the bile canaliculi. Normally only trace amounts of monohydroxy cholic acids are present in the bile. However, in pathologic conditions there may be a considerable increase. Therefore, variations in the concentration or type of bile acid synthetized disturb micelle formation resulting in abnormal accumulation and production of liquid crystals. The abnormal mixture of cholesterol, lecithin, and bile salts form these liquid crystals and sometimes amorphous materials. These structures precipitate in intracanalicular spaces and produce thrombi leading to fragmentation of the microvilli and pericanalicular cell membranes, with altered cytoplasmic constituents including the endoplasmic reticulum and mitochondria.[224,389,482] Disturbances are probably associated with the metabolic capacity of these cellular organelles.

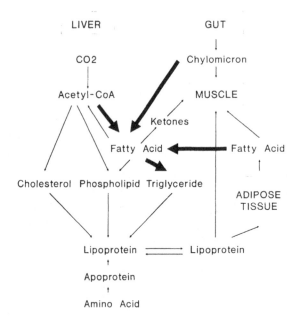

FIGURE 4.   Pathways of fatty liver production by impairment of lipid transport and metabolism. Major defects include increased fat mobilization from adipose tissue or dietary sources, or enhanced synthesis as indicated by thicker arrows, or decreased lipoprotein synthesis and transport of lipids from the liver, and decreased oxidation of lipids as indicated by broken lines.

Microsomal enzymes are responsible for the transformation of cholesterol to bile acids and mitochondrial enzymes for the side chain cleavage of this molecule, providing more sites for further hydroxylation.[145,213,225,341,491,553] Inhibition of these processes and particularly impairment of the microsomal enzyme system have been reported as the principal causative factors in cholestasis. Due to faulty hydroxylation, the process of bile acid production is incomplete. Following this defect, excess amounts of mono- and dihydroxy bile acids are formed at the expense of cholic acid. The excretion of lithocholic acid may damage the entire excretory apparatus from the microvilli to the ductules. The accumulating monohydroxy bile acids, such as lithocholic acid, are poor micelle formers, and therefore, these components may be involved in the development of cholestasis. In these circumstances the activity of hepatic hydroxylating enzymes and cytochrome P-450 are reduced. The conversion of dihydroxy acids to monohydroxy derivatives by intestinal bacteria can also be considered as a secondary factor. The prevalence of chenodeoxycholic acid in the intestines enhances the formation of lithocholic acid which is then reabsorbed via the enterohepatic circulation in abnormally high amounts. This condition is characterized in human extrahepatic cholestasis brought about by anabolic steroids or ethynyl estradiol. In experimental animals, the time related increase of these changes runs parallel with the extrahepatic biliary obstruction, indicating that perhaps they represent the consequences rather than the cause of cholestasis.

B. FATTY LIVER

The liver can accumulate various lipids, the major component being triacylglycerol. If lipid accumulation in extensive, pathological conditions set in[271] (Figure 4). Fatty liver can develop when the supply of lipids to the liver is excessive or lipid disposition is disturbed (Figure 5). Lipid accumulation originates from three main sources: (1) dietary lipids reaching the bloodstream as chylomicra, (2) lipids from adipose tissue degradation which are trans-

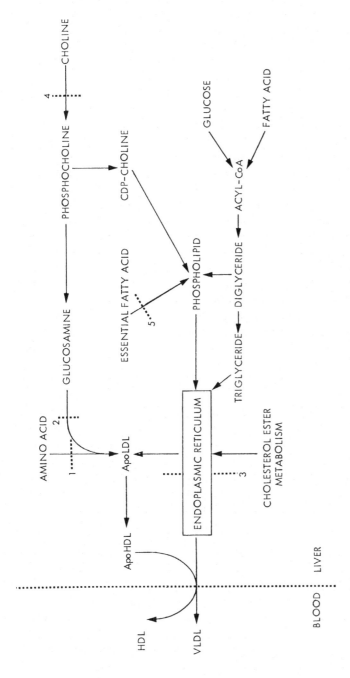

FIGURE 5. Mechanism of fatty degeneration of the liver brought about by various factors. The sites where various compounds or lack of lipotropic factor cause fatty degeneration are marked, hepatotoxins (carbon tetrachloride, ethionine, puromycin) (1), orotic acid (2), lack of phospholipid synthesis or direct effect on endoplasmic reticulum membranes by hepatotoxins (3), choline or methyl donor deficiency (4), and essential fatty acid deficiency (5).

ported to the liver as free fatty acids, and (3) lipids synthesized in the liver itself. Due to various metabolic disturbances, these fatty acids can accumulate in the liver. The major disturbances are (1) increased fat mobilization from peripheral tissues, (2) enhanced lipid synthesis in the liver, (3) decreased hepatic lipid oxidation, and (4) decreased production and release of hepatic lipoproteins. Two major types of fatty liver can be distinguished. In one type, the free fatty acid content of the plasma is increased as the consequence of enhanced mobilization of fat from peripheral adipose tissue or from accelerated hydrolysis of triacylglycerol content of chylomicrons or lipoproteins by lipoprotein lipase in extrahepatic tissues. Part of the free fatty acid produced in this way is taken up and esterified in the liver. If the influx of free fatty acids into the liver is not complete and due to the reduced level of lipoproteins, triacylglycerol accumulates causing fatty degeneration. Starvation or the consumption of a high-fat diet causes impaired metabolism of neutral fats and changes in normal lipoprotein secretion by the liver. Fatty infiltration and liver enlargement occur in uncontrolled diabetes and toxemia of pregnancy.

The production of lipoprotein responsible for lipid transport can be inhibited usually by a metabolic block. The inhibition is frequently associated with the lack of a lipotropic factor. The deficiency of this factor results in accumulation of triacylglycerol, even if the rates of fatty acid production and uptake are normal. Choline, methionine, and betaine act as lipotropic factors.[240] The lack of these agents, such as in choline deficiency, is associated with fatty liver. This condition may be cured by the administration of methionine, since the methyl group in methionine contributes to important methyl transfer reactions. However, if the utilization of methyl groups is excessive or the diet is poor in methyl donors, fatty degeneration can occur. The role of choline as lipotropic agent is important in the function of low density lipoproteins. Choline is also essential in the synthesis of intracellular membranes, and choline deficiency may impair membrane synthesis.[3,405,411,423,523] Several hepatotoxins induce fatty liver, including carbon tetrachloride, chloroform, phosphorus, ethionine, or puromycin. The action of these compounds results in abnormal changes in important cellular processes. It can be caused by an impairment of protein synthesis, reduction of the availability of adenosine triphosphate, inhibition of methyl transfer, mostly related to an interference with the endoplasmic reticulum function. Administration of orotic acid brings about fatty change due to a specific block in the synthesis of the low density lipoprotein apoproteins. The possible mechanism and site of these effects is illustrated (Figure 6). Vitamin E deficiency enhances choline deficiency, protein deficiency enhances lack of essential fatty acids, and pyridoxine or pantothenic acid can cause hepatic fatty change. Alcoholism can also lead to hepatic fat accumulation, hyperlipidemia, dyslipoproteinemia, and ultimately, cirrhosis. This latter condition occurs when the accumulation of lipids in the liver becomes chronic, associated with fibrotic changes and progressively impaired functions.[437,535]

IV. DISEASES OF PORPHYRIN SYNTHESIS

Porphyrias comprise a group of diseases associated with an abnormality of porphyrin-heme biosynthesis.[143,151] Recent advances have shed light on the pathogenic mechanism by the elucidation of factors regulating the formation of these compounds.[119,213,341,439,541] Porphyrins are red pigments with a cyclic tetrapyrrole structure. Their biosynthesis takes place in the bone marrow, liver, and reticulo-endothelial system. The total daily porphyrin production amounts approximately to a few hundred micrograms.

Some types of porphyrias are common in some areas of the world. Most of these are inherited diseases, and they are not easy to diagnose. Certain drugs provoke the onset of porphyria and may even cause a fatal outcome. Porphyrias may be conveniently divided into two main groups: one group manifests mainly in the liver and the other in the erythropoietic system. In some porphyrias both sites participate. Since various deficiencies of

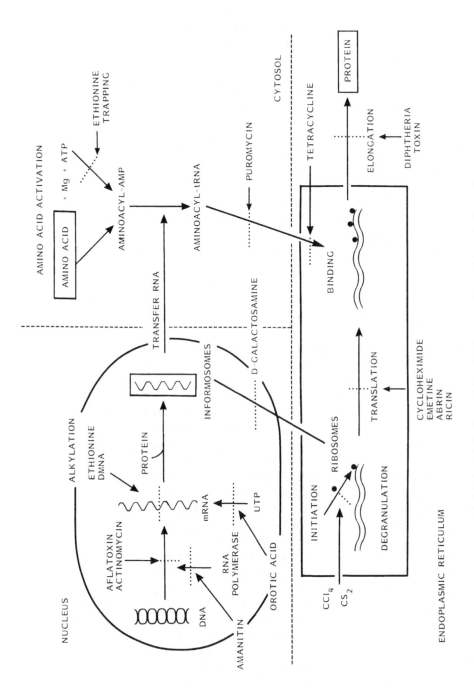

FIGURE 6. Mechanism and site of action on various toxins on the liver cell.

hepatic porphyrin biosynthesis are responsible for the most frequent causes, the entire group will be discussed under liver diseases.

The sites of porphyrin metabolism are the red blood cells, the reticuloendothelial system: spleen, bone marrow, lymph nodes, and liver.[267] The major pathway of porphyrin excretion is from the liver into the bile; a minor pathway is the elimination of porphyrins into the urine. Only 1 to 50 μg amounts of uroporphyrin I and II and coproporphyrin I and III are excreted into the feces and urine when the liver function is normal and the synthesis proceeds undisturbed to the formation of heme (Figure 7).

A. CELLULAR CONTROL OF HEME SYNTHESIS

The pathway of heme formation has been demonstrated a long time ago.[414, 510, 511] All nitrogen atoms and eight carbon atoms of the heme molecule are derived from glycine, the remaining carbon atoms derive from succinate via the Krebs' cycle. In the first step, glycine and succinate are combined, and two of the resulting δ-aminolevulinic acid molecules are condensed to give monopyrrole porphobilinogen. The next step is an enzymatic polymerization of four porphobilinogen units leading to the formation of uroporphyrinogen. Subsequently, decarboxylation yields coproporphyrinogen; a side chain modification transforms this compound to protoporphyrinogen IX and finally, the incorporation of ferrous ion gives rise to heme and the addition of a globin leads to hemoglobin[459] (Figure 8). The heme molecule is the prostetic group of a variety of hemoproteins such as hemoglobin, myoglobin, cytochromes, catalase, peroxidase, and others.

In the overall heme synthesis, δ-aminolevulinic acid production is the rate-limiting step. There are marked differences in the synthesis of heme, however, between various cells within one organism. Red blood cells contain 1000 times more heme molecules than hepatic cells, indicating probably the action of a nonenzymatic mechanism besides enzyme effects in the regulation of heme synthesis pathway.[141,142] The intra- and extramitochondrial localization of participating enzymes suggests the existence of such a regulation mediated through differential permeability of mitochondrial membranes to key intermediates or differences in compartmentalization, end-product repression, or direct inhibition. The availability of the precursors glycine and succinyl-CoA, limitation of pyridoxal phosphate, and a reciprocal end-product feedback action of hemoprotein appears to be essential in the synthesis control mechanism. Another important regulating mechanism may be associated with the fact that mitochondrial δ-aminolevulinic acid synthetase is an inducible enzyme, and its levels are influenced by inducers of drug metabolism.[242,243] Hydrocortisone stimulates the activity of this enzyme in adrenalectomized animals. This hepatic effect may be associated with alterations in the endoplasmic reticulum necessary for hepatic enzyme induction. The increased mitochondrial enzyme production is also mediated by changes in the endoplasmic reticulum.[120,121,554,555] In contrast to the rise in porphyrin synthesis, the presence of additional enzyme pathways metabolizing intermediates may decrease heme formation. The oxidation of porphobilinogen to 5-oxo-porphobilinogen by porphobilinogen oxidase,[186] or a protease which specifically breaks down pyridoxal phosphate requiring enzymes,[317] may play such a role. Inhibition of heme biosynthesis is caused by hemin, hemoglobin, or bilirubin.[214-216,421] These substances block the conversion of the soluble δ-aminolevulinic acid synthetase into the mitochondrial bound form. Drug-induced porphobilinogenuria could be prevented by increased intake of glucose in the diet. Glucose inhibits the induction of δ-aminolevulinic acid synthetase.[456,488] The action of glucose is probably related to the transformation to uridine diphosphate glucuronic acid which converts porphyria-inducing substances such as corticosteroids to inactive glucoronide conjugates.

δ-Aminolevulinic acid can be converted along two pathways besides being precursor of the heme molecule; it can be transformed to formyl moiety, which is incorporated into purines, or to succinate, which participates in the Krebs' cycle. The δ-carbon atom of the

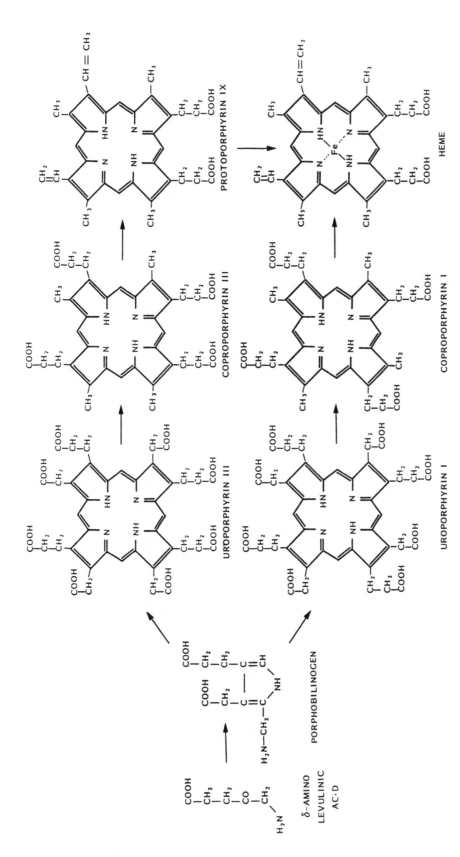

FIGURE 7. Structure of some intermediates of heme synthesis.

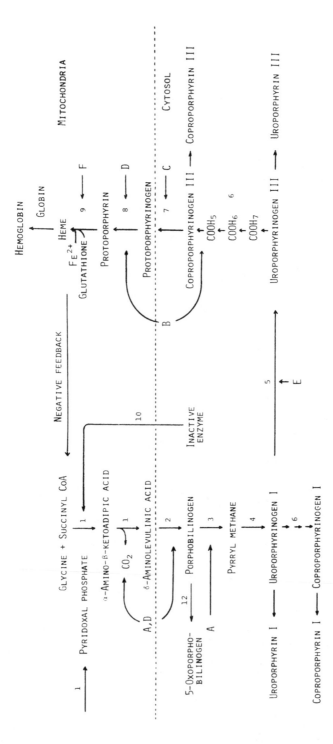

FIGURE 8.   Biosynthesis of porphyrins and hemoglobin. Enzymes which catalyze the sequence are aminolevulinic acid synthetase (1), aminolevulinic acid dehydrase (2), porphobilinogen deaminase (3), urogen synthetase (4), uroporphyrin isomerase or urogen cosynthetase (5), urogen decarboxylase (6), coprogenase or coproporphyrin dehydrogenase (7), protogen oxidase (8), and heme synthetase or FeII-chelatase (9). Side reactions lead to the formation of various types of porphyria; the probable sites are acute intermittent porphyria (A) and porphyria (B), hereditary coproporphyria (C), porphyria cutanea tarda and drug-induced porphyria (D), erythropoietic protoporphyria and lead induced porphyria (F). The rate of synthesis is under a negative feedback control by the end-product heme. There are several regulatory steps including the activation of the cytosomal aminolevulinic acid synthetase (10), the reduction of the essential coenzyme by hydrolytic breakdown of the apoenzyme by apoenzyme protease (11), or the reduction of intermediates by side reactions catalyzed by porphobilinogen oxidase (12).

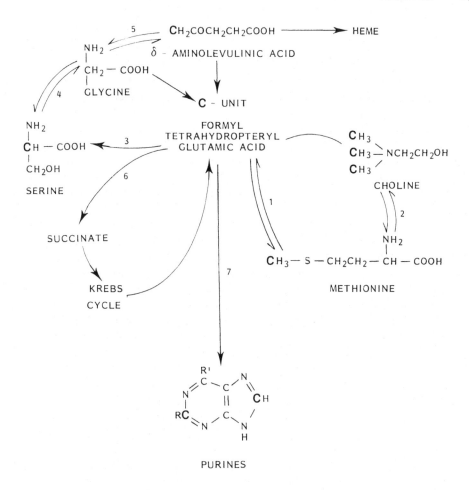

C = incorporated into various intermediates

FIGURE 9. Utilization of the one carbon unit in the biosynthesis of aminolevulinic acid and related processes. The one carbon unit, formyl-tetrahydropteryl glutamic acid provides the methyl group to methionine (1) and further methyl transfer reactions (2) producing choline. It is incorporated into serine (3) and glycine (4), and further forms aminolevulinic acid (5). One carbon unit also takes part in the synthesis of succinate (6) and purines (7).

aminolevulinic acid is used for the synthesis of serin β-carbon and methionine methyl group. The existence of these pathways (Figure 9) has been clearly established, but it is not yet known to what extent these reactions may be important in the development of porphyria or other diseases.

B. HEPATIC DISORDERS OF PORPHYRIN SYNTHESIS

Acute intermittent porphyria is the most important and commonest of the porphyrias, occurring mostly in Sweden and Britain. In acute porphyria, an inherited autosomal dominant disease, attacks of severe colicky abdominal pains and constipation are accompanied by lesions of the nervous system. These may be present as peripheral neuritis or as a progressive paralysis of the lower limbs and reaching the trunk, arms, neck, and finally, the respiratory system. Lesions may occur in the brain, brain stem, spinal cord, and in the autonomic nervous system.

Characteristic abdominal pains and neurological symptoms are the main clinical features of this disease, and probably caused by lesions of the nervous system. The axon or the myelin sheath are primarily affected and the gastrointestinal pain is probably caused by lesions of the preganglionic motor fibers that innervate the viscerae. Some cases may present abdominal or neurological symptoms only. In some cases, the disease is latent and only biochemical findings are noted without clinical signs. An abnormal mental state is associated with acute porphyria, and these symptoms are exemplified by abnormal behavioral responses including fear or painful illness.

During an acute attack in acute intermittent porphyria the main defect is in the liver. Remissions are also associated with moderate increases of several components of the porphyrin pathway. Earlier observations revealed increased δ-aminolevulinic acid synthetase activity. More recent evidence, however, indicated both aminolevulinic acid and porphobilinogen excreted in excess in the urine. The hepatic metabolic abnormality is either due to an enzyme deficiency causing a block in the conversion of porphobilinogen to porphyrins due to decreased uroporphyrin synthetase and porphobilinogen deaminase, or to the increased activity of δ-aminolevulinic acid synthetase and dehydrase is just incidental.[163,206,528] Uroporphyrin synthetase activity is concomitantly diminished in erythrocytes.[335,540]

The excretion of the excess δ-aminolevulinic acid and porphobilinogen and the changes in the nervous system are separate manifestations of the same metabolic event. The metabolic abnormality must always be present although its clinical manifestation usually becomes apparent between the ages of 30 to 40 years. The acute attacks are frequently precipitated by the administration of barbiturates, sulphonamides, griseofulvin, and other drugs, including oral contraceptives. However, the action of drugs is not essential for the onset of an acute crisis. Pregnancy is also often associated with an increased frequency of episodes. If unexplained peripheral neuritis, abdominal pains, psychosis, or neurosis occurs, tests for porphobilinogen may reveal the abnormality in hepatic porphyrin synthesis.

Cutaneous hepatic porphyria is also inherited as an autosomal dominant disease usually beginning in early adulthood and clinical symptoms appear in the 30- to 40-year age group. The photosensitivity observed in the cutaneous form is less severe than in the congenital form and does not lead usually to deformities or scarring. In addition, neurological signs also occur. In this condition hepatic δ-aminolevulinic acid synthetase is enhanced, whereas liver and erythrocyte uroporphyrin synthetase are normal. The defect is mainly hepatic; laboratory findings show increased urinary levels of δ-aminolevulinic acid, porphobilinogen, uro-, and coproporphyrins. In the feces, the excretion of uro- and coproporphyrins and protoporphyrin is also elevated. In remission, urinary porphyrins may be normal, but the fecal excretion remains increased. In addition to the previous defect, there is also an abnormality in the oxidation-reduction system in the liver and other functions.[430] Uroporphyrinogens may be oxidized in this condition to the corresponding porphyrins which cannot reversibly return to the biosynthetic pathway and accumulate in the tissue or the excess is excreted.

Acquired hepatic porphyria or porphyria cutanea tarda usually occurs in the adult middle age mainly among South African Bantus. Women are more frequently affected than men.[96,132] However, it is not a hereditary disease, but it is probably associated with genetic abnormality. The onset of porphyria is usually provoked by hepatotoxic agents such as alcohol[388] or by the ingestion of other toxins such as hexachlorobenzene. Acute attacks are usually harmless. A marked increase in urinary porphyrin excretion, mostly uroporphyrin, is the evidence of the biochemical abnormality. Fecal porphyrin levels are normal or only slightly elevated. Porphobilinogen and δ-aminolevulinic acid are not present in quantities.

Protocoproporphyria (porphyria variegata) occurs in relatively greater numbers in South Africa. It shows many common features with acute intermittent porphyria. Inherited as a dominant characteristic, it manifests only after puberty. Skin lesions of varied severity are common and acute attacks are associated with abdominal or neurological symptoms which may be precipitated by drugs. The main biochemical finding is the excessive fecal excretion of porphyrins with persisting elevated levels. During an acute attack porphobilinogen, δ-aminolevulinic acid and porphyrin are present in the urine, but these disappear shortly after the attack.

Hereditary coproporphyria is inherited as an autosomal dominant disorder. The neurologic-visceral symptoms in some cases are similar to the acute intermittent porphyria and photosensitivity rarely occurs.[76] In several instances, no clinical symptoms appear at all. However, the disease may be provoked by drugs or other chemicals which induce aminolevulinic acid synthetase in the liver.[208,240] The major laboratory finding is an increased fecal coproporphyrin excretion. Additionally, urinary levels of δ-aminolevulinic acid, porphobilinogen, and coproporphyrin are elevated. In remission the only biochemical sign of the disease is increased fecal coproporphyrin. This indicates that the major deficiency lies in the activity of coproporphyrin dehydrogenase.

Hereditary coproporphria resembles acute intermittent porphyria with mild photosensitivity. Acute attacks develop through the action of drugs. This condition is inherited and the major biochemical abnormality is an increased fecal coproporphyrin. During the acute phase various precursors are present in the urine.

C. ERYTHROPOIETIC DISORDERS OF PORPHYRIN SYNTHESIS

Erythropoietic porphyrias are very rare; the defect is in the red blood cell related to a genetically determined abnormality in porphyrin synthesis. Congenital erythropoietic porphyria is a recessive disease characterized by severe photosensitivity, which starts at birth or soon after, and persists throughout life. It leads sometimes to very severe scarring and deformities. Large quantities of porphyrins are deposited in the bones, teeth, and skin, and they become pigmented showing a characteristic red fluorescence in ultraviolet light. Hemolysis often occurs. This form of porphyria is not accompanied by lesions of the abdomen or nervous system.

The enzyme abnormality is present in the conversion of porphobilinogen to Type I and III porphyrins in the bone marrow. This abnormality is associated with a deficiency or absence of uroporphyrin isomerase.[104,219] Normally the synthesis is shifted to the dominant formation of Type III porphyrins, which are used in heme synthesis. In congenital porphyria, since uroporphyrin isomerase is reduced, the amount of Type I porphyrin produced is very great, 100 mg or more per day. The Type I porphyrins are useless for the synthesis of the prosthetic groups; by not being degraded to bile pigments, they are excreted or deposited in the body. Therefore, pigmentation is a well recognized feature of the disease. In addition, photosensitivity of the skin due to porphyrins leads to various skin injuries. Compensatory mechanisms may allow the formation of normal heme, but uroporphyrin I and coproporphyrin I are markedly increased. The increase of uroporphyrin in the red cells causes hemolysis due to photosensitivity. The enhanced rate of hemolysis is compensated by an increased heme synthesis which further aggravates the condition through an increased production of Type I porphyrins as byproducts of the disease mechanism.

Erythropoietic protoporphyria is characterized by a dominant inheritance. A great excess of protoporphyrins is excreted in the feces, often 10 mg or more per day. The urine usually contains little protoporphyrins, but during periods of impaired liver function, the plasma levels increase together with excess amounts of porphyrin excreted in the urine. Increased photosensitivity occurs from childhood onwards. The concentrations of free protoporphyrin and coproporphyrin are markedly raised in red blood cells from 50 μg/dl to 2 mg/dl or more of protoporphyrin and from 2.5 μg/dl to 400 to 500 μg/dl of coproporphyrin.

D. DRUG-INDUCED PORPHYRIA

Several substances cause episodes of toxic porphyria by inducing abnormalities in porphyrin biosynthesis and excretion. This phenomenon is apparently benign and originates in

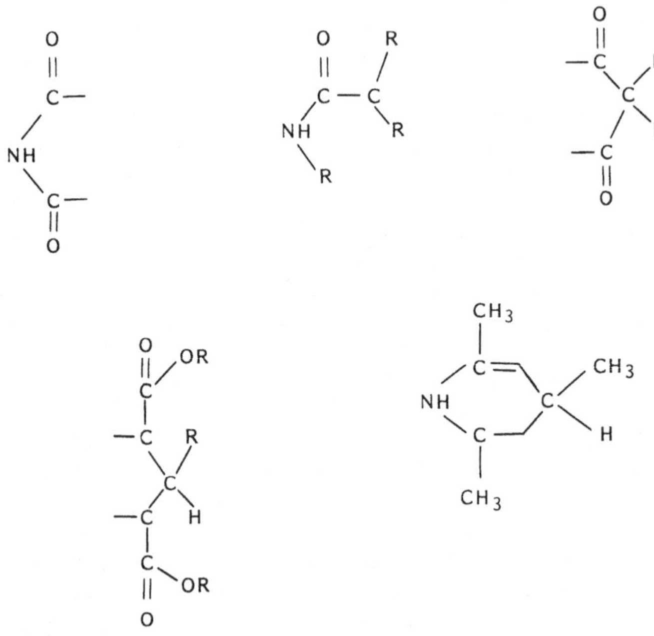

FIGURE 10.   Chemical structures associated with the induction of porphyria.[212,215,385]

the liver.[52,122,207] Major biochemical changes of the drug-induced porphyria are the excretion of uroporphyrin and coproporphyrin, mainly Type III, and porphyrins with 5, 6, and 7 carboxyl groups. Sometimes δ-aminolevulinic acid excretion is also elevated. Coproporphyrin and uroporphyrin are increased in the liver. Abdominal pains and neurological signs are the major clinical symptoms in very severe cases.

Many drugs are involved casually in this condition: barbiturates, halogenated insecticides, steroids, alcohol, collidin, allylisopropylacetamide, theophyllin, griseofulvin, and others. In barbiturates, characteristic chemical groups are associated with the induction (Figure 10). The most potent porphyria-inducing steroids are 5β-steroids, 5β-androstane (C19), and 5β-pregnane (C21).[301] The wide structural variety of chemicals which modify the hepatic formation of porphyrins suggests that either they act on different sites or that some nonspecific receptor provides a common site of action. Lead poisoning is also a condition resulting in porphyria. The action of lead is probably related to inhibition of ferrochelatase activity, which requires glutathione. The enzyme is inactivated by lead through binding to the sulfhydryl groups.

Animal experiments have established that in drug-induced porphyria the only common features clearly seen are liver hypertrophy and an effect on hepatic drug metabolism associated with increased microsomal phospholipids. The rate of cytochrome P-450 formation is, however, decreased. In chronic administration of many drugs, δ-aminolevulinic acid synthetase activity is increased not only in the mitochondria, but in the microsomes and soluble fraction.[370,412,457] These events can be explained by postulating that the porphyria-inducing substances cause a transient increase in microsomal enzyme activity. Subsequently, they may damage the microsomal structure, resulting in more labile heme pools sensitive to peroxidation. In normal hepatocytes more than half the heme molecules produced are used in the synthesis of cytochrome P-450. The enhanced although transient turnover of cytochrome P-450, following the administration of porphyria-inducing drugs, may divert heme from its role as repressor of δ-aminolevulinic acid synthetase, resulting in increased enzyme synthesis and the subsequent rise of intermediates. The action of steroids may be related to their effect on lysosomes (Figure 11).

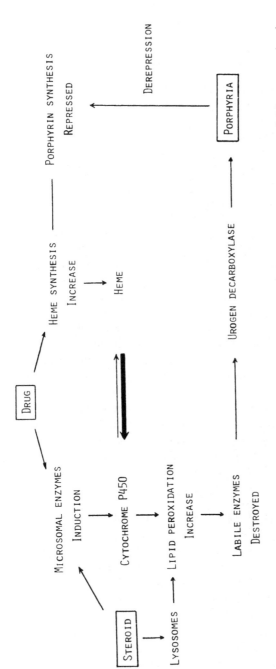

FIGURE 11. Possible mechanism of the action of drugs and steroids on porphyrin synthesis. In the sequence of events, a link between continued stimulation of drug metabolizing enzymes, a shift between heme and cytochrome P-450, and increased lipid peroxidation are related to the increased porphyrin accumulation. The enzyme defects show certain similarities to porphyria cutanea tarda reflecting a similar mechanism of the biochemical lesion.[141,142,459]

E. EFFECT OF CARBOHYDRATES

Diet has marked effects on the clinical symptoms and levels of porphyrin precursors in both acute intermittent and variegata porphyria. Drug-induced porphyria in experimental animals can be inhibited by concurrent sucrose feeding. In many patients, the abdominal pain and confused mental state have cleared up within hours of high carbohydrate administration. In some instances, the lack of response was related to the lack of glucose going into the liver to an acceptable extent. The glucose remains in the blood compartment indicating a diabetic-like response resembling that seen in adult-onset diabetes.

The mechanism of the glucose effect has not been established. It may reflect a catabolite repression. Since there is no catabolite common in the pathways between glucose metabolism and heme synthesis, the catabolic repression is probably linked with cyclic AMP. The effect of glucose in porphyria is remarkably similar to the effect of glucose on the synthesis of cyclic AMP. The related δ-aminolevulinic acid synthetase formation is lowered by glucose because it represses the intracellular levels of cyclic AMP. Consequently, reduced levels of cyclic AMP reduce the rate of enzyme synthesis. The relationship of this effect to the disappearance of the neurological symptoms is not clear.

F. ACTIONS OF DRUGS

At present the treatment of all forms of porphyria can only be symptomatic. Treatments include the reduction of photosensitivity by avoiding sunlight, sunscreens, and antibiotic treatment of infected lesions. The hepatic involvement can be moderated by abstaining from alcohol, drugs (particularly barbiturates), estrogens, and oral contraceptives.

Knowledge of the molecular mechanism in porphyria makes it possible to attempt influencing the frequency of episodes. One such possibility is the alteration of the coenzyme level. In acute intermittent porphyria where δ-aminolevulinic acid synthesis is disturbed, it would be logical to diminish the pyridoxine-dependent synthesis of this intermediate by using pyridoxine antagonists. Several substances have been tested, and deoxypyridoxine has been applied successfully. A structurally unrelated pyridoxine antagonist, penicillamine causes no improvement in the neurological symptoms and is associated with no clinical or biochemical changes. Another alternative lies in the inhibition of increased enzyme activity. Chlorpromazine and other drugs block the activity of several enzymes and therefore reduce the excess δ-aminolevulinic acid and porphobilinogen production and excretion. However, on returning to the proper feeding regime, porphyria reoccurs. Chloroquine has also been reported to have a beneficial effect on cutaneous hepatic porphyria, but this compound produces liver dysfunction, and this certainly argues against its use.

V. DISEASES OF HEPATIC SECRETORY FUNCTION

A. BILE FORMATION

Our present knowledge of the mechanism of bile secretion is still limited due to the wide anatomic variations of the biliary tract and marked differences in bile composition and flow.[168,545] Nevertheless, some diseases show causal relationship with the loss of hepatic secretory function.[297] Jaundice is a manifestation of hepatic disease due to the failure of bile secretory activity. Changes in bile secretion and composition as caused by liver injury produce various types of jaundice. These changes are also important in the pathogenesis of gallstones.

There is a distinction between the formation of bile and the secretion of other substances in the bile. Bile production is independent of the hydrostatic pressure of the blood perfusing the liver and is only related to the various chemical processes providing energy for bile secretion. Bile acids play a primary role in this process.

In a man, about 700 to 1200 ml of bile is excreted daily, and the normal bile contains between 8 to 28 g/dl of total solids. The major constituents are bile acids (53 to 71%) and lipids (23 to 29%), while other components include bile pigments, electrolytes, and proteins comprising less than 15%. Some constituents, such as bilirubin, are actively secreted against a concentration gradient occurring in the bile at a higher level then in the plasma. Other components are present at approximately the same levels such as electrolytes. The biliary salt concentration varies, and in conditions where the amounts of chloride and bicarbonate are low, bile salt anions are dominant. Human gall bladder bile is virtually a pure bile salt solution. The majority of bile salts is secreted in the bile. Cholic and chenodeoxycholic acids are the major bile acids and form micellar solutions in bile and intestinal contents. These compounds are synthetized by the degradation of cholesterol via a β- and ω-oxidation associated with the hepatic microsomal hydroxylating enzyme system (Figure 12.)[245] The onset of drug-induced cholestasis underlines the importance of this biotransformation and the participation of the drug metabolizing enzyme system in bile acid synthesis.[110,235,553] Bile acids are further altered by conjugation either with glycine or taurine. In the bile, glycine conjugates are predominantly present and the ratio of glycine to taurine conjugated bile acids is about 3:1. The daily production of bile acids is about 350 mg and the half-life is 3 d. The synthesis is homeostatically controlled by the concentration of bile acids in the portal blood.

Bile acids are the main end-products of cholesterol metabolism (Figure 12); significant amounts are converted to coprosterol in the stool, and smaller amounts are used to the production of steroid hormones (Figure 13). The majority of bile acids is eliminated in the feces and small amounts, about 5%, are excreted in the urine. The fecal bile acid fraction represents a complex mixture of bile acids derived from the liver and of metabolites produced by the gut flora. The bile acid composition depends upon the intestinal flora and is influenced by changes brought about by diet, antibiotics, or other drugs. Some of these bile acids are reabsorbed from the distal portion of the small intestines and processed again in the liver. During enterohepatic circulation of the bile, primary metabolites are modified by intestinal microorganisms in the cecum and colon (Figure 14). Starting with the removal of the 7α-hydroxyl group, hydrolysis yields free bile acids, mainly deoxycholic and lithocholic acids. These components are then reabsorbed from the gut in various amounts. Deoxycholic acid constitutes about 20% of bile acids in human bile, while lithocholic acid is poorly reabsorbed under normal circumstances, because it is trapped intracellularly in bacteria or firmly bound to water-insoluble structures.

The bile salts are surface active agents, and essentially lipophilic molecules with strongly polar side chains represented by the carboxyl or sulfonate groups, depending on whether they are conjugated with glycine or taurine. At high concentrations, bile salts form poly-molecular aggregates termed micelles. The hydroxyl group of the steroid nucleus is essential for the stability of bile salt micelles. Thus when hepatic hydroxylating activity is disturbed, inadequate micelle formation may be a contributing factor to the stagnation of bile. With the addition of lecithin or triglycerides containing unsaturated fatty acids and cholesterol, very stable micelles are formed. Altogether, large polyanionic aggregates are produced; however, the exact size, arrangement, and water content is uncertain. There is considerable attraction of cations forming an outer layer of positive charges around the negatively charged aggregates. This structural arrangement is probably the major reason that the solubilizing capacity of micelles for any cell component greatly exceeds that of pure bile salt solutions.

B. FAT ABSORPTION

Bile salt-lecithin-cholesterol micelles are secreted into the intestines during the digestion of fats. Fat absorption is associated with partition of fat soluble materials into the micellar and the oil phase. The micelles undergo some changes; part of the fatty acids in lecithin is cleaved by pancreatic phospholipase and thus lysolecithin, a water-soluble compound is formed. The fatty acids thus released are then readily absorbed into the intestinal wall by the micelles, while di- and triglycerides remain emulsified in the oil phase.[56,258,260] Subse-

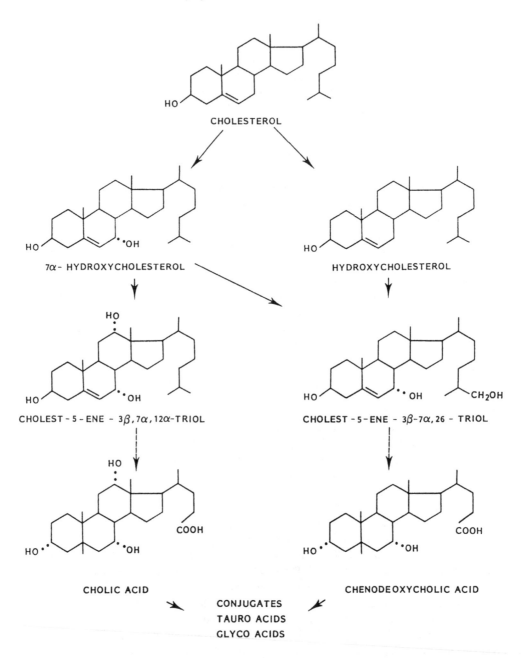

FIGURE 12. Mechanism of bile acid synthesis in the liver. Cholesterol is converted to hydroxy intermediates and bile acids by an enzyme system bound to the endoplasmic reticulum. Some steps may be connected with β- and ω-oxidation as CoA derivatives. The final step leads to glycine and taurin conjugates. In man, the ratio of glyco:tauro-bile acids is about 3:1.

quently, when micelles solubilize the monoglycerides and fatty acids, these are also incorporated into the micelle complex structure. Bile salt-monoglyceride-fatty acid micelles are formed which in turn can further dissolve more cholesterol and fat-soluble vitamins in the hydrophobic regions.

An association exists between the micelles and microvilli. There is a direct action of bile salts on the intestinal wall, but the exact mechanism has not yet been established. The action of micelles on the intestinal mucosa resides in the reconstitution of triglycerides. It

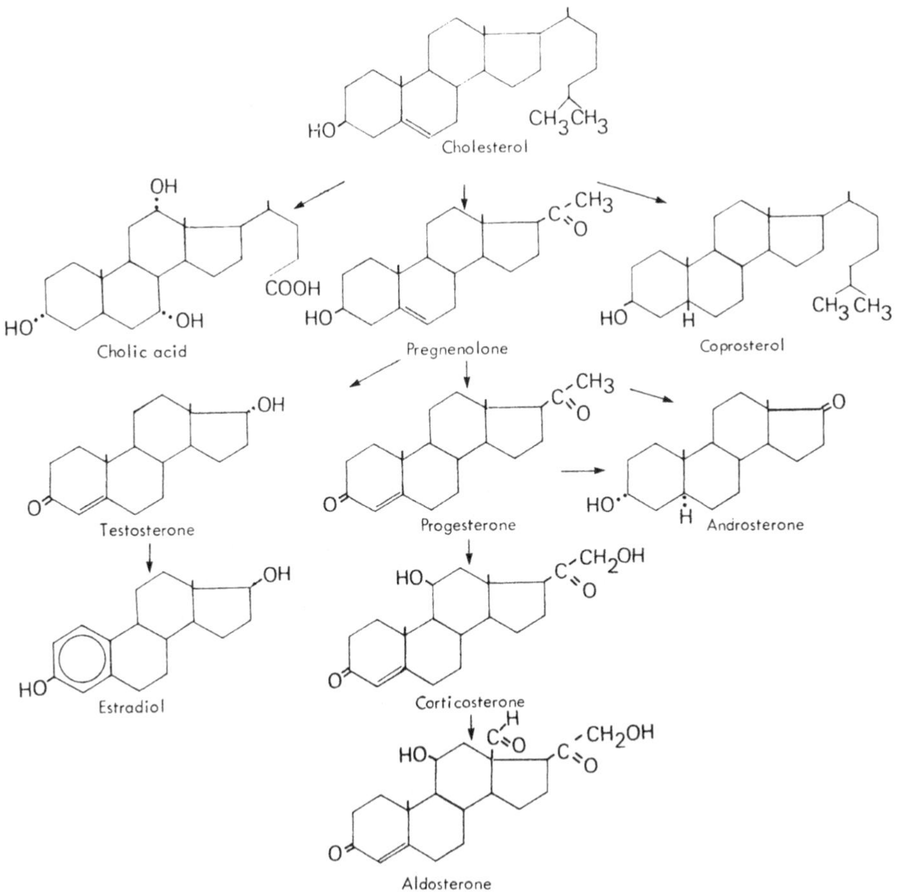

FIGURE 13.   Transformation of cholesterol into various steroid derivatives. The majority is converted to bile acids or fecal sterols and eliminated. Fragment of total cholesterol is used in the synthesis of essential hormonal steroids.

has been suggested that bile salts stimulate the ability of the mucosa to esterify fatty acids. In particular, taurocholate exerts some control on the amount of fatty acids esterified and transported and also influences the ultimate route of absorbed fat and fat soluble components. It is probable that under physiological conditions the bile salt micelle is the final common path in the uptake of dietary fat and other water-insoluble molecules. Abnormalities in the production of micelles are related to diseases in the absorption of fats and fat-soluble components. A compensatory mechanism may exist because some fat can be absorbed even in the absence of bile.

C. GALLSTONE FORMATION

Gallstones are produced when losses occur in the solvent phase of the bile solution. This leads to the alteration of the chemical composition which is the most important factor in the pathogenesis of cholelithiasis. The changes in chemical constitution cause an impairment in micellar solubilization that is considered the primary cause of gallstone formation. Investigations on the chemical composition of bile in a group of patients with gallstones revealed low total bile acid and lecithin concentration, low tri:dihydroxy acid and glycine:taurine conjugation ratio. There is also a significant increase in calcium concentration. Under these circumstances, cholesterol approaches a saturation level and at this unbalanced stage, factors such as stasis or gallbladder infection may precipitate gallstone formation.

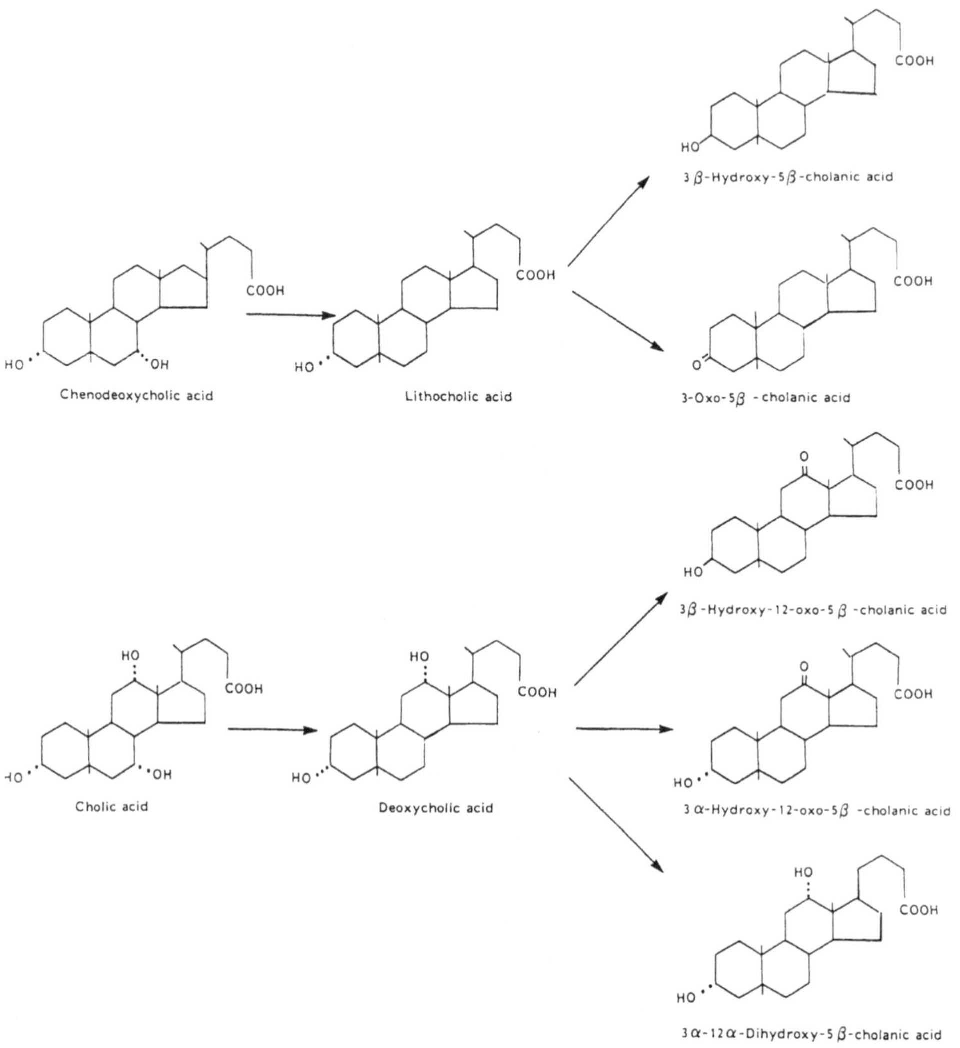

FIGURE 14.   Mechanism of bile acid degradation in the feces. The main bile acids in human feces are lithocholic, 3β-hydroxy-12-oxo-5β-cholanic, and 3β, 12-dihydroxy-5β cholanic acid. Minor components are deoxycholic and 3-oxo-5β cholanic acid.

Once the nucleus is formed, additional layers readily deposit. Various bacterial infections such as *Escherichia coli, Salmonella typhi,* and *Streptococcus* are found to be further possible contributing factors.

Biliary lipids contain mostly phospholipids and cholesterol. Cholesterol esters, triglycerides, and free fatty acids are present only in trace amounts.[419] Lecithin accounts for more than 80% of bile phospholipids, cholesterol constitutes only about 4% of the solids. Cholesterol concentration in liver bile is 120 to 220 mg/dl; in gallbladder bile, it is 400 to 800 mg/dl. In the latter, cholesterol is mainly present as an unstable complex held in micellar solution by phospholipids and bile salts, primarily dihydroxycholic acid conjugates. Changes in the production and distribution of these substances lead to cholelithiasis.

Most gallstones consist of cholesterol monohydrate crystals combined with the calcium salt of bilirubin or sometimes only contain calcium bilirubinate.[49,71,84,259] Dietary manipulations in animal experiments have shown that gallstones are formed when the ratio of bile salts to cholesterol is altered. These conditions decrease the micellar solubility of cholesterol and increase the concentration of unbound calcium and bilirubin.

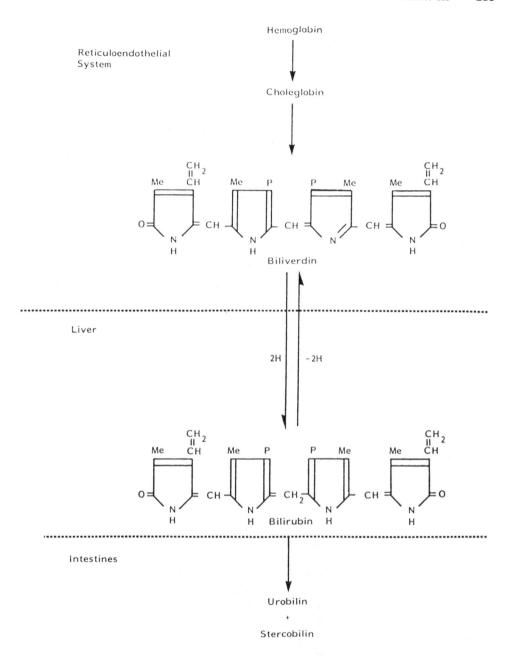

FIGURE 15. Mechanism of hemoglobin degradation. Hemoglobin is converted to choleglobin (verdohemo-globin) in the reticuloendothelial system. This green iron-globin-containing complex is further metabolized to biliverdin with the loss of iron and protein. From the plasma, the circulating ferrous ions are concentrated in the iron stores of the liver and globin is reutilized in the amino acid pool. By hydrogenation, biliverdin is converted to bilirubin and some minor products.

VI. ABNORMALITIES IN BILIRUBIN METABOLISM

A. HEMOGLOBIN DEGRADATION

From the breakdown of hemoglobin, the tetrapyrrole derivative, bilirubin, is formed and secreted by the liver into the gut.[594] The hemoglobin of aged or damaged red blood cells is metabolized to bilirubin by a complex series of reactions (Figure 15). The average life of the red blood cell is 120 d, and about 6 g of hemoglobin is released each day from the disintegration of aged cells. The reticuloendothelial system, especially the cells in the spleen, liver, and bone marrow, destroy the erythrocytes by phagocytosis and then convert the released hemoglobin into bilirubin.[218,333,339]

The catabolism of hemoglobin to bilirubin proceeds rapidly. Whereas the basic major pathway of hemoglobin breakdown is known, all of the intermediate steps have not yet been established. Fatty acids may exert a control over bilirubin levels in the blood.[99] During this process, bile pigments are the only products eliminated from the body.[144,473] Part of the iron is stored locally as hemosiderin in the endothelial cells, while the rest is transported to other tissues, mainly to the liver by transfer where it is stored as ferritin. The globin molecule enters the body protein pool and is used again for the resynthesis of hemoglobin.

In the mechanism of hemoglobin breakdown to bilirubin, several intermediates have been suggested (Figure 16). Hematin is considered to be a normal intermediary. In intravascular hemolysis such as hematin icterus, the production of hematin is increased without bilirubin elevation. Lack of hyperbilirubinemia suggests a shift in the normal metabolism to the accumulation of hematin. Animal experiments using labeled hemin are in agreement with the formation of this intermediate. The formation of choleglobin or verdohemoglobin, a green iron-containing protein complex, has also been proposed. By successive oxidation, the α-methene bridge is replaced by an ether bond. The next step leads to loss of iron and protein, and the biliverdin formed is reduced to bilirubin. The presence of biliverdin reductase and heme-α-methenyl oxygenase in the liver and kidney provides evidence for the existence of this pathway. Verdoglobinuria occurs in *Pseudomonas* septicemia, indicating that the bacterial toxin interferes with the complete metabolism of hemoglobin, resulting in the accumulation of verdoglobin.[418,533]

Approximately 300 mg of bilirubin is produced daily from the breakdown of hemoglobin. Minor amounts are synthetized directly and bound to albumin in the liver and bone marrow. Bilirubin is transported in the blood from the reticuloendothelial system to the liver. At the surface of the liver cell it is released from albumin and internalized. Within the cell, bilirubin is attached to ligandin and carried to the endoplasmic reticulum, where it is conjugated with glucuronic acid. The conjugated bilirubin is excreted into the intestines via the bile. Further conversion of bilirubin in the large intestines into urobilinogen, to urobilin and stercobilinogen, and then to stercobilin, is mainly bacterial. Some of these bile pigments are reabsorbed from the gut and again taken up by the liver. About 90 to 350 mg of urobilin is excreted daily in the feces and less than 4 mg is eliminated by the kidney (Figure 17).

B. DIRECT BILIRUBIN SYNTHESIS

Minor amounts of bilirubin are derived from direct synthesis and from the degradation of a number of nonhemoglobin tetrapyrrole compounds such as myoglobin and cytochromes. Using labeled precursor of heme synthesis, 15 *N*-glycine, most of the label appeared in fecal stercobilin at the end of the normal 120 d life of the erythrocytes.[220,363] Moreover, two stercobilin components were also present at earlier intervals, at 10 d and between 20 to 100 d after isotope administration. This indicates the contribution of other hemes to the total bile pigment or the *de novo* synthesis of bilirubin. The amount of stercobilins is twice as much in newborns as compared with adults, and it is highly elevated in various disorders of erythrocyte formation such as pernicious anemia, thalassemia minor and erythropoietic porphyria. In these diseases, the early components take up about 80% of the total excreted stercobilin as compared with 10% of the total in normals. In contrast, the extent of the labeling in the circulating hemoglobin, protoporphyrin, and breakdown products is greatly reduced. These disorders are related to the ineffective production of red blood cells, or dyserythropoiesis.[221] In these circumstances, young cells appear in the circulation which are rapidly destroyed and their metabolites probably contribute to the early pigment. In man, when bone marrow activity is stimulated by bleeding, the initial peak is increased. Investigations of a family showing enhanced bile pigment production, but normal erythrocyte

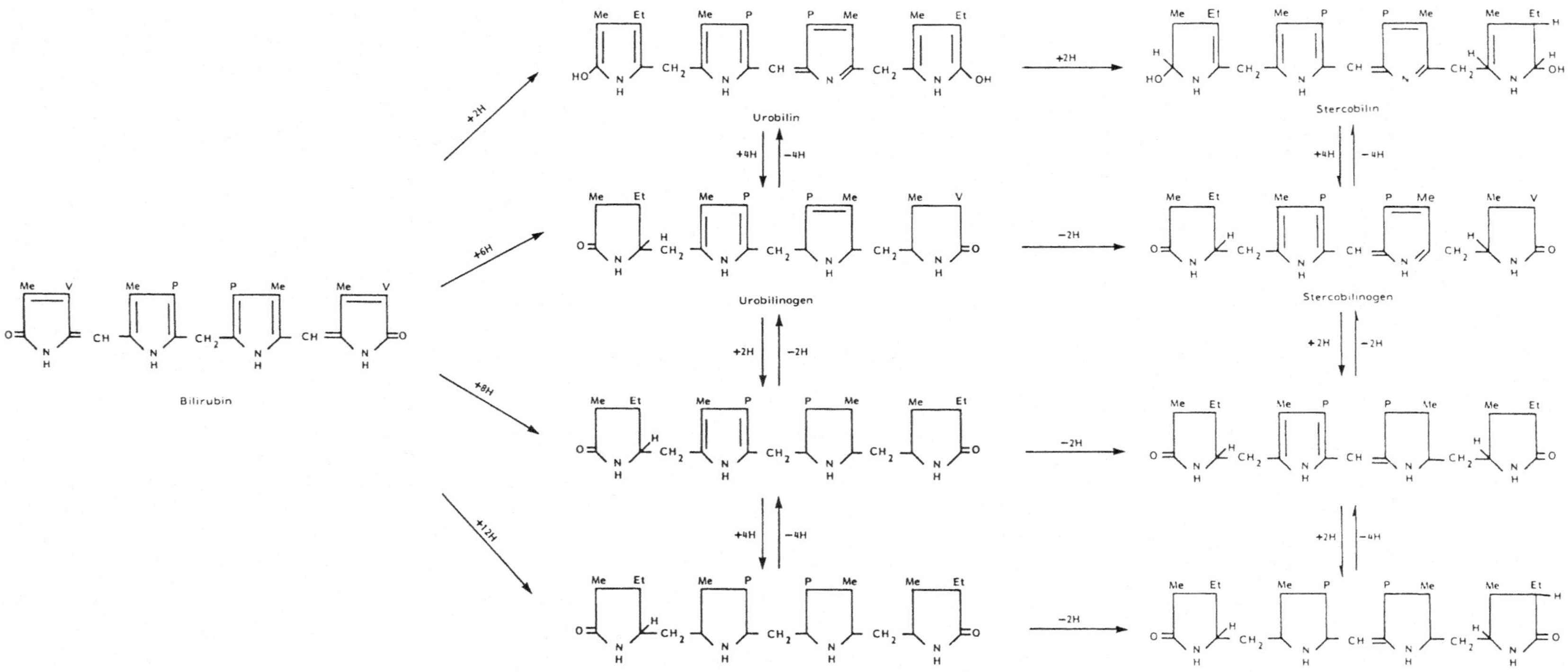

FIGURE 16. Transformation of bilirubin to various urobilins by reductive reactions.

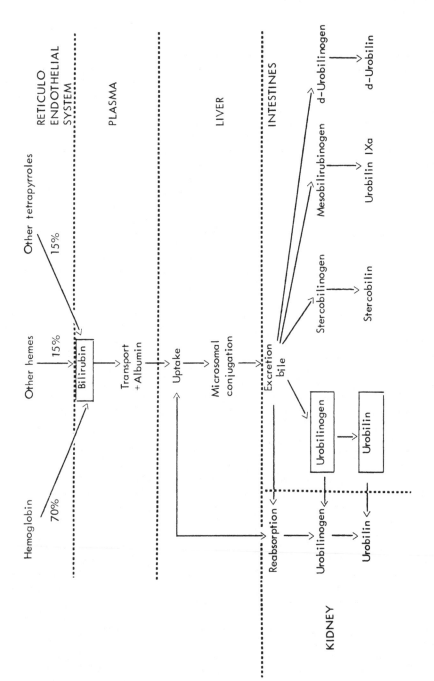

FIGURE 17.   Various routes of bilirubin excretion. These include plasma transport, hepatic metabolism, reabsorption by enterohepatic circulation, and elimination in the urine and feces. The total production of bilirubin, daily 300 mg, is mainly excreted as urobilinogen, daily 90 to 350 mg.

formation and breakdown, revealed a large increase of the early fecal stercobilin component. In a patient suffering from the condition of idiopathic dyserythropoietic jaundice, an early labeling of fecal urobilin was apparent with low incorporation rate in hemoglobin proto-porphyrin. In general, the more ineffective the erythrocyte formation, the more marked is the disproportion between the increase of early labeled component and the decrease of bile pigment derived from the circulating hemoglobin. This impairment indicates a shift away from the normal erythrocyte toward earlier pathways. This concept is supported by the study of a patient with aplastic anemia. The labeled glycine was not incorporated into the he-moglobin of the circulating red blood cells, although the rate of incorporation into fecal stercobilin was normal or increased, suggesting that the early bile pigment originated outside the bone marrow.

C. BILIRUBIN TRANSPORT AND UPTAKE

Normal levels of bilirubin in the serum are between 0.2 and 0.8 mg/dl. The bilirubin level is determined by the relative rate at which bile pigments enter or leave the circulation. Bilirubin is tightly bound to albumin, 2 mol of pigment to each protein molecule, corre-sponding to the normal amount of unconjugated bilirubin in the serum of adults.[429,591] Minor amounts are found in globulin fractions. The excess bilirubin is rapidly metabolized, first to yellow oxidation products which are still partly associated with albumin, then further to colorless derivatives which bind preferably to globulins. The bilirubin phenolic hydroxyl groups and the protein amino groups play a part in the bond between the pigment and albumin. Probably, lysine residues provide the free amino groups. If these lysin residues are blocked by reactions with methylisourea, the binding capacity of the albumin is consid-erably reduced. Other properties of the albumin molecule are also important since other proteins with high lysine content, for example, γ-globulin, show no affinity to bilirubin. Bilirubin diglucuronide is also bound to serum albumin. There are four absorption sites for the conjugate per albumin molecule. Similarly to free bilirubin, an interaction between hydroxyl and amino groups takes place in the binding of bilirubin diglucuronate.[68, 227]

During uptake of the pigment by the liver cell, the bilirubin-albumin complex molecules are first concentrated at the surface of the membranes. After passing into the cell, the bilirubin is separated from albumin inside the membrane with the subsequent formation of glucuronides in the microsomal region. These molecules move across the cell and are concentrated at the canalicular membrane before they are excreted into the bile. The uni-directional nature of this process is essential (Figure 18). Any disturbance of this mechanism produces leaks from the bile canaliculi back into the sinusoids, resulting in jaundice. From the bile canaliculi network, the bile is transported to the common bile duct and then to the gallbladder where it is concentrated and emptied into the duodenum. The bilirubin glucu-ronide is carried to the large intestine and converted to urobilinogen under the influence of reducing enzymes of chronic bacteria. Most of this urobilinogen is oxidized to urobilin and finally excreted into the stool. The remainder is carried back to the liver by the portal vein and may either be converted to bilirubin glucuronides by the liver cells or excreted into the bile canaliculi unchanged. The glucuronides, as well as any unchanged urobilinogen and urobilin, are carried back to the intestine by the bile, and thus the enterohepatic circulation is completed (Figure 19).

In the presence of hepatic dysfunction or partial biliary obstruction, urobilinogen can be diverted from the bile and excreted in the urine. The enterohepatic circulation is impaired and elevated urobilinogen and urobilin appear in the urine of patients with hepatitis and other forms of primary liver damage unless obstructive jaundice interferes with bilirubin transport. These pigments are present after severe hemolytic processes associated with ex-cessive heme degradation or after liver poisoning with hepatotoxins. Urobilinuria also occurs in diseases connected with secondary liver damage, such as congestive heart failure. In the

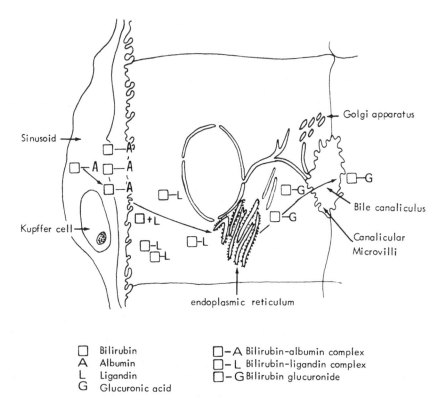

□	Bilirubin	□–A Bilirubin-albumin complex
A	Albumin	□–L Bilirubin-ligandin complex
L	Ligandin	□–G Bilirubin glucuronide
G	Glucuronic acid	

FIGURE 18.   Bilirubin transport through the liver cell. In the plasma, bilirubin is bound to albumin and this complex molecule enters the cell by the sinusoids, Within the cell the bilirubin-albumin association breaks off, the intracellular bilirubin becomes bound to ligandin, and it is transported to the microsomal region. There bilirubin is conjugated with glucuronide by the enzyme UDP-glucuronyl transferase and the conjugate is eliminated through the bile canaliculi.

presence of a liver disease, reexcretion of these pigments is inhibited, so urobilinogen passes to the kidney and it is excreted. If there is a bacterial invasion in the small intestine, urobilinogenuria may follow. This is due to increased chromogen absorption as well as to diminished hepatobiliary function. In contrast, broad-spectrum antibiotics suppress the function of the intestinal flora and prevent the transformation of bilirubin to urobilinogen, thereby eliminating urobilinogen from the urine.

The small amount of urobilinogen that is not taken up by the liver cells is transported to the kidney and excreted in the urine. On the other hand, unconjugated bilirubin is not eliminated by the kidney and is absent in the urine while conjugated bilirubin is only excreted by the kidney tubules if present in abnormal concentrations.

D. BILIRUBIN CONJUGATION

The synthesis of the mono- and diglucuronides occurs mainly in the liver catalyzed by the microsomal enzyme uridine 5′-diphosphate glucuronyltransferase (UDPGT).[135,136,276] Conjugation is a prerequisite for the excretion of bilirubin into the bile and may itself be the limiting factor in transport, since conjugated bilirubin is excreted in the bile more rapidly than the unconjugated pigment. Conjugate formation occurs in kidney, intestines, lung, and skin. The renal cortex and the gastrointestinal mucosa contain UDPGT and a microsomal nicotinamide adenine dinucleotide-dependent oxidative enzyme which catalyzes bilirubin conjugation in a manner similar to hepatic microsomes. In the liver of the embryo and newborn, UDPGT levels are very low. However, in the gastrointestinal tract in the early

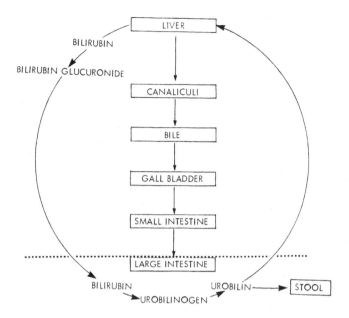

FIGURE 19.   Enterohepatic circulation. Bilirubin conjugates are excreted from the liver via canaliculi into the bile and through the gall bladder into the intestines. In the intestines, two processes are involved: catabolism by enzymes leading to the release of free bilirubin and the production of several derivatives. The second process is the reabsorption of bilirubin and derivatives back into the liver. Bilirubin glucuronides are hydrolyzed at alkaline pH of the intestinal content by β-glucuronidase derived from the liver, intestinal epithelial cells, and intestinal bacteria. The various catabolic processes include hydrolysis, reduction, and oxidation.[143]

fetal period this enzyme is present at adult levels. The inadequate synthesis of bilirubin conjugates in the human neonatal liver is responsible for the physiologic jaundice of the newborn. In contrast, various glucuronides, including glucuronides of injected foreign substances, are formed in the gastrointestinal tract, so this site may be important in the detoxication mechanism of the neonate.[129] The regulation of glucuronide formation depends on many factors[10,223,442] (Figure 20).

The relative amount of conjugated and unconjugated bilirubin can be used for the differential diagnosis of various liver diseases. Early investigations described a test involving the coupling of bilirubin with diazotized sulfanilic acid in the presence of alcohol. In the serum of patients with hemolytic jaundice, this reaction gave a red color. Van der Bergh found that alcohol is not necessary in estimating bilirubin in the serum of patients with obstructive jaundice. These two types of reactions are known as indirect and direct bilirubin indicating that the former reaction required alcohol, but the latter did not. The difference between the two measurements represents the relative amounts of bilirubin conjugates (direct) and nonconjugated bilirubin (indirect) present in the serum of jaundiced patients.

The direct reacting pigment can be separated into two components.[41,43,89,444] When bilirubin obtained from serum is passed through a column containing silicon-treated Kieselguhr, three different bands are distinguished on reverse phase chromatography. The diazo products from each band reveal only two separate compounds. Subsequent analysis established that Pigment I is the monoglucuronide and Pigment II is the diglucuronide of bilirubin (Figure 21).

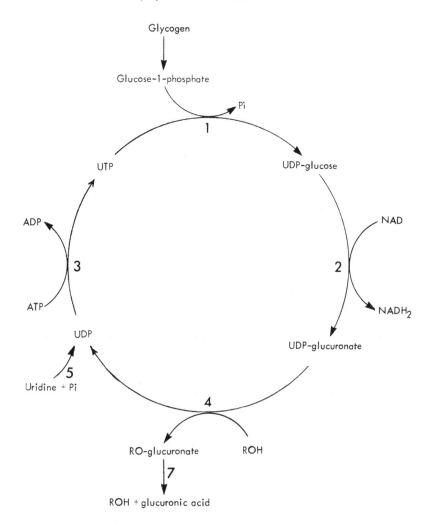

FIGURE 20.   Regulation of glucuronide formation. Carbohydrate, oxygen, and energy are required to operate this cycle. It is catalyzed by enzymes located in the cytoplasm, such as glucose 1-phosphate uridyltransferase (1), uridyldiphosphoglucose dehydrogenase (2), and nucleoside diphosphate kinase (3), or bound to the endoplasmic reticulum, such as uridine-diphosphate glucuronyltransferase (4) and nucleoside diphosphatase (5). The level of uridine triphosphate is dependent on the amount of adenosine triphosphate (6) and on the activity of nucleoside diphosphate kinase (3). The maintenance of uridinediphosphate, glucose 1-phosphate from glycogen by the glycolytic pathway by β-glucuronidase (7) are also regulatory valves of this cycle.

VII. JAUNDICE

Abnormalities in the hepatic processing of bilirubin usually result in jaundice, a condition characterized by an increase of bilirubin in the blood and brownish-yellow pigmentation of the skin, sclera, and mucous membranes.[542] Jaundice may be associated with (1) an over-production of bilirubin due to increased hemolysis, (2) impairment of the shunt mechanism which controls the utilization of glycine for the synthesis of either heme or bilirubin directly, (3) defects of uptake or retention of the unconjugated bilirubin in the hepatocyte, (4) defect in detoxication or regurgitation of conjugated bilirubin, and (5) failure of excretion from the liver cell into bile or from the bile into the intestine due to various lesions (Figure 22). Under normal conditions, the serum bilirubin concentration is about 1 mg/dl, but apparently

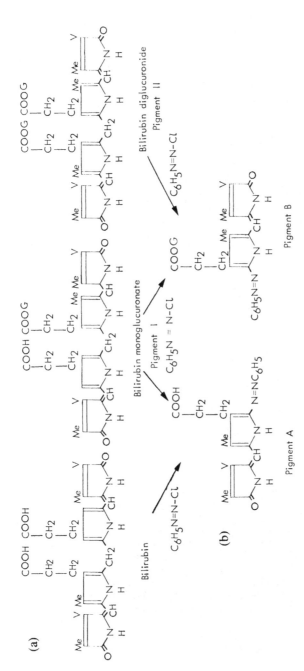

FIGURE 21. Separation of bilirubin and conjugates by column chromatography and diazo derivatives. Serum bilirubin is separated into three different bands (a). One band corresponds to bilirubin, the other two bands are named Pigment I and II. Diazotation of these bands only produced two separate compounds (b). This reaction indicates a cleavage of the bilirubin skeleton into two parts in the middle, and the subsequent formation of the diazo derivatives of the free acid, Pigment A, or the glucuronic ester containing moiety, Pigment B.

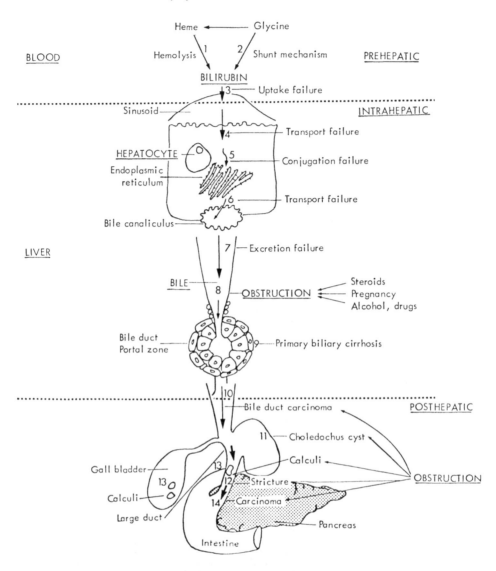

FIGURE 22. Diseases related to defects in bilirubin transport or metabolism in the liver cell. The various causes of jaundice may be prehepatic due to over production of bilirubin by overt hemolysis (1), or defect of the shunt mechanism and shunt bilirubinemia (2). Intrahepatic causes are connected with failure of uptake (3) and transport through the sinusoids (4) associated with inadequate binding to albumin such as Gilbert disease, conjugation failure (5) related to the deficiency of UDP-glucuronyl transferase activity of the endoplasmic reticulum characterized by the retention of unconjugated bilirubin such as neonatal jaundice or Crigler-Najjar disease, failure of conjugated transport into bile canaliculi (6) such as Dubin-Johnson disease, or failure of excretion into the bile (7). Some steroids can produce a block in the canaliculi associated with inflammation. The two latter causes are linked with regurgitation of bilirubin by the liver. Similarly, periductular inflammation induced by promazine and other drugs, alcoholic cholestasis and obstructive jaundice of pregnancy are associated with lesions in the bile duct (8). Primary biliary cirrhosis affects the portal zone (9). Extrahepatic causes are connected with obstruction of the large duct, including bile duct carcinoma (10), choleduchus cyst (11) stricture (12), calculi (13) and ascaris infection in the duct or in the gall bladder, and pancreatic and ampullary carcinoma (14).

normal levels may reach 2 to 3 mg/dl. Whereas no bilirubin is excreted in the urine, 0.5 to 4.0 mg urobilinogen is eliminated daily. In disease, the serum concentration is raised and invariably bilirubin is excreted; urobilinogen can be increased, decreased, or even be absent from the stool. Several mechanisms can lead to jaundice (Table 1), and various types can be distinguished relative to the localization of the defect (Table 2).

TABLE 1
Defects in Bilirubin Metabolism Leading to Jaundice

Production	Impairment
Excessive	Uptake
Decreased erythrocyte half-life	Benign hyperbilirubinemia
Congenital	Albumin level low
Acquired	Carrier — ligandin level low
Increased bilirubin level	Metabolic clearance impaired
Increased synthesis	Secondary to cholestasis
Decreased incorporation	Feedback inhibition
Into heme	Conjugation
	Temporary
	Immature neonatal enzymes
	Lucey-Driscoll syndrome
	Nursing, inhibitor in milk
	Partial, relatively benign
	Complete
	Total enzyme absence
	Excretion
	Transport defect
	Accumulation of conjugates
	Rotor syndrome
	Dubin-Johnson syndrome
	Intrahepatic elimination
	Hepatitis
	Canaliculi obstruction
	Enlarged regenerating cells
	Cholangiole lesions
	Inflammation
	Cell proliferation
	Drugs
	Allergy
	Genetic
	Intrahepatic duct lesions
	Biliary cirrhosis
	Infectious cholangitis
	Carcinoma
	Extrahepatic Transport
	Stones
	Strictures
	Neoplasm

A. PREHEPATIC JAUNDICE

1. Hemolytic Conditions in Adults

This condition is usually associated either with production of deficient erythrocytes or with the hemolysis of the normal red cells due to antibodies or other hemolytic substances. The abnormalities leading to hemolytic anemias may be congenital, acquired, or associated with Rh-factor incompatibility. Hemolysis of normal red cells may occur following the transfusion of incompatible blood or the exposure to hemolytic substances such as poisons, sulphonamides, phenylhydrazines, snake venom, bacterial or protozoal toxins, and malaria. The serum of patients with excessive hemolysis often shows a mild to moderate unconjugated hyperbilirubinemia as the result of bilirubin overproduction. This mechanism, however, rarely causes severe jaundice unless the liver function is also impaired. Hemoglobinuria and excessive excretion of fecal urobilin and stercobilin, however, may occur (Figure 23). An overload of hemoglobin alone is generally insufficient to cause jaundice, and it may be necessary to have the preexistence of some degree of liver damage. Hepatic damage may be due to fatty infiltration associated with anemia or can be the result of direct toxic damage.

TABLE 2
Relationship Between Serum Bilirubin and Type of Jaundice

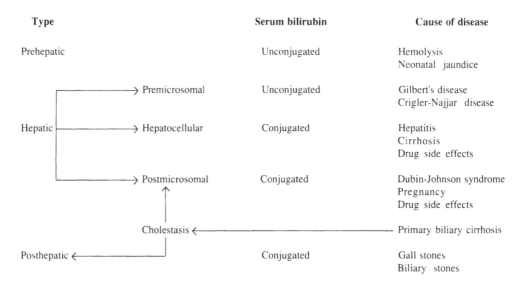

Type	Serum bilirubin	Cause of disease
Prehepatic	Unconjugated	Hemolysis Neonatal jaundice
Hepatic → Premicrosomal	Unconjugated	Gilbert's disease Crigler-Najjar disease
Hepatic → Hepatocellular	Conjugated	Hepatitis Cirrhosis Drug side effects
Hepatic → Postmicrosomal	Conjugated	Dubin-Johnson syndrome Pregnancy Drug side effects
Cholestasis ←		← Primary biliary cirrhosis
Posthepatic ←	Conjugated	Gall stones Biliary stones

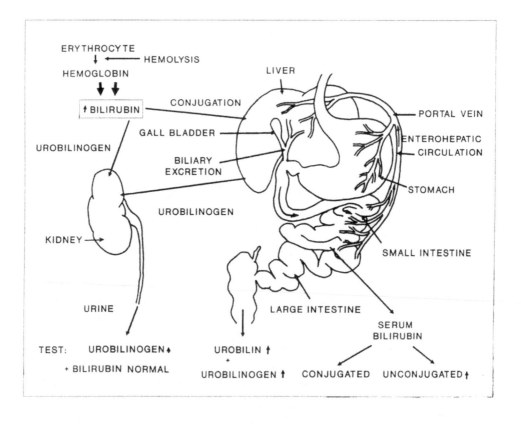

FIGURE 23.   Mechanism of bilirubin metabolism and elimination in hemolytic jaundice. Excessive hemolysis of erythrocytes leads to the overproduction of bilirubin. The hepatic processing reactions and the enterohepatic circulation are normal, but due to the bilirubin overload, the serum level of unconjugated bilirubin is elevated. Abnormal amounts of urobilinogen are excreted in the urine with urobilinogen and urobilin in the feces.

TABLE 3
Causes of Neonatal Hyperbilirubinemia

| Mechanism | Serum bilirubin | |
	Unconjugated	Conjugated
Immaturity	Physiologic jaundice	
Inhibition	Breast milk	
	Maternal serum inhibitor	
	Vitamin K	
Metabolism	Maternal diabetes	
	Cretinism	
	Mongolism	
Erythrocyte	Hemoglobinopathies	
Lesions	Enzyme deficiencies	
	Hereditary spherocytosis	
Immunology	Hemolytic disorders	Excretion failure
Infections	Bacterial hemolysis	Bacterial sepsis, secondary
		Diarrhea
		Viral hepatitis

Normally, about 6.25 g of hemoglobin is broken down daily, disposed readily by a specialized network of cells in the reticuloendothelial system. This amount does not exceed the bilirubin processing ability of the body. In normal subjects, the reticuloendothelial system can degrade up to 45 g of hemoglobin per day leading to a total bilirubin load of about 1.5 g, which is six times greater than the normal body burden. The excess bilirubin is mainly conjugated, but this function may also be increased through the activity of renal conjugating enzymes or from hepatic recycling. Only 3 to 3.5 mg/dl of excess serum unconjugated bilirubin is produced because the liver has a substantial reserve of additional excretory capacity to remove the pigment.[105,339,340,586] In more severe forms of hemolytic anemia, the pigment production may be large enough to cause significant retention of unconjugated bilirubin without the coexistence of an additional liver defect. If serum bilirubin levels are greater than 4 to 5 mg/dl, hepatocellular dysfunction may be present. In hemolytic jaundice, bilirubin is not excreted in the urine since the unconjugated compound is water insoluble. The excretion of the pigment in bile is enhanced and hence, large amounts of stercobilinogen are found in the feces and urobilinogen in the urine.

In hemolytic jaundice, laboratory tests show increased serum unconjugated bilirubin, anemia with reticulocytosis, abnormal erythrocytes, and the presence of hemolytic antibodies. Due to the large bilirubin load, urinary excretion of urobilinogen and coproporphyrin is elevated, but there is no bilirubin in urine. The excretion of fecal pigments, urobilinogen, and urobilin is also increased. Liver function tests are normal since the liver cells are not involved in the pathologic process.

2. Hemolytic Diseases of the Newborn

Neonatal jaundice may be linked with a congenital disorder or transient conditions such as obstruction of the bile ducts, umbilical sepsis, Rh-blood group incompatibility, or delayed synthesis of liver microsomal conjugating enzymes. The major causes are related to hepatic immaturity, presence of inhibitory substances, metabolic or immunological defects, or increased hemoglobin catabolism (Table 3). The liver of the newborn has a limited ability to excrete bilirubin in the bile, capable of eliminating only about 1 to 2% of the amount produced by the adult liver. In these circumstances, even the normal bilirubin production will result in jaundice. The pigment thus accumulated is unconjugated bilirubin, since the liver of the newborn has a low capacity to conjugate bilirubin due to the delayed formation of UDP-glucuronyltransferase. This enzyme is almost completely absent at birth, but rapidly increases during the first few days of life.[608] Virtually all infants show this transient hyper-bilirubinemia for several days. The hemolytic process produces more bilirubin than can be conjugated, due to the immaturity of the enzyme.

Newborn infants become jaundiced during the first week after birth. In most cases, the jaundice is transient and never intense. No other signs of illness are present and the condition is termed "physiologic jaundice" when the bilirubin concentration is less than 10 mg/dl. However, with the maturation of conjugating mechanism proceeding in the first 2 weeks after birth, the serum bilirubin levels fall progressively.

Prematurity is the most common cause of unconjugated hyperbilirubinemia. More than 5% of premature babies develop bilirubin levels greater than 20mg/dl. The smaller and more premature infants show a greater degree of elevated serum bilirubin level than full-term babies. Hypoxia at birth also brings about a transient rise of serum bilirubin. Infants of diabetic mothers and cretins may have elevated bilirubin levels.[265] Recently, it was suggested that in plasma various amino acid ratio can be used as an index of hepatocellular maturity in the neonate.[203]

The jaundice is due to defective conjugation caused by the delayed or absent development of the UDP-glucuronyltransferase or to inhibitory substances. These substances include various steroids, novobiocin, and male fern extract.[236,237,261]

During pregnancy there is a shift in steroid metabolism from hydroxylation to the reductive pathway.[5] As a result, more reduced progesterone metabolites were formed (Figure 24), inhibiting microsomal enzyme activity in the liver of the mother. These compounds were probably also responsible for the delay in the development of the fetal or newborn enzyme system. On the other hand, hydroxylated progesterone derivatives induced hepatic drug metabolism and enhanced conjugation.[9,11] The effects of various progesterones were related to the production of endoplasmic reticulum membranes rich in phosphatidylcholine (Figure 25). Prolonged neonatal hyperbilirubinemia is sometimes associated with breast milk feeding (Figure 26). This marked neonatal jaundice appears 8 to 10 d postpartum and is probably due to factors which block conjugation, mainly maternal steroids, including progesterone derivatives. Feeding pregnanediol to full-term infants causes a reversible unconjugated hyperbilirubinemia unrelated to hemolysis or hepatic damage.[174,303]

3. Kernicterus

Sometimes in the newborn, the jaundice is severe and persistent. At serum concentrations exceeding 20 to 30 mg/dl of bilirubin damage may develop in the brain. Thus, excessive unconjugated hyperbilirubinemia causes a special encephalopathy, called kernicterus, involving the deposit of pigment in the nucleus of the brain with subsequent damage to the nerve cells.[103,116] The clinical signs vary from mild lethargy and spasticity to loss of reflexes and respiratory irregularity leading frequently to death. In the acute stage, many parts of the brain contain unconjugated bilirubin, namely the basal ganglia, the nuclei of hypothalamus, thalamus, dentate, hippocampus, and part of cerebellum. The survivors show spastic paralysis, deafness, and mental retardation.

The development of kernicterus is due to the presence of high amounts of unbound bilirubin crossing the blood-brain barrier. Consequently, the amount of pigment transferred into the brain is related to the amount of free and not to the total bilirubin. In the mechanism of action of free bilirubin on the brain cells, the inhibition of mitochondrial function is probably essential. Mitochondria accumulate bilirubin and the highly pigmented area contains decreased adenosine triphosphate. Bilirubin causes mitochondrial swelling and interferes with the oxidative phosphorylation.[128,150,426,492] These developments can be prevented by the infusion of albumin; thus reducing the amount of free bilirubin in the serum by binding and protecting cellular respiration from interference by bilirubin. Conversely, in the presence of some compounds such as salicylate, oleate, the free bilirubin concentration is increased. These compounds bind competitively to albumin, release bilirubin into the medium, and

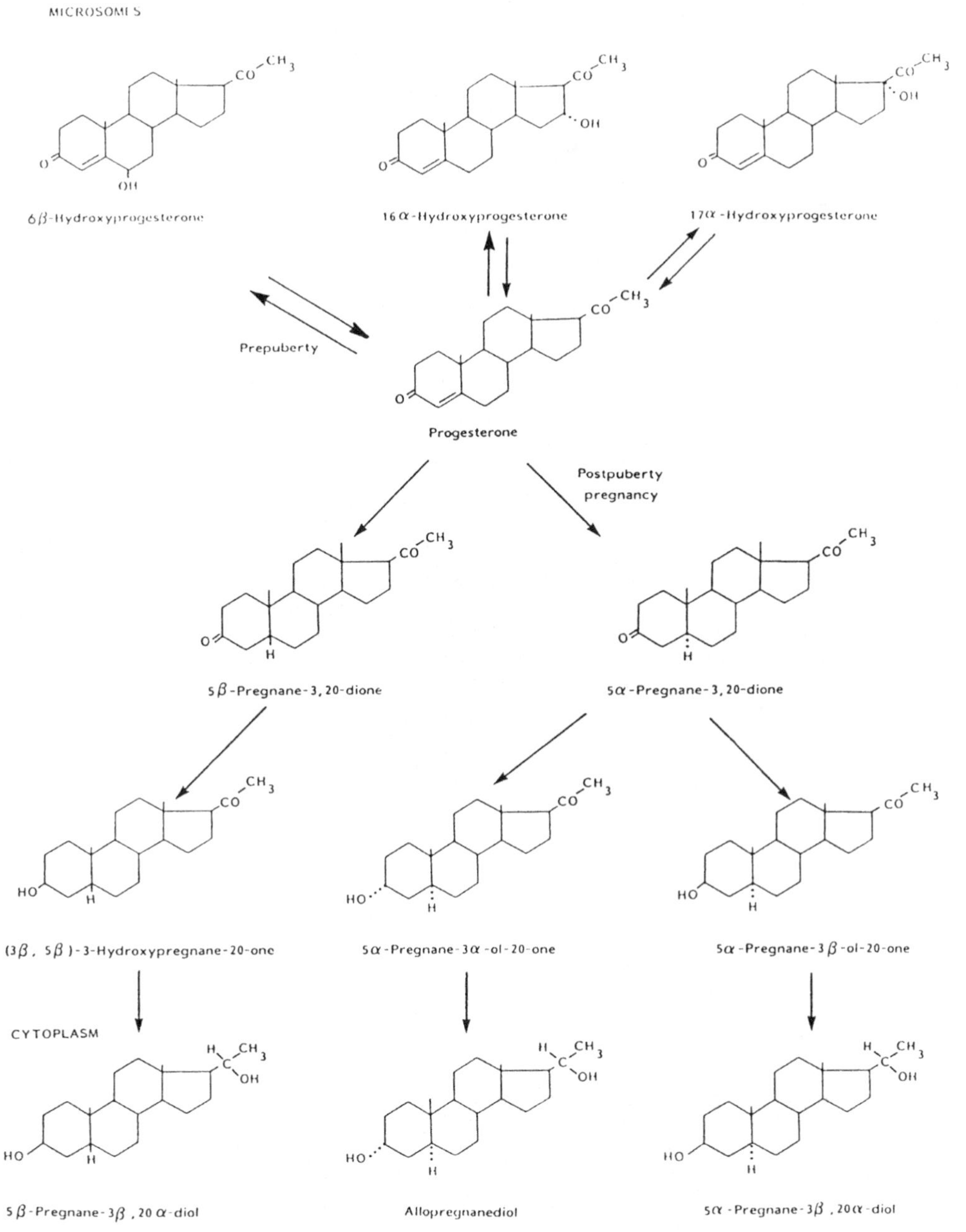

FIGURE 24. Simplified scheme of hepatic progesterone metabolism during pregnancy and in the newborn, and its possible effect on enzyme activities of the endoplasmic reticulum. Besides the overall rise of progesterone biosynthesis during late pregnancy, there is a shift in the metabolic pathways of progesterone from the hydroxylating to the reductive route. Puberty causes a reversal; it shifts progesterone metabolism to the hydroxylating pathways.[170,303]

increase the amount of bilirubin passing into the brain. Some drugs, such as sulfisoxazole, decrease serum bilirubin, but enhance the incidence of kernicterus. This action is probably associated with competition for albumin binding sites, and thus more bilirubin can cross the blood-brain barrier.

In the diagnosis and treatment of neonatal hyperbilirubinemia and kernicterus, the measurement of serum bilirubin levels provides a useful guide to assess this risk factor and helps

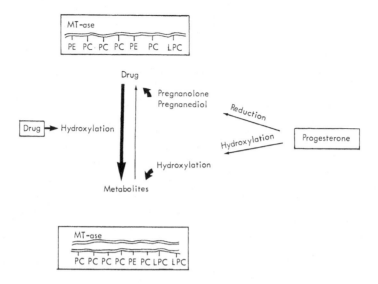

FIGURE 25. The effect of progesterone metabolism on bilirubin elimination. The increased level of pregnanolone and pregnanediol causes an inhibition of drug metabolizing enzymes including UDP-glucuronyltransferase. Elevated amounts of hydroxyprogesterones bring about an induction. These activity changes are probably associated with the synthesis of membrane-bound phosphatidylcholine from phosphatidylethanolamine by stepwise methylation. This process is catalyzed by the S-adenosyl-L-methionine:microsomal-phospholipid methyl transferase. When drug metabolism is induced by drugs, more endoplasmic reticulum membranes are formed together or as the consequence of elevated methyl transferase level and subsequently increased microsomal phosphatidyl- and lysophosphatidyl-choline contents.[170,174]

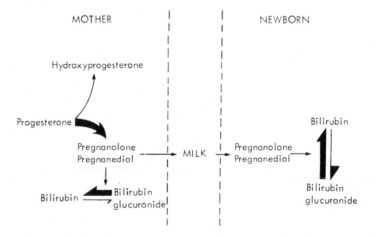

FIGURE 26. Effects of maternal progesterones on the metabolism of bilirubin in the newborn. During pregnancy progesterone metabolism is shifted to the reductive pathway resulting in the formation of greater amounts of pregnanolone and pregnanediol. These progesterone metabolites cause a reduction of drug metabolism by the hepatic endoplasmic reticulum of the mother. With the milk, these compounds are transported into the newborn, and subsequently, they are probably responsible for the inhibition of bilirubin conjugation in the liver.[10,263]

treatments aimed at avoiding bilirubin levels above 20 mg%. Exchange transfusion applied to the newborn or certain drug treatments given to the pregnant mother or newborn are the usual therapeutic measures. Recent developments in this field include the sampling of amniotic fluid before birth. The bilirubin content of this fluid gives a good indication of the severity of the hemolytic process and may even indicate the need for an intrauterine transfusion.

4. Rh-Factor Incompatibility

This prehepatic icterus is due to the absence of Rh factor in the blood of pregnant women. The condition is not infrequent since 12% of marriages match a Rh-negative woman with a Rh-positive man. The difference in blood subgroups has an adverse effect on the children, resulting in a disorder termed erythroblastosis fetalis. This is due to the transplacental passage of maternal antibodies directed against fetal blood cells containing the Rh antigens. The consequence of this transplacental transfer is the destruction of red blood cells leading to severe anemia, accumulation of bilirubin and toxic substances causing fetal death. The reason for the antibody production and for the loss of erythrocytes is the exposure of the mother to the Rh-positive fetal blood which leaks across the placenta and enters the maternal blood stream as a result of hemorrhage during the first delivery. Consequently, the Rh-negative mother becomes sensitized or immunized against the Rh-positive fetus producing antibodies during subsequent pregnancies. The transplacental passage of antibodies thus destroys the fetal red cells. Accordingly, the firstborn child is usually not affected, unless the mother has been sensitized by previous transfusions.

In Rh-factor incompatibility, the antibody coats the surface of the red cells and these cells then are sequestered in the spleen and, to a lesser extent, in other organs. The clumping of erythrocytes occurs probably in the splenic circulation which slows down the blood flow leading eventually to substrate deprivation and anemia. Liver and lymph nodes may take part in hemolysis.

Mildly affected babies may be only somewhat anemic and recover from the jaundice. In more serious erythroblastosis fetalis cases, too many immature red blood cells are formed which are unable to carry oxygen to the tissues, subsequently causing an attempt to compensate by other blood-producing organs, mainly the liver and spleen, and swelling develops. This series of events progress to congestive heart failure and eventual death. Most of the seriously afflicted babies are stillborn.

The earlier treatment of Rh disease consisted of massive blood transfusion before or shortly after birth replacing virtually the entire fetal blood volume. Nowadays, Rh immune globulin is administered to the Rh-negative mother a few days prior to delivery and before every abortion or miscarriage. In this fusion, the formation of Rh antibodies in the mother is prevented, and thus the baby develops normally.

B. HEPATIC JAUNDICE

Within the boundaries of the hepatocellular plasma membrane, this type of jaundice is associated with premicrosomal, microsomal, postmicrosomal, or general cytoplasmic defects. In the premicrosomal form, bilirubin conjugation is impaired resulting in an increased unconjugated pigment level in the serum. Jaundice also may be due to a familial hereditary abnormality of bilirubin metabolism as in Gilbert's syndrome. This autosomal dominant disease is not uncommon and probably represents a heterogenous group of benign disorders or may be the final outcome of several unrelated lesions. This syndrome is characterized by failure of bilirubin transport indicated by mild unconjugated hyperbilirubinemia between 1 to 4 mg/dl. There is an impaired bilirubin uptake by the hepatocytes, the bile composition is normal, and the fecal urobilinogen excretion is either unaltered or only slightly reduced. Liver function tests are normal and there are no significant structural abnormalities. The

Gunn strain of rat exhibits similarities to the symptoms of Gilbert's syndrome.[12] This mutant strain of rats develops a hereditary jaundice with autosomal recessive characteristics.

Microsomal defects are related to conjugation failure as the consequence of absent UDP-GT activity. The hyperbilirubinemia in Crigler-Najjar syndrome represents a form of congenital nonhemolytic jaundice which is genetically controlled and may be transmitted as a Mendelian dominant. The Crigler-Najjar syndrome is very rare.[116] In these patients, the primary enzyme defect involves the complete absence of UDPGT from birth and therefore, only unconjugated bilirubin is found in the serum. Bilirubin is formed continuously from hemoglobin, but the degree of jaundice is fairly constant, indicating that alternate metabolic pathways partly compensate the defect in the hepatic conjugation system. Infants suffering from this disease develop severe jaundice and usually die from kernicterus.

In postmicrosomal hyperbilirubinemia bilirubin conjugation is normal, but the conjugated derivative is not transported to the large bile ducts. In the serum, elevated amounts of conjugated and unconjugated bilirubin appear, and this combination is known as Dubin-Johnson syndrome. The pigment is mainly accumulated in the centrilobular areas of the parenchymal cells and, to a lesser extent, in Kupffer cells. Bilirubin deposition within the hepatocyte is found in the lysosomes of the pericanalicular area. In biopsy specimens, the dark appearance of the liver is of useful diagnostic value.

The Dubin-Johnson syndrome is often seen in young people and is familial in most cases, originating from an inborn error. The presence of mild and asymptomatic jaundice may be detected in early childhood. The severe form is precipitated by chronic physical exhaustion, alcoholism, infectious diseases, and pregnancy. Abdominal pain in the liver region is the major clinical sign of the disease. Serum bilirubin levels fluctuate from normal values up to 19 mg/dl. The amounts of conjugated bilirubin show variations although glucuronide production is normal. The usual liver tests are also normal or slightly impaired. The abnormality leading to this disorder lies in a primary defect of the hepatic excretory mechanism, since in normal circumstances lipofuscin-type pigments are eliminated from the liver via the bile.

A similar hepatic excretory defect is found in the Rotor syndrome except that there are no pigment bodies in hepatocytes. The liver structure is apparently normal although the number of pericanalicular lysosomes is increased. Rotor syndrome is a familial disorder and is associated with elevation of conjugated serum bilirubin. There is a mild jaundice which may be worsened with physical stress, chronic emotional problems, and infections. Abdominal pain is absent.

In hepatocellular jaundice, all the functions of the liver are affected to some degree, although bilirubin conjugation is usually normal. In these conditions, bilirubin appears in the urine, which is normally not excreted through the kidney (Figure 27). Infectious hepatitis is the most familiar example of this disorder. The main pathological findings include centrilobular necrosis and swelling of the liver cells which cause blockade of the sinusoids and lymphatics. In severe cases, the whole architecture of the lobule may be destroyed affecting the function of bilirubin transport through the intrahepatic bile channels.[5,116,192]

The causes of intrahepatic icterus are numerous, including virus hepatitis (epidemic infective hepatitis), homologous serum jaundice, cholangiolytic hepatitis, cirrhosis, and toxic hepatitis from drugs and from bacterial toxins.[571,576] In viral hepatitis and cirrhosis, the jaundice is associated with diffuse parenchymal damage.[406,490] The serum contains significant amounts of bilirubin due to the reduced mass of functional hepatic parenchyma. Cholestatic jaundice is also related to infection, and in the newborn, bacterial sepsis brings about severe conjugated hyperbilirubinemia indicating an excretory defect. These conditions show no apparent extrahepatic obstruction, but histopathologic examinations reveal bile stasis and dilatation of bile canaliculi. Bacterial toxins cause a local inflammatory reaction, and thus partial closure of the canaliculi or various products of inflammation prevent the elimination

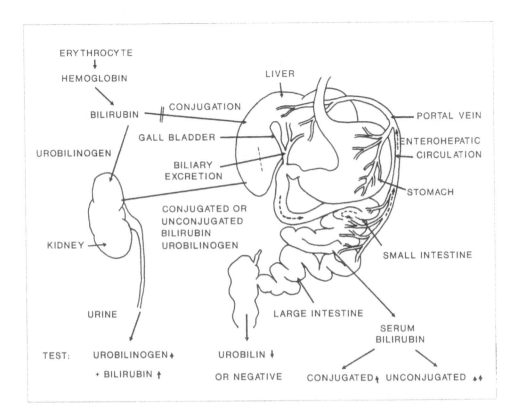

FIGURE 27.   Mechanism of bilirubin metabolism and elimination in hepatocellular jaundice. In this disease, the elimination of bilirubin is blocked and due to liver defect, both unconjugated and conjugated bilirubin are increased in the serum; the level of unconjugated is greater than conjugated. Elevated amounts of urobilinogen are excreted in the urine. Small amounts of bilirubin also pass through the kidney. The enterohepatic circulation is not functioning, therefore no or very small amounts of urobilinogen are present in the small intestines and small amounts of urobilin are excreted in the feces.

of conjugated bilirubin from the liver cell. Cholestatic jaundice occasionally follows a surgical intervention as a possible consequence of acute infection. This complicated jaundice develops on the first or second postoperative day. In this case, the transient hepatic insufficiency following surgery is causing a temporary defect in the conjugated bilirubin excretion.

Cholestatic jaundice occurs during pregnancy in some cases, usually during the last trimester, probably representing an unusual liver response to some steroids produced by the pregnant mother. Drug treatment may potentiate the severity of jaundice due to reduced hepatic drug metabolism during pregnancy.[101,173,282] Bile duct proliferation and inflammatory processes at the portal spaces are the usual morphological findings. Electron microscopy shows dilation and vacuolization of the endoplasmic reticulum. The serum bilirubin concentration is usually less than 4 mg/dl, and both conjugated and unconjugated forms are present. At parturition, the recurrent jaundice completely disappears.

C. POSTHEPATIC JAUNDICE

The cause of posthepatic jaundice is a mechanical blockade in the bile canaliculi or bile duct (Figure 28). Due to this obstacle, bile canaliculi are distended, and the bile usually regurgitates into the blood stream. Obstruction of the main routes most frequently is caused by gallstones, tumors, or local metastic invasion.

Biochemical tests show increased, mainly conjugated, bilirubin in the serum; bilirubin, urobilin and bile salts appear in the urine, whereas they are diminished or absent in the

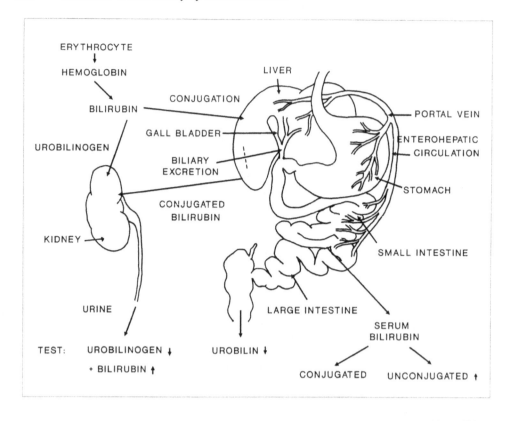

FIGURE 28. Mechanism of bilirubin metabolism and elimination in obstructive jaundice. In this condition, due to a failure of biliary excretion of bilirubin, both unconjugated and conjugated are elevated in the serum; the conjugated in greater extent. Enterohepatic circulation is inhibited, no or very small amounts of urobilinogen are present in the small intestines and eliminated in the feces or urine. Considerable amounts of bilirubin are excreted through the kidney.

stool. Further abnormalities include elevated serum cholesterol, phospholipid, and serum enzyme levels. Serum proteins are normal and variable changes in liver function tests have been reported.

VIII. DETOXIFICATION OF FOREIGN COMPOUNDS

One of the major functions of the liver cell is to metabolize and eliminate drugs and other foreign compounds from the body.[27,332,574] During this process, biologically or pharmacologically active substances are converted to inactive metabolites by the drug metabolizing enzyme system also termed the microsomal mixed function oxidase system.[53,580] This system provides a natural protection against adverse reactions to drugs. Without these enzymes catalyzing the conversion of lipid-soluble compounds to more polar and therefore less lipid-soluble derivatives, many drugs could exert their action for an unnecessarily long time. This intrahepatic metabolism also prevents reabsorption by rendering the drugs water-soluble, allowing metabolites to be filtered through the glomerulus in the kidney. There are drugs giving rise to metabolites which remain as active as the original compounds. Occasionally, the pharmacological effect of metabolites is even greater than that of the parent compound indicating metabolic activation.

The ability of the liver to metabolize foreign compounds is used to measure hepatic function in man in a noninvasive fashion.[44,63,64,384,471] In normal circumstances, the metabolism and disposition of drugs are adequate, and thus therapeutic doses have no harmful

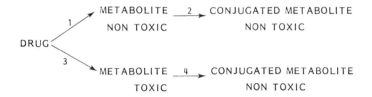

FIGURE 29.   Scheme of hepatic metabolism of foreign compounds leading to their detoxification. The mechanism of deactivation involves in the first phase various nonsynthetic reactions (1), including oxidation, hydrolysis, oxidative deamination, oxidative dealkylation, and in the second phase synthetic reactions (2), including conjugation with glucuronic acid, glycine, S-acetylcysteine (mercapturic acid), sulfation, alkylation, and acylation. Foreign compounds can be activated by these processes to form toxic derivatives by the first phase reactions (3), and further inactivated by the second phase reactions (4). The metabolism of drugs often leads to change of activity or to the production of toxic compounds which may be incorporated into normal metabolic processes. The latter reactions are called lethal syntheses.

effects on hepatic function. The efficiency and duration of the drug effect depend on the rate at which drugs are activated or inactivated. Under certain conditions, however, adverse reactions occur related either to hepatic dysfunction or to the toxic nature of the foreign compound.[517] These reactions result in hepatic disorders which may be reversible, like drug-induced jaundice, or irreversible causing long-term damage, like cirrhosis.

The processes leading to the conversion of drugs to more polar compounds take place in the endoplasmic reticulum or microsomal fraction of the liver cell (Figure 29). Drug metabolizing enzymes are bound to smooth membranes and transform foreign compounds through various routes, which include oxidation, hydroxylation, reduction, hydrolysis, alkylation, and conjugation. Many cofactors are involved in hepatic microsomal drug metabolism, including cytochrome P-450, cytochrome b_5, glutathione, regenerating enzymes, and phospholipids.[343,394] In several cases, the transformation of foreign compounds in the liver leads to metabolites possessing altered pharmacological activity or to the production of toxic derivatives (Table 4).

Microsomal enzymes do not generally metabolize endogenous compounds such as phenylalanine and tryptophan which are hydroxylated by specific enzymes occurring in other parts of the cell, although tryptamine and tyramine have been shown to be catabolized by hepatic microsomal enzymes. However, various steroids are hydroxylated by the liver microsomal mixed function oxidase system. Postnatal developments of drug detoxification mechanisms and steroid metabolism show close parallelism. On the other hand, some foreign compounds may also undergo changes catalyzed by some of the enzymes of the intermediary metabolism, such as alcohol dehydrogenase, aldehyde dehydrogenase, xanthine oxidase, and esterases.

It is beyond the scope of this book to describe the mechanism of drugs metabolism and factors influencing enzyme activities.[302] We will address the relationship between the function of the endoplasmic reticulum and hepatic disease. The response of the liver cell to foreign compounds may be grouped into two categories (Table 5). Drugs usually evoke a beneficial response leading to the proliferation of the endoplasmic reticulum membranes and increased activity of drug metabolizing enzymes with subsequent enhanced detoxication. In contrast, hepatotoxins damage the endoplasmic reticulum membranes, impair the activity of normal membrane-bound enzymes, and thus inhibit drug metabolism. Hepatotoxins bring about decreased detoxification leading to pathological lesions and eventual death of the cell.[140] Drug side effects may be associated with adverse reactions similar to the effect of hepatotoxins. Chronic administration of drugs can affect steroid metabolism.[168] Hepatic drug me-

TABLE 4

Changes Occurring in Pharmacological or Biological Activity of Foreign Compounds Associated with Hepatic Detoxication Processes

Process	Foreign compound	Metabolic reaction	Metabolite	Activity changes
Inactivation	Butylated hydroxytoluene	Oxidation	BHT-alcohol, acid	Loss of antioxidant activity
	Pentobarbital	Oxidation	Hydroxypentobarbital	Loss of hypnotic activity
	Phenobarbital	Hydroxylation	4-Hydroxyphenobarbital	Loss of hypnotic activity
	Procain	Hydrolysis	p-Aminobenzoic acid diethyl-aminoethanol	Loss of anesthetic activity
Activation	Prednisone	Reduction	Prednisolone	Immunosuppressive action
	Acetanilide	Hydroxylation	p-Hydroxyacetanilide	Analgesic and antipyretic action
	2-Naphtylamine	Hydroxylation	2-Amino-1-naphtol	Carcinogen
	Prontosil	Azo reduction	Sulfanylamide	Antibacterial action
Modification	Codeine	O-demethylation	Morphine	Analgesic → narcotic
	Iproniazid	N-dealkylation	Isoniazid	Antidepressive → antitubercular
	Prominal	N-demethylation	Phenobarbital	Short acting → long acting hypnotic
	Pyramidon	N-demethylation	4-Aminoantipyrine	Analgesic and antipyretic → reduced activity
Lethal synthesis	Amygdalin	Hydrolysis	HCN	Cytotoxic action
	Fluoroethanol	Metabolism	Fluorocitrate	Neurotoxic action
	Methanol	Oxidation	Formaldehyde	Toxic action
	Parathion	Oxidation	Paraoxon	Enzyme inhibition

TABLE 5
Major Changes in the Hepatic Endoplasmic Reticulum Following the Administration of Foreign Compounds

| | Endoplasmic reticulum | | | |
| | Structure | | Function | |
Substance	Rough	Smooth	Rough	Smooth
Hepatotoxins	Cisternae dilated Dense bodies appear Polysome loss	Parallelism disturbed Disorientation Fragmentation	Normal enzymes impaired Protein synthesis inhibited Phospholipid synthesis inhibited Lipid infiltration	Drug metabolism inhibited or no effect
Drug	No apparent change	Proliferation	No apparent change Protein synthesis increased Phospholipid synthesis increased	Enzyme induction Drug metabolism increased Cytochrome P-450 increased

tabolism can be altered by different liver diseases, diabetes, congestive heart failure, and other conditions[2,172,300,374,383,420,475,487] Inherited defects and polymorphism also occur in hepatic drug oxidation,[54,327,572] and some pancreatic disease may modulate hepatic detoxification.[60] Racial and genetic differences also influence drug metabolism.[115,187,293,294,295,422] The relationship between detoxication and drug-induced disease will be discussed later.

A. DRUG-INDUCED LIVER DISORDERS

Hepatic side effects of drugs present a wide-ranging picture.[6,87,162,316,323] Morphological and biochemical studies demonstrate lipid metabolic disturbances, similar to many diseases mainly manifest in liver disorders. Coronary heart disease, as well as various inherited defects leading to lipidosis, can be potentiated by various foreign compounds via hepatic metabolic processes. Liver abnormalities are caused by the accumulation of iron in hepatocytes (Plate 1).

A variety of occupational diseases or chronic drug effects cause impaired lipid metabolism. These lipid metabolic alterations can be categorized into (1) disorders connected with pathological lipid accumulation in the liver resulting from absorption of hepatotoxins or excessive amounts of otherwise nontoxic drugs, (2) drug-induced hepatitis, and (3) atherosclerotic vascular lesions pertaining to the long-term effects of various occupational agents. Individuals with varying susceptibilities can develop idiosyncratic jaundice from a particular drug. Differences in microsomal drug metabolizing enzymes and genetic variations may be responsible for these different susceptibilities.[431] Genetic factors seem to be particularly important in jaundice produced by oral contraceptives, chlorpromazine, and alcohol.

Chemically induced liver injury can manifest in various morphological entities. The acute effects may appear as accumulation of lipids. In that case, the results are fatty liver or degenerative processes leading to necrosis connected with cell death. Liver injury resulting from chronic exposure to chemicals can cause pronounced alterations of the liver architecture with simultaneous proliferative and degenerative changes as seen in different forms of cirrhosis. Biochemical changes reflecting the disrupted lipid metabolism include excessive triglyceride deposition and lipidoses characterized by abnormal accumulation of cholesterol or phospholipids. These can not only be induced by hepatotoxic substances, but by nutritional deficiency of certain lipotropic agents and other essential dietary factors. Clinical symptoms are varied.[127,140,374] Some are similar to those seen in conditions reflecting impaired bilirubin metabolism or intrahepatic cholestasis,[594] some show similarities to virus-induced hepatitis, some produce fatty degeneration and necrosis, and some cause acute cytotoxic injury.[87,316]

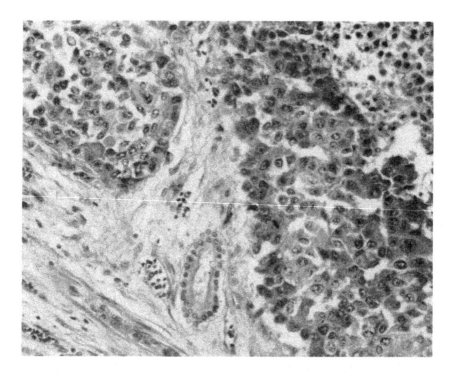

PLATE 1.   Hepatocellular carcinoma, the histogram shows nests of tumor cells with foci of necrosis. At the top of the micrograph there is a surviving bile duct.

Changes in liver function and signs of hepatic injury are similar to symptoms of mild or severe liver diseases of nonchemical origin (Table 6). Acute cytotoxic injury is also associated with drugs (Table 7).

B. DRUG-INDUCED CHOLESTASIS

Drug-induced cholestasis results in the stagnation of bile formed by hepatocytes and with the retention of biliary substances in the blood due to a failure of clearance. Several drugs produce this type of cholestasis as an adverse effect and drug hypersensitivity manifests also in cholestasis.[83,449,453,454,512]

The effect of many drugs is associated with cholestatic reactions in experimental animals. α-Naphthylisothiocyanate and taurolithocholic acid produce cholestatic responses such as bile stasis, hyperbilirubinemia, and sulfobromophthalein retention, and affect several other hepatocyte functions. A single intoxicating dose of ethanol or its continuous ingestion can cause elevation of hepatic triglycerides. Hypertriglyceridemia also occurs with high frequency among chronic alcoholics. The basic biochemical process responsible for this abnormal fat accumulation is not known. The mechanisms underlying fatty liver formation in alcohol addicts can be connected with (1) enhanced mobilization of lipids from adipose tissues, (2) decreased intrahepatic metabolism by oxidation, (3) increased lipogenesis by greater rate of esterification of free fatty acids in the liver, and (4) impairment of hepatic triglyceride secretion connected with transport defects. Carbon tetrachloride and chloroform disrupt the lipoprotein secretory mechanism. Many other toxic chemicals cause an inhibition of hepatic lipoprotein synthesis due to defects of intrahepatic utilization of neutral fats and faulty incorporation of fatty acids with subsequent reduced secretion into the circulation. Abnormal production of β-lipoprotein in very low density lipoprotein fractions occupies a key position in the development of fatty liver.

The adverse action of many chemicals is linked with metabolic biotransformation. Toxic

TABLE 6
Some Representatives of Drugs or Hepatotoxic Compounds Associated with Various Types of Liver Lesions

Effect	Compound	Compound
Intrahepatic cholestasis	Carbutamide	Methandrolone
	Chlorpromazine	Phenindone
	Chlorpropamide	Propylthiouracil
	Chlorthiazide	Sulfanilamide
	Mestranol	Trifluoperazine
Virus-like hepatitis	Halothane	Phenelzine
	Indomethacine	Phenylbutazone
	Iproniazid	6-Mercaptopurine
	Isoniazid	Tranylcypromine
	Nialamide	Zoxazolamine
Chronic active hepatitis	Dantrolene	
	Methyldopa	
	Nitrofurantoin	
Fatty liver	Alcohol	Cycloheximide
	Allyl alcohol	Dichloroethylene
	Amanita phalloides	Dimethylhydrazine
	Azacytidine	Ethionine
	Azaserine	Methotrexate
	Bleomycin	Puromycin
	Carbon tetrachloride	Pyrrolizidine alkaloids
	Chloroform	Tetracycline
	Cerium	Valproic acid
		Warfarin
Necrosis	Aflatoxin	Carbon tetrachloride
	Allyl alcohol	Chloroform
	Amanita phalloides	Ethyl alcohol
	Azaserine	Tannic acid
	Bromobenzene	Thioacetamide

liver responses in several instances are due to the formation of toxic metabolites. This has been shown with pyrrolizidine alkaloids present in "bush teas", allyl alcohol, dimethyl-nitrosamine, and α-naphthylisothiocyanate. Metabolism of carbon tetrachloride, chloroform, or bromobenzene is also determinant of the development of hepatic lesions. These compounds are metabolized by liver microsomes, and stimulation of their biotransformation enhances their hepatotoxicity if not connected with faster elimination.[65-67,193,370,381,391,468-470,476] Generally, these metabolites can interact with various steps of the normal detoxication process (Figure 30).

There are conditions when cholestasis occurs more frequently, such as in the newborn and in pregnancy. Most detoxication reactions are not present in early postnatal liver. Particularly important is the low activity of glucuronidation. Glucuronidase activity has not been found in human placenta, and therefore, the maternal liver UDP-glucuronyltransferase takes care of the elimination of many endogenous and exogenous metabolites. Bilirubin conjugation appears after birth. Drugs compete with bilirubin for the conjugation site and for transport and secretion. Thus the low conjugating capacity of the newborn is the cause for direct poisoning by drugs and for the development of cholestasis and jaundice at that age.

Drug metabolizing capability of the maternal liver in late pregnancy is reduced, and at

TABLE 7
Drug Side Effects Associated with Acute Cytotoxic Injury

Anesthetics	Halothane	Cancer chemotherapy	Chlorambucil
	Methoxyflurane		Cyclophosphamide
	Fluroxene		Mercaptopurine
			Methramycin
Anti-inflammatory agents	Allopurinol		Nitrosoureas
	Colchicine		Streptozotocin
			Thioguanine
Antimicrobials	Amodiaquine	Urethane	
	Ampicillin		
	Antimonials	Cardiovascular drugs	Furosemide
	Chloramphenicol		Methyldopa
	Clindamycin		Nicotinic Acid
	Ethionamide		Papaverine
	Griseofulvin		Perihexiline Maleate
	Hycanthone		Procainamide
	Hydroxystilbamidine		Pyridoxal carbamate
	Idoxuridine		Quinidine
	Isoniazid		Verapamil
	Mepacrine		
	Novobiocin	Hormonal agents	Acetohexanide
	PAS		Azepinamide
	Penicillin G		Carbutamide
	Pyrazinamide		Metahexamide
	Rifampicin		Propylthiouracil
	Sulfonamides		
	Thiosemicarbazone	Neuropsychotropics	Hydrazine
			Anticonvulsives
Antispasm agents	Dantrolene		
	Fenclozic Acid	Miscellaneous drugs	Acetaminophen
	Fenoprofen		Azulfidine
	Gold compounds		Lergotrile mesylate
	Indomethacin		Carbamazepine
	Phenylbutazone		Disulfiram
	Oxybutazone		Phenazopyridine
	Ketobutazone		Vitamin A
	Probenecid		
	Salicylates		
	Zoxazolamine		

the same time, there are increased demands that drain some of the energy needed in detoxication reactions. This event results in the more frequent occurence of drug-induced side effects and cholestasis during pregnancy. The adverse cholestatic response during pregnancy may be due to the significant increase in steroid hormones;[83] anabolic steroids or oral contraceptives also cause cholestasis.[590,607]

C. DRUG-INDUCED JAUNDICE

Drugs cause liver damage with or without jaundice by a variety of mechanisms.[48,102,204,334,403,526,550] Often the first clinical sign of hepatotoxicity is jaundice. This condition indicates an excessive production of bilirubin or an interference with normal metabolism and elimination. The mechanism of adverse action can occur at many sites (Figure 31).

Prehepatic drug-related jaundice may be produced directly by the administration of drugs such as phenylhydrazine, which causes hemolytic anemia by its action on red blood cells. The effects can be indirect, as with drugs such as primaquine, which induces hemolysis due to a genetically determined enzyme defect. There is a glucose 6-phosphate dehydrogenase

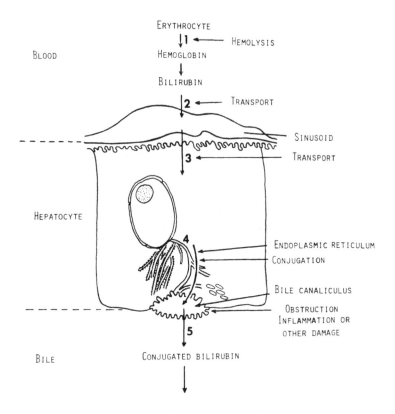

FIGURE 30.   Sites of drug interaction with bilirubin metabolism and transport. Drug-induced jaundice may be due to (1) increased degradation of erythrocytes, increased hemolysis yielding excessive production of bilirubin, (2) interference with transport into hepatocytes associated with competition for the transport protein, albumin, (3) interference with uptake by the cell associated with competition for intracellular transport protein, ligandin, and (4) interference with the function of the endoplasmic reticulum. This could be primary: direct inhibition of conjugation due to substrate competition for the processing sites on the membrane, or direct hepatotoxicity associated with reduced enzyme activity, or secondary to generalized parenchymal cell damage; (5) interference with excretion from the cell linked with obstruction of the bile canaliculi and (6) interference with biliary transport due to inflammatory lesions or any other damage brought about by the drug.[37]

deficiency in the erythrocytes of primaquine-sensitive individuals. In addition, the red blood cells are also deficient in glutathione and nicotinamide adenine dinucleotide. These cofactors are essential for the maintenance of cellular integrity. The metabolic consequence of the defect is that glutathione cannot be kept in the reduced state. This mechanism is implicated in the direct action of phenylhydrazine. Indirect effects causing hemolysis and bilirubin overload can occur when drugs are bound to the erythrocyte membrane. The effects of phenacetine and para-aminosalicylate are probably associated with this mechanism; these drugs also initiate the formation of antibodies and promote red blood cell agglutination and hemolysis.

Hepatic jaundice may be caused by the generalized toxic action of powerful hepatotoxins. Certain chemicals act directly on the liver cells and cause hepatocellular necrosis. The resulting inflammatory reaction is often slight, but an intense fatty infiltration develops. Iproniazid derivatives cause hepatitis-like jaundice, due to a hypersensitivity reaction clinically and pathologically undistinguishable from infectious hepatitis. Often it is difficult to rule out the possibility of coincidental viral infections. Cholestatic-type response occurs with many drugs such as chlorpromazine and derivatives, C^{17}-alkyl steroids, such as methyltes-

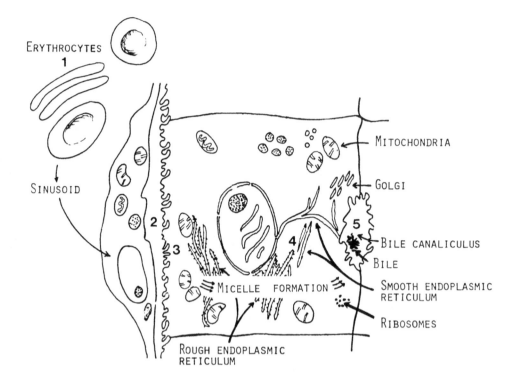

CAUSES OF FAILURE

(1) EXTRACELLULAR CARRIER PROTEIN (ALBUMIN)
(2) INTRACELLULAR CARRIER PROTEIN (LIGANDIN)
(3) INHIBITION OF ENDOPLASMIC RETICULUM FUNCTION (METABOLISM)
(4) OBSTRUCTION OF BILE CANALICULI

FIGURE 31.   Schematic representation of the mechanism of cholestasis. Mild action of foreign compound on the liver cell causes intrahepatic cholestasis. Bilirubin level may be increased due to enhanced hemolysis of erythrocytes (1). The site of defect in the hepatocyte may represent an interaction or competition for the extracellular carrier protein, albumin (2), or a competition for the intracellular carrier protein, ligandin (3), inhibition of metabolism by the endoplasmic reticulum (4), or obstruction of bile canaliculi (5).

tosterone, and oral contraceptive hormones containing progestogens of C^{17}-type structure. This cholestatic-type response may also represent a hypersensitivity reaction, although steroids inhibit conjugation indicating a block in bilirubin metabolism. Posthepatic jaundice may be associated with a competition for bilirubin transport. Novobiocin and bunamiodyl retard the removal of bilirubin from the serum.

IX. HEPATITIS

Acute liver disease is usually related to bacterial or viral infection, or it is caused by drugs and other chemicals.[37] The most important forms of acute hepatitis are viral, alcoholic, and drug-induced. The most common form is the acute infectious hepatitis caused by viruses.[406,577] A differential diagnosis can be made between these disease forms by means of light microscopy, and liver injury details can be obtained by electronmicroscopy. A case of

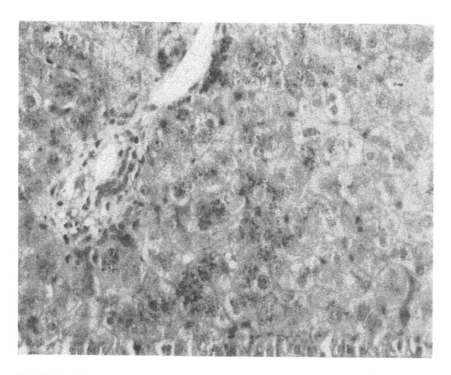

PLATE 2.   Metabolic liver abnormality, the photo micrograph shows iron load in hepatocytes indicated by the Prussian blue reaction.

hepatitis is seen in Plate 2. Ultrastructural studies show that hepatic insufficiency can occur because of the endoplasmic reticulum injury in viral hepatitis and mitochondrial damage in alcoholic liver disease. In drug-induced hepatitis, mitochondrial damage can be noted in some cases (halothane)[125] and endoplasmic reticulum injury in others (methyldopa).[124,126] The mitochondrial damage involves both the inner and outer membranes, but not enlargement or crystalloid formation. Clinical manifestations may be the same irrespective of the target organelle. The compensatory and regenerative aspects of the disease process can be evaluated from the status of the endoplasmic reticulum membranes and ribosomes, and mitochondria.

Inflammatory reactions reflecting systemic symptoms of hepatitis originated as a result of cytoplasmic injury. Necrosis and shedding of cytoplasmic structures attract macrophages, leukocytes, lymphocytes, and plasma cells, constituting the inflammatory aspect of all forms of hepatitis.[212] The ensuing inflammation alters the microcirculation by restricting the size of sinusoids and by altering Disse's space forming a barrier to the blood-hepatocyte interface due to edema. Cholestasis occurs in all types of hepatitis and is connected with canalicular dilatation and loss of microvilli. Cell to cell variations are reflected in differences in the amounts of water, lipids, and glycogen within each cell.[385] Differences in the degree of hepatocellular organelle damage, inflammation, and cholestasis explain readily the heterogeneous and often overlapping clinical aspect of the various forms of hepatitis. The development of chronicity is associated with the persistence of the original disease cause and the inflammatory response from lymphoid cells relating to immunological abnormalities.

A. ACUTE INFECTIOUS HEPATITIS

Acute infectious hepatitis is by far the most predominant form of hepatitis.[72,559] It occurs sporadically and in endemic proportions. By and large it is a benign disease, seldom ending fatally, although the recovery is very slow. Epidemiologic and experimental observations indicate that two specific viruses account for most of the acute viral hepatitis cases. These agents have been designated viral hepatitis Type A (infectious hepatitis or epidemic jaundice)

TABLE 8

Epidemiologic and Clinical Characteristics of Hepatitis Virus Infections

Characteristics	Type A	Type B
Incubation period	15—50 days	43—180 days
Route of infection	Predominantly fecal—oral	Predominantly parenteral
Type of onset	Acute	Insidious
Age distribution	Children and young adults	All ages
Seasonal variation	Autumn and winter	All year
Occurrence of virus/antigen		
Blood	Days	Months—years
Stool	Early, weeks—months	Present
Urine	?	Present
Virus	HAV	HBV
Antigen	HA Ag	HBAg, HB$_s$Ag
Antibody	HA Ab	Anti-HB$_c$, Anti-HB$_s$
Clinical and laboratory features		
Fever > 38°C	Common early	Less common
Duration of transaminase elevation	1—3 weeks	1—6 months or more
Immunoglobulins (IgM levels)	Significantly elevated	Normal to slightly elevated
HB antigen (HBAg, Australia antigen)	Not present	Present
Immunity		
Homologous	Yes	Yes
Heterologous	No	No
Duration	IgM anti-HAV, short	Anti-HB$_c$ relatively short
	IgG anti-HAV, long high level	Anti-HB$_s$ long low level
γ - Globulin therapy	Regularly prevents or modifies hepatitis	Prevents or modifies hepatitis if specific HB immune serum globulin of sufficient potency is given

and viral hepatitis Type B (serum hepatitis or homologous serum jaundice). Pertinent epidemiologic and clinical features of viral hepatitis A and B are seen in Table 8. Liver biopsy shows a characteristic histologic picture but does not distinguish between the two diseases.[39] Occasionally, other viruses such as yellow fever, herpes simplex, infectious mononucleosis and cytomegalic disease have been incriminated in the pathogenesis of viral hepatitis.

B. VIRAL HEPATITIS A AND B

Historically, hepatitis A was regarded to be an enteric infection spread by fecal-oral contact with contaminated milk or shellfish as vehicles. In contrast, hepatitis B was considered to be infectious only following the innoculation of virus-infected blood or blood products. Usually contracted by the parenteral route, recently it was found that hepatitis A may also be spread by infected blood.[324] Hepatitis B infection can be the consequence of ingesting contaminated foodstuffs or water and is transmitted by oral as well as parenteral routes.[249,315,463] In the blood of an Australian aborigine infected with hepatitis B virus, an antigen was first identified and designated as Australia antigen.[47] The frequency of distribution of Australia antigen is low in the normal population in North America and Europe, more prevalent in people living in the tropics and Southeast Asia, and among patients with Down's syndrome, leukemia and leprosy.[46,196,464] Although these diseases have distinct clinical, immunologic, and epidemiologic features (Table 8), the specific diagnosis is dependent on the presence or absence of the responsible antigen.

Before clinical symptoms develop, a virus-like particle 27 nm in diameter has been identified in the stool of hepatitis A patients. Hepatitis A antigen can be measured quantitatively. The virus survives 56°C for 30 min, but is inactivated following a 1-min exposure to 98°C.[241,325] Hepatitis A is probably a RNA virus since it is destroyed by ribonuclease. An antibody is produced against the antigen and is present in the serum during the resolution of the disease. The virus disappears from the stool as a consequence of anti-HAV production which appears in the serum initially as IgM and later as IgG. This IgG persists for a long time and confers immunity against subsequent viral attacks.

In the development of viral hepatitis immunologic mechanisms appear to play a significant role. Among the hepatitis viruses (hepatitis A, hepatitis B, or other viruses), the immunologic features associated with hepatitis B virus infection have been studied extensively. Two phases have been distinguished in the course of chronic hepatitis B infection. In the early replicative phase, the hepatitis B virus DNA in episomal form reacts with the hepatocyte nuclei and infectious viral particles are formed. Simultaneously hepatitis B core antigen (HB^{c}Ag) is produced and becomes detectable in serum. This replicative phase is associated with chronic active hepatitis. In the later, nonreplicative phase, the hepatitis B virus DNA is in integrated form and anti-HB^c and noninfectious hepatitis B surface (HB^{s}Ag) antigens are present in the serum. This nonreplicative phase of the virus is accompanied by inactive liver disease. Hepatitis B virus is not cytotoxic, but leads to immunologically mediated liver injury. Cytotoxic T cells are formed and their action is directed against the core antigen. The cytotoxic action of T cells is expressed on the hepatocyte membrane resulting in liver cell necrosis. Differences in the progress and severity of the chronic hepatitis may depend partly on the modulatory factors which include circulating antibodies to HB^{c}Ag, immune mediators, and lymphoid cells.

Electron microscopic studies revealed that hepatitis B antigen exists in the form of three distinct particles that can be aggregated by specific hepatitis B antibodies and thus share a common surface antigen (HB^{s}Ag)[396] The most numerous HB^{s}Ag particles are spherical, 20 nm in diameter. Larger, more complex double-membraned complete virions are present, measuring 40 to 45 nm in diameter with a 28 nm central core surrounded by an inner membrane 2 nm thick. The inner core of the larger particles, also known as Dane particles, is synthesized in the nuclei of the affected liver cells. Dane particles contain double-stranded DNA, DNA-polymerase, and core antigen (HB^{c}Ag). Occasionally, tubular or filament forms are found in the serum with varying length from 22 to 30 nm in diameter and 100 to 700 nm long. These particles are almost entirely built from excess surface antigen. The surface antigen is present in the serum before the first clinical symptoms are apparent and persists through the whole course of the disease. The incubation period is 43 to 180 d. Administration of contaminated blood or blood products often causes hepatitis B, and this is why it has been named serum or posttransfusion hepatitis. Other clinical procedures such as dialysis and organ transplantation procedures unintentionally may also lead to this disease.[137,404]

The antibody to the core antigen (HB^{c}Ab) rises in the serum at the onset of the acute disease and gradually decreases to undetectable levels after 1 to 2 years. The antibody to the surface antigen (HB^{s}Ab) is present during the resolution of the illness and in the convalescent period and persists for a long time providing immunity to reinfection. When the disease abates, the surface antigen disappears from the serum. If this antigen does not develop, the disease will not resolve and the patient will remain a carrier with persisting HB^{c}Ab and HB^{s}Ab serum levels. The occurrence of carrier state is about 5 to 10% in North America. A high percentage of these patients develop chronic active liver disease.[462] Since the duration of the carrier state is unknown, chronic carriers also represent serious health hazards to the population. Persons who have had hepatitis should not be considered as blood donors.

C. OTHER HEPATITIS-CAUSING VIRUSES

A number of viruses have been implicated in hepatitis. Yellow fever is a viral disease affecting many systems in the body, mainly the liver and kidneys. The virus is an arbovirus (arthropod-borne) and carried by mosquitoes as intermediate hosts. This disease is endemic in Central and South America and tropical Africa. In most instances, yellow fever is mild and can go unnoticed. The incubation period is 3 to 6 d followed by a sudden clinical attack of chills, fever, headache, backache, and prostration. Several days later jaundice develops, indicating liver involvement, and proteinuria appears, associated with kidney disease. In 7 to 10 d, the symptoms diminish and the patients recover. Mortality rate is usually 5 to 10% and may be higher during an epidemic. In fatal cases, midzonal necrosis is extensive in the liver, and the kidneys show extensive tubular damage and necrosis.

The Epstein-Barr virus is a common cause of hepatitis and is probably related to the development of infectious mononucleosis. In this disease, the liver is involved, with pathologic changes resembling those of infectious hepatitis. Only a few patients develop jaundice or other evidence of severe hepatocellular disease. The biochemical changes are similar to hepatitis A or B and the diagnosis is based on clinical findings which include a characteristic blood picture (monocytosis with aberrant cells), generalized splenomegaly and lymphadenopathy, and positive heterophil antibodies (Paul-Bunnell test). The recovery of Epstein-Barr virus infectious mononucleosis is slow. Herpex simplex virus occasionally produces a highly fatal generalized infection with prominent liver inflammation and necrosis in infants. The Coxsackie B virus group produces hepatitis occasionally.[46]

Posttransfusion hepatitis is also caused by viral agents. This condition is fairly common. The virus has not been identified, but it is distinct from hepatitis A or B virus. During the neonatal period, hepatitis develops occasionally by a number of viruses, including herpes simplex, rubella, and cytomegalovirus. In neonatal hepatitis, the virus can be isolated from the placenta or from liver biopsy. Viral antibody titers can also be used to confirm the diagnosis.

Some bacterial infections result in specific forms of hepatitis, including brucellosis and syphilis. Leptospiral infection leading to Weil's disease occurs rarely. In these cases the death rate is very high preceded by acute hepatitis, renal failure, and hemorrhage. Sepsis also causes secondary liver failure partly due to the direct action of bacteria and their toxins on the hepatocyte. Amebic infections can cause hepatocellular necrosis and large abscesses in the liver. Some parasitic diseases are also connected with hepatitis, such as malaria and toxoplasmosis in newborns.

D. BIOCHEMICAL FEATURES OF VIRAL HEPATITIS

The early symptoms of hepatitis A and B resemble those of influenza together with nausea, occasional abdominal pain, diarrhea, and vomiting. The onset of jaundice is followed by abdominal pain. The duration of jaundice is variable. In hepatitis A it usually lasts for 2 weeks, although about three quarters of the patients show no apparent jaundice (subclinical hepatitis), and thus the disease remains unrecognized as hepatitis. Hepatitis B is more severe; the jaundice persists for about 4 weeks with complete recovery lacking in 8 to 10% of the cases. Due to edema caused by the inflammatory process, the liver is often enlarged and splenomegaly occurs occasionally.

Mild hyperbilirubinemia is present and the urine is often dark containing conjugated bilirubin excreted by the kidney. The extracting ability of the liver to remove further bilirubin metabolites is impaired and thus urobilin appears in the urine. In 10% of viral hepatitis patients cholestasis develops. Due to cholestasis, bilirubin and bile acid excretion in the stool is decreased and fat elimination is increased. Steatorrhea is present in about half of the hepatitis cases. The duration of the biliary stasis varies from a few days to 4 weeks or longer. When urobilinogen reappears in the urine, it indicates the beginning of the recovery followed by the reversal of bilirubin elimination via the urine. Serum bilirubin levels also return to normal.

Pathological tissue changes are apparent in severe cases. Spotty necrosis occurs, and in more advanced cases widespread necrosis damages the architecture of the liver leading to impairment of hepatic function and release of parenchymal enzymes. Dramatic increases occur in aminotransferases in the serum ranging from 10 to 100 times of normal range. Elevated serum aminotransferases may be found in patients with only mild symptoms. These enzyme measurements can be used for screening hepatitis patients, for monitoring the status of the disease, and in epidemiological studies. Prodromal increased aminotransferase activity may occur. Since the amount of AST is greater in the liver, the serum levels of AST are always more elevated than that of ALT. ALT is cleared more slowly from the blood, and in most cases, shows the dominant changes. In chronic persistent hepatitis, ALT usually remains higher than AST. In case of postnecrotic cirrhosis, AST is the dominant enzyme. High levels of AST indicate continuing cirrhosis with unfavorable prognosis.

Biliary stasis may occur in viral hepatitis as the consequence of inflammation and edema and general destruction of the liver function. Necrotic debris sometimes plug the bile canaliculi followed by intrahepatic cholestasis with modest increases of serum enzymes such as aminotransferases, γ-glutamyltranspeptidase, leucine aminopeptidase, and 5'-nucleotidase. The levels of these enzymes are usually lower than those in extrahepatic obstruction or in primary intrahepatic cholestasis.

Destruction of the liver cells causes the release of other cellular constituents in the blood. In viral hepatitis, serum concentrations of iron and glucose are elevated. Iron is released from stores, and glucose is released from the breakdown of glycogen. In severe forms of the disease, hepatic glycogen stores are exhausted causing hypoglycemia. In hepatitis, the protein synthesis is also impaired. In acute liver disease, serum albumin may be reduced, but it never reaches pathologically low values. The serum level of blood coagulation enzymes is low, due to their much shorter half-life than albumin. Measurement of prothrombin concentrations (prothrombin time) shows abnormalities in acute hepatitis and cannot be restored by parenteral administration of vitamin K. The 2-h postprandial bile acid level or exogenous overload of organic anions such as BSP or indocyanine green can be used for establishing an overall estimation of disturbed hepatic function.

In hepatitis due to various viral agents other than hepatitis A or B, less reaction and necrosis is found in the liver. The increase of serum aminotransferases is usually only five to ten times greater than the normal range. The inflammatory response, however, may be quite pronounced, and giant cells are formed. Cholestasis may be present usually accompanied by moderate increases of alkaline phosphatase. In neonatal hepatitis, the serum concentrations of total bilirubin are very high.

X. CIRRHOSIS

This disease is due to chronic progressive destruction of liver cells and accompanied by diffuse fibrosis.[450] Elevated serum bile acids and increased collagen formation due to enhanced enzyme activity are significant landmarks.[153,427,478,513,551] The symptoms of liver cirrhosis have been well known for a long time, but the etiopathogenesis of cirrhosis still remains largely unresolved.[449] A considerable length of time is required to produce the final stages in man, indicating that the initial stages of this disease can never be precisely established. The results of animal experiments where the early phases may be seen can be extrapolated to the disease process in man. Biliary cirrhosis may be sex related.[481]

Cirrhosis is the end-stage of numerous diseases, including (1) viral infections such as epidemic infective hepatitis, homologous serum jaundice, and yellow fever, (2) bacterial infections such as pneumonia, septicemia, and coli-typhoid infections, (3) protozoal infections such as leptospirosis, malaria, and syphilis, and (4) chronic exposure to various toxic compounds including inorganic compounds, arsenicals, phosphorus, gold, alcohol, other organic solvents, sulphonamides, tannic acid, mushroom poisoning, and mycotoxins. These actions may be associated with chronic biliary obstruction, cholangiolytic hepatitis, (5) nutritional deficiencies such as Kwashiorkor, a condition of protein deficiency in childhood,

Laennec's cirrhosis, and malnutrition associated with alcoholism. Many experimental conditions, such as low protein containing diets, choline deficiency, and cystine deficiency, also cause cirrhosis; (6) several other circumstances are associated with this disorder such as anoxia, impaired copper metabolism,[520] severe infection, and shock.

Since the etiological factors of this disease are variable, it is not easy to understand how such a variety of causes can produce a similar end-stage condition. The interpretation of the development of cirrhosis is even more complicated since very similar experimental conditions may lead to distinct major types: diffuse hepatic cirrhosis and postnecrotic scarring and some minor types related to secondary liver damage.

Diffuse hepatic cirrhosis is produced by diets deficient in lipotropic choline, and it is always preceded by a long period of extensive fatty change. The nature of this factor in preventing fatty infiltration was first described as a result of fatty liver degeneration developed in dogs after pancreatectomy. Methionine was found to protect against the production of diffuse hepatic cirrhosis caused by choline deficiency. Choline and methionine are important methyl donors for lecithin biosynthesis. The progress of hepatic cirrhosis is therefore probably linked with the failure of phospholipid formation (Figure 32). This form of hepatic cirrhosis is associated with diffuse fine fibrous septa throughout the liver. Concomitantly, there is altered collagen and elastin synthesis.[570] Experimental diffuse cirrhotic livers show small nodules of fairly uniform size which correspond to multilobular cirrhosis in man. Poisoning with some powerful compound results in similar pathological features.

Postnecrotic scarring is the sequel to a massive necrosis of the liver. In experimental animals, low protein diets lead to this condition. Cystine, tocopherol, and certain antibiotics are essential protective factors. Methionine also provides protection, but this may be due to its conversion to cystine as precursor. In contrast to diffuse fibrosis, the characteristic pathological picture of postnecrotic scarring includes large irregular hyperplastic nodules often associated with liver atrophy. In man, a similar condition may follow an attack of acute hepatitis and as the consequence of prolonged inflammation.

Hepatic cirrhosis and fibrosis occur occasionally in association with heart failure, syphilis, cholangitis, malaria, and hemochromatosis. Cirrhosis is accompanied by a reduction of many metabolic functions of the liver.[222] The regular consumption of "bush teas" in Jamaica, Indonesia, and Africa causes an unusual type of cirrhosis. Senecio alkaloids present in the "bush teas" have been identified as the causative factors.[494,495] If the disease is present in childhood, the outcome may result in early death. The high incidence of liver carcinoma in Africa may be attributed to other "bush teas" or to trace amounts of aflatoxin contaminants in ground-nut meal. Perhaps the occurrence of liver carcinoma in other countries is also associated with mycotoxin contamination of the diet.

The major role of the liver in detoxification processes explains why this organ is often involved secondarily in various diseases. Some of the conditions which lead to secondary liver damage and subsequent cirrhosis are burns, dermatitis, diabetes mellitus, gastroenteritis, glandular fever, sickle cell anemia, meningitis, obesity, peptic ulcer, pneumonia, tuberculosis, rheumatoid arthritis, and thyrotoxicosis. In most conditions, the liver damage is coincidental, but in others it is intimately connected with the pathology of the disease indicating a causal relationship: diabetes leads to fatty infiltration. This may ultimately lead to cirrhosis, particularly in childhood.

XI. HEPATIC FAILURE

Massive hepatic necrosis leading to fulminant hepatic failure represents the most serious complication of viral hepatitis. Severe necrosis is often connected with severe lactic acidosis, hypoglycemia, failure of urea production, renal failure with increasing serum creatinine concentrations, encephalopathy, and high blood ammonia levels. Bleeding diathesis is present

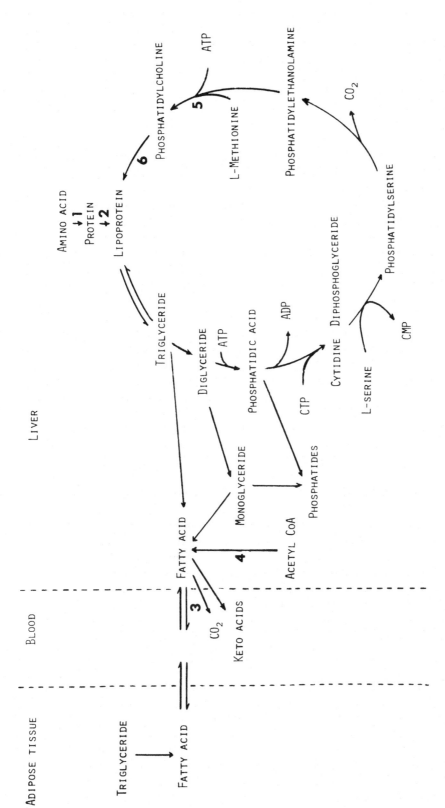

FIGURE 32. Mechanism of fatty liver production and subsequent cirrhosis. Deficiencies due to reduced amino acid intake (1) are associated with the inhibition of protein synthesis probably by interference with the endoplasmic reticulum. This is followed by a reduced lipoprotein synthesis (2) and accumulation of fat as triglyceride, due to lack of transport protein (3). Mitochondrial injury leads to impaired oxidation of fatty acid (4), and necrosis sets in. Lipotropic factors are important in the synthesis of phosphatidylcholine (5). In the absence of these factors, the synthesis of very low density lipoprotein becomes insufficient (6), and more chylomicron triglycerides remain in the liver rather than be transported into the blood. Reduced phospholipid synthesis causes an impairment of membrane bound enzymes, since phospholipids represent integral parts required for catalytic activity.

and may be aggravated by disseminated intravascular coagulation; the final outcome of liver failure may be respiratory or cardiac failure.

Chronic liver failure is characterized by hepatomegaly which tends to be firm and irregular in cirrhosis. Portal hypertension develops with many secondary manifestations such as enlarged spleen, dilatation of collateral veins in the esophagus, anterior abdominal wall and rectum, and ascites. Ascites occurs when portal hypertension develops due to reduced albumin synthesis and continued intake of salts. There is an associated decreased oncotic pressure and blood volume, resulting in excess secretion of aldosterone and antidiuretic hormone.

Many metabolic abnormalities develop including impaired appetite, disturbed absorption and digestion, and subsequent weight loss. Depletion of proteins leads to a failure of synthesis of many constituents such as albumin, clotting factors, and essential enzymes such as pseudocholine esterase, lecithin:cholesterol acyltransferase. Final consequences of impairment of protein metabolism are the defect of urea production in final stages.

Carbohydrate and fat metabolism are also modified. Detoxication processes are also disturbed. This represents a change in the induction of drug metabolizing enzymes followed by an impairment of Phase II components of the cytochrome P-450 system. Reduction of conjugation and altered protein binding cause a defective steroid elimination leading to hirsutism and gynecomastia.

Effects on several organs are associated with chronic hepatic failure, such as the central nervous, cardiovascular, and hematopoietic systems. Neuropsychiatric abnormalities are the major manifestations of this condition. These central nervous system abnormalities include increased sensitivity to antidepressant drugs, hypoxia and acid-base disturbances, and changes in ammonia metabolism. Cardiovascular effects include increased cardiac output, tachycardia, and increased peripheral vasodilatation. Bleeding or ascites causes hypovolemic shock with associated renal failure. The hematologic abnormalities include excessive red blood cell destruction connected with increased spleen weight. Erythrocyte formation is impaired due to defects in vitamin B_{12} and folate metabolism. Impaired synthesis of clotting factors stimulates an increased bleeding tendency.

XII. HEPATIC ACTIONS OF ALCOHOL

The major action of ethanol manifests in the liver cell which exerts an essential role in ethanol metabolism.[358,549] These effects include alcoholic hepatitis, alcoholic fatty liver, and alcoholic cirrhosis (Figure 33). There are, however, other organs which are involved in alcohol-induced disease and the onset and prognosis of many nonhepatic conditions such as gastritis, peptic ulcer, heart and arterial diseases, cancer of the larynx, stomach, mouth, and throat, are greatly influenced by the excessive consumption of alcoholic drinks. Alcoholic beverages contain ethyl alcohol and many other congeners. Some of the additional beverage congeners may be inherently toxic and other constituents are beneficial such as essential minerals, nutrients, and vitamins, as in wine and beer.[329,330,602]

A. ABSORPTION AND METABOLISM OF ALCOHOL

The absorption of alcohol is rapid, passing quickly through mucous membranes.[522] Alcohol vapors are also taken up directly by the lung. With an empty stomach the alcohol-water mixture is absorbed from the upper alimentary tract. With the ingestion of food, absorption from the stomach is delayed, and alcohol is taken up further down the gastrointestinal tract. The rate of absorption varies according to the concentration of alcohol in the given beverage. The higher concentration of alcohol is faster to be absorbed. There is also a difference between the absorption rate of pure alcohol and alcoholic drinks. A 12% aqueous solution of alcohol is absorbed faster than 4% as in beer. These differences are related to

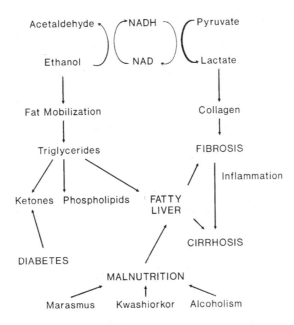

FIGURE 33. Possible mechanism suggesting the interrelation between ethanol oxidation, mitochondrial respiratory chain, and collagen synthesis in the liver. Some of the NADH produced in the oxidation of ethanol to acetaldehyde is used for shifting lactate synthesis by mitochondria. Increased acidity enhances collagen synthesis and production of fibrosis. Inflammatory conditions may be involved in the progression of fibrosis to cirrhosis. The effects of malnutrition and diabetes are indicated.

the nonalcoholic components of the respective beverage. Following absorption, alcohol diffuses very rapidly across capillaries and other membranes and ultimately, it is distributed uniformly throughout the body in the extra- and intracellular water. The time to attain equilibrium depends on the blood flow of the various tissues. Blood flow is fast in brain, heart, lungs, and kidneys and slow in skeletal muscle.

Two enzyme systems are involved in the metabolism of alcohol; one is cytosolic, and the other is microsomal. Alcohol and aldehyde dehydrogenases are cytosolic components mainly responsible for the first two steps of alcohol oxidation.[57,233,288,544] The second alcohol oxidizing enzyme complex is bound to the microsomal fraction.[36,549] Alcohol dehydrogenase is found mainly in the liver. This enzyme is the rate-limiting step in the metabolism of alcohol (Figure 34). In the human liver, there are three to seven active alcohol dehydrogenase isoenzyme fractions with variable activity.[280,565,610] The isoenzymes composition varies widely from and with different turnover rates, thus explaining the individual and ethnic variations. Aldehyde dehydrogenase is present in many tissues,[564] and several isoenzymes have been identified.[234,246,425,474] Animal experiments have shown that with alcohol pretreatment the activity of alcohol dehydrogenase increases. This adaptive change may be important in the development of tolerance in alcoholism.

The microsomal ethanol oxidizing system constitutes part of the drug metabolizing enzymes which detoxify drugs.[350,351,408] Normally, this system is capable of metabolizing and eliminating many drugs including barbiturates. This finding offers an explanation for the resistance of many alcoholics to drugs. However, upon excessive alcohol intake, the drug metabolizing system is utilized for the elimination of the alcohol overload, thus the ability to metabolize barbiturates is exhausted. This fact may explain the increased suscep-tibility of alcohol addicts to anesthetics and other drugs in the drunken state.

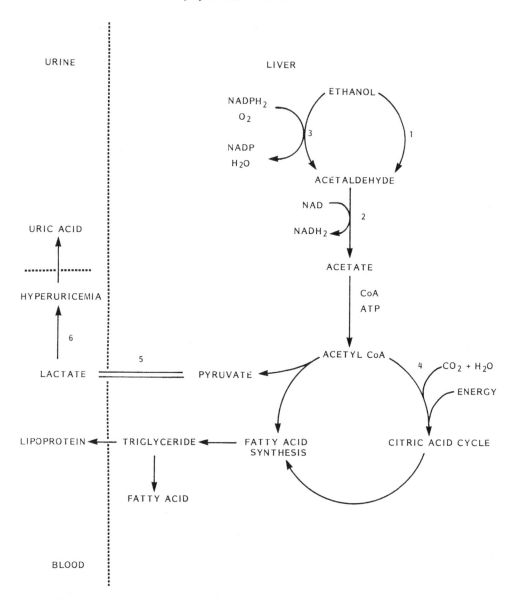

FIGURE 34. Metabolism of ethanol in the hepatocyte and its relationship with intermediary metabolism. Ethanol is metabolized by oxidation via cytosol enzymes alcohol dehydrogenase (1) and acetaldehyde dehydrogenase (2) to yield acetate. Endoplasmic reticular oxidation (3) is also essential.[111,349] Ethanol metabolism interferes with the citric acid cycle (4) and with the reduction of pyruvate to lactate (5). The latter leads to increased blood lactate level and possible aggravation of lactic acidosis. Hyperlactacidemia reduces urinary uric acid excretion leading to alcoholic hyperuricemia (6). This may represent a link between gout and alcoholism.[352] An overall result of ethanol action is an increased fatty acid and triglyceride synthesis and the production of fatty liver.

The potentiality of increased toxicity of hepatotoxins in alcoholics is also related to hypoxia producing a hypermetabolic state[273,275,398,548] and to the impairment of the drug metabolizing enzymes.[599] For example, a high level of alcohol exceeding the capacity of this enzyme system to detoxify and the simultaneous carbon tetrachloride may cause transient liver damage and general intoxication. Conversely, carbon tetrachloride induces hepatic damage, and the resulting dysfunction potentiates the action of alcohol.

An additional aspect of alcohol metabolism is connected with the breakdown of serotonin,

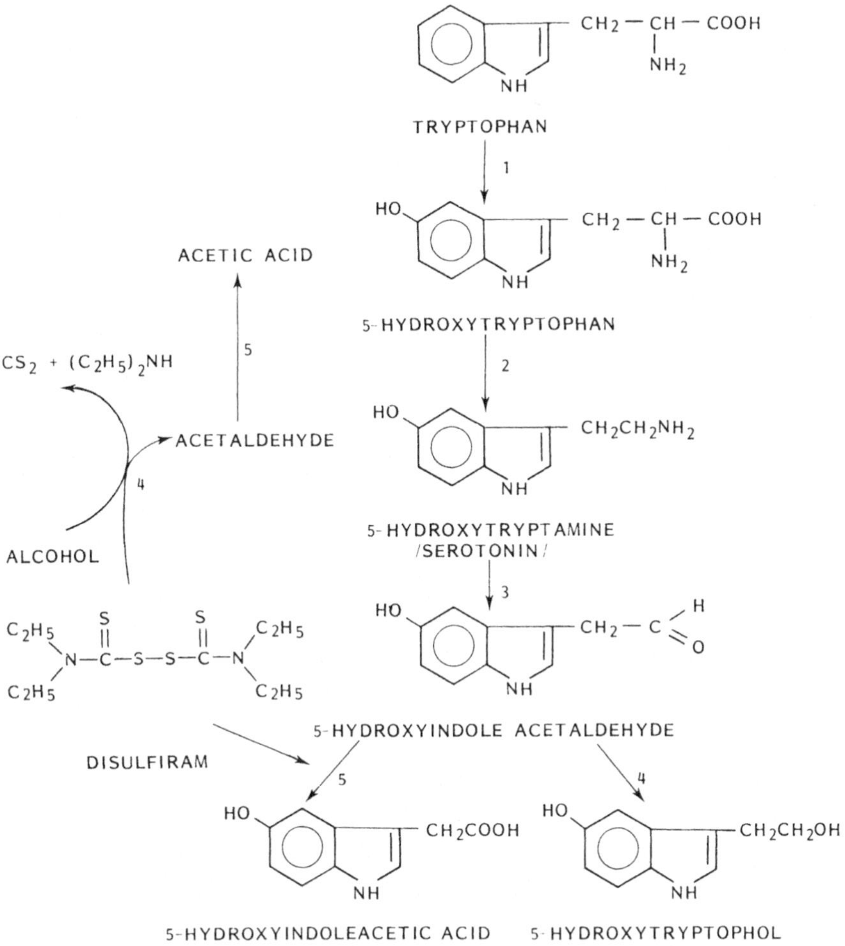

FIGURE 35. Relationship between the metabolism of serotonin and alcohol. Serotonin is derived from tryptophan by the action of several enzymes: hydroxylase (1), decarboxylase (2), and monoamine oxidase (3). Serotonin is further degraded by alcohol dehydrogenase (4) or aldehyde dehydrogenase (5). Antabuse (disulfiram) inhibits the activity of aldehyde dehydrogenase; it is slowly metabolized in the body. However, in the presence of alcohol, its metabolism is greatly accelerated.[4,165,199]

an important neurohumoral transmitter involved in the autonomic reactions of stress.[1,226,443,458] This compound is metabolized primarily to 5-hydroxyindole acetic acid (Figure 35). In this mechanism, both alcohol and aldehyde dehydrogenase enzymes take part. Drugs may affect serotonin function by altering intraneuronal uptake and release by storage granule membranes. Ethanol blocks the uptake of serotonin and inhibits the efflux of 5-hydroxytryptamine and 5-hydroxyindole acetic acid. Ethanol causes a reduction of 5-hydroxyindole acetic acid production, but since alcohol stimulates dehydrogenase activity, more serotonin is broken down to 5-hydroxytryptophane. This compound resembles the ethanol molecule and probably competitively blocks the ethanol induced behavioral effects. Therefore, more and more alcohol is necessary to achieve similar behavioral effects to that produced previously by lower doses. This may be a factor in accounting for acquired tolerance.

In the metabolism of norepinephrine, both alcohol and aldehyde dehydrogenases participate (Figure 36). This action affects behavior which depends on whether norepinephrine is increased at the receptor site associated with excitation or decreased and linked with

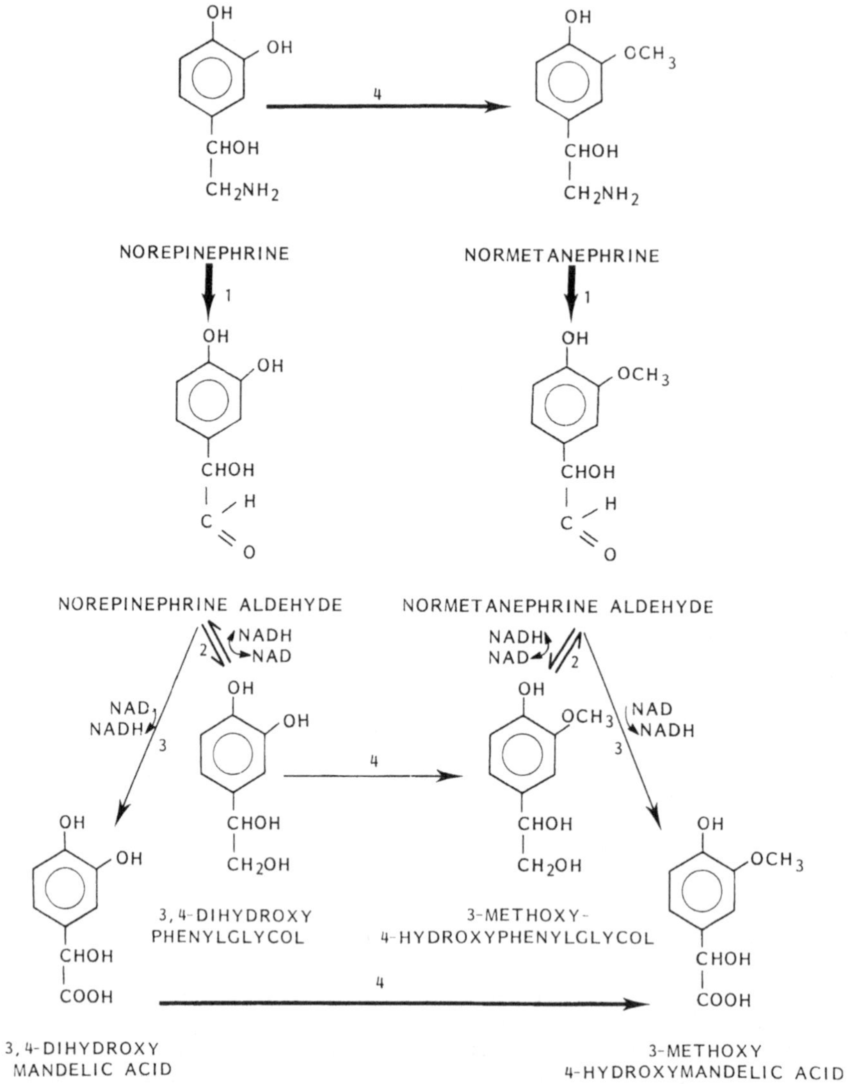

FIGURE 36. The effect of ethanol on the metabolism of norepinephrine. Enzymes participating in this pathway are monoamine oxidase (1), alcohol dehydrogenase (2), aldehyde dehydrogenase (3), and catechol O-methyl transferase (4). Ethanol inhibits norepinephrine reuptake by the neuronal membranes and brings about a shift in the product formation away from the oxidative toward the reductive pathway, resulting in a decreased 3-methoxy-4-hydroxymandelic acid and decreased glycol production. These processes cause an increased electrical reactivity of the brain and facilitate synaptic transmission which may be linked with the feeling of well-being and euphoria.[112-114]

sedation. The inactivation of norepinephrine is related to the neuronal membrane reuptake process which is blocked by alcohol, and therefore, the norepinephrine effect is prolonged.

Metabolic derangements in alcoholism are partly connected with the direct action of ethanol and acetaldehyde on the hepatocyte and other cells.[79,282,345,472,539,557,574,601] and partly with the lack of essential dietary components, vitamins, and cofactors.[109,575,614] The presence of elevated amounts of ethanol metabolites increases fat production and fat infiltration.[73,133,531] Acetaldehyde is regarded as the major factor of alcohol toxicity in association with dietary deficiencies.[77,78,82,85,185,232, 283,319,329,330,428,546,556,582,602,603]

Certain symptoms of hangover have been attributed to acetaldehyde, such as headache, profuse perspiration, nausea, and vomiting. This aldehyde has also been identified as the

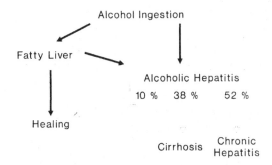

FIGURE 37. Major clinical forms of alcoholic liver damage. The percentage distribution of the various conditions is given.

principal mediator of the disulfiram-ethanol reaction. Acetaldehyde is responsible for the interference of alcohol with the pyruvate-stimulated oxidative phosphorylation in brain mitochondria, inactivation of coenzymes, and the production of hyperglycemia.[552] The mobilization of peripheral fat accompanying very large doses of ethanol may be mediated by acetaldehyde through an adrenergic mechanism.

Alcoholism affects many organs.[139,184,291,313,338,372,378,386,465,496,506,573] Among them, the liver is the most vulnerable to heavy drinking. Fat accumulates rapidly due to impairment of the endoplasmic reticulum function. Chronic exposure to alcohol leads to fragmentation of the endoplasmic reticulum and to subsequent damage to all organelles of the liver cell.[69,138,191,346,435] Eventually, large portions of the liver are lost and replaced by scar tissue (Figure 37). A major consequence of this chain of events is diffuse cirrhosis, in addition to the enhanced lipid synthesis due to hepatotoxic action.[347,354,357] This condition is associated with the dietary deficiency of lipotropic factors.[411] The reduced choline intake potentiates liver damage, always preceded by a long period of fatty change. The fatty infiltration in alcoholism can be prevented by lipotropic factors. Choline or methionine can protect against this type of fatty liver, probably serving as methyl donors.

Acute alcoholism elicits multiple actions on carbohydrate metabolism. It alters the metabolism, transport, and disposition of carbohydrate intermediates. Secondary influences are associated with changes of cofactor levels, hemodynamic modifications, and induction of hormone secretion.[277,530] Chronic exposure to alcohol brings about structural changes in the liver and pancreas. Abnormalities in hepatic carbohydrate hemostasis are related to the degree of liver damage.[561] Chronic alcoholics frequently show glucose intolerance and frank diabetes. Chronic pancreatitis probably contributes to these symptoms. People with this disorder have reduced insulin reserves.[277] However, the exaggerated insulin response to oral glucose does not reflect a deficiency in the function of the pancreatic β-cells.

Some symptoms of chronic alcoholism are due to the inadequate intake of essential nutrients.[82,85,232, 283,329,330,347,354,357,546,556,602,603] The unbalanced diet of the alcoholic leads to nutritional deficiencies which may progress to frank clinical manifestations. This may suggest that alcohol acts as a conditioning agent rather than the primary cause of the nutritional complications. The influence of dietary deficiency is seen particularly in cirrhosis and is quite common in Africa. On this continent, cirrhosis often occurs in the native population who live mainly on maize-meal, beans, and fermented cows milk. The clinical and pathological consequences are mostly due to vitamin deficiency (nicotinic acid and pyridoxine), subnormal intake of choline or other methyl donors, and subnormal protein intake. The low protein diet is probably responsible for the postnecrotic scarring which occurs in the liver of some alcoholic patients. (Figure 33).

Other organs affected by alcoholism include the brain, heart, and stomach.[13,205,472]

Alcohol exerts its immediate effects upon the central nervous system. Alcohol influences behavior first by its excitatory action on the nervous system, and second by acting at high doses as a central nervous system depressant. It is difficult to assess the effects of alcohol upon specific areas of the brain. However, recent works have shown that the initial action of alcohol is not primarily a depression of the cerebral cortex in general, but rather a selective action on some part of the structure of the reticular system. Small doses of alcohol may improve certain intellectual functions by impairment of the alerting function of the reticular system with subsequent disregard of distracting external stimuli.

Chronic alcoholism, however, evokes more serious changes in the central nervous system. After two or more drinks, judgement, memory, and cognitive functions obviously deteriorate. The more serious consequences of drunkeness are changes occurring in the blood and blood vessels. These changes affect the blood supply to the brain, causing the death of thousands of brain cells. The brain contains about 18 billion cells, but the cumulative effect of several years' drinking may result in irreversible damage because of the loss of neurons.

In some social drinkers the muscle fibers of the heart become flabby and weakened. This form of heart damage, or cardiomyopathy, is a complication of alcoholism. Alcoholism also has hemodynamic consequences.[274] Excessive drinking of concentrated spirits often produces an inflammation of the stomach lining and alcoholic gastritis, and sometimes bleeding occurs. A beer drinkers' epidemic in Quebec causing cardiomyopathy was first thought to be due to heavy beer drinking. Later, it was found that the heart muscle damage was caused by the large amounts of cobalt contaminating the beer rather than to the alcohol content.

B. ALCOHOLIC HEPATITIS

Excess drinking of alcoholic beverages over a long period combined with poor food intake is followed by various liver diseases in many people.[100,181,525] Among these conditions alcoholic hepatitis is fairly common with frequency of about one in ten alcoholics. Alcoholic hepatitis is a morphological entity characterized by an inflammatory reaction of polymorphonuclear leukocytes and hepatocellular necrosis.[406] The lesions are mainly localized in the centrolobular area, but in more severe cases it may be more diffuse across the liver lobule. Irregular clumps of hyalin, so-called Mallory bodies, may be present in damaged cells. The severity of the lesions is usually associated with the presence of Mallory bodies.[197] Similar structures have been, however, described in hepatocytes in other conditions such as primary biliary cirrhosis,[380] hepatocellular carcinoma,[304] following griseofulvin treatment,[123] and in patients who had bypass operations for morbid obesity.[238]

The pathogenesis of alcoholic hyalin is not known, but there are experimental conditions where hyalin bodies can be produced by agents which interfere with protein synthesis. Immune reactions are involved in the pathogenesis of alcoholic liver injury and hyalin formation.[189] Typical alcoholic hyalin can be found in patients with jaundice, fever, ascites, and hepatomegaly, but it is also associated with nonspecific conditions.[33] Generally, severe clinical symptoms are usually associated with severe histological changes.

The mechanism of alcoholism leading to hepatic necrosis has not been fully elucidated. A variety of causes are involved, such as toxic effects of acetaldehyde,[552] consequences of lesions occurring in mitochondria,[482] endoplasmic reticulum,[307] and microtubules,[389] and metabolite damage due to fat and proteins accumulation and subsequent swelling of the hepatocytes.[271,308,313,537]

Several tests can be applied for the diagnosis of alcoholic hepatitis.[592] Due to the characteristic histological lesions, liver biopsy represents the most accurate way of determining the extent of liver cell necrosis. This is, however, not always practical and the leakage of liver enzymes into the blood, especially transaminases, is used commonly to determine the degree of hepatic damage. Serum transaminases are only moderately elevated

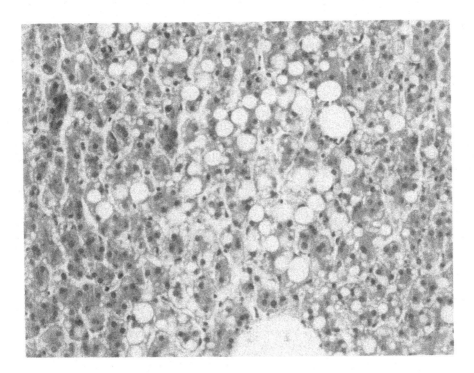

PLATE 3.   Fatty change of the liver showing large and small vacuoles where lipids were deposited.

in alcoholic hepatitis in contrast to viral hepatitis.[292] Alkaline phosphatase is often increased and leukocytosis also occurs. Elevated bilirubin, low serum albumin, and prolonged prothrombin time may be present to a variable degree. Some correlation has been reported between γ-glutamyltranspeptidase and liver cell necrosis.[604] Increases of γ-glutamyltranspeptidase from nonhepatic origin are also common, and even in alcoholics the increased serum levels may be due to microsomal induction by ethanol.[190,272,285] A recent study indicated that glutamate dehydrogenase reflects more accurately the degree of cell necrosis underlying alcoholic hepatitis.[567] This is a highly liver-specific enzyme and derives from mitochondria mainly located in centrolobular areas.[229]

C. ALCOHOLIC FATTY LIVER

Milder forms of alcoholic liver disease are characterized by the accumulation of excess fat in hepatocytes, representing the so-called fatty liver.[74] Lipid deposition originates from three major sources: (1) dietary lipids transported in the blood stream as chylomicrons, (2) adipose tissue lipids transferred from adipocytes to the liver as free fatty acids, and (3) lipids produced in the liver from basic precursors. Fats derived from these sources can accumulate in the liver as a consequence of various metabolic disturbances such as (1) decreased hepatic metabolism with decreased oxidative processes, (2) increased hepatic synthesis of lipids, (3) decreased synthesis of lipid carrier proteins, (4) decreased elimination of lipids by decreased hepatic release of lipoproteins due to reduced receptor synthesis, (5) increased mobilization of peripheral fat depots, and (6) increased uptake of circulating lipids into the liver. The mechanism of fatty liver production is illustrated in Figure 33. A case illustrating fatty change of the liver is shown on Plate 3.

When ethanol is given with lipid-containing diets, there is increased accumulation of lipids in the liver from dietary fatty acids. When ethanol is consumed with low-fat diets, endogenously synthesized fatty acids accumulate in hepatocytes.[357] Some of these actions are connected with the metabolism of ethanol. Ethanol actually competes with fatty acids as normal fuel for hepatic mitochondria. This results in a decreased fatty acid oxidation, and fatty acids derived from adipose tissue depots also accumulate in hepatocytes when the ethanol concentration is high in the cells. In this initial stage, the transport mechanism that eliminates lipids into the blood stream is through the release of lipoproteins and is activated by ethanol. In addition to the functional changes, chronic alcoholism causes more persistent damage to mitochondria, associated with functional abnormalities as reflected in reduced fatty acid oxidation. In short-term human investigations, ethanol intake produced a fall in the level of circulating free fatty acids by affecting fat release from adipose tissue.[284] Moreover, free fatty acid turnover was reduced and circulating glycerol decreased.[161] The effect of ethanol on the mobilization of free fatty acids is mediated by acetate which is actually the end-product of ethanol metabolism in the liver.[568] With progression of the liver injury, lipoprotein secretion falls below normal levels, and this altered lipoprotein secretion aggravates liver damage even further.

The development of alcoholic fatty liver is influenced by dietary factors[354,357] In normal volunteers given measured amounts of alcohol, more fatty change developed with normal fat diets than with low-fat diets. Replacement of triglycerides containing long-chain fatty acids with triglycerides containing medium-chain fatty acids showed that the ability of alcohol to produce liver fat accumulation is markedly reduced.

Lipotropic factors (choline and methionine) and protein influence alcohol-induced steatosis. In growing rats, the lack of protein or lipotropic factors produces fatty liver.[38] Primates, however, are less susceptible to protein and lipotrope deficiency than rodents.[257] Treatment of patients suffering from alcoholic liver disease with choline is ineffective.[483] The reason for this discrepancy is that primate and human liver contain very little choline oxidase activity as compared to rodent liver. Protein deficiency also affects the liver. In children, protein deficiency leads to steatosis. In volunteers, however, excess protein cannot prevent fat accumulation brought about by ethanol consumption.[355] Ethanol impairs methionine conservation in circumstances of protein deficiency by increasing the activities of hepatic cystathionine synthetase and 5-methyltetrahydrofolate-homocysteine methyltransferase.[178] In baboons and alcoholic patients, the alcohol-induced liver injury is associated with increased branched-chain amino acids and γ-amino-n-butyric acid. Following intestinal bypass for obesity, the absorption of dietary protein is reduced and plasma γ-amino-n-butyric acid branched-chain amino acids and essential amino acids, such as threonine, lysine and phenylalanine, are decreased, whereas nonessential amino acids such as glycine and serine are elevated.[413] In alcoholics characteristically, the plasma level of γ-amino-n-butyric acid is enhanced.[508]

D. ALCOHOLIC CIRRHOSIS

The majority of deaths due to alcoholism is associated primarily with liver cirrhosis. Typical cellular changes characterizing alcoholic cirrhosis are shown on Plate 4. Irreversible cirrhosis is characteristic of the end-stage of alcoholic liver disease in contrast to the fully reversible fat accumulation which can occur after a few days of excessive alcohol drinking. In man, the progression of fatty liver to cirrhosis may take from 5 to 20 years. In the development of this condition, several transitional stages occur between fatty liver and end-stage cirrhosis. Extensive necrosis and polymorphonuclear cell infiltration are characteristic precursor lesions of cirrhosis. Delineation at such a stage is not always possible. Extensive hepatitis is less common than fatty liver or cirrhotic changes as determinants of irreversible liver injury. Milder forms of necrosis and inflammation are also associated with striking lesions of mitochondria and endoplasmic reticulum.

In addition to fat accumulation, changes in deposition and nature of proteins are also frequent, especially in early stages.[24,25,55] Protein accumulation contributes to hepatomegaly. Although enhanced formation of protein is manifest in these circumstances, the major proteins deposited in hapatocytes are cytosolic and mainly transport proteins, such as albumin and

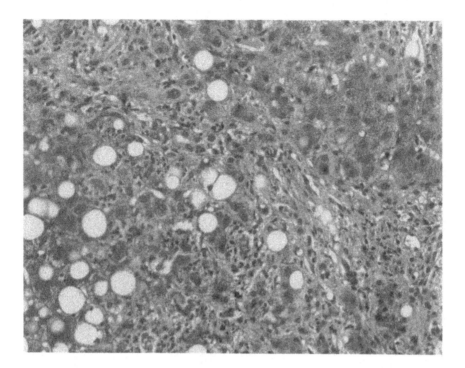

PLATE 4. In alcoholic cirrhosis, regenerating nodules of liver cells are separated by wide fibrous bands. Large vacuolar fatty change is present.

transferrin. Decreased hepatic microtubulin is connected with the reduced export of proteins from the liver. Ethanol metabolites such as acetaldehyde, a known hepatotoxicant, is probably responsible for this effect. Protein retention may contribute to the ballooning effect of hepatocytes, a common morphological change observed in alcoholic liver injury.[331]

Lipoprotein release is also altered in the liver of alcoholics with or without cirrhosis.[367] Chronic alcohol administration causes hyperlipidemia in volunteers.[353] After 2 to 3 weeks, with progressing liver injury, however, blood lipid content declines as a consequence of a fall in lipoprotein output. Peak serum lipid values are associated with the stage of fatty change. During the subsequent stages of steatosis and chronic hepatitis, serum lipids are progressively reduced, predominantly in triglyceride and cholesterol fractions. In well-established cirrhosis serum lipoprotein levels are low[28] or even absent, and abnormal lipoproteins may be present.[18,486] Progressive deterioration of liver function, including failure of lipoprotein synthesis and release into the blood, is responsible for the aggravation of fat accumulation and the onset of swelling. In turn, swelling and stagnation of metabolism are connected with necrosis and cell death.

E. HEPATIC FIBROSIS

Hepatic fibrosis representing excess formation of connective tissue in the liver is a widespread alteration of metabolic processes and occurs in acute and more often in chronic liver disease.[448] In many instances, the morphologic manifestation of connective tissue alteration has little functional significance due to the large reserve capacity of the liver. There are, however, conditions where hepatic fibrosis compromises liver function and represents a defect of metabolic homeostasis followed by the possible progression of fibrosis into cirrhosis. Fibrosis is the most common consequence of alcoholic fatty liver, hepatitis, and cirrhosis.[399] This condition is mainly responsible for cirrhotic disfiguration of the organ and the resulting clinical aberrations. The build-up of collagen, normally only 1 to 2% of the total liver mass, can increase several fold in alcoholic liver disease.[397]

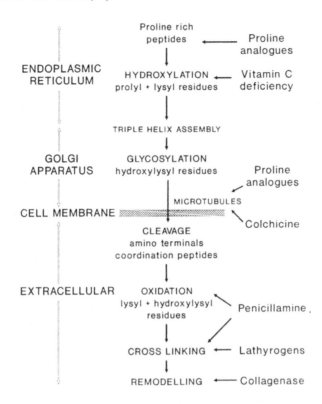

FIGURE 38.   Scheme of the intracellular collagen biosynthesis, extracellular assembly of collagen fibers, and the
possible site of action of various antifibroblastic agents.

Fibrosis used to be thought of as a simple collapse of the preexisting reticulin framework
following hepatocyte necrosis, but now it is believed to be the result of a dynamic process.
Connective tissue is essentially made up of scleroproteins embedded in a ground substance
or matrix. Scleroproteins include elastin and several collagens.[344] Five main types of collagen
are now characterized and include collagen I, II, and III, all rich in proline and lysine.
These are the interstitial collagens, displaying a characteristic periodicity due to their stag-
gered triple helices in tissue. Collagen IV and V species are basement membrane components
with no observable periodicity. Collagens I and III are present in vessel walls of the central
and portal canals with collagen III representing a matrix in which collagen I can form both
during normal development and under pathological conditions. Basement membrane collagens IV and V (V to a lesser extent) interact with ground substance glycoproteins to form
a three-dimensional network. This is not visible under normal circumstances, but only when
they are increased around bile ducts, ductules, and portal capillaries, in disease conditions.[348,612]

Various biochemical events occur in collagen biosynthesis (Figure 38). The complex
molecular structure of collagen determines its unique supporting function. The rough endoplasmic reticulum is the intracellular site of procollagen synthesis, a precursor containing
proline-rich peptide chains.[87] This process is dependent on the free proline pool which is
increased in chronic liver injury. The next step is hydroxylation of proline and lysine already
bound in the peptide chain. The procollagen moves then to the Golgi apparatus where
glycosidation of the lysyl radicals takes place. Two a_1 chains and one a_2 chain are assembled,
and the procollagen leaves the cell in triple helix form with the aid of microtubules. After
the extrusion of the collagen molecules from the cell, amino terminal coordination peptides
are cleared, and the fiber is formed. In further steps, specific lysyl and hydroxylysyl residues

are oxidized to aldehydes, and the maturation and growth of the fibrils to fibers leads to stable intermolecular cross-linkages. Vitamin C and copper are involved in collagen synthesis. In alcoholic hepatitis, the collagen turnover is reversibly enhanced.[399] Procollagen proline hydroxylase is elevated and the urine hydroxyproline content is increased. A variety of agents influence collagen production including proline analogs, penicillamine, colchicine, lathyrogens, and vitamin C deficiency (Figure 38).[448]

The accumulation of collagen represents a sign of fibrosis and cirrhosis. In simple fatty liver it is barely detectable, but when collagen deposition is visible by light microscopy, usually it appears around the central vein first, and so-called perivenular sclerosis is produced.[434] It is possible that alcohol exerts a direct effect on collagen metabolism, independent of inflammation or necrosis. It was suggested that the liver injury may be a consequence of malnutrition rather than the alcohol per se. In experiments carried on in baboons given doses of alcohol comparable to that of alcoholics, it was indicated that the alcohol itself resulted in the development of typical complications observed in alcoholics. Also, an adequate diet was judged not sufficient to prevent the development of lesions in the liver of alcoholics unless alcohol consumption was controlled.[566] This effect could be due to alcohol producing malabsorption. Nutritional deficiencies potentiated the effects of alcohol and dietary cholesterol drastically altered the development of cirrhosis.[433]

Morphological studies have shown that laminin and fibronectin are significantly enriched around hepatocytes in alcoholic steatosis. Laminin is a rigid, elongated cross-shaped glycoprotein of the basement membrane. Fibronectin is a U-shaped glycoprotein surrounding normal hepatocytes which plays a role in binding to macromolecules, cellular adhesion, and in fibroblast chemotaxis. When this fibrotic stage has been reached, portal tracts and septa show diffuse deposition of laminin and basement membrane collagens IV and V. This feature is highly reflective of active fibroplasia with subsequent deposition of collagens I and III around the hepatocytes and collagenization of Disse's space. This anatomical change then results in poor exchange between hepatocytes and blood, further disrupting the integrity of the hepatocyte.

Breakdown of collagen is increased in early fibrosis, but reduced in later stages. However, collagen still remains susceptible to collagenase actions suggesting that a faulty breakdown and not excessive synthesis is the cause of increased formation of connective tissue in hepatocytes. The process of fibroplasia is elusive. Hepatocellular necrosis was considered the main stimulus, but it now appears that lymphocytes and granulocytes can also stimulate fibroplasia due to the release of mediators. In addition, hepatocellular enlargement may also stimulate fibroplasia by increasing pressure. Experimental hepatocellular injury can lead to attraction and proliferation of cells, probably by chemotactic mechanisms. During the process, fat storing cells are possibly transformed to fibroblasts and macrophages.

Fibroplasia can be divided into three biochemical processes: synthesis, maturation, and degradation.[344,612] When baboons and rats were fed ethanol as 36% of the calories in an adequate diet for 2 months, the incorporation of ^{14}C-proline into collagen by liver slices was increased.[161] Similarly, serum proline and hydroxyproline concentrations were high in patients with alcoholic hepatitis and cirrhosis.[348] The greater collagen synthesis after ethanol ingestion could be due to more lactic acid, resulting from the higher $NADH/NAD^+$ ratio found after ethanol oxidation. Lactic acid inhibits proline oxidation *in vitro*,[131,337] while it simultaneously activates collagen prolyl hydroxylase in fibroblasts.[397] The enhancement of this enzyme activity or its substrate (proline) could also promote collagen synthesis. Collagen prolyl hydroxylase activity is especially increased in liver biopsy specimens of patients with alcoholic hepatitis, but not in those with fatty liver or cirrhosis.[322,612] In addition, any further build-up of lactate is known to inhibit proline oxidase which results in increased free proline and hydroxyproline pool size,[131,547] playing a key role in collagen synthesis and regulation.

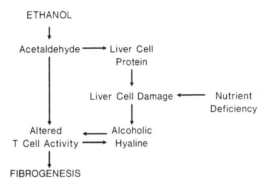

FIGURE 39.   Interrelationship between alcoholic hyaline, T-cell
activity, and fibrogenesis.

F. ALCOHOL EFFECTS ON IMMUNE LIVER DISEASE

An increase in the overall immune response brought by the onset of alcoholic liver
disease may play a significant role in the further deterioration of hepatic function along with
fibrogenesis.[35,452] Patients with alcoholic liver disease exhibit depressed cell-mediated immune responses to foreign antigens, and increased responses to liver tissue components via
humoral or cellular pathways.[298,397,432,613,615] The depressed cell-mediated response is due
primarily to fewer circulating T lymphocytes, and B lymphocytes remain relatively unaltered.
Conditions such as malnutrition, diarrhea, and vitamin deficiencies (i.e., folic acid and
pyridoxine) are largely responsible for the immune effects. In addition, hypergammaglob-
ulinemia is common in patients with alcoholic hepatitis.[547] High levels of antibodies against
dietary protein and Gram-positive bacteria have also been found. Alcoholic hyalin antigen
appears early in the serum during the course of alcoholic hepatitis (Figure 39).[615] When
drinking is discontinued, the level of this antigen decreases while alcoholic hyalin antibody
appears. Serum IgA in alcoholic cirrhotic patients binds to necrotic hepatocytes containing
alcoholic hyalin. The deposition of immune complexes may play a significant role in hepatocellular damage. The decreased number of circulating T cells in alcoholic hepatitis may
be due to their infiltration and subsequent accumulation in the liver.[397] In addition, the
circulating lymphocytes undergo transformation to fibroblasts and release migration inhibition factor (MIF) in the presence of either alcoholic hyalin or autologous liver.[401] The
synthesis and release of MIF can be enhanced by acetylaldehyde exposure. High levels of
MIF cause monocytes to remain in the liver and transform into cells with a high degree of
phagocytosis potential, thus causing more hepatocellular damage. The cytotoxicity is induced
by a nonrossetting lymphocyte [B or K (null) lymphocyte]. It has also been shown that
alcoholic hyalin by itself has no cytotoxic potential, but when it is added to serum, it becomes
strongly chemotactic, suggesting that this may be due to the interaction with antibodies.[397]
In addition, suppressor T cell activity which plays a key role in dampening an overreactive
immune response is significantly reduced in lymphocytes of patients with active alcoholic
liver disease, again supporting an explanation for this hyperactivity. A summary of both
humoral and cellular immunological abnormalities of alcoholic liver disease is given in Table
9.

G. ALCOHOL EFFECTS ON ALIMENTARY TRACT CANCER

Excess alcohol intake is connected with various types of cancer, mainly esophagus,
pharynx, larynx, and, to a lesser extent, liver. There is no evidence that absolute ethanol
per se is carcinogenic; some alcoholic beverages may be carcinogenic by containing some
carcinogens. Possible carcinogens in beverages are fusel oil,[198] some aromatic hydrocar-

TABLE 9
Immunological Abnormalities in Alcoholic Liver Disease

Humoral mediated immunity	Expression of disease		
	Fatty liver	**Alcoholic hepatitis**	**Alcoholic cirrhosis**
B lymphocytes (peripheral blood)	N	N	N
Ig-forming cells (spontaneous activation)	—	I	I
IgA serum level	N or I	I	I
Secretory IgA, serum level	—	—	I
IgE serum level	—	I	I
IgG serum level	N or I	N	I
IgM serum level	N or I	I	I
IgD serum level	N	N	I
Anti-liver membrane Ab	I	I	I
Anti-alcoholic hyaline Ab	—	N, I	I
Anti-smooth muscle Ab	—	I	I
Anti-liver specific lipoproteins	—	I	—
Anti-fibroblast Ab	—	—	I
Immune complexes	N	—	—
2 Cell-mediated immunity			
T lymphocytes, liver	N	D	N, D
Suppressor T-cell activity	—	N, D	D
Lymphocytes sensitization to:			
Liver extract	—	I	N
Alcoholic hyaline	N	N, I	N
Liver-specific antigen	—	I	—
Cytotoxicity to:			
Autologous hepatocytes	N, I	I	N
Xenogenetic hepatocytes	N	I	N, I
Chang cells	N	I	N
Lymphocytes stimulation			
by phytohemagglutinin	D	D	D
by concanavalin A	D	—	—

Note: I = increased; D = decreased; N = normal.

bons,[328] or nitrosamines. The mechanism of primary liver cancer associated with alcohol consumption has not been established. There is a close correlation between cancer and cirrhosis of the liver,[306] and 60 to 90% of primary liver cancers have a history of excessive alcohol intake.[80] Liver cancer may result from nutritional deficiencies that are commonly associated with alcoholism.[336] The diet of a chronic alcoholic is nutritionally inadequate. Cancers of the upper alimentary tract also occur most commonly in individuals who do not eat a balanced diet.[499] Alcohol consumption can lead to impaired absorption of nutrients and vitamins.[579] Decreasing vitamin A levels are particularly important since this vitamin participates in the regulation of epithelial cell differentiation.[569]

According to a World Health Organization's survey on alcoholism and cancer, it was found that an association exists between the excessive consumption of alcoholic beverages and cancer of the mouth, larynx, and esophagus.[600] In heavy drinkers, the risk of developing cancer of the mouth is tenfold higher than in nondrinkers. Subjects who drink heavily often smoke heavily.[180] A risk association was established between alcohol and tobacco in tumors of the oral cavity larynx and esophagus, sites that come directly in contact with alcohol.[479] Actually the risk for heavy drinkers who smoke to develop oral cancer is about 15-fold greater than for nondrinkers and nonsmokers.[164,188] It seems that alcohol plays a role more important than smoking in the development of esophagus cancer, whereas smoking is more strongly associated with cancer of the pharynx and mouth.[180] Alcohol may affect other sites where cancer develops, such as the pancreas, stomach, and colon.[70,254,596]

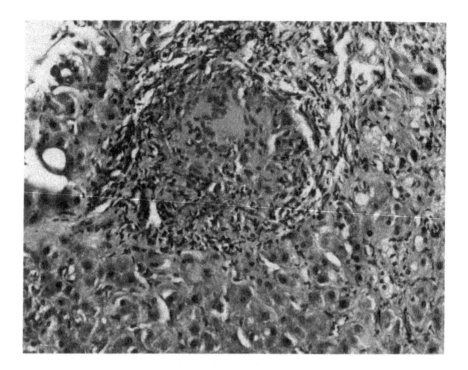

PLATE 5.   In granulomatous hepatitis, increased amounts of fibrous tissue and a well-defined granuloma composed of epitheloidal cells and multinucleated giant cell are seen in the portal area.

XIII. LIVER CANCER

Liver neoplasia in man is not one of the most common forms of cancer.[239,305,361,417] An example for primary hepatocellular carcinoma is seen on Plate 5. A close association exists between exposure to hepatitis B and liver cancer; the exact role of the virus in the pathogenesis is not known. The possible importance of other agents such as mycotoxins or parasites is uncertain. The pattern of tumor development in man and the steps required in the production of cancer in experimental animals with chemical carcinogens appear to be similar. Experimental studies established various steps in tumor formation such as initiation and promotion. In the initiation phase, many processes take place indicating the importance of the carcinogen metabolism into active compounds, the nature of these active forms, the interaction of carcinogens with DNA and other cellular constituents, the modifications of DNA structure and function, and the repair of DNA alterations. Some of these steps in the pathogenesis of hepatocellular cancer are physiological and represent adaptive responses to the environmental chemicals involved in the process.[155]

There are age differences in the onset of primary liver cancer and in the regeneration of nodular hyperplasia in the liver.[409,410,529] The geographic distribution of primary liver cancer or hepatoma is also uneven. It is not frequent in North America or in Europe as compared to secondary metastatic cancer. It is particularly frequent in many African and Asian countries. The incidence rate in Mozambique, Africa is 107 people in contrast with the U.S. at 6 to 7 people and in Norway 1 person per 100,000 people.[134] Primary hepatocellular carcinoma is the leading malignant neoplasm in Taiwan, in Canada and the U.S., it is 22nd.[239] The increased frequency of hepatoma in China is blamed upon the infestation with the liver flukes *Clonorchis sinensis* or *Opisthorchis felineus*. These parasites get into the small bile ducts where they cause dilatations which are followed by liver damage contributing to cholangiocarcinoma. Hepatocellular carcinoma accounts for 70 to 90% of liver cancer in most parts of Asia free of liver fluke. It is considered therefore, that environmental carcinogens may represent an etiologically important contribution to the development of liver cancer.

Diagnosis of primary liver cancer is mainly based on clinical observations, X-ray, or liver scan. Hepatoma cells frequently contain bilirubin, possibly because they lose the ability to conjugate and excrete this pigment. Bilirubin is retained in the tumor cells since there is no connection with bile ducts to allow for normal flow. Cholangiocarcinomas do not show bile pigment. In the serum of many hepatoma patients α-fetoglobulin is found.[7,130] Hepatitis and cirrhosis patients do not have this protein. The finding of a positive test for α-fetoglobulin is of great diagnostic value. In some cases, severe metabolic abnormalities are found, including serious reductions of blood glucose, which are difficult to treat,[376] and large quantities of glucose are necessary to maintain the concentration near normal. In primary human liver tumor, enzyme changes can be detected. These include glutathione S-transferase and UDP-glucuronyltransferase,[489] glucose 6-phosphatase,[400] intestinal-type alkaline phosphatase,[609] ATP-ase,[179] thymidine phosphorylase,[318] prolyl hydroxylase,[51] and galactosyltransferase.[46] Aberrant porphyrin metabolism[560] and calcitonin[93] are also observed in hepatocellular carcinoma. Changes in aldolase isoenzyme pattern are found in human cancer.[16] Alterations in sex steroid receptor protein are connected with malignancy of liver tissue.[50,268]

Primary tumors frequently occur singly in the liver, and the detection of hepatic masses usually represents metastases, the primary tumor being from other organs (lung, gastrointestinal tract, breast, and many others). Liver metastases are the most common consequence of cancer with the exception of the lymph nodes in drainage areas where the frequency of secondary manifestations is equally great.[166] Extensive invasion and replacement of the liver tissue by metastatic tumor is usually asymptomatic with a few metabolic disturbances. A large proportion of the liver has to be replaced by the malignancy before jaundice or other signs of liver failure become apparent. Increased alkaline phosphatase activity in the serum represents one of the earliest biochemical changes. This finding has diagnostic importance. Elevated alkaline phosphatase activity without jaundice or other evidence of hepatocellular disease may strongly point to metastatic liver or bone tumor. Liver lectins are suggested as mediators for metastases.[562] Occasionally, blockage of one main intrahepatic bile duct by invasion or pressure by the tumor mass causes jaundice.

A. VIRAL HEPATITIS AND PRIMARY LIVER TUMOR

Epidemiologic studies have shown a strong correlation between hepatitis B virus infection and the development of hepatocellular carcinoma.[14,29,30-32,364,446,461] A relationship has also been found with related viruses.[451] Infection with hepatitis B virus may have several consequences. Transient infection can cause subclinical disease, anicteric hepatitis, acute icteric hepatitis, or fulminant hepatitis. Persistent infections may lead to chronic conditions, such as chronic persistent hepatitis, chronic active hepatitis, or postnecrotic cirrhosis. Any of these conditions may lead to liver neoplasia. There is, however, a long incubation period lasting from 20 to 40 years between the onset of persistent hepatitis B virus infection and the development of primary hepatocellular carcinoma.[356,365]

The virus-tumor association is supported by (1) common geographic distribution of high incidence of hepatocellular carcinoma and markers of hepatitis B viral infection in most countries;[356,365,461] (2) case-control studies have shown a higher frequency of hepatitis B virus surface antigen (HB$_S$Ag) among primary carcinoma patients;[581] and (3) excess HB$_S$Ag positivity is greater among mothers than fathers of primary carcinoma patients, indicating a direct transmission of the disease from the mother with later development of cancer in the child.[159,195,440] A Taiwan study shows that most primary liver carcinomas that arise from hepatitis B virus infections occur in infancy and childhood. (4) The relative risk of hepatitis B virus producing a HB$_S$Ag carrier state is inversely related to age.[29] (5) The incidence of hepatocellular carcinoma is considerably higher in males than in females throughout the world.

Molecular hybridization studies revealed the integration of hepatitis B virus DNA into one or a discrete number of sites in the vast majority of tumors as evidenced by the viral DNA sequence in the tumor DNA.[62,320,501] Each tumor displays a unique banding pattern of integrated hepatitis B virus DNA molecules suggesting monoclonal or oligoclonal origin of tumor cell preparations. In regions of the liver surrounding the tumor, integrated hepatitis B virus DNA is found with hybridization patterns identical or partly related to DNA present in the tumor cells.[502-504,516] Integration of hepatitis B virus DNA into unique or multiple sites has also been reported in the liver genome of hepatitis B carriers without the development of hepatocellular carcinoma.[61,231,296,320] Hepatitis B virus replicates through a reverse transcription mechanism,[502,503] but unlike many known RNA tumor viruses (retroviruses), a specific viral oncogene has not yet been identified as hepatitis B virus.

B. HEPATOCELLULAR CARCINOMA IN ALCOHOLICS

Liver cancer is fairly common and associated with cirrhosis in alcoholics.[103,278] Hepatocellular carcinoma also occurs in noncirrhotic alcoholics. Alcohol is considered as a cocarcinogen. In addition to the direct effects of ethanol, indirect consequences of malnutrition are associated with carcinogenesis. These include deficient intake of vitamins, riboflavin, pyridoxine, pantothenic acid, and essential trace metals. The effect of malnutrition in promoting cancer is very common. It is associated with oral, head, and neck cancer.[314,387,606] In these cases, deficiencies are reported in iron, zinc, thiamin, riboflavin, ascorbic acid, and vitamin A. Alcohol may cause malnutrition and influence the absorption, distribution, metabolism, storage, and elimination of various essential nutrients.

Specific nutritional deficiencies in alcoholics are involved in abnormal metabolic processes. Low serum carotene and vitamin A contents associated with impaired hepatic synthesis of retinol-binding protein have been found in alcoholics.[269,521] Vitamin A is essential in the differentiation of epithelial tissue and deficiency of this vitamin affects the induction of lung,[91,117] colon,[477] bladder,[88] and uterine cervix tumors.[86] Epidemiological surveys confirm these observations.

Experimental evidence shows the effect of riboflavin deficiency on skin tumors.[356] Pyridoxine deficiency occurs in alcoholics, probably attributable to the formation of acetaldehyde; pyridoxine derivatives enhance the destruction of this compound.[373] Pyridoxine deficiency is connected with increased formation of liver cancer.[605] In addition to the key role of vitamin B_6 in hematopoiesis, it also participates in the antibody response to various antigens,[19] thus indirectly modifying the development of various tumors. In alcoholics, blood levels of vitamin E are very low.[368,416] Vitamin E and other antioxidants, such as butylated hydroxytoluene and propyl gallate, reduce the incidence of tumors induced by certain carcinogens.[563,584]

Alcoholics show deficiencies of essential trace elements such as iron, magnesium, and zinc.[182,287,536] Zinc deficiency has been associated with esophageal carcinoma in Iran.[314] Molybdenum deficiency is also connected with increased incidence of this tumor.[558]

C. CHEMICAL CARCINOGENESIS

Many chemicals cause liver cancer in man. These include aflatoxin, 4-amino-biphenyl, arsenic compounds, auramine and benzidine, steroids, oxymeltholone, and vinylchloride monomer.[392,532,543] 2-Naphthylamine induces hepatic tumors in experimental animals and bladder tumors in man.[424] The development of cancer involves many sequential steps and as the process advances probability to grow into a malignant tumor increases. The process often takes from 10 to 30 years before manifestations of the cancer are apparent. Many factors contribute to this process and these may interact with one or more human host factors including age, sex, hormone balance, genetic structure, and immune status. We know now that many cancers would not develop if certain chemicals were not present in the environment. It is generally accepted that environmental factors contribute to about 80% of cancers. These environmental factors can be grouped into several categories including (1) occupational exposure at the work place, (2) lifestyle habits including eating, drinking, and smoking, (3) exposure to iatrogens, and (4) general environmental effects.

In chemical carcinogenesis, the hepatic microsomal cytochrome P-450 dependent enzyme system is involved by catalyzing the metabolic conversion of many structurally diverse chemicals to metabolites with electrophilic characteristics.[167,431] These electrophiles are responsible for the carcinogenic effects of the parent compounds by reacting with nucleic acids and proteins. Activation of many procarcinogens by microsomal enzymes is an obligatory event in tumor production. Components of the cytochrome P-450 system and associated enzymes such as UDP-glucuronidase, glutathione S-transferase, glutathione peroxidase, glutathione reductase, and epoxide hydrase and progesterone binding are modified by tumor inducing chemicals.[156,157,177,309,438] Recent experimental data have shown that enzymic retrodifferentiation occurs during hepatocarcinogenesis.[106]

Cytochrome P-450 dependent reactions which lead to carcinogen production include (1) epoxide formation from polycyclic aromatic hydrocarbons,[108,519] furosemide,[597] and aflatoxins,[407] (2) dealkylation of alkylnitrosamines,[107,230,407] (3) N-hydroxylation of aromatic amines such as 2-aminofluorene, 2-acetylaminofluorene,[22,210,407] and hydrazines.[587] In man, the major site of the cytochrome P-450 system is the liver.[42,112,493] but it also occurs in skin,[342] placenta,[92] lungs,[534] colon,[17] intestines,[255] and lymphocytes.[593] The metabolism of foreign compounds in tissues which have direct contact with the environment is important for carcinogenesis. Target organs are skin, lungs, and intestines, since metabolism in these tissues can influence absorption, reactivity, metabolism, and systemic distribution.[538]

1. Various Stages of Carcinogenesis

The development of cancer in man takes many years, and during the latent period, progressive cellular and tissue changes occur.[157] New cell populations emerge from normal cells and through initiated preneoplastic and premalignant stages until the manifestation of highly malignant neoplasia.[155,159,440] From animal experiments, conceptually, two early steps are distinguished in chemical carcinogenesis: initiation and promotion.[159,402,440] The validity of this concept has been established for the development of human tumor growth. Limited exposure to vinyl chloride gas many years later may produce hepatic angiosarcoma.[371,382,500] Similarly, a short exposure to diethylstilbestrol during pregnancy may lead to the development of vaginal neoplasia in the offspring.[589] Oral contraceptives may be also responsible for the occurrence of hepatocellular carcinoma.[247]

Cancer development with chemical agents can start with a short exposure to an activated form of a carcinogen, and the chemical may not be present again in the organism. Initiation of tumor production occurs in the liver, but also in other organs such as skin, mammary gland, kidney, brain, and urinary bladder.[159,440,498] The brief effects of the carcinogen stimulate some cells and subsequently results in focal proliferations.[467]

This action is connected with metabolic activation of the chemical agents to highly reactive metabolites.[402] Usually, a positively charged molecule is formed as an electrophilic reactant, interacting with various cellular components such as DNA, RNA, proteins, and glutathione.[22,23,160,326,359,369,505,578] It is known that some chemical carcinogens do not need metabolic activation to more reactive metabolites such as nitrogen mustard, alkylnitrosoureas, and alkylnitrosamines. In the conversion of precarcinogens to carcinogen, the liver is the most active organ. Beside activation, this organ and some others can also detoxify potential carcinogens. The final outcome of these reactions depends on the balance between activation and inactivation which is influenced by many drugs and other chemicals, hormones, nutrition, age, strain, and genetic factors.[21,34,175,497,585]

Following the exposure to an initial dose of carcinogen, the process of initiation begins. During promotion, the initiated tissue develops focal proliferations which may act as intermediate in the subsequent steps of the carcinogenic process leading to tumor formation and frank cancer development. In experimental models of hepatocarcinogenesis, a relatively short exposure of 2 to 3 weeks is needed for the formation of hyperplastic nodules.[524] In other models, the promoting agent has to be applied for many months.[436,441,514]

In the progression of the cancer, one or more of the focal proliferations formed during promotion or selection may represent the sites where further changes can occur. Few cells proliferate without any apparent external influence. This rare event repeats itself until the malignant tumor develops. Subsequent sequences of progression in man include various types of precancerous lesions such as carcinoma *in situ,* atypical hyperplasia, and displasia.[158,321,393] These lesions appear later than focal proliferations, and at present, we do not know how these lesions relate to each other. Precancerous or cancerous lesions can arise in the area of focal proliferation in the liver of experimental animals and in many sites in humans.[595] Many chemicals can induce hyperplastic nodules which are further transformed to malignant lesions. These chemicals include diethylnitrosamine, 3'-methyl-4'-dimethylaminoazobenzene, aramite, and ethionine.[147,209,455,524]

2. Effects of Extrahepatic Tumors on the Liver

Another important aspect of carcinogenesis is the effect of extrahepatic tumorigenesis on liver function. This action is essential since it is well known that cancer patients often die from impaired function of vital organs, including the liver. Derangement of hepatic function is involved in the breakdown of the homeostatic regulation of metabolic and endocrine functions leading to death. The cachexia syndrome cannot be explained only by the location, size, and type of tumor and the burden it represents. The systemic effects of neoplasia on the host could result from (1) competition of the tumor with normal tissue for essential cofactors and metabolites; exhaustion of these constituents causing changes in metabolism and hormone balance. (2) Tumor effects from distant sites manifesting in decreased differentiation, impairment of regulatory functions, changes in enzyme pattern, and disruption of the feedback system which coordinates the activities of endocrine glands.[507] (3) Since the liver is the major site of homeostatic control of metabolism,[171] and the hepatic endoplasmic reticulum has a number of functions in maintaining homeostasis,[431] this organ plays a central role in the development of cachexia. (4) Factors released from the tumor into circulation may be responsible for the remote action of the tumor on other organs.[97,98]

Many investigations on experimental animals bearing extrahepatic tumors have shown that the liver is a very sensitive organ responding with changes to distant neoplasms.[106,250,251,253] In some cases, the enzymatic pattern of histologically normal liver in the host shifts in the direction of the immature liver.[130,250,252] Evidence of hepatic dedifferentiation has been found as early as a few days after subcutaneous transplantation of neoplasms and became more marked as the tumor progressed. Recently, we have shown that the growth of transplanted R3230AC mammary adenocarcinoma in rats is connected with changes in the metabolic functions of hepatocytes.[169] Cytochrome P-450 dependent enzymes are decreased; glutathione-S-acyltransferase, γ-glutamyltranspeptidase, and glutathione are increased. Microsomal progesterone content and receptor binding in hepatic microsomes are also increased.[176] Similar changes were observed in liver microsomes isolated from nodules produced by diethylnitrosamine-2-acetylaminofluorene treatment.[148,177,438] These data indicate that the enzymatic abnormalities in the liver cell are connected with the initiating phase of cancer production and the hepatic dedifferentiation appears to be indistinguishable in hepatocarcinoma from those seen with extrahepatic neoplasms.

XIV. METABOLIC DISEASES

Since one of the major roles of the liver is the maintenance of metabolic homeostasis, hepatic diseases are often connected with impairments of one or several metabolic functions. These changes are varied and include altered protein synthesis and metabolism,[15,90,152,282,345,360,415,509,588,601] amino acid composition,[81,281,362,509,583] nucleoside metabolizing enzymes,[395] lipid synthesis and metabolism,[8,58,95,118,133,152] carbohydrate synthesis and metabolism,[266,583] effects on the production of various blood components,[58,94,211,256,390,539,598] disturbance of hormone balance,[26,289,290,472,527,530,603] cofactor utilization,[109] and drug disposition.[248,264,430,599] Many disease conditions in various organs are also associated with changes in normal hepatic metabolic processes such as inflammation, recurrent Reye-like syndrome, preeclampsia, hepatic encephalopathy, heartstroke, and obesity.[45,154,217,286,299,377,480]

A. INBORN ERRORS OF METABOLISM

Inborn errors frequently cause clinical symptoms indicating primary liver involvement. The clinical features of many deficiencies involving inborn errors of amino acid, peptide, and protein synthesis and carbohydrate and lipid metabolisms often include hepatic changes. Here only diseases with primary hepatic origin will be discussed. Examples are some amino acid disorders related to abnormal hepatic tyrosine metabolism, like tyrosyluria and tyrosinemia,[200,202] and the impaired biosynthesis of carnitine and cystathionein.[201] Inborn errors of plasma proteins, congenital coagulation defects, although most plasma proteins are synthetized in the liver, were dealt with in Volume I.

1. Tyrosyluria and Tyrosinemia

Tyrosyluria and tyrosinemia are diseases of abnormal tyrosine metabolism. In tyrosyluria or tyrosinosis elevated amounts of tyrosine and its derivatives, particularly *p*-hydroxyphenylpyruvic acid, are excreted. If the diet contains large amounts of tyrosine, other tyrosyl metabolites, *p*-hydroxyphenyllactic and *p*-hydroxyphenyl acetic acid, also occur in the urine. Tyrosyluria is characterized by cirrhosis of the liver, and the patient is dying from liver failure during the first week of life, but some cases have survived for months or years. In these cases, multiple renal tubular defects develop. The renal changes may affect to a greater or lesser extent the reabsorption of water, potassium, and bicarbonate ions, uric acid, glucose, amino acids, phosphate, and even protein. Other tubular functions are inconsistent and show variations.

This inborn error is related to the defect of *p*-hydroxyphenylpyruvic acid oxidase or tyrosine transaminase[194,200-202,460] (Figure 40). Elevated *p*-hydroxypyruvic acid excretion is also present in other liver disease and following splenectomy. Treatment with a diet low in tyrosine and phenylalanine can normalize the plasma tyrosine level and reverse the other biochemical abnormalities.

The major biochemical defect manifesting in tyrosinemia patients is the elevated blood tyrosine level and excessive urinary elimination of tyrosine and tyrosyl compounds. The clinical features include enlargement of the liver and spleen, nodular cirrhosis of the liver, and multiple renal tubular reabsorption defects. Slight mental retardation is seen in some cases, but mental deficiency is not a constant symptom in tyrosinemia. This inborn error is probably also derived from the lack of *p*-hydroxyphenylpyruvic acid oxidase.

2. Carnitine Deficiency

Carnitine is synthesized in the liver and enters the tissues via the circulation. Tissue levels greatly exceed serum levels, which implies that tissue uptake is dependent on an active transport mechanism. Thus, carnitine deficiency might be caused by an impaired

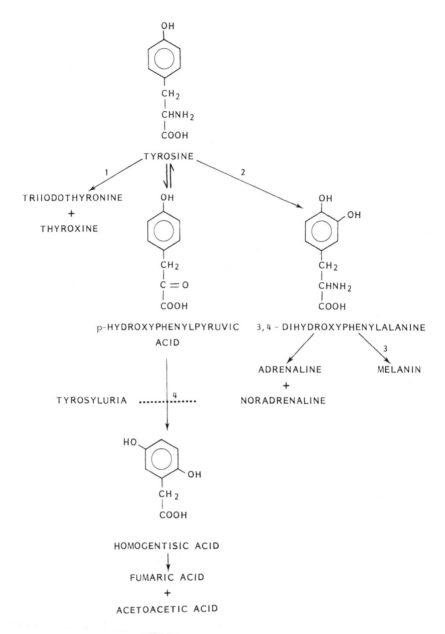

FIGURE 40.   Metabolism of tyrosine. Tyrosine is essential in the synthesis of thyroid hormones (1), catecholamines (2), and melanine (3). In tyrosyluria *p*-hydroxyphenylpyruvic acid oxidase (4) is deficient.

hepatic biosynthesis or a defective active transport.[146,270] Some cases of carnitine deficiency are due to a transport defect since hepatic synthesis is intact and the serum levels are within normal limits. In other cases, hepatic biosynthesis is faulty, and serum, muscle, and liver carnitine levels are below normal. Carnitine concentration is highest in skeletal and cardiac muscle, while the brain and liver have the lowest.

The clinical features of patients suffering from carnitine deficiency are due to fluctuating hepatomegaly, muscle weakness, and triglyceride accumulation in the muscle fibers. This syndrome is referred to as Type I lipid storage myopathy. Besides abnormal lipid deposits, mitochondrial volume is increased probably as a compensation for the decreased fatty acid oxidation.

XV. LIVER FUNCTION TESTS

These tests provide an indication of various hepatic functions necessary for diagnosis, and they are generally useful guides to therapy. These biochemical tests demonstrate functional disturbances of the liver, and therefore they are based on specific functions. Accordingly, they can be grouped into classes: (1) tests on excretory function: serum bilirubin determinations, measurement of bile derivatives, and dye excretion tests such as bromsulphthalein; (2) tests on metabolic function and indirect indicators of synthesis: serum proteins, flocculation tests, serum enzymes, serum cholesterol, and prothrombin time; (3) tests on biotransformation of various compounds; and (4) tests on detoxication mechanisms. The latter group contains many noninvasive methods.[44,63,64,384,471,604]

Liver function tests are important in the assessment and prognosis of suspected primary or secondary hepatic disorders, the diagnosis of cholestasis, jaundice, and cirrhosis, and also in other diseases with hepatic participation such as anemias, and porphyrias. Alterations of hepatic function as a result of disease or the adverse effect of foreign compounds is reflected in abnormal concentration of plasma constituents. Qualitative and quantitative changes that occur in many components of blood and urine provide the basis of these tests used to detect pathological processes manifest in the liver or mediated by this organ. Some liver function tests reveal disorders of hormone producing glands since the liver plays an important part in the regulation of hormone metabolism. Many hormones are processed in this organ which are essential in homeostasis.

Many hepatic function tests are being used in the laboratory as valuable indices of disease, but a large number are now of historical interest only. Moreover, some liver function tests have limited value because mild and prolonged effects are often occurring while these tests give positive results only in case of severe damage and functional impairment. Therefore, it is very important to detect other responses of the liver. Several tests depend upon the summation of many integrated enzymatic actions taking place within the liver cells. Enzyme actions, however, are influenced by the intracellular supply of substrates, oxygen and energy, presence or absence of inhibitors, accelerators, cofactors, composition of the intracellular milieu, pH, electrolytes, and blood flow. Many of these factors may be altered qualitatively or quantitatively without visible histological changes in the liver. The correlation between liver function tests abnormalities and demonstrable morphological changes is often difficult, but should be pursued. The liver has large functional reserves that can mask the value of the tests. The liver has a significant power of regeneration and it is not known with exactitude to what extent the parenchyma has to be damaged for enzyme changes to appear in the serum.

REFERENCES

1. **Abu-Murad, C., Griffiths, P. J., and Littleton, J. M.,** The induction and study of physical dependence on ethanol in mice, *Br. J. Pharmacol.*, 56, 377, 1976.
2. **Acheampong-Mensah, D. and Feuer, G.,** Dietary-induced liver ailment and drug metabolism, *Clin. Chem.*, 21, 960, 1975.
3. **Acheampong-Mensah, D. and Feuer, G.,** Enhanced utilization of methylated drugs for the synthesis of hepatic phospholipids during methyl deficiency, *Nutr. Rep. Int.*, 10, 297, 1974.
4. **Adamson, A. R., Grahame-Smith, D. G., Peast, W. S., and Starr, M.,** Pharmacological blockade of carcinoid flushing provoked by catecholamines and alcohol, *Lancet*, 2, 293, 1969.
5. **Adlercreutz, H., Svanborg, A., and Anberg, A.,** Recurrent jaundice in pregnancy. I. A clinical and ultrastructural study, *Am. J. Med.*, 42, 335, 1967.
6. **Alberti-Flor, J. J., Iskandarani, M., Jeffers, L., Zeppa, R., and Schiff, E. R.,** Focal nodular hyperplasia associated with the use of a synthetic anabolic androgen, *Am. J. Gastroenterol.*, 79, 150, 1984.

7. **Alpert, M. E., Uriel, J., and de Nechaud, B.,** Alpha-1 fetoglobulin in the diagnosis of human hepatoma, *N. Engl. J. Med.,* 278, 984, 1968.
8. **Aly, A., Carlson, K., Johansson, C., Kirstein, P., Rossner, S., and Wallentin, L.,** Lipoprotein abnormalities in patients with early primary biliary cirrhosis, *Eur. J. Clin. Invest.,* 14, 155, 1984.
9. **Arias, I. M. and Gartner, L. M.,** Production of unconjugated hyperbilirubinemia in full-term new-born infants following administration of pregnane-3 (alpha), 20 (beta)-diol, *Nature (London),* 203, 1292, 1964.
10. **Arias, I. M., Gartner, L. M., Seifter, S., and Furman, M.,** Neonatal unconjugated hyperbilirubinemia associated with breast feeding, *J. Clin. Invest.,* 42, 913, 1963.
11. **Arias, I. M., Gartner, L. M., Seifter, S., and Furman, M.,** Prolonged neonatal unconjugated hyperbilirubinemia associated with breast feeding and a steroid, pregnane-3 (alpha), 20 (beta)-diol, in maternal milk that inhibits glucuronide formation in vitro, *J. Clin. Invest.,* 43, 2037, 1964.
12. **Arias, I. M., Johnson, L., and Wolfson, S.,** Biliary excretion of injected conjugated and unconjugated bilirubin by normal and Gunn rats, *Am. J. Physiol.,* 200, 1091, 1961.
13. **Aronson, D. C., Heymans, H. S., and Bijlmer, R. P.,** Cor pulmonale and acute liver necrosis due to upper airway obstruction as part of pycno-dysostosis, *Eur. J. Pediatr.,* 141, 251, 1984.
14. **Arthur, M. J., Hall, A. J., and Wright, R.,** Hepatitis B, hepatocellular carcinoma and strategies for prevention, *Lancet,* 1, 607, 1984.
15. **Artur, Y., Wellman-Bednawska, M., Jacquier, A., and Siest, G.,** Associations between serum gamma-glutamyltransferase and apolipoproteins: relationship with hepatobiliary diseases, *Clin. Chem.,* 30, 1318, 1984.
16. **Asaka, M., Nagase, K., and Alpert, E.,** Biochemical and clinical studies of aldolase isozymes in human cancer, *Isozymes Curr. Top. Biol. Med. Res.,* 11, 183, 1983.
17. **Autrup, H., Harris, C. C., Stoner, G. D., Jesudason, M. L., and Trump, B. F.,** Binding of chemical carcinogens to macromolecules in cultured human colon, *J. Natl. Cancer Inst.,* 59, 351, 1977.
18. **Avogaro, P. and Cazzolato, G.,** Changes in the composition and physicochemical characteristics of serum lipoproteins during ethanol-induced lipaemia in alcoholic subjects, *Metabolism,* 24, 1231, 1975.
19. **Axelrod, A. E. and Trakatellis, A. C.,** Relationship of pyridoxine to immunologic phenomena, *Vitam. Horm.,* 22, 591, 1964.
20. **Back, P.,** Identification and quantitative determination of urinary bile acids excreted in cholestasis, *Clin. Chim. Acta,* 44, 199, 1973.
21. **Bannasch, P.,** Strain and species differences in susceptibility to liver tumour induction, *Int. Agency Res. Cancer Sci. Publ.,* 51, 9, 1983.
22. **Baranyi-Furlong, B. L. and Goodman, J. I.,** Damage to a specific hepatic DNA base sequences following exposure to the hepatocarcinogen 2-acetylaminofluorene, *Dev. Toxicol. Environ. Sci.,* 11, 363, 1983.
23. **Baranyi-Furlong, B. L. and Goodman, J. I.,** Non-random interaction of N-2-acetylaminofluorene and its N-hydroxy metabolite with DNA of rat hepatic parenchymal and non-parenchymal cell nuclei following in vivo administration of carcinogen, *Chem. Biol. Interact.,* 48, 15, 1984.
24. **Baraona, E., Leo, M. A., Borowsky, S. A., and Lieber, C. S.,** Alcoholic hepatomegaly: accumulation of protein in the liver, *Science,* 190, 794, 1975.
25. **Baraona, E., Leo, M. A., Borowsky, S. A., and Lieber, C. S.,** Pathogenesis of alcohol-induced accumulation of protein in the liver, *J. Clin. Invest.,* 60, 546, 1977.
26. **Barreca, T., Franceschini, R., Messina, V., Bottaro, P., and Rolandi, E.,** Changes in pituitary secretion after administration of branched-chain amino acids to patients with hepatic cirrhosis, *Eur. J. Clin. Pharmacol.,* 25, 763, 1983.
27. **Bass, L.,** Models of hepatic drug eliminations, *J. Pharm. Sci.,* 72, 1229, 1983.
28. **Baumgartner, H. P. and Filippini, L.,** Alkoholinduzierte Hyperlipoproteinamien, *Schweiz. Med. Wochenschr.,* 107, 1406, 1977.
29. **Beasley, R. P.,** Hepatitis B virus as the etiologic agent in hepatocellular carcinoma — epidemiologic considerations, *Hepatology,* 2, 21, 1980.
30. **Beasley, R. P. and Hwang, L. Y.,** Hepatocellular carcinoma and hepatitis B virus, *Semin. Liver Dis.,* 4, 113, 1984.
31. **Beasley, R. P., Hwang, L. Y., Lin, C. C., and Chien, C. S.,** Hepatocellular carcinoma and hepatitis B virus. A prospective study of 22,707 men in Taiwan, *Lancet,* 2, 1129, 1981.
32. **Beasley, R. P., Hwang, L. Y., Lin, C. C., Stevens, C. E., Wang, K. Y., Sun, T. S., Hsieh, F. J., and Szmuness, W.,** Hepatitis B immune globulin efficacy in the interruption of perinatal transmission of hepatitis B virus carrier state, *Lancet,* 2, 388, 1981.
33. **Beckett, A. G., Livingston, A. V., and Hill, K. R.,** Acute alcoholic hepatitis without jaundice, *Br. Med. J.,* 2, 580, 1962.
34. **Bentley, P. and Oesch, P.,** Enzymes involved in activation and inactivation of carcinogens and mutagens, in *Primary Liver Tumors,* Remmer, H., Bolt, H. M., Bannasch, P., and Popper, H., Eds., MTP Press, Lancaster, 1978, 239-252.

35. **Bernstein, I. M., Webster, K. H., Williams, R. C., and Strickland, R. G.,** Reductions in circulating T lymphocytes in alcoholic liver disease, *Lancet,* 2, 488, 1974.
36. **Berry, M. N., Grivell, A. R., and Wallace, P. G.,** Biological significance of compartmentation of hepatic ethanol oxidation, *Pharmacol. Biochem. Behav.,* 18(Suppl. 1), 201, 1983.
37. **Berthelot, P., Sicot, C. C., Benhasson, J. P., and Fauvert, R.,** Les hepatites medicamenteuses. I. Considerations generales, *Rev. Franc. Etud. Clin. Biol.,* 10, 39, 1965.
38. **Best, C. H., Hartroft, W. S., Lucas, C. C., and Ridout, J. H.,** Liver damage produced by feeding alcohol or sugar and its prevention by choline, *Br. Med. J.,* 2, 1001, 1949.
39. **Bianchi, L.,** Morphologic features in biopsy diagnosis of acute viral hepatitis, *Progress in Liver Diseases,* Vol. 3, Popper, H. and Schaffner, F., Eds., Grune & Stratton, New York, 1970, 236—251.
40. **Biempica, L., Gutstein, S., and Arias, I. M.,** Morphological and biochemical studies of benign recurrent cholestasis, *Gastroenterology,* 52, 521, 1967.
41. **Billing, B. H.,** Chromatographic method for determination of 3 bile pigments in serum, *J. Clin. Pathol.,* 8, 126, 1955.
42. **Billing, B. H. and Black, M.,** The action of drugs on bilirubin metabolism in man, *Ann. N.Y. Acad. Sci.,* 179, 403, 1971.
43. **Billing, B. H., Cole, P. G., and Lathe, G. H.,** The excretion of bilirubin as a diglucuronide giving the direct van den Bergh reaction, *Biochem. J.,* 65, 774, 1957.
44. **Bircher, J.,** Non-invasive methods for the assessment of hepatic drug disposition, *Int. J. Clin. Pharmacol. Res.,* 3, 415, 1983.
45. **Bjorkhem, I., Angelin, B., Backman, L., Liljeqvist, L., Nilsell, K., and Einarsson, K.,** Triglyceride metabolism in human liver: studies on hepatic phosphatidic acid phosphatase in obese and non-obese subjects, *Eur. J. Clin. Invest.,* 14, 233, 1984.
46. **Blumberg, B. S., Gerstley, B. J. S., Sutnick, A. I., Millman, I., and London, W. T.,** Australia antigen, hepatitis virus and Down's syndrome, *Ann. N.Y. Acad. Sci.,* 171, 486-499, 1970.
47. **Blumberg, B. S., Sutnick, A. I., London, W. T., and Millman, I.,** The discovery of Australia antigen and its relation to viral hepatitis, *Perspect. Virol.,* 7, 223, 1971.
48. **Bocker, R., Estler, C. J., Gotz, H., and Pesch, H. J.,** Investigation into the combined hepatotoxicity of rolitetracycline and ethinyloestradiol, *Arch. Int. Pharmacodyn. Ther.,* 264, 168, 1983.
49. **Bogren, H. and Larsson, K.,** Crystalline components of biliary calculi, *Scand. J. Clin. Lab. Invest.,* 15, 457, 1963.
50. **Bojar, H., Petzinna, D., Staib, W., and Brolsch, C.,** Steroid receptor status of focal-nodular hyperplasia of the human liver, *Klin. Wochenschr.,* 62, 446, 1984.
51. **Bolarin, D., Andy, J. J., and Alabi, Z. O.,** Liver immunoreactive prolyl hydroxylase protein in human primary hepatocellular carcinoma, *Hepatogastroenterology,* 30, 230, 1983.
52. **Bonkowsky, H. L., Tschudy, D. P., and Collins, A.,** Control of 5-aminolevulinic acid synthetase and tyrosine aminotransferase in tumors and livers of tumor-bearing rats, *J. Natl. Cancer Inst.,* 50, 1215, 1973.
53. **Boobis, A. R. and Davies, D. S.,** Human cytochromes P-450, *Xenobiotica,* 14, 151, 1984.
54. **Boobis, A. R., Murray, S., Hampden, C. E., and Davies, D. S.,** Genetic polymorphism in drug oxidation: in vitro studies of human debrisoquine 4-hydroxylase and bufuralol 1'-hydroxylase activities, *Biochem. Pharmacol.,* 34, 65, 1985.
55. **Booth, N. A., Anderson, J. A., and Bennett, B.,** Plasminogen activators in alcoholic cirrhosis: demonstration of increased tissue type and urokinase type activator, *J. Clin. Pathol.,* 37, 772, 1984.
56. **Borgstrom, B., Lundh, G., and Hoffmann, A.,** The site of absorption of conjugated bile salts in man, *Gastroenterology,* 45, 229, 1963.
57. **Bosron, W. F., Crabb, D. W., and Li, T. K.,** Relationship between kinetics of liver alcohol dehydrogenase and alcohol metabolism, *Pharmacol. Biochem. Behav.,* 18(Suppl. 1), 223, 1983.
58. **Bouillon, R., Auwerx, J., Dekeyser, L., Fevery, J., Lissens, W., and De Moor, P.,** Serum vitamin D metabolites and their binding protein in patients with liver cirrhosis, *J. Clin. Endocrinol. Metab.,* 59, 86, 1984.
59. **Boyer, J. L. and Klatskin, G.,** Pattern of necrosis in acute viral hepatitis. Prognostic value of bridging subacute hepatic necrosis, *N. Engl. J. Med.,* 283, 1063, 1970.
60. **Braganza, J. M.,** Pancreatic disease: a casualty of hepatic "detoxification"?, *Lancet,* 2, 1000, 1983.
61. **Brechot, C., Hadchouel, M., Scotto, J., Fonck, M., Potet, F., Vyas, G. N., and Tiollais, P.,** State of hepatitis B virus DNA surface antigen-positive and -negative liver diseases, *Proc. Natl. Acad. Sci. U.S.A.,* 78, 3906, 1981.
62. **Brechot, C., Pourcel, C., Louise, A., Rain, B., and Tiollais, P.,** Presence of integrated hepatitis B virus DNA sequences in cellular DNA of human hepatocellular carcinoma, *Nature (London),* 286, 533, 1980.
63. **Breen, K. J., Bury, R. W., Calder, I. V., Desmond, P. V., Peters, M., and Mashford, M. L.,** A [14C] phenacetin breath test to measure hepatic function in man, *Hepatology,* 4, 47, 1984.
64. **Breyer-Pfaff, V., Seyfert, H., Weber, M., and Egberts, E. H.,** Assessment of drug metabolism in hepatic disease: comparison of plasma kinetics of oral cyclobarbital and the intravenous aminopyrine breath test, *Eur. J. Clin. Pharmacol.,* 26, 95, 1984.

65. **Brodie, B. B., Krishna, G., Reid, W. D., and Cho, A. K.,** Drug metabolism in man: past, present and future, *Ann. N.Y. Acad. Sci.,* 179, 11, 1971.

66. **Brodie, B. B., Reid, W. D., and Cho, A. K.,** Possible mechanism of liver necrosis caused by aromatic organic compounds, *Proc. Natl. Acad. Sci., U.S.A.,* 68, 160, 1971.

67. **Brodie, B. B., Reid, W. D., Cho, A. K., Sipes, G., Krishna, G., and Gillette, J. R.,** Possible mechanism of liver necrosis caused by aromatic organic compounds, *Proc. Natl. Acad. Sci., U.S.A.,* 68, 160, 1971.

68. **Brown, W. R., Grodsky, G. M., and Carbone, J. V.,** Intracellular distribution of tritiated bilirubin during hepatic uptake and excretion, *Am. J. Physiol.,* 207, 1237, 1964.

69. **Brunt, P. W., Kew, M. C., Scheuer, P. J., and Sherlock, S.,** Studies in alcoholic liver disease in Britain. I. Clinical and pathological patterns related to natural history, *Gut,* 15, 52, 1974.

70. **Burch, G. E. and Ansari, A.,** Chronic alcoholism and carcinoma of the pancreas: a correlative hypothesis, *Arch. Intern. Med.,* 122, 273, 1968.

71. **Burnett, W.,** The pathogenesis of gall stones, in *The Biliary System,* Taylor, W., Ed., Blackwell Scientific, Oxford, 1965, 601—614.

72. **Burrell, C. J., Gowans, E. J., Rowland, R., Hall, P., Jilbert, A. R., and Marmion, B. P.,** Correlation between liver histology and markers of hepatitis B virus replication in infected patients, *Hepatology,* 4, 20, 1984.

73. **Cairns, S. R. and Peters, J. J.,** Biochemical analysis of hepatic lipid in alcoholic, diabetic and control subjects, *Clin. Sci.,* 65, 645, 1983.

74. **Cairns, S. R. and Peters, J. J.,** Isolation of micro- and macro-droplet fractions from needle biopsy specimens of human liver and determination of the subcellular distribution of accumulation liver lipids in alcoholic fatty liver, *Clin. Sci.,* 67, 337, 1984.

75. **Cairns, S. R., Thomson, M., Lawson, A. M., Madigan, M. J., Variend, S., and Peters, T. J.,** Biochemical and histological assessment of hepatic lipid in sudden infant death syndrome, *J. Clin. Pathol.,* 36, 1188, 1983.

76. **Casali, C., Lo Monaco, M., D'Allessandro, L., Griso, D., Amanta, A., Topi, G. C., and Tonali, P.,** Hereditary coproporphyria: unusual nervous system involvement in two cases, *J. Neurol.,* 231, 99, 1984.

77. **Cederbaum, S. D., Lieber, C. S., and Beattie, D. S.,** Effect of chronic ethanol ingestion on fatty acid oxidation by hepatic mitochondria, *J. Biol. Chem.,* 250, 5122, 1975.

78. **Cederbaum, A., Lieber, C. S., and Rubin, E.,** Effects of chronic ethanol treatment of mitochondrial functions damage to coupling site, *Arch. Biochem. Biophys.,* 165, 560, 1974.

79. **Cederbaum, A. I. and Rubin, E.,** Molecular injury to mitochondria produced by ethanol and acetaldehyde, *Fed. Proc.,* 34, 2045, 1975.

80. **Chan, C. H.,** Primary carcinoma of the liver, *Med. Clin. North Am.,* 59, 989, 1976.

81. **Chawla, R. K., Lewis, F. W., Kutner, M. H., Bate, D. M., Roy, R. G., and Rudman, D.,** Plasma cysteine, cystine and glutathione in cirrhosis, *Gastroenterology,* 87, 770, 1984.

82. **Cherrick, G. R., Baker, H., Frank, O., and Leevy, C. M.,** Observations on hepatic avidity for folate in Laennec's cirrhosis, *J. Lab. Clin. Med.,* 66, 446, 1965.

83. **Chiarantini, E.,** Hepatocyte taurocholic acid uptake in the regression of ethinyl estradiol cholestasis, *Boll. Soc. Ital. Biol. Sper.,* 60, 523, 1984.

84. **Christenson, F., Prange, I., and Dam, H.,** Alimentary production of gallstones in hamsters. Influence of highly unsaturated fats and certain minerals on gallstone production, *Z. Ernaehrungswiss.,* 4, 186, 1964.

85. **Christoffersen, P., Eghoje, K. N., and Juhl, E.,** Mallory bodies in liver biopsies from chronic alcoholics. A comparative morphological, biochemical, and clinical study of two groups of chronic alcoholics with and without Mallory bodies, *Scand. J. Gastroenterol.,* 8, 341, 1973.

86. **Chu, E. W. and Malmgren, R. A.,** Inhibitory effect of vitamin A on the induction of tumors of forestomach and cervix in the Syrian hamster by carcinogenic polycyclic hydrocarbons, *Cancer Res.,* 25, 884, 1965.

87. **Chvapil, M. and Ryan, J. N.,** The pool of free proline in acute and chronic liver injury and its effect on the synthesis of collagen and globular proteins, *Agents Actions,* 3, 38, 1973.

88. **Cohen, S. M., Wittenberg, J. F., and Bryan, G. T.,** Effect of hypo- and avitaminosis A on urinary bladder carcinogenicity of N-(4-(5-nitro-2-furyl)-2-thiazolyl)formamide, *Fed. Proc.,* 33, 602, 1974.

89. **Cole, P. G., Lathe, G. H., and Billing, B. H.,** Separation of bile pigments of serum, bile and urine, *Biochem. J.,* 57, 514, 1954.

90. **Colombo, M., Annoni, G., Donato, M. F., Fargion, S., Tiribelli, C., and Dioguardi, N.,** Serum marker of type III procollagen in patients with idiopathic hemochromatosis and its relationship to hepatic fibrosis, *Am. J. Clin. Pathol.,* 80, 499, 1983.

91. **Cone, M. V. and Nettesheim, P.,** Effects of vitamin A and 3-methylcholanthrene induced squamous metaplasias and early tumors in the respiratory tract of rats, *J. Natl. Cancer Inst.,* 50, 1599, 1973.

92. **Conney, A. H., Welch, R., Kuntzman, R., Poland, R., Poppers, P. J., Finster, M., Wolff, J. A., Munro-Faure, A. D., Peck, A. W., Bye, A., Chang, R., and Jacobson, M.,** Effects of environmental chemicals on the metabolism of drugs, carcinogens, and normal body constituents in man, *Ann. N.Y. Acad. Sci.,* 179, 155, 1971.

93. **Conte, N., Cecchettin, M., Manente, P., Valmachino, G., Roiter, I., and Pavan, P.,** Calcitonin in hepatoma and cirrhosis, *Acta Endocrinol.,* 106, 109, 1984.

94. **Cordova, C., Musca, A., Violi, F., Alessandri, C., Ferro, D., Piromalli, A., and Balsano, F.,** Prekallikrein behaviour in chronic active hepatitis and in cirrhotic patients, *Haemostasis,* 14, 218, 1984.

95. **Cordova, C., Musca, A., Violi, F., Alessandri, C., and Iuliano, L.,** Apolipoproteins A-I, A-II, and B in chronic active hepatitis and in liver cirrhotic patients, *Clin. Chim. Acta,* 137, 61, 1984.

96. **Cortes, J. M. and Salata, H.,** Hepatic pathology in porphyria cutanea tarda, *Liver,* 3, 413, 1983.

97. **Costa, G.,** Cachexia, the metabolic component of neoplastic diseases, *Cancer Res.,* 37, 2327, 1977.

98. **Costa, G.,** Determination of nutritional needs, *Cancer Res.,* 37, 2419, 1977.

99. **Cowan, R. E. and Thompson, R. P.,** Fatty acids and the control of bilirubin levels in blood, *Mol. Hypotheses,* 11, 343, 1983.

100. **Crapper, R. M., Bhathaland, P. S., and Mackay, I. R.,** Chronic active hepatitis in alcoholic patients, *Liver,* 3, 327, 1983.

101. **Crawford, J. S. and Rudofsky, S.,** Some alterations in the pattern of drug metabolism associated with pregnancy, oral contraceptives, and the newly-born, *Br. J. Anaesth.,* 38, 446, 1966.

102. **Cresteil, T., Celier, C., Kremers, P., Flinois, J. P., Beaune, P., and Leroux, J. P.,** Induction of drug-metabolizing enzymes by tricyclic antidepressants in human liver: characterization and partial resolution of cytochromes P-450, *Br. J. Clin. Pharmacol.,* 16, 651, 1983.

103. **Crigler, J. F. and Najjar, V. A.,** Congenital familial nonhemolytic jaundice with kernicterus, *Pediatrics,* 10, 169, 1952.

104. **Cripps, D. J., Hawgood, R. S., and Magnus, I. A.,** Iodine tungsten fluorescence microscopy for porphyrine fluorescence. A study on erythropoietic protoporphyria, *Arch. Derm.,* 93, 129, 1966.

105. **Crosby, W. H. and Akeroyd, J. H.,** Limit of hemoglobin synthesis in hereditary hemolytic anemia; its relation to excretion of bile pigment, *Am. J. Med.,* 13, 273, 1952.

106. **Curtin, N. J. and Snell, K.,** Enzymic retrodifferentiation during hepatocarcinogenesis and liver regeneration in rats in vivo, *Br. J. Cancer,* 48, 495, 1983.

107. **Czygan, P., Greim, H., Garro, A. J., Hutterer, F., Schaffner, F., Popper, H., Rosenthal, O., and Cooper, D. Y.,** Microsomal metabolism of dimethylnitrosamine and the cytochrome P-450 dependency of its activation to a mutagen, *Cancer Res.,* 33, 2938, 1973.

108. **Daly, J. W., Jerina, D. M., and Witkop, B.,** Arene oxides and the NIH shift: the metabolism, toxicity and carcinogenicity of aromatic compounds, *Experientia (Basel),* 28, 1129, 1972.

109. **Dancy, M., Evans, G., Gaitonde, M. K., and Maxwell, J. D.,** Blood thiamine and thiamine phosphate ester concentrations in alcoholic and non-alcoholic liver disease, *Br. Med. J.,* 289, 79, 1984.

110. **Danielsson, H. and Sjovall, J.,** Bile acid metabolism, *Annu. Rev. Biochem.,* 44, 233, 1975.

111. **Daughaday, W. H., Lipicky, R. J., and Rasinski, D. C.,** Lactic acidosis as a cause of nonketotic acidosis in diabetic patients, *N. Engl. J. Med.,* 267, 1010, 1962.

112. **Davies, D. S. and Thorgeirsson, S. S.,** Mechanism of hepatic drug oxidation and its relationship to individual differences in rates of oxidation in man, *Ann. N.Y. Acad. Sci.,* 179, 411, 1971.

113. **Davis, V. E., Brown, H., Huff, J. A., and Cashaw, J. L.,** Ethanol-induced alterations of norepinephrine metabolism in man, *J. Lab. Clin. Med.,* 69, 787, 1967.

114. **Davis, V. E., Brown, H., Huff, J. A., and Cashaw, J. L.,** The alteration of serotonin metabolism to 5-hydroxytryptophol by ethanol ingestion in man, *J. Lab. Clin. Med.,* 69, 132, 1968.

115. **Dayer, P., Balant, L., Courvoisier, F., Kupfer, A., Kubli, A., Gorgia, A., and Fabre, J.,** The genetic control of bufuralol metabolism in man, *Env. J. Drug Metab. Pharmacokin.,* 7, 73, 1982.

116. **DeBrito, T., Borges, M. A., and Da Silva, L. C.,** Electron microscopy of the liver in nonhemolytic acholuric jaundice with Kernicterus (Crigler-Najjar) and in idiopathic conjugated hyperbilirubinemia (Rotor), *Gastroenterologia,* 106, 325, 1968.

117. **DeLuca, L., Maestri, N., Bonanni, F., and Nelson, D.,** Maintenance of epithelial cell differentiation: the mode of action of vitamin A, *Cancer (Philadelphia),* 30, 1326, 1972.

118. **De Martiis, M., Barlattani, A., Parenzi, A., and Sebastiani, F.,** Pattern of lecithin-cholesterol-acyl-transferase (L-CAT) activity in the course of liver cirrhosis, *J. Int. Med. Res.,* 11, 232, 1983.

119. **De Matteis, F.,** Disturbances of liver porphyrin metabolism caused by drugs, *Pharmacol. Rev.,* 19, 523, 1968.

120. **De Matteis, F.,** Increased synthesis of L-ascorbic acid caused by drugs which induce porphyria, *Biochem. Biophys. Acta,* 82, 641, 1964.

121. **De Matteis, F.,** Rapid loss of cytochrome P-450 and haem caused in the liver microsomes by the porphyrogenic agent 2-allyl-2-isopropyl-acetamide, *FEBS Letters,* 6, 343, 1970.

122. **De Matteis, F.,** Toxic hepatic porphyrias, *Sem. Hematol.,* 5, 409, 1968.

123. **Denk, H., Gschnait, F., and Wolff, K.,** Hepatocellular hyalin (Mallory bodies) in long term griseofulvin-treated mice: a new experimental model for the study of hyalin formation, *Lab. Invest.,* 32, 773, 1975.

124. **Desmet, V.,** Morphologic aspects of intrahepatic cholestasis, in *Intrahepatic Cholestasis,* Gentilini, P., Teodori, V., Gorini, S., and Popper, H., Eds., Raven Press, New York, 1975, 7—16.

125. **Desmet, V., Bullens, A. M., and De Groot, J.,** A clinical and histochemical study of cholestasis, *Gut,* 11, 516, 1970.
126. **Desmet, V. and De Groot, J.,** Histological diagnosis of viral hepatitis, *Clin. Gastroenterol.,* 3, 337, 1974.
127. **de Wolff, F. A., Vermeij, P., Ferrari, M. D., Buruma, O. J., and Breimer, D. D.,** Impairment of phenytoin parahydroxylation as a cause of severe intoxication, *Ther. Drug Monitoring,* 5, 213, 1983.
128. **Diamond, I. and Schmid, R.,** Experimental bilirubin encephalopathy. The mode of entry of bilirubin 14C in the central nervous system, *J. Clin. Invest.,* 45, 678, 1966.
129. **Diczfalusy, E., Cassmer, O., Alonso, C., de Miguel, M., and Westin, B.,** Oestrogen metabolism in the human foetus. II. Oestrogen conjugation by foetal organs in vitro and in vivo, *Acta Endocrinol.,* 37, 516, 1961.
130. **Dolezalova, V., Stratil, P., Simickova, M., Kocent, A., and Nemecek, R.,** Alpha-fetoprotein and alpha-2-macroglobulin as the markers of distinct responses of hepatocytes to carcinogens in the rat, Carcinogenesis, *Ann. N.Y. Acad. Sci.,* 417, 294, 1984.
131. **Domschke, S., Domschke, W., and Lieber, C. S.,** Hepatic redox state: attenuation of the acute effects of ethanol induced by chronic ethanol consumption, *Life Sci.,* 15, 1327, 1974.
132. **Doss, M., Sauer, H., von Tieparmann, R., and Colombi, A. M.,** Development of chronic hepatic porphyria (porphyria cutanea tarda) with inherited uroporphyrinogen decarboxylase deficiency under exposure to dioxin, *Int. J. Biochem.,* 16, 369, 1984.
133. **Duhamel, G., Nalpas, B., Goldstein, S., Laplaud, P. M., Berthelot, P., and Chapman, M. J,** Plasma lipoprotein and apolipoprotein profile in alcoholic patients with and without liver disease: on the relative roles of alcohol and liver injury, *Hepatology,* 4, 577, 1984.
134. **Dunham, L. J. and Bailar, J. C.,** World maps of cancer mortality notes and frequency ratios, *J. Natl. Cancer Inst.,* 41, 155, 1968.
135. **Dutton, G. J.,** Comparison of glucuronide synthesis in developing mammalian and avian liver, *Ann. N.Y. Acad. Sci.,* 111, 259, 1963.
136. **Dutton, G. J. and Storey, I. D. E.,** Uridine compounds in glucuronic acid metabolism; formation of glucuronides in liver suspensions, *Biochem. J.,* 57, 275, 1954.
137. **Edgington, T. S. and Ritt, D. J.,** Intrahepatic expression of serum hepatitis virus-associated antigens, *J. Exp. Med.,* 134, 871, 1971.
138. **Edmondson, H. A., Peters, R. L., Reynolds, T. B., and Kuzma, O. T.,** Sclerosing hyaline necrosis of the liver in the chronic alcoholic. A recognizable clinical syndrome, *Ann. Intern. Med.,* 59, 646, 1963.
139. **Egana, E. and Rodrigo, R.,** Some biochemical effects of ethanol on CNS, *Int. J. Neurol.,* 9, 143, 1974.
140. **Eichelbaum, M.,** Defective oxidation of drugs: pharmacokinetic and therapeutic implications, *Clin. Pharmacokin.,* 7, 1, 1982.
141. **Elder, G. H.,** Identification of a group of tetracarboxylate porphyrins containing one acetate and three propionate substituents, in faeces from patients with symptomatic cutaneous hepatic porphyria and from rats with porphyria due to hexachlorobenzene, *Biochem. J.,* 126, 877, 1972.
142. **Elder, G. H., Evans, J. O., and Matlin, S. A.,** The effect of the porphyrogenic compound, hexachlorobenzene, on the activity of hepatic uroporphyrinogen decarboxylase in the rat, *Clin. Sci. Mol. Med.,* 51, 71, 1976.
143. **Elder, G., Gray, C. H., and Nicholson, D. C.,** The porphyrias: a review, *Sem. J. Clin. Pathol.,* 25, 1013, 1972.
144. **Elek, G., Rockenhauer, A., Kovacs, L., and Balint, G.,** Free radical signal of bile pigment in paraffin embedded liver tissue, *Histochemistry,* 79, 405, 1983.
145. **Elliot, W. H. and Hyde, P. M.,** Metabolic pathways of bile acid synthesis, *Am. J. Med.,* 51, 568, 1971.
146. **Engel, A. G., Banker, B. Q., and Eiben, R. M.,** Carnitine deficiency: clinical, morphological and biochemical observations in a fatal case, *J. Neurol. Neurosurg. Psychiat.,* 40, 313, 1977.
147. **Epstein, S., Ito, N., Merkow, L., and Farber, E.,** Cellular analysis of liver carcinogenesis: the induction of large hyperplastic nodules in the liver with 2-fluorenylacetamide or ethionine and some aspects of their morphology and glycogen metabolism, *Cancer Res.,* 27, 1702, 1967.
148. **Eriksson, L. C., Torndal, U. B., and Andersson, G. N.,** Isolation and characterization of endoplasmic reticulum and Golgi apparatus from hepatocyte nodules in male Wistar rats, *Cancer Res.,* 43, 3335, 1983.
149. **Erlinger, S., Dhumeaux, D., Berthelot, P., and Dumont, M.,** Effect of inhibitors of sodium transport in bile formation in the rabbit, *Am. J. Physiol.,* 219, 416, 1970.
150. **Ernster, L.,** The mode of action of bilirubin on mitochondria, in *Kernicterus,* Sass-Kortsak, A., Ed., University of Toronto Press, Toronto, 1961, 174—181.
151. **Eubanks, S. W., Patterson, J. W., May, D. L., and Aeling, J. L.,** The porphyrias, *Int. J. Dermatol.,* 22, 337, 1983.
152. **Evensen, S. A.,** Incorporation of precursors into sterols and proteins in liver biopsies from patients with liver disorders, *Scand. J. Gastroenterol.,* 19, 6, 1984.
153. **Fallon, A., Bradley, J. F., Burns, J., and O'D McGee, J.,** Collagen stimulating factors in hepatic fibrinogenesis, *J. Clin. Pathol.,* 37, 542, 1984.

154. **Faraj, B. A., Camp, V. M., Kutner, M., and Ahmann, P. A.**, Abnormal regulation of pyridoxal 5'-phosphate in Reye's syndrome, *Clin. Chem.*, 29, 1832, 1983.

155. **Farber, E.**, Pre-cancerous steps in carcinogenesis: their physiological adaptive nature, *Biochim. Biophys. Acta*, 738, 171, 1984.

156. **Farber, E.**, The biochemistry of the preneoplastic liver: a common metabolic pattern in hepatocyte nodules, *Can. J. Biochem. Cell Biol.*, 62, 486, 1984.

157. **Farber, E.**, The multistep nature of cancer development, *Cancer Res.*, 44, 4217, 1984.

158. **Farber, E.**, The resistance of putative premalignant liver cell populations, hyperplastic nodules to the acute cytotoxic effects of some hepatocarcinogens, *Cancer Res.*, 36, 3879, 1976.

159. **Farber, E. and Cameron, R.**, The sequential analysis of cancer development, *Adv. Cancer Res.*, 31, 125, 1980.

160. **Faustman-Watts, E. M. and Goodman, J. I.**, DNA-purine methylation in hepatic chromatin following exposure to dimethylnitrosamine or methylnitrosourea, *Biochem. Pharmacol.*, 33, 585, 1984.

161. **Feinman, L. and Lieber, C. S.**, Effect of ethanol on plasma glycerol in man, *Am. J. Clin. Nutr.*, 20, 400, 1967.

162. **Felding, I. and Rane, A.**, Congenital liver damage after treatment of mother with valproic acid and phenytoin, *Acta Paediatr. Scand.*, 73, 565, 1984.

163. **Feldman, D. S., Levere, R. D., Lieberman, J. S., Cardinal, R. A., and Watson, C. J.**, Presynaptic neuromuscular inhibition by porphobilinogen and porphobilin, *Proc. Natl. Acad. Sci., U.S.A.*, 68, 383, 1971.

164. **Feldman, J. G., Hazan, M., Nagaranjan, M., and Kissin, B.**, A case control investigation of alcohol, tobacco and diet in head and neck cancer, *Prev. Med.*, 4, 444, 1975.

165. **Feldstein, A. and Sidel, C. M.**, The effect of ethanol on the in vivo conversion of 5-HTP-14C to serotonin-14C, 5-hydroxyindoleacetaldehyde-14C and its metabolites in rat brain, *Int. J. Neuropharmacol.*, 8, 347, 1969.

166. **Fenster, L. F. and Klatskin, G.**, Manifestations of metastatic tumors of the liver, *Am. J. Med.*, 31, 238, 1961.

167. **Feuer, G.**, Carcinogenesis and cytochrome P-450, in *Cytochrome P-450, Biochemistry, Biophysics and Induction. Proc. 5th Int. Conf. Cytochrome P-450*, Vereczkey L. and Magyar, K., Eds., Akademia Kiado, Budapest, 1985, 509—515.

168. **Feuer, G.**, Drug control of steroid metabolism by the hepatic endoplasmic reticulum, *Drug Metab. Rev.*, 14, 1119, 1983.

169. **Feuer, G.**, Hepatic metabolism and carcinogenesis: its role in hepatoma and adenocarcinoma, in *Proc. Int. Conf. Occupational and Environmental Significance of Industrial Carcinogens*, Bologna, October 8—10, 1985.

170. **Feuer, G.**, The link between the mother and fetus in drug metabolism, *Rev. Canad. Biol.*, 32(Suppl.), 113, 1973.

171. **Feuer, G. and de la Iglesia, F. A.**, *Molecular Biochemistry of Human Disease*, Vol. 1, CRC Press, Inc., Boca Raton, FL, 1985.

172. **Feuer, G., de la Iglesia, F. A., and Sosa-Lucero, J. C.**, Effect of dietary hepatic necrosis on the metabolism of foreign compounds in rat liver, *Nutr. Reports Int.*, 11, 199, 1975.

173. **Feuer, G. and Kardish, R.**, Hormonal regulation of drug metabolism during pregnancy, *Int. J. Clin. Pharmacol. Biopharm.*, 11, 366, 1975.

174. **Feuer, G., Kardish, R., and Farkas, R.**, Differential action of progesterones on hepatic microsomal activities in the rat, *Biochem. Pharmacol.*, 26, 1495, 1977.

175. **Feuer, G. and Kellen, J. A.**, Link between carcinogenecity and hepatic metabolism of 7, 12-dimethyl-benz(a)anthracene, *Oncology*, 30, 499, 1974.

176. **Feuer, G. and Kellen, J. A.**, The effect of experimental rat tumours on progesterone binding in the host liver, *Clin. Science*, 64, 303, 1983.

177. **Feuer, G., Stuhne-Sekalec, L., Roomi, M. W., and Cameron, R. G.**, Changes in progesterone binding and metabolism in liver microsomes from persistent hepatocyte nodules and hepatomas in male rats, *Cancer Res.*, 46, 76, 1986.

178. **Finkelstein, J. D., Cello, J. P., and Kyle, W. E.**, Ethanol-induced changes in methionine metabolism in rat liver, *Biochem. Biophys. Res. Comm.*, 61, 525, 1974.

179. **Fischer, G., Katz, N., Fischer, W., and Schauer, A.**, Biochemical quantification of ATPase activities during liver carcinogenesis, *Cancer Detect. Pres.*, 6, 363, 1983.

180. **Flamant, R., Lasserre, O., Lazar, P., Leguerinais, J., Denoix, P., and Schwartz, D.**, Differences in sex ratio according to cancer site and possible relationship with use of tobacco and alcohol. Review of 65,000 cases, *J. Natl. Cancer Inst.*, 32, 1309, 1964.

181. **Fleming, K. A. and McGee, J. O.**, Alcohol-induced liver disease, *J. Clin. Pathol.*, 37, 721, 1984.

182. **Flink, E. B.**, Mineral metabolism in alcoholism, in *The Biology of Alcoholism*, Vol. 1, Kissin, B. and Begleiter, H., Eds., Plenum Press, New York, 1971, 377—395.

183. **Fraser, I. H., Coolbear, T., Sarkar, M., and Mookerjea, S.,** Increase of sialyltransferase activity in the serum and liver of inflamed rats, *Biochim. Biophys. Acta,* 799, 102, 1984.

184. **Freinkel, N., Singer, D. L., Arky, R. A., Bleicher, S. J., Anderson, J. B., and Silbert, C. K.,** Alcohol hypoglycemia. I. Carbohydrate metabolism of patients with clinical alcohol hypoglycemia and the experimental reproduction of the syndrome with pure ethanol, *J. Clin. Invest.,* 42, 1112, 1963.

185. **Freund, G. and O'Hollaren, P.,** Acetaldehyde concentrations in alveolar air following a standard dose of ethanol in man, *J. Lipid Res.,* 6, 471, 1965.

186. **Frydman, R. B., Tomaro, M. L., Wanschelbaum, A., and Frydman, B.,** The enzymatic oxidation of porphobilinogen, *FEBS Lett.,* 26, 203, 1972.

187. **Forsman, A. O.,** Individual variability in response to haloperidol, *Proc. R. Soc. Med.,* 69(Suppl. 9), 1976.

188. **Fortier, R. A.,** Etude sur le facteurs etiologiques des cancers buccauxpharynges dans la province de Quebec, *J. Can. Dent. Assoc.,* 41, 235, 1975.

189. **Fox, R. A.,** Immune mechanisms in alcoholic liver disease, in *Alcohol and the Liver,* Vol. 3, Fisher, M. M. and Rankin, J. G., Eds., Plenum Press, New York, 1977, 309—322.

190. **Freer, D. E. and Statland, B. E.,** Effects of ethanol (0.75 g/kg body weight) on the activities of selective enzymes in sera of healthy young adults. II. Inter-individual variations in response of γ-glutamyltransferase to repeated ethanol challenges, *Clin. Chem.,* 23, 2099, 1977.

191. **Galambos, J. T.,** Natural history of alcoholic hepatitis, *Gastroenterology,* 63, 1026, 1972.

192. **Gall, E. A. and Dobrogorski, O.,** Hepatic alterations in obstructive jaundice, *Am. J. Clin. Pathol.,* 41, 126, 1965.

193. **Garner, R. C. and McLean, A. E. M.,** Increased susceptibility to carbon tetrachloride poisoning in the rat after pretreatment with oral phenobarbitone, *Biochem. Pharmacol.,* 18, 648, 1969.

194. **Gentz, J., Jagenburg, R., and Zetterstrom, R. J.,** Tyrosinemia, an inborn error of tyrosine metabolism with cirrhosis of the liver and multiple renal tubular defect (de Toni-Debre-Fanconi syndrome), *J. Pediatr.,* 66, 670, 1965.

195. **Gerber, M. A.,** Immunology of liver disease, *Semin. Liver Dis.,* 4, 69, 1984.

196. **Gerber, M. A., Brodin, A., Steinberg, D., Vernace, S., Yang, C. P., and Paronetto, F.,** Periarteritis nodosa, Australia antigen and lymphatic leukemia, *N. Eng. J. Med.,* 286, 14—17, 1972.

197. **Gerber, M. A., Orr, W., Denk, H., Schaffner, F., and Popper, H.,** Hepatocellular hyalin in cholestasis and cirrhosis: its diagnostic significance, *Gastroenterology,* 64, 89, 1973.

198. **Gibel, W., Wildner, G. P., and Lohs, K.,** Untersuchungen zur Frage einer kanzerogenen und hepatotoxischen Wirkung von Fuselol, *Arch. Geschwulstforsch.,* 32, 115, 1968.

199. **Girard, J. P.,** Action of ethyl alcohol on serotonin metabolism, *Med. Exp.,* 7, 287, 1962.

200. **Gjessing, L. R.,** Studies on urinary phenolic compounds in man. II. Phenolic acids and amines during a load of alpha-methyl-dopa and disulfiram in periodic catatonia, *Scand. J. Clin. Lab. Invest.,* 17, 549, 1965.

201. **Gjessing, L. R. and Mauritzen, K.,** Cystathioninuria in hepatoblastoma, *Scand. J. Clin. Lab. Invest.,* 17, 513, 1965.

202. **Gjessing, L. R., Nishimura, T., and Borud, O.,** Studies on urinary phenolic compounds in man. I. Excretion of p-hydroxy-mandelic acid by man, *Scand. J. Clin. Lab. Invest.,* 17, 401, 1965.

203. **Glasgow, J. F. and Moore, R.,** Plasma amino acid ratio as an index of hepatocellular maturity in the neonate, *Biol. Neonate,* 44, 146, 1983.

204. **Glazer, S. D., Roenigk, H. H., Jr., Yokoo, H., Sparberg, M., and Paravicini, U.,** Ultrastructural survey and tissue analysis of human livers after a 6-month course of etretinate, *J. Am. Acad. Dermatol.,* 10, 632, 1984.

205. **Gluud, C., Bahnsen, M., Bennett, P., Brodthagen, U. A., Dietrichson, O., Johnsen, S. G., Nielsen, J., Micic, S., Svendsen, L. B., and Svenstrup, B.,** Hypothalamic-pituitary-gonadal function in relation to liver function in men with alcoholic cirrhosis, *Scand. J. Gastroenterol.,* 18, 939, 1983.

206. **Goldberg, A.,** Acute intermittent porphyria, *Quart. J. Med.,* 28, 183, 1959.

207. **Goldberg, A.,** Experimental porphyria, *Biochem. Soc. Sympos.,* 28, 35, 1968.

208. **Goldberg, A., Rimington, C., and Lochhead, A. C,** Hereditary coproporphyria, *Lancet,* 1, 632, 1967.

209. **Goldfarb, S.,** A morphological and histochemical study of carcinogenesis of the liver in rats fed 3-methyl-4-dimethylaminoazobenzene, *Cancer Res.,* 33, 1119, 1973.

210. **Goldfarb, S., Pugh, T. D., and Koen, H.,** Hepatocellular injury, hyperplasia and putative premalignancy in rats fed 2-acetylaminofluorene, *Adv. Enzyme Regul.,* 22, 123, 1984.

211. **Graber, D., Giuliani, D., Leevy, C. M., and Morse, B. S.,** Platelet-associated IgG in hepatitis and cirrhosis, *J. Clin. Immunol.,* 4, 108, 1984.

212. **Granick, S.,** The induction in vitro of the synthesis of delta-aminolevulinic acid synthetase in chemical porphyria: a response to drugs, sex hormones and foreign chemicals, *J. Biol. Chem.,* 241, 1359, 1966.

213. **Granick, S. and Kappas, A.,** Steroid control of porphyrin and heme biosynthesis: a new biological function of steroid hormone metabolites, *Proc. Natl. Acad. Sci. U.S.A.,* 57, 1463, 1967.

214. **Granick, S. and Kappas, A.,** Steroid induction of porphyrin synthesis in liver cell culture. I. Structural basis and possible physiological role in the control of heme formation, *J. Biol. Chem.,* 242, 4587, 1967.

215. **Granick, S. and Sassa, S.,** Steroids and porphyrin synthesis in Metabolic Pathways, Vol. 5, Vogel, H. J., Ed., Academic Press, New York, 1971, 77.

216. **Granick, S. and Urata, G.,** Increase in activity of 5-aminolevulinic acid in liver mitochondria induced by feeding of 3,5-dicarbethoxy-1,4-dihydrocollidin, *J. Biol. Chem.,* 238, 821, 1963.

217. **Granot, E., Deckelbaum, R. J., Judd, R., Jr., Slonim, A. E., and Gutman, A.,** Recurrent Reye-like syndrome: possible association with Krebs cycle abnormality, *Isr. J. Med. Sci.,* 20, 148, 1984.

218. **Gray, C. H.,** *Bile Pigments in Health and Disease,* Am. Lecture Series No. 422, Charles C Thomas, Springfield, IL, 1961.

219. **Gray, C. H., Kulczycka, A., Nicholson, D. C., Magnus, I. A., and Rimington, C.,** Isotope studies on a case of erythropoietic protoporphyria, *Clin. Sci.,* 26, 7, 1964.

220. **Gray, C. H., Neuberger, A., and Sneath, P. H. A.,** Studies in congenital porphyria; incorporation of 15 N into coproporphyrin, uroporphyrin and hippuric acid, *Biochem. J.,* 47, 87, 1950.

221. **Gray, C. H. and Scott, J. J.,** The effect of hemorrhage on the incorporation of (alpha-C14) glycine into stercobilin, *Biochem. J.,* 71, 38, 1959.

222. **Greco, A. V., Bentoli, A., Caputo, S., Altomonte, L., Manna, R., and Ghirlanda, G.,** Decreased insulin binding to red blood cells in liver cirrhosis, *Acta Diabetol. Lat.,* 20, 251, 1983.

223. **Greenwood, D. T. and Stevenson, I. H.,** The stimulation of glucuronide formation in vitro and in vivo by a carcinogen, diethylnitrosamine, *Biochem. J.,* 96, 37, 1965.

224. **Gregg, J. A.,** Urinary excretion of bile acids in patients with obstructive jaundice and hepatocellular disease, *Am. J. Clin. Pathol.,* 49, 404, 1968.

225. **Greim, H., Trulzsch, D., Czygan, P., Rudick, J., Hutterer, F., Schaffner, F., and Popper, H.,** Bile acids in human livers with or without biliary obstruction, *Gastroenterology,* 63, 846, 1972.

226. **Griffiths, P. J., Littleton, J. M., and Ortiz, A.,** Evidence of a role for brain monoamines in ethanol dependence, *Br. J. Pharmacol.,* 48, 354, 1973.

227. **Grodsky, G. M., Cantopoulous, A. N., Fanska, R., and Carbone, J. V.,** Distribution of bilirubin-H3 in the fetal and maternal rat, *Am. J. Physiol.,* 204, 837, 1963.

228. **Guarino, A. M., Gram, T. E., Schroeder, D. H., Call, J. B., and Gillette, J. R.,** Alterations in kinetic constants for hepatic microsomal aniline hydroxylase and ethylmorphine N-demethylase associated with pregnancy in rats, *J. Pharmacol. Exp. Ther.,* 168, 224, 1969.

229. **Guder, W. G., Habicht, A., Kleissl, J., Schmidt, U., and Wieland, O. H.,** The diagnostic significance of liver cell inhomogeneity: serum enzymes in patients with central liver necrosis and the distribution of glutamate dehydrogenase in normal human liver, *Z. Klin. Chem. Klin. Biochem.,* 13, 311, 1975.

230. **Guttenplan, J. B., Hutterer, F., and Garro, A. J.,** Effects of cytochrome P-448 and P-450 inducers on microsomal dimethylnitrosamine demethylase activity and the capacity of isolated microsomes to activate dimethylnitrosamine to a mutagen, *Mutat. Res.,* 35, 415, 1976.

231. **Hadziyannis, S. J., Lieberman, H. M., Karvountzis, G. G., and Shafritz, D. A.,** Analysis of liver disease, nuclear HBcAg, viral replication, and hepatitis B virus DNA in liver and serum of HBeAg vs. anti-HBe positive carriers of hepatitis B virus, *Hepatology,* 3, 656, 1983.

232. **Halstead, C. H., Robles, E. A., and Mezey, E.,** Decreased jejunal uptake of labeled folic acid (3H-PGA) in alcoholic patients: roles of alcohol and nutrition, *N. Engl. J. Med.,* 285, 701, 1971.

233. **Harada, S., Agarwal, D. P., and Goedde, H. W.,** Human liver alcohol dehydrogenase isoenzyme variations. Improved separations methods using prolonged high voltage starch-gel electrophoresis and isoelectric focusing, *Hum. Genet.,* 40, 215, 1978.

234. **Harada, S., Misawa, S., Agarwal, D. P., and Goedde, H. W.,** Liver alcohol dehydrogenase and aldehyde dehydrogenase in Japanese: isoenzyme variation and its possible role in alcohol intoxication, *Am. J. Hum. Genet.,* 32, 8, 1980.

235. **Hardison, W. G. M.,** Bile salts and the liver, *Prog. Liver Dis.,* 4, 83, 1972.

236. **Hargreaves, T.,** The effect of diethylaminoethyl diphenylpropyl-acetic acid (SKF 525A) on uridine 5-pyrophosphate glucuronyltransferase, *Biochem. Pharmacol.,* 16, 1481, 1967.

237. **Hargreaves, T. and Holton, J. B.,** Jaundice of the newborn due to novobiocin, *Lancet,* 1, 839, 1962.

238. **Harinasuta, U. and Zimmerman, H. J.,** Alcoholic steatonecrosis. I. Relationship between severity of hepatic disease and presence of Mallory bodies in the liver, *Gastroenterology,* 60, 1036, 1971.

239. **Harris, C. C. and Sun, T.,** Multifactoral etiology of human liver cancer, *Carcinogenesis,* 5, 697, 1984.

240. **Hartroft, W. S. and Ridout, J. H.,** Pathogenesis of cirrhosis produced by choline deficiency, *Am. J. Pathol.,* 27, 951, 1951.

241. **Havens, W. P., Jr. and Paul, J. R.,** Infectious hepatitis and serum hepatitis, in *Viral and Rickettsial Infections of Man,* Horsfall, F. L. and Tamm, I., Eds., J.B. Lippincott, Philadelphia, 1965, 965—993.

242. **Hayashi, N., Kurashima, Y., and Kikuchi, G.,** Mechanism of allylisopropylacetamide-induced increase of 5-aminolevulinate synthetase in liver mitochondria, *Arch. Biochem. Biophys.,* 148, 10, 1972.

243. **Hayashi, N., Yoda, B., and Kikuchi, G.,** Difference in molecular size of delta-aminolevulinate synthetases in the soluble and mitochondrial fractions of rat liver, *J. Biochem. Tokyo,* 67, 859, 1970.

244. **Heard, G. S., Hood, R. L., and Johnson, A. R.,** Hepatic biotin and the sudden infant death syndrome, *Med. J. Aust.,* 2, 305, 1983.

245. **Hellstrom, K. and Sjovall, J.,** Conjugation of bile acids in patients with hypothyroidism (bile acids and steroids, 105), *J. Atheroscler. Res.,* 1, 205, 1961.

246. **Hempel, J., Von Bahr-Lindstrom, H., and Jornvall, H.,** Structural relationships among aldehyde dehydrogenases, *Pharmacol. Biochem. Behav.,* 18(Suppl. 1), 117, 1983.

247. **Henderson, B. E., Preston-Martin, S., Edmondson, H. A., Peters, R. L., and Pike, M. C.,** Hepatocellular carcinoma and oral contraceptives, *Br. J. Cancer,* 48, 437, 1983.

248. **Hepner, G. W., Piken, E., and Lechago, J.,** Abnormal aminopyrine metabolism in patients with chronic hepatitis, *West. J. Med.,* 134, 390, 1981.

249. **Hersh, T., Meinick, J. L., Goyal, R. K., and Hollinger, F. B.,** Nonparenteral transmission of viral hepatitis type B (Australia antigen-associated serum hepatitis), *N. Engl. J. Med.,* 285, 1363—1364, 1971.

250. **Herzfeld, A. and Greengard, O.,** The differentiation pattern of enzymes in livers of tumor-bearing rats, *Cancer Res.,* 32, 1826, 1972.

251. **Herzfeld, A. and Greengard, O.,** The effect of other neoplasms on hepatic and plasma enzymes in the host rat, *Cancer Res.,* 37, 231, 1977.

252. **Herzfeld, A., Greengard, O., and McDermott, W. V.,** Enzyme pathology of the liver in patients with and without non-hepatic cancer, *Cancer,* 45, 2383, 1980.

253. **Herzfeld, A., Greengard, O., and Warren, S.,** Tissue enzyme changes in parabiotic rats with subcutaneous lymphoma or fibrosarcoma, *J. Natl. Cancer Inst.,* 60, 825, 1978.

254. **Hillman, R. W.,** Alcoholism and malnutrition, in *Biology of Alcoholism,* Vol. 3, Kissin, B. and Begleiter, H., Eds., Plenum Press, New York, 1974, 513—560.

255. **Hoensch, H., Schmid, A., Hartmann, F., and Dolle, W.,** Drug metabolizing enzymes in human small intestinal biopsies: influence of exocrine pancreatic function, *Gastroenterology,* 74, 1045, 1978.

256. **Hofeler, H. and Klingemann, H. G.,** Fibronectin and factor VIII-related antigen in liver cirrhosis and acute liver failure, *J. Clin. Chem. Clin. Biochem.,* 22, 15, 1984.

257. **Hoffbauer, F. W. and Zaki, F. G.,** Choline deficiency in baboon and rat compared, *Arch. Pathol.,* 79, 364, 1965.

258. **Hoffmann, A. F. and Borgstrom, B.,** The intraluminal phase of fat digestion in man: the lipid content of the micellar and oil phases of intestinal content obtained during fat digestion and absorption, *J. Clin. Invest.,* 43, 247, 1964.

259. **Hoffmann, A. F. and Mosbach, E.,** Identification of allodeoxycholic acid as the major component of gallstones induced in the rabbit by 5d-cholestan-3β-ol, *J. Biol. Chem.,* 239, 2813, 1964.

260. **Holt, P. R., Haessler, H. A., and Isselbacher, K. J.,** Effects of bile salts on glucose metabolism by slices of hamster small intestine, *J. Clin. Invest.,* 42, 777, 1963.

261. **Holton, J. B. and Lathe, G. H.,** Inhibitors of bilirubin conjugation in new-born infant serum and male urine, *Clin. Sci.,* 25, 499, 1963.

262. **Horak, W., Grabner, G., and Paumgartner, G.,** Inhibition of bile salt-independent bile formation by indocyanine green, *Gastroenterology,* 64, 1005, 1973.

263. **Hsia, D. Y. Y., Riabov, S., and Dowben, R. M.,** Inhibition of glucuronosyl transferase by steroid hormones, *Arch. Biochem. Biophys.,* 103, 181, 1963.

264. **Huet, P. M. and Villeneuve, J. P.,** Determinants of drug disposition in patients with cirrhosis, *Hepatology,* 3, 913, 1983.

265. **Hugh-Jones, K., Slack, J., Simpson, K., Grossman, A., and Hsia, D. Y. Y.,** Clinical course of hyperbilirubinemia in premature infants, a preliminary report, *N. Engl. J. Med.,* 263, 1223, 1960.

266. **Hultberg, B., Isaksson, A., Joelsson, B., Alwmark, A., Gullstrand, P., and Bengmark, S.,** Pattern of serum beta-hexosaminidase in liver cirrhosis, *Scand. J. Gastroenterol.,* 18, 877, 1983.

267. **Ibraham, N. G., Friedland, M. L., and Levere, R. D.,** Heme metabolism in erythroid and hepatic cells, *Prog. Hematol.,* 13, 75, 1983.

268. **Iqbal, M. J., Wilkinson, M. L., Johnson, P. J., and Williams, R.,** Sex steroid receptor proteins in foetal, adult and malignant liver tissue, *Br. J. Cancer,* 48, 791, 1983.

269. **Insunza, I. and Ugarte, G.,** Esteatorrea en alcoholicos con y sin cirrosis hepatica, *Rev. Med. Chile,* 98, 669, 1970.

270. **Isaacs, H., Heffron, J. J. A., and Badenhorst, M.,** Weakness associated with the pathological presence of lipid in skeletal muscle: a detailed study of a patient with carnitine deficiency, *J. Neurol. Neurosurg. Psychiat.,* 39, 1114, 1976.

271. **Iseri, O. A., Lieber, C. S., and Gottlieb, L. S.,** The ultrastructure of fatty liver induced by prolonged ethanol ingestion, *Am. J. Pathol.,* 48, 535, 1966.

272. **Ishii, H., Kanno, T., Shigeta, Y., Takagi, S., Yasuroka, S., Kano, S., Takeshit, E., and Tsuchiya, M.,** Hepatic gamma glutamyl transpeptidase (GGTP) activity: its activation by chronic ethanol administration, *Gastroenterology,* 71:A20, 913, 1976.

273. **Israel, Y. and Orrego, H.,** Hypermetabolic state and hypoxic liver damage, *Recent Dev. Alcohol., 2,* 119, 1984.

274. **Israel, Y. and Orrego, H.,** On the characteristic of alcohol-induced liver enlargement and its possible hemodynamic consequences, *Pharmacol. Biochem. Behav.,* 18(Suppl. 1), 433, 1983.

275. **Israel, Y., Videla, L., and Bernstein, J.,** Liver hypermetabolic state after chronic ethanol consumption: hormonal interrelations and pathogenic implications, *Fed. Proc.,* 34, 2052, 1975.

276. **Isselbacher, K. J., Chrabas, M. F., and Quinn, R. C.,** The solubilization and partial purification of glucuronyl transferase from rabbit liver microsomes, *J. Biol. Chem.,* 237, 3033, 1962.

277. **Iversen, J., Vilstrup, H., and Tygstrup, N.,** Insulin sensitivity in alcoholic cirrhosis, *Scand. J. Clin. Lab. Invest.,* 43, 565, 1983.

278. **Jakobovits, A., Dudley, F. J., and Allen, P.,** Primary liver cell carcinoma complicating secondary biliary cirrhosis, *Br. Med. J. Clin. Res.,* 289, 227, 1984.

279. **Javitt, N. B., Fortner, J. G., and Shiu, M. H.,** Bile salt synthesis in transplanted human liver, *Gastroenterology,* 60, 405, 1971.

280. **Jenkins, W. J. and Peters, T. J.,** Subcellular localization of acetaldehyde dehydrogenase in human liver, *Cell Biochem. Funct.,* 1, 37, 1983.

281. **Joelsson, B., Hultberg, B., Alwmark, A., Gullstrand, P., and Bengmark, S.,** Pattern of serum amino acids in patients with liver cirrhosis, *Scand. J. Gastroenterol.,* 19, 547, 1984.

282. **Joelsson, B., Hultberg, B., Alwmark, A., Gullstrand, P., and Bengmark, S.,** Total serum bile acids, gamma-glutamyl transferase, prealbumin and tyrosine: sensitive serum markers of hepatic dysfunction in alcoholic liver cirrhosis, *Scand. J. Gastroenterol.,* 18, 497, 1983.

283. **Joliffe, N. and Jelinek, E. M.,** Vitamin deficiencies and liver cirrhosis in alcoholism: cirrhosis of liver, *Quart. J. Stud. Alcohol,* 2, 544, 1941.

284. **Jones, D. P., Losowsky, M. S., Davidson, C. S., and Lieber, C. S.,** Effects of ethanol on plasma lipids in man, *J. Lab. Clin. Med.,* 62, 675, 1963.

285. **Jones, D. P., Perman, E. S., and Lieber, C. S.,** Free fatty acid turnover and triglyceride metabolism after ethanol ingestion in man, *J. Lab. Clin. Med.,* 66, 804, 1965.

286. **Jones, E. A.,** The enigma of hepatic encephalopathy, *Postgrad. Med. J.,* 59(Suppl. 4), 42, 1983.

287. **Jones, J. E., Shane, S. R., Jacobs, W. H., and Flink, E. B.,** Magnesium balance studies in chronic alcoholism, *Ann. N. Y. Acad. Sci.,* 162, 934, 1969.

288. **Jornvall, H., Hempel, J., Vallee, B. L., Bosron, W. F., and Li, T. K.,** Human liver alcohol dehydrogenase, *Proc. Natl. Acad. Sci. U.S.A,* 81, 3024, 1984.

289. **Kabadi, U. M., Eisenstein, A. B., Tucci, J., and Pellicone, J.,** Hyperglucagonemia in hepatic cirrhosis: its relation to hepatocellular dysfunction and normalization on recovery, *Am. J. Gastroenterol.,* 79, 143, 1984.

290. **Kabadi, U. M. and Premachandra, B. N.,** Serum T3 and reverse T3 levels in hepatic cirrhosis: relation to hepatocellular damage and normalization on improvement in liver dysfunction, *Am. J. Gastroenterol.,* 78, 750, 1983.

291. **Kalant, H.,** Ethanol and the nervous system: experimental neurophysiological aspects, *Int. J. Neurol.,* 9, 111, 1974.

292. **Kallai, K., Hahn, A., Roder, V., and Zupanic, V.,** Correlation between histological findings and serum transaminase values in chronic diseases of the liver, *Acta Med. Scand.,* 175, 49, 1964.

293. **Kalow, W.,** Ethnic differences in drug metabolism, *Clin. Pharmacokin.,* 7, 373, 1982.

294. **Kalow, W.,** Pharmacoanthropology: drug metabolism, *Fed. Proc.,* 43, 2326, 1984.

295. **Kalow, W.,** Pharmacoanthropology: outline, problems and the nature of case histories, *Fed. Proc.,* 43, 2314, 1984.

296. **Kam, W., Rall, L. B., Smuckler, E. A., Schmid, R., and Rutter, W. J.,** Hepatitis B viral DNA in liver and serum of asymptomatic carriers, *Proc. Natl. Acad. Sci. U.S.A.,* 79, 7522, 1982.

297. **Kamath, P. S.,** Haemodynamics of the liver and its alteration in disease, *Trop. Gastroenterol.,* 4, 79, 1983.

298. **Kanagasundaram, N., Kakumu, S., Chen, T., and Leevy, C. M.,** Alcoholic hyaline antigen (AHAg) and antibody (AHAb) in alcoholic hepatitis, *Gastroenterology,* 73, 1368, 1977.

299. **Kaplan, H. A., Woloski, B. M., Hellman, M., and Jamieson, J. C.,** Studies on the effect of inflammation on rat liver and serum sialyltransferase, *J. Biol. Chem.,* 258, 11505, 1983.

300. **Kaplan, H. A., Woloski, B. M., and Jamieson, J. C.,** Studies on the effect of experimental inflammation on rat liver nucleotide sugar pools, *Comp. Biochem. Physiol. A,* 77, 207, 1984.

301. **Kappas, A. and Granick, S.,** Experimental hepatic porphyria: studies with steroids of physiological origin in man, *Ann. N.Y. Acad. Sci.,* 151, 842, 1968.

302. **Kappas, A. and Song, C. S.,** Enzyme induction in the liver, *Gastroenterology,* 55, 731, 1968.

303. **Kardish, R. and Feuer, G.,** Relationship between maternal progesterones and the delayed drug metabolism in the neonate, *Biol. Neonate,* 20, 58, 1972.

304. **Keeley, A. F., Iseri, O. A., and Gottlieb, L. S.,** Ultrastructure of hyaline cytoplasmic inclusions in a human hepatoma: relationship to Mallory's alcoholic hyalin, *Gastroenterology,* 62, 280, 1972.
305. **Kew, M. C.,** Hepatocellular carcinoma, *Postgrad. Med. J.,* 59(Suppl. 4), 78, 1983.
306. **Kew, M. C. and Popper, H.,** Relationship between hepatocellular carcinoma and cirrhosis, *Semin. Liver Dis.,* 4, 136, 1984.
307. **Khawaja, J. A., Lindholm, D. B., and Hilska, P.,** Production of a lesion on liver rough endoplasmic reticulum after prolonged ethanol ingestion and its reversal through abstinence, *Toxicol. Lett.,* 3, 197, 1979.
308. **Kiessling, K. H., Pilstrom, L., Strandberg, B., and Lindgren, L.,** Ethanol and the human liver: correlation between mitochondrial size and degree of ethanol abuse, *Acta Med. Scand.,* 178, 633, 1965.
309. **Kitahara, A., Yamazaki, T., Ishikawa, T., Camba, E., and Sato, K.,** Changes in activities of glutathione peroxidase and glutathione reductase during chemical hepatocarcinogenesis in the rat, *Gann,* 74, 649, 1983.
310. **Klaassen, C. D.,** Does bile acid secretion determine canalicular bile production in rats?, *Am. J. Physiol.,* 220, 667, 1971.
311. **Klaassen, C. D.,** Effects of phenobarbital on the plasma disappearance and biliary excretion of drugs in rats, *J. Pharmacol. Exp. Ther.,* 175, 289, 1970.
312. **Klaassen, C. D. and Watkins, J. B.,** Mechanisms of bile formation, hepatic uptake, and biliary excretion, *Pharmacol. Rev.,* 36, 1, 1984.
313. **Klion, F. M. and Schaffner, F.,** Ultrastructural studies in alcoholic liver disease, *Digestion,* 1, 2, 1968.
314. **Kmet, J. and Mahboubi, E.,** Esophageal cancer in the Caspian littoral of Iran: initial studies, *Science,* 175, 846, 1972.
315. **Koff, R. S. and Isselbacher, K. J.,** Changing concepts in the epidemiology of viral hepatitis, *N. Engl. J. Med.,* 278, 1371, 1968.
316. **Kolts, B. E. and Langfitt, M.,** Drugs and the liver, *Compr. Ther.,* 10, 55, 1984.
317. **Kominami, E., Kobayashi, K., Kominami, S., and Katunuma, N.,** Properties of a specific protease for pyridoxal enzymes and its biological role, *J. Biol. Chem.,* 247, 6848, 1972.
318. **Kono, A., Hara, Y., Sugata, S., Matsushima, Y., and Ueda, T.,** Substrate specificity of a thymidine phosphorylase in human liver tumor, *Chem. Pharm. Bull. (Tokyo),* 32, 1919, 1984.
319. **Korsten, M. A., Matsuzaki, S., Feinman, L., and Lieber, C. S.,** High blood acetaldehyde levels after ethanol administration. Difference between alcoholic and nonalcoholic subjects, *N. Engl. J. Med.,* 292, 386, 1975.
320. **Koshy, R., Maupas, P., Muller, R., and Hofschneider, P. H.,** Detection of hepatitis B virus-specific DNA in the genomes of human hepatocellular carcinoma and liver cirrhosis tissues, *J. Gen. Virol.,* 57, 95, 1981.
321. **Koss, I. G.,** Precancerous lesions, in *Persons at High Risk of Cancer,* Fraumeni, J. F., Ed., Academic Press, New York, 1975, 85—101.
322. **Kowaloff, E. M., Phang, J. M., Granger, A. S., and Downing, S. J.,** Regulation of proline oxidase activity by lactate, *Proc. Natl. Acad. Sci. U.S.A.,* 74, 5368, 1977.
323. **Kronborg, I. J., Evans, D. T., Mackay, I. R., and Bhathal, P. S.,** Chronic hepatitis after successive halothane anaesthetics, *Digestion,* 27, 123, 1983.
324. **Krugman, S. and Giles, J. P.,** Viral hepatitis. New light on an old disease, *JAMA,* 212, 1019, 1970.
325. **Krugman, S., Giles, J. P., and Hammond, J.,** Hepatitis virus: effect of heat on the infectivity and antigenicity of the MS-1 and MS-2 strains, *J. Infect. Dis.,* 122, 432—436, 1970.
326. **Kulkarni, M. S. and Anderson, M. W.,** Persistence of benzo(a)pyrene metabolite: DNA adducts in lung and liver of mice, *Cancer Res.,* 44, 97, 1984.
327. **Kupfer, A. and Preisig, R.,** Inherited defects of hepatic drug metabolism, *Semin. Liver Dis.,* 3, 341, 1983.
328. **Kuratsune, M., Kohchi, S., and Horie, A.,** Carcinogenesis in the esophagus. I. Penetration of benzo(a)pyrene and other hydrocarbons into the esophageal mucosa, *Gann,* 56, 177, 1965.
329. **Labadarios, D., Roussouw, J. E., McConnell, J. B., Davis, M., and Williams, R.,** Thiamine deficiency in fulminant hepatic failure and effects of supplementation, *Int. J. Vitam. Nutr. Res.,* 47, 17, 1977.
330. **Labadarios, D., Roussouw, J. E., McConnell, J. B., Davis, M., and Williams, R.,** Vitamin B6 deficiency in chronic liver disease-evidence for increased degradation of pyridoxal-5'-phosphate, *Gut,* 18, 23, 1977.
331. **Lamy, J., Aron, E., and Weill, J.,** Profil biologique des premieres etapes de la cirrhose alcoolique: IgA, transferrine, haptoglobine, orosomucoide et α_1-antitrypsine, *Pathol. Biol.,* 22, 401, 1974.
332. **Larrey, D. and Brunch, R. A.,** Clearance by the liver: current concepts in understanding the hepatic disposition of drugs, *Semin. Liver Dis.,* 3, 285, 1983.
333. **Lathe, G. H. and Tovey, L. A.,** Caeruloplasmin and green plasma in women taking oral contraceptives, in pregnant women and in patients with rheumatoid arthritis, *Lancet,* 2, 596, 1968.
334. **Lee, R. G., Avner, D. L., and Berenson, M. M.,** Structure-function relationships of protoporphyrin-induced liver injury, *Arch. Pathol. Lab. Med.,* 108, 744, 1984.
335. **Lees, R. S., Song, C. S., Levere, R. D., and Kappas, A.,** Hyperbeta-lipoproteinemia in acute intermittent porphyria: preliminary report, *N. Engl. J. Med.,* 282, 432, 1970.

336. **Leevy, C. M., Baker, H., TenHove, W., et al.,** B-complex vitamins in liver disease of the alcoholic, *Am. J. Clin. Nutr.*, 16, 339, 1965.

337. **Lehninger, A. L.,** *Biochemistry*, Worth Publishers, New York, 3rd ed., chap. 20, 1982, 543—558.

338. **Lelbach, W. K.,** Relation between alcohol digestion and liver damage, *Gastroenterology*, 53, 670, 1967.

339. **Lester, R. and Schmid, R.,** Intestinal absorption of bile pigments. II. Bilirubin absorption in men, *N. Engl. J. Med.*, 270, 779, 1964.

340. **Lester, B., Schuner, W., and Schmid, R.,** Intestinal absorption of bile pigments. IV. Urobilinogen absorption in man, *N. Engl. J. Med.*, 272, 939, 1965.

341. **Levere, R. D. and Kappas, A.,** Biochemical and clinical aspects of the porphyrias, *Adv. Clin. Chem.*, 11, 133, 1968.

342. **Levin, W., Conney, A. H., and Alvares, A. P.,** Induction of benzo(a)pyrene hydroxylase in human skin, *Science*, 176, 419, 1972.

343. **Levine, W. G.,** Glutathione and hepatic mixed function oxidase activity, *Drug Metab. Rev.*, 14, 909, 1983.

344. **Lieber, C. S.,** Alcohol and the liver, in *Liver Annual, A Series of Critical Surveys of the International Literature*, Vol. 3, Arias, I. M., Frenkel, M., and Wilson, J. H. P., Eds., 1983, 104—120.

345. **Lieber, C. S.,** Alcohol, liver injury and protein metabolism, *Pharmacol. Biochem. Behav.*, 13(Suppl. 1), 17, 1980.

346. **Lieber, C. S.,** Liver disease and alcohol: fatty liver, alcoholic hepatitis, cirrhosis, and their interrelationships, *Ann. N.Y. Acad. Sci.*, 252, 63, 1975.

347. **Lieber, C. S.,** Metabolic effects produced by alcohol in the liver and other tissues, *Adv. Intern. Med.*, 14, 151, 1968.

348. **Lieber, C. S.,** Metabolism and metabolic effects of alcohol. Symposium on ethyl alcohol and disease, *Med. Clin. North Am.*, 68:1, 3, 1984.

349. **Lieber, C. S. and DeCarli, L. M.,** Effect of drug administration on the activity of the hepatic microsomal ethanol oxidizing system, *Life Sci.*, 9(Part 2), 267, 1970.

350. **Lieber, C. S. and DeCarli, L. M.,** Hepatic microsomal ethanol oxidizing system: in vitro characteristics and adaptive properties in vivo, *J. Biol. Chem.*, 245, 2505, 1970.

351. **Lieber, C. S. and DeCarli, L. M.,** The role of hepatic microsomal ethanol oxidizing system (MEOS) for ethanol metabolism in vivo, *J. Pharmacol. Exp. Ther.*, 181, 279, 1972.

352. **Lieber, C. S., Jones, D. P., Losowsky, M. S., and Davidson, C. S.,** Interrelation of uric acid and ethanol metabolism in man, *J. Clin. Invest.*, 41, 1863, 1962.

353. **Lieber, C. S., Jones, D. P., Mendelson, J., and DeCarli, L. M.,** Fatty liver, hyperlipemia and hyperuricemia produced by prolonged alcohol consumption despite adequate dietary intake, *Trans. Assoc. Am. Physicians*, 1:289, 1963.

354. **Lieber, C. S. and Rubin, E.,** Alcoholic fatty liver, *N. Engl. J. Med.*, 280, 705, 1969.

355. **Lieber, C. S. and Rubin, E.,** Alcoholic fatty liver in man on a high protein and low fat diet, *Am. J. Med.*, 44, 200, 1968.

356. **Lieber, C. S., Seitz, H. K., Garro, A. J., and Worner, T. M.,** Alcohol-related diseases and carcinogenesis, *Cancer Res.*, 39, 2863, 1979.

357. **Lieber, C. S., Spritz, N., and DeCarli, L. M.,** Fatty liver produced by dietary deficiencies: its pathogenesis and potentiation by ethanol, *J. Lipid Res.*, 10, 283, 1969.

358. **Lieber, C. S., Teschke, R., Hasumura, Y., and DeCarli, L. M.,** Differences in hepatic and metabolic changes after acute and chronic alcohol consumptions, *Fed. Proc.*, 34, 2060, 1975.

359. **Lindamood, C., III, Bedell, M. A., Billings, K. C., Dyroff, M. C., and Swenberg, J. A.,** Dose-response for DNA and 06-methylguanine-DNA methyltransferase activity in hepatocytes of rats continuously exposed to dimethylnitrosamine, *Cancer Res.*, 44, 196, 1984.

360. **Linnet, K., Kelbaeck, H., and Bahnsen, M.,** Diagnostic values of fasting and postprandial concentrations in serum of 3-alpha-hydroxy-bile acids and gamma-glutamyl transferase in hepatobiliary disease, *Scand. J. Gastroenterol.*, 18, 49, 1983.

361. **Lithner, F. and Wetterberg, I.,** Hepatocellular carcinoma in patients with acute intermittent porphyria, *Acta Med. Scand.*, 215, 271, 1984.

362. **Loda, M., Clowes, G. H., Jr., Nespoli, A., Bigatello, L., Birkett, D. H., and Menzoian, J. O.,** Encephalopathy, oxygen consumption, visceral amino acid clearance, and mortality in cirrhotic surgical patients, *Am. J. Surg.*, 147, 542, 1984.

363. **London, I. M., West, R., Shemin, D., and Rittenberg, D.,** On origin of bile pigment in normal man, *J. Biol. Chem.*, 184, 351, 1950.

364. **London, W. T. and Blumberg, B. S.,** A cellular model of the role of hepatitis B virus in the pathogenesis of primary hepatocellular carcinoma, *Hepatology*, 2, 10S, 1082.

365. **London, W. T. and Blumberg, B. S.,** Hepatitis B and related viruses in chronic hepatitis cirrhosis and hepatocellular carcinoma in man and animals, in *Chronic Active Liver Disease*, Soloway, R. D., Ed., Churchill-Livingstone, New York, 1982, 58—73.

366. **London, W. T. and Blumberg, B. S.,** Hepatitis B virus and primary hepatocellular carcinoma, *Cancer: Achievements, Challenges and Prospects for the 1980's,* Vol. 1, Burchenal, J. H. and Oettgen, H. F., Eds., Grune & Stratton, New York, 1981, 161—183.

367. **Losowsky, M. S., Jones, D. P., Davidson, C. S., and Lieber, C. S.,** Studies of alcoholic hyperlipemia and its mechanism, *Am. J. Med.,* 35, 794, 1963.

368. **Losowsky, M. S. and Leonard, P. J.,** Evidence of vitamin E deficiency in patients with malabsorption or alcoholism and the effects of therapy, *Gut,* 8, 539, 1967.

369. **Lotlikar, P. D., Jhee, E. C., Insetta, S. M., and Clearfield, M. S.,** Modulation of microsome-mediated aflatoxin B1, binding to exogenous and endogenous DNA by cytosolic glutathione S-transferases in rat and hamster livers, *Carcinogenesis,* 5, 269, 1984.

370. **Lottsfeldt, F. I. and Labbe, R. F.,** Some cytologic changes of rat liver in experimental porphyria, *Proc. Soc. Exp. Biol. Med.,* 119, 226, 1965.

371. **Louagie, Y. A., Gianello, P., Kestens, P. J., Bonbled, F., and Haot, J. G.,** Vinylchloride induced hepatic angiosarcoma, *Br. J. Surg.,* 71, 322, 1984.

372. **Lowenfels, A. B., Masih, B., Lee, T. C., and Rohman, M.,** Effect of intravenous alcohol on the pancreas, *Arch. Surg.,* 96, 440, 1968.

373. **Lumeng, L. and Li, T.,** Vitamin B6 metabolism in chronic alcohol abuse, *J. Clin. Invest.,* 53, 693, 1974.

374. **Lunde, P. K. M., Frislid, K., and Hansteen, V.,** Disease and acetylation polymorphism, *Clin. Pharmacokin.,* 2, 182, 1977.

375. **Luxon, B. A. and Forker, E. L.,** Determining hepatic transport kinetics by mathematical modeling, *Fed. Proc.,* 43, 161, 1984.

376. **McFadzean, A. J. S. and Yeung, R. T. T.,** Further observations on hypoglycemia in hepatocellular carcinoma, *Am. J. Med.,* 47, 220, 1969.

377. **MacKenna, J., Dover, N. L., and Brame, R. G.,** Preeclampsia associated with hemolysis, elevated liver enzymes and low platelets — an obstetric emergency?, *Obstet. Gynecol.,* 62, 751, 1983.

378. **McLaughlan, J. M., Noel, F. J., and Moodie, C. A.,** Hypoglycemia in humans induced by alcohol and a low carbohydrate diet, *Nutr. Rep. Int.,* 8, 331, 1973.

379. **McLean, A. E.,** The effect of protein deficiency and microsomal enzyme induction by DDT and phenobarbitone on the acute toxicity of chloroform and pyrrolizidine alkaloide, retrorsine, *Br. J. Exp. Pathol.,* 51, 317, 1970.

380. **MacSween, R. N. M.,** Mallory's (alcoholic) hyaline in primary biliary cirrhosis, *J. Clin. Pathol.,* 26, 340, 1973.

381. **Magee, P. N.,** Possible mechanisms of carcinogenesis by N-nitroso compounds and alkylating agents, *Food Cosmet. Toxicol.,* 6, 572, 1968.

382. **Maltoni, C., Clini, C., Vicini, F., and Masina, A.,** Two cases of liver angiosarcoma among polyvinyl chloride (PVC) extruders of an Italian factory producing PVC bags and other containers, *Am. J. Ind. Med.,* 5, 297, 1984.

383. **Mangiantini, M. T., Leoni, S., Spagnuolo, S., and Trentalance, A.,** Modulation of metabolic activity in hepatocytes of proliferating systems, *Boll. Soc. Ital. Biol. Sper.,* 60(Suppl. 4), 115, 1984.

384. **Manolis, A.,** The diagnostic potential of breath analysis. *Clin. Chem.,* 29, 5, 1983.

385. **Marks, G. S., Hunter, G. S., Terner, U. K., and Schneck, D. W.,** Studies of the relationship between the chemical structure and porphyria-inducing activity, *Biochem. Pharmacol.,* 21, 2509, 1972.

386. **Marks, V. and Chakraborty, J.,** The clinical endocrinology of alcoholism, *J. Alcohol,* 8, 94, 1973.

387. **Martinez, I.,** Retrospective and prospective study of carcinoma of the esophagus, mouth and pharynx in Puerto Rico, *Bol. Assoc. Med. Puerto Rico,* 62, 170, 1970.

388. **Marver, H. S. and Schmid, R.,** The porphyrias, in *The Metabolic Basis of Inherited Disease,* 3rd ed., Stanbury, J. B., Wyngaarden, J. B., and Fredrickson, D. S., Eds., McGraw-Hill, New York, 1972, 1087.

389. **Matsuda, Y., Baranoa E., and Salaspuro, M.,** Effects of ethanol on liver microtubules and golgi apparatus, *Lab. Invest.,* 41, 455, 1979.

390. **Matsuo, T., Matsuo, C., and Matsuo, O.,** Characterization of the biological activity of antithrombin III in patients with hepatic cirrhosis, *Clin. Chem. Acta,* 140, 125, 1984.

391. **Mattocks, A. R.,** Toxicity of pyrrolizidine alkaloids, *Nature (London),* 217, 723, 1968.

392. **Mays, E. T. and Christopherson, W.,** Hepatic tumors induced by sex steroids, *Semin. Liver Dis.,* 4, 147, 1984.

393. **Medline, A. and Farber, E.,** Multi-step theory of neoplasia, *Rec. Adv. Histopathol.,* 11, 19, 1981.

394. **Meister, A.,** New developments in glutathione metabolism and their potential application in therapy, *Hepatology,* 4, 739, 1984.

395. **Mejer, J. and Reinicke, V.,** Changes in some nucleoside metabolizing enzymes of lymphocytes and granulocytes from patients with cirrhosis of the liver, *Scand. J. Clin. Lab. Invest.,* 43, 227, 1983.

396. **Melnick, J. P. and Hollinger, B. F.,** Hepatitis virology, in *Progress in Liver Diseases,* Vol. 4, Popper, H. and Schaffner, F., Eds., Grune & Stratton, New York, 1972, 345—352.

397. **Mezey, E.,** Alcoholic liver disease, in *Progress in Liver Disease,* Vol. 7, Popper, H. and Schaffner, F., Eds., Grune & Stratton, Toronto, 1982, 226—231.

398. **Mezey, E.,** Commentary on the hypermetabolic state and the role of oxygen in alcohol-induced liver injury, *Rev. Dev. Alcohol.,* 2, 135, 1984.

399. **Mezey, E., Potter, J. J., and Maddrey, W. C.,** Collagen turnover in alcoholic liver disease, *Gastroenterology,* 65A-36, 560, 1973.

400. **Michals, K., Pringle, K., Pang, E. J., and Matalon, R.,** Glucose-6-phosphatase as a marker for tumors of liver and kidney origin, *Biochem. Med.,* 30, 127, 1983.

401. **Mihas, A. A., Bull, D. M., and Davidson, C. S.,** Cell-mediated immunity to liver in patients with alcoholic hepatitis, *Lancet,* 1, 951, 1975.

402. **Miller, E. C.,** Some current perspectives on chemical carcinogenesis in humans and experimental animals, *Cancer Res.,* 38, 1479, 1978.

403. **Miller, W. I., Souncy, P. F., and Chang, J. T.,** Hepatic dysfunction following nafc, !in and cephalothin therapy in a patient with a history of oxacillin hepatitis, *Clin. Pharm.,* 2, 465, 1983

404. **Mirick, G. S., Ward, R., and McCollum, R. W.,** Modification of post-transfusion hepatitis by gamma globulin, *N. Engl. J. Med.,* 273, 59—65, 1965.

405. **Mishkel, M. A. and Morris, B.,** The metabolism of free fatty acids and chylomicron triglycerides by the perfused choline-deficient rat's liver, *Quart. J. Exp. Physiol.,* 49, 21, 1964.

406. **Mistilis, S. P. and Barr, G. D.,** Alcohol and the liver. I. Acute alcoholic hepatitis, *Med. J. Aust.,* 2, 182, 1980.

407. **Mitchell, J. R. and Jollow, D. J.,** Role of metabolic activation in chemical carcinogenesis and in drug induced hepatic injury, in *Drug and Liver,* Gerok, W. and Sickinger, K., Eds., 3rd Int. Symp., Schattauer Verlag, Stuttgart, 1975, 395—416.

408. **Miwa, G. T., Levin, W., and Thomas, P. E.,** The direct oxidation of ethanol by a catalase and alcohol dehydrogenase-free reconstituted system, containing cytochrome P-450, *Arch. Biochem. Biophys.,* 197, 464, 1979.

409. **Mones, J. M. and Saldana, M. J.,** Nodular regenerative hyperplasia of the liver in a 4-month-old infant, *Am. J. Dis. Child.,* 138, 79, 1984.

410. **Mones, J. M., Saldana, M. J., and Alboves-Saavedra, J.,** Nodular regenerative hyperplasia of the liver, *Arch. Pathol. Lab. Med.,* 108, 741, 1984.

411. **Mookerjea, S.,** Action of choline in lipoprotein metabolism, *Fed. Proc.,* 30, 143, 1971.

412. **Moses, H. L., Stein, J. A., and Tschudy, D. P.,** Hepatocellular changes associated with allylisopropylacetamide-induced hepatic porphyria in rats, *Lab. Invest.,* 22, 432, 1970.

413. **Moxley, R. T., Pozefsky, T., and Lockwood, D. H.,** Protein nutrition and liver disease after jejunoileal bypass for morbid obesity, *N. Engl. J. Med.,* 290, 921, 1974.

414. **Muir, H. M. and Neuberger, A.,** Biogenesis of porphyrins; origin of methyne carbon atoms, *Biochem. J.,* 47, 97, 1950.

415. **Myara, I., Myara, A., Mangeot, M., Fabre, M., Charpentier, C., and Lemonnier, A.,** Plasma prolidase activity: a possible index of collagen catabolism in chronic liver disease, *Clin. Chem.,* 30, 211, 1984.

416. **Myerson, R. M.,** Acute effects of alcohol on the liver with special reference to the Zieve syndrome, *Am. J.Gastroenterol.,* 49, 304, 1968.

417. **Nagasue, N., Yukaya, H., Hamada, T., Hirose, S., Kanashima, R., and InoKuchi, K.,** The natural history of hepatocellular carcinoma. A study of 100 untreated cases, *Cancer,* 54, 1461, 1984.

418. **Nakajima, H., Takemura, T., Nakajima, O., and Yamaoka, K.,** Studies on heme alpha-methenyl oxydase. I. The enzymatic conversion of pyridine-hemochromogen and hemoglobin into a possible precursor of biliverdin, *J. Biol. Chem.,* 238, 3784, 1963.

419. **Nakayama, F. and Johnston, C. G.,** Fractionation of bile lipids with silicic acid column chromatography, *J. Lab. Clin. Med.,* 59, 364, 1962.

420. **Narang, A. P., Datta, D. V., and Mathur, V. S.,** In vitro drug metabolism in humans with different liver diseases, *Int. J. Clin. Pharmacol. Ther. Toxicol.,* 21, 496, 1983.

421. **Narisawa, K. and Kikuchi, G.,** Effect of inhibitors of DNA synthesis on allylisopropylacetamide-induced increases of delta-aminolevulinic acid synthetase and other enzymes in rat liver, *Biochim. Biophys. Acta,* 99, 580, 1965.

422. **Nebert, D. W., Eisen, H. J., Negishi, M., Lang, M. A., Hjelmeland, L. M., and Okey, A. B.,** Genetic mechanisms controlling the induction of polysubstrate monooxygenase (P-450) activities, *Annu. Rev. Pharmacol. Toxicol.,* 21, 431, 1981.

423. **Nestel, P. J., Carroll, K. F., and Havenstein, N.,** Plasma triglyceride response to carbohydrates, fats and caloric intake, *Metabolism,* 19, 1, 1970.

424. **Newberne, P. M.,** Chemical carcinogenesis: mycotoxins and other chemicals to which humans are exposed, *Semin. Liver Dis.,* 4, 122, 1984.

425. **Nilius, R., Zipprich, B., and Krabbe, S.,** Aldehyde dehydrogenase in chronic alcoholic liver diseases, *Hepatogastroenterology,* 30, 134, 1983.

426. **Odell, G. B.,** The distribution of bilirubin between albumin and mitochondria, *J. Pediatr.,* 68, 164, 1966.

427. **Ohkubo, H., Okuda, K., Iida, S., Ohnishi, K., Ikawa, S., and Makino, I.,** Role of portal and splenic vein shunts and impaired hepatic extraction in the elevated serum bile acids in liver cirrhosis, *Gastroenterology*, 86, 514, 1984.

428. **Ortiz, A., Griffiths, P. J., and Littleton, J. M.,** A comparison of the effects of chronic administration of ethanol and acetaldehyde to mice: evidence for a role of acetaldehyde in ethanol dependence, *J. Pharm. Pharmacol.*, 26, 249, 1974.

429. **Ostrow, J. D. and Schmid, R.,** The protein binding of C-14-bilirubin in human and murine serum, *J. Clin. Invest.*, 42, 1286, 1963.

430. **Ostrowski, J., Kostrzewska, E., Michalak, T., Zawirska, B., Medrzejewski, W., and Gregor, A.,** Abnormalities in liver function and morphology and impaired aminopyrine metabolism in hereditary hepatic porphyrias, *Gastroenterology*, 85, 1131, 1983.

431. **Parke, D. V.,** The endoplasmic reticulum: its role in physiological functions and pathological situations, in *Concepts in Drug Metabolism*, Part B, Jenner, P. and Testa, B., Eds., Marcel Dekker, New York, 1981, 1—52.

432. **Paronetto, F.,** Immunologic factors in alcoholic liver disease, *Semin. Liver Dis.*, 1, 232, 1981.

433. **Patek, A. J., Bowry, S., and Hayes, K. C.,** Cirrhosis of choline deficiency in the Rhesus monkey. Possible role of dietary cholesterol, *Proc. Soc. Exp. Biol. Med.*, 148, 370, 1975.

434. **Patek, A. J., Jr., Bowry, S. C., and Sabesin, S. M.,** Minimal hepatic changes in rats fed alcohol and a high casein diet, *Arch. Pathol. Lab. Med.*, 100, 19, 1976.

435. **Pequignot, H., Cocheton, J., and Christorofov, B.,** Transparietal puncture biopsy of the liver. A review of 464 cases, *Mater. Med. Pol.*, 5, 99, 1973.

436. **Peraino, C., Fry, R. J. M., and Grube, D. D.,** Drug-induced enhancement of hepatic tumorigenesis, in *Carcinogenesis: Mechanisms of Tumor Promotion and Cocarcinogenesis*, Vol. 2, Slaga, T. J., Sivak, A., and Boutwell, R. K., Raven Press, New York, 1978, 421—432.

437. **Phillips, M. J. and Steiner, J. W.,** Electron microscopical studies on the liver cells in hyperplastic nodules of human cirrhosis, *Rev. Int. Hepat.*, 16, 307, 1966.

438. **Pickett, C. B., Williams, J. B., Cameron, R. G., and Lu, A. Y.,** Regulation of glutathione transferase and DT-diaphorase in MRNAs in persistent hepatocyte nodules during chemical hepatocarcinogenesis, *Proc. Natl. Acad. Sci. U.S.A.*, 81, 5091, 1984.

439. **Pindyck, J., Kappas, A., and Levere, R. D.,** Recent advances in porphyrin metabolism, *CRC Crit. Rev. Clin. Lab. Sci.*, 2, 639, 1971.

440. **Pitot, H. C.,** Biological and enzymatic events in chemical carcinogenesis, *Annu. Rev. Med.*, 30, 25, 1979.

441. **Pitot, H. C., Baraness, L., and Kitagawa, T.,** Stages in the process of hepatocarcinogenesis in rat liver, in *Carcinogenesis: Mechanisms of Tumor Promotion and Cocarcinogenesis*, Vol. 2, Slaga, T. J., Sivak, A., and Boutwell, R. K., Eds., Raven Press, New York, 1978, 421—432.

442. **Pogell, B. M. and Leloir, L. F.,** Nucleotide activation of liver microsomal glucuronidation, *J. Biol. Chem.*, 236, 293, 1961.

443. **Pohorecky, L. A., Jaffe, L. S., and Berkeley, H. A.,** Effects of ethanol on serotonergic neurons in the rat brain, *Res. Commun. Chem. Pathol. Pharmacol.*, 8, 1, 1974.

444. **Polonovski, M. and Bourillon, R.,** Les phospholipides de la bille, *Bull. Soc. Chim. Biol.*, 34, 712, 1952.

445. **Popper, H.,** Cholestasis, *Annu. Rev. Med.*, 19, 39, 1968.

446. **Popper, H.,** Concerning particularly delta agent infection, chronic hepatitis, and relation of hepatitis B infection to hepato-cellular carcinoma, *Prog. Clin. Biol. Res.*, 143, 397, 1983.

447. **Popper, H.,** Gallensauren und Cholestase, *Leber Magen Darm.*, 2, 205, 1972.

448. **Popper, H.,** Overview of past and future of hepatic collagen metabolism, in *Collagen Metabolism in the Liver*, Popper, H. and Becker, K., Eds., Stratton Intercontinental Medical Book Corporation, New York, 1975, 227—242.

449. **Popper, H., Barka, T., and Goldfarb, S.,** Factors determining chronicity of liver disease, *J. Mt. Sinai Hosp. N.Y.*, 30, 336, 1963.

450. **Popper, H. and Berk, P. D.,** Lessons from the study of cirrhosis and other fibrotic diseases of the liver, *Prog. Clin. Biol. Res.*, 154, 405, 1984.

451. **Popper, H., Gerber, M. A., and Thung, S. N.,** The relation of hepatocellular carcinoma to infection with hepatitis B and related viruses in man and animals, *Hepatology*, 2, 1-S, 1982.

452. **Popper, H., Gerber, M. A., and Vernace, S.,** Immunologic factors in liver disease, *Isr. J. Med. Sci.*, 9, 103, 1973.

453. **Popper, H. and Schaffner, F.,** Fine structural changes of the liver, *Ann. Intern. Med.*, 59, 674, 1963.

454. **Popper, H., Schaffner, F., Rubin, E., Barka, T., and Pasonetto, F.,** Mechanisms of intrahepatic cholestasis in drug-induced hepatic injury, *Ann. N.Y. Acad. Sci.*, 104, 988, 1963.

455. **Popper, H., Sternberg, S. S., Oser, B. L., and Oser, M.,** The carcinogenic effect of aramite in rats. A study of hepatic nodules, *Cancer*, 13, 1035, 1960.

456. **Porra, R. J. and Irving, E.,** The detection of delta-aminolaevulinic acid synthetase in anaerobically grown torulopsis utilis, *Arch. Biochem. Biophys.*, 149, 563, 1972.

457. **Posalaki, Z. and Barka, T.,** Alterations of hepatic endoplasmic reticulum in porphyric rats, *J. Histochem. Cytochem.*, 16, 337, 1968.
458. **Post, M. E. and Sun, A. Y.,** The effect of chronic ethanol administration on the levels of catecholeamines in different regions of the rat brain, *Res. Commun. Chem. Pathol. Pharmacol.*, 6, 887, 1973.
459. **Poulson, R. and Polglase, W. J.,** Evidence for the identification of P-503 with prototetrahydroporphyrin IX, *Biochim. Biophys. Acta*, 329, 256, 1973.
460. **Prensky, A. L. and Moser, H. W.,** Brain lipids, proteolipids and free amino acids in maple syrup urine disease, *J. Neurochem.*, 13, 863, 1966.
461. **Prince, A. M.,** Hepatitis B virus and hepatocellular carcinoma: molecular biology provides further evidence for an etiologic association, *Hepatology*, 1, 73, 1981.
462. **Prince, A. M.,** Role of serum hepatitis virus in chronic liver disease, *Gastroenterology*, 60, 913—921, 1971.
463. **Prince, A. M., Hargrove, R. L., Szmuness, W., Cherubin, C. E., Fontanta, V. J., and Jeffries, G. H.,** Immunologic distinction between infectious and serum hepatitis, *N. Engl. J. Med.*, 282, 987, 1970.
464. **Prince, A. M., Szmuness, W., Hargrove, R. L., Jeffries, G. H., Cherubin, C. E., and Kellner, A.,** The serum hepatitis virus specific antigen (SH): a status report, *Perspect. Virol.*, 7, 241—292, 1971.
465. **Evans, J. G., Prior, I. A. M., and Harvey, H. P. B.,** Relation of serum uric acid to body bulk haemoglobin and alcohol intake in two South Pacific polynesian populations, *Ann. Rheumatic Dis.*, 27, 319, 1968.
466. **Qian, G. X., Liu, C. K., and Waxman, S.,** Abnormal isoelectric focusing patterns of serum galactosyltransferase activity in patients with liver neoplasia, *Proc. Soc. Exp. Biol. Med.*, 175, 21, 1984.
467. **Rabes, H. M.,** Development and growth of early preneoplastic lesions induced in the liver by chemical carcinogens, *J. Cancer Res. Clin. Oncol.*, 106, 85, 1983.
468. **Rees, K. R. and Tarlow, M. J.,** The hepatotoxic action of allyl formate, *Biochem. J.*, 104, 757, 1967.
469. **Reid, W. D., Cho, A. K., Krishna, G., and Brodie, B. B.,** On the mechanism by which organic compounds produce tissue lesions. I. Hepatotoxicity of aromatic hydrocarbons and enhancement by phenobarbital, *Pharmacologist*, 12, 208, 1970.
470. **Reid, W. D., Christie, B., Krishna, G., Mitchell, J. R., Moskowitz, J., and Brodie, B. B.,** Bromobenzene metabolism and hepatic necrosis, *Pharmacology*, 6, 41, 1971.
471. **Renner, E., Wahlander, A., Huguenin, P., Wietholtz, H., and Preisig, R.,** Caffeine: a model compound for measuring liver function, *Hepatology*, 4, 74, 1984.
472. **Renner, I. G., Rinderknecht, H., and Wisner, J. R., Jr.,** Pancreatic secretion after secretion and cholecystokinin stimulation in chronic alcoholics with and without cirrhosis, *Dig. Dis. Sci.*, 28, 1089, 1983.
473. **Ricci, G. L., Michiels, R., Fevery, J., and De Groote, J.,** Enhancement by secretion of the apparently maximal hepatic transport of bilirubin in the rat, *Hepatology*, 4, 651, 1984.
474. **Ricciardi, B. R., Saunders, J. B., Williams, R., and Hopkinson, D. A.,** Hepatic ADH and ALDH isoenzymes in different racial groups and in chronic alcoholism, *Pharmacol. Biochem. Behav.*, 18(Suppl. 1), 61, 1983.
475. **Rissam, H. S., Nair, C. R., Anard, I. S., Madappa, C., and Wahi, P. L.,** Alteration of hepatic drug metabolism in female patients with congestive cardiac failure, *Int. J. Clin. Pharmacol. Ther. Toxicol.*, 21, 602, 1983.
476. **Roberts, R. J. and Plaa, G. L.,** Potentiation and inhibition of alpha-naphthyl-isothiocyanate-induced hyperbilirubinemia and cholestasis in rats, *J. Pharmacol. Exp. Ther.*, 150, 499, 1965.
477. **Rogers, A. E., Herndon, B. J., and Newberne, P. M.,** Induction by dimethylhydrazine of intestinal carcinoma in normal rats and rats fed high or low levels of vitamin A, *Cancer Res.*, 33, 1033, 1973.
478. **Rojkind, M. and Perez-Tamayo, R.,** Liver fibrosis, *Int. Rev. Connect. Tissue Res.*, 10, 333, 1983.
479. **Rothman, K. and Keller, A.,** The effect of joint exposure to alcohol and tobacco on risk of cancer of the mouth and pharynx, *J. Chronic Dis.*, 25, 711, 1972.
480. **Rubel, L. R.,** Hepatic injury associated with heatstroke, *Ann. Clin. Lab. Sci.*, 14, 130, 1984.
481. **Rubel, L. R., Rabin, L., Seeff, L. B., Licht, H., and Cuccherini, B. A.,** Does primary biliary cirrhosis in men differ from primary biliary cirrhosis in women?, *Hepatology*, 4, 671, 1984.
482. **Rubin, E., Beattie, D. S., Toth, A., and Lieber, C. S.,** Structural and functional effects of ethanol on hepatic mitochondria, *Fed. Proc.*, 31, 131, 1972.
483. **Rubin E. and Lieber, C. S.,** Alcohol-induced hepatic injury in non-alcoholic volunteers, *N. Engl. J. Med.*, 278, 869, 1968.
484. **Rubin, E. and Lieber, C. S.,** Early fine structural changes in the human liver induced by alcohol, *Gastroenterology*, 52, 1, 1967.
485. **Ruffolo, R. and Covington, H.,** Matrix inclusion bodies in the mitochondria of the human liver: evidence of hepatocellular injury, *Am. J. Pathol.*, 51, 101, 1967.
486. **Sabesin, S. M., Hawkins, H. L., Kuiken, L., and Ragland, J. B.,** Abnormal plasma lipoproteins and lecithin-cholesterol acyltransferase deficiency in alcoholic liver disease, *Gastroenterology*, 72, 510, 1977.
487. **Salmela, P. I.,** Association between liver histological changes and hepatic monooxygenase activities in vitro in diabetic patients, *Horm. Metab. Res.*, 16, 7, 1984.

488. **Sassa, S. and Granick, S.,** Induction of delta-aminolevulinic acid synthetase in chick embryo liver in culture, *Proc. Natl. Acad. Sci. U.S.A.,* 67, 517, 1970.

489. **Sato, K., Kitahara, A., Yin, Z., Ebina, T., Satoh, K., Tsuda, H., Ito, N., and Dempo, K.,** Molecular forms of glutathione S-transferase and UDP-glucuronyltransferase as hepatic preneoplastic marker enzymes, *Ann. N.Y. Acad. Sci.,* 417, 213, 1983.

490. **Schaffner, F.,** Intralobular changes in hepatocytes and the electron microscopic mesenchymal response in acute viral hepatitis, *Medicine,* 45, 547, 1966.

491. **Schaffner, F., Bacchin, P. G., Hutterer, F., Scharnbeck, H. H., Sarkozi, L. L., Denk, H., and Popper, H.,** Mechanism of cholestasis 4. Structural and biochemical changes in the liver and serum in rats after bile duct ligation, *Gastroenterology,* 60, 888, 1971.

492. **Schenker, S., McCandless, D. W., and Zollman, P. E.,** Studies of cellular toxicity of unconjugated bilirubin in kernicteric brain, *J. Clin. Invest.,* 45, 1213, 1966.

493. **Schmidt, E. and Schmidt, F. W.,** Methode und Wert der Bestimmung der Glutaminsaure-Dehydrogenase-Aktivitat im Serum ein Beitrag zur Bedeutung der Untersuchung von Enzym-Relationen im Serum, *Klin. Wochenschr.,* 40, 962, 1962.

494. **Schoental, R.,** Hepatotoxic activity of retrorsine, senkirkine and hydroxysenkirkine in newborn rats and the role of epoxides in carcinogenesis by pyrrolizidine alkaloids and aflatoxins, *Nature (London),* 227, 401, 1970.

495. **Schoental, R. and Bensted, J. P.,** Gastro-intestinal tumours in rats and mice following various routes of administration on N-methyl-N-nitroso-N'-nitroguanidine and N-ethyl-N-nitroso-N'-nitroguanidine, *Br. J. Cancer,* 23, 757, 1969.

496. **Schreiber, S. S., Oratz, M., and Rothschild, M. A.,** Alcoholic cardiomyopathy. II. The inhibition of cardiac microsomal protein synthesis by acetaldehyde, *J. Mol. Cell. Cardiol.,* 6, 207, 1974.

497. **Schulte-Hermann, R.,** *Reactions of the Liver to Injury: Adaptation in Toxic Liver Injury,* Farber, E. and Fisher, M. M., Eds., Marcel Dekker, New York, 1979, 285.

498. **Scribner, J. D. and Suss, R.,** Tumor initiation and promotion, *Int. Rev. Exp. Pathol.,* 18, 137, 1978.

499. Second Special Report to the U.S. Congress on Health, New Knowledge from the Secretary of Health, Education and Welfare, DHEW Publication No. (ADM) 74-124, United States Government Printing Office, Washington, D.C., 1974.

500. **Selikoff, I. J. and Hammond, E. C., Eds.,** Toxicity of vinyl-chloride-polyvinyl chloride, *Ann. N.Y. Acad. Sci.,* 246, 1, 1975.

501. **Shafritz, D. A. and Kew, M. C.,** Identification of integrated hepatitis B virus DNA sequences in human hepatocellular carcinomas, *Hepatology,* 1, 1, 1981.

502. **Shafritz, D. A. and Lieberman, H. M.,** The molecular biology of hepatitis B virus, *Annu. Rev. Med.,* 35, 219, 1984.

503. **Shafritz, D. A. and Rogler, C. E.,** Molecular characterization of viral forms observed in persistent hepatitis infections, chronic liver disease and hepatocellular carcinome in woodchucks and humans, in *Viral Hepatitis and Liver Disease,* Vyas, G., Dienstag, J., and Hoofnagle, J., Eds., Grune & Stratton, New York, 1984, 225—243.

504. **Shafritz, D. A., Shouval, D., Sherman, H. I., Hadziyannis, S. J., and Kew, M. C.,** Integration of hepatitis B virus DNA into the genome of liver cells in chronic liver disease and hepatocellular carcinoma, *N. Engl. J. Med.,* 305, 1067, 1981.

505. **Shank, R. C.,** Evidence for indirect genetic damage as methylation of DNA guanine in response to cytotoxicity, *Dev. Toxicol. Environ. Sci.,* 11, 145, 1983.

506. **Shapiro, H., Wruble, L. D., and Britt, L. G.,** The possible mechanism of alcohol in the production of acute pancreatitis, *Surgery,* 60, 1108, 1966.

507. **Shapot, V. S.,** On the multiform relationships between the tumor and the host, *Adv. Cancer Res.,* 30, 89, 1979.

508. **Shaw, S., Lue, S. L., and Lieber, C. S.,** Biochemical tests for the detection of alcoholism: comparison of plasma alpha amino-n-butyric acid with other available tests, *Alcoholism,* 2, 3, 1978.

509. **Shaw, S., Worner, T. M., and Lieber, C. S.,** Frequency of hyperprolinemia in alcoholic liver cirrhosis: relationship to blood lactate, *Hepatology,* 4, 295, 1984.

510. **Shemin, D. and Rittenberg, D.,** Utilization of glycine for synthesis of porphyrin, *J. Biol. Chem.,* 159, 567, 1945.

511. **Shemin, D. and Rittenberg, D.,** Life span of human red blood cell, *J. Biol. Chem.,* 166, 627, 1946.

512. **Sherlock, S.,** Advances in the treatment of diseases of the liver, *Practitioner,* 195, 485, 1966.

513. **Sherlock, S.,** Chronic hepatitis and cirrhosis, *Hepatology,* 4(Suppl. 25), S, 1984.

514. **Shinozuka, H., Sells, M. A., Katyal, S. L., Sell, S., and Lombardi, B.,** Effects of choline-devoid diet on the emergence of γ-glutamyltranspeptidase-positive foci in the liver of carcinogen-treated rats, *Cancer Res.,* 39, 2515, 1979.

515. **Shires, G. T., III, Albert, S. A., Illner, H., and Shires, G. T.,** Hepatocyte dysfunction in thermal injury, *J. Trauma,* 23, 899, 1983.

516. **Shouval, D., Chakraborty, P. R., Ruiz-Opazo, N., et al.,** Chronic hepatitis in chimpanzee carriers of hepatitis B virus: morphologic, immunologic and viral DNA studies, *Proc. Natl. Acad. Sci. U.S.A.,* 77, 6147, 1980.

517. **Sies, H., Brigelius, R., Wefers, H., Muller, A., and Cadenas, E.,** Cellular redox changes and response to drugs and toxic agents, *Fundam. Appl. Toxicol.,* 3, 200, 1983.

518. **Simon, F. R. and Arias, I. M.,** Alteration of bile canalicular enzymes in cholestasis. A possible cause of bile secretory failure, *J. Clin. Invest.,* 52, 765, 1973.

519. **Sims, P. and Grover, P. L.,** Epoxides in polycyclic aromatic hydrocarbons metabolism and carcinogenesis, *Adv. Cancer Res.,* 20, 165, 1974.

520. **Singh, S., Malhotra, R. S., Nagpal, B. L., and Lal, H.,** The role of copper in Indian childhood cirrhosis, *Ind. Pediatr.,* 20, 663, 1983.

521. **Smith, F. R. and Lindenbaum, J.,** Human serum retinol transport in malabsorption, *Am. J. Clin. Nutr.,* 27, 700, 1974.

522. **Smuckler, E. A.,** Alcoholic drink, its production and effects, *Fed. Proc.,* 34, 2038, 1975.

523. **Smuckler, E. A. and Barker, E. A.,** Effects of drugs on amino acid incorporation in the liver, *Proc. Eur. Soc. Study Drug Toxic.,* 7, 83, 1966.

524. **Solt, D. B., Medline, A., and Farber, E.,** Rapid emergence of carcinogen-induced hyperplastic lesions in a new model for the sequential analysis of liver carcinogenesis, *Am. J. Pathol.,* 88, 595, 1977.

525. **Sorensen, T. I., Orholm, M., Bentsen, K. D., Hoybye, G., Eghoje, K., and Chistoffersen, P.,** Prospective evaluation of alcohol abuse and alcoholic liver injury in men as predictors of development of cirrhosis, *Lancet,* 2, 241, 1984.

526. **Sotaniemi, E. A., Sutinen, S., Arranto, A. J., Sotaniemi, K. A., Lehtola, J., and Pelkonen, R. O.,** Liver damage in nurses handling cytostatic agents, *Acta Med. Scand.,* 214, 181, 1983.

527. **Speroni, G., Pezzarossa, A., Bonora, E., and Capretti, L.,** Effect of TRH on plasma glucagon in cirrhotic patients, *Horm. Metab. Res.,* 15, 619, 1983.

528. **Stein, J. A., Tschudy, D. P., Corcoran, P. L., and Collins, A.,** Delta-aminolevulinic acid synthetase, 3. Synergistic effect of chelated iron on induction, *J. Biol. Chem.,* 245, 2213, 1970.

529. **Stevens, R. G., Merkle, E. J., and Lustbader, E. D.,** Age and cohort effects in primary liver cancer, *Int. J. Cancer,* 33, 453, 1984.

530. **Stewart, A., Johnston, D. G., Alberti, K. G., Nattrass, M., and Wright, R.,** Hormone and metabolite profiles in alcoholic liver disease, *Eur. J. Clin. Invest.,* 13, 397, 1983.

531. **Stigendal, L. and Olsson, R.,** Alcohol consumption pattern and serum lipids in alcoholic cirrhosis and pancreatitis. A comparative study, *Scand. J. Gastroenterol.,* 19, 582, 1984.

532. **Stoloff, L.,** Aflatoxin as a cause of primary liver-cell cancer in the United States, a probability study, *Nutr. Cancer,* 5, 165, 1983.

533. **Stone, H. H., Martin, J. D., Jr., and Graber, C. D.,** Verdoglobinuria: an ominous sign of pseudomonas septicemia in burns, *Ann. Surg.,* 159, 991, 1964.

534. **Stoner, G. D., Harris, C. C., Autrup, H., Trump, B. F., Kingsbury, E. W., and Myers, G. A.,** Explant culture of human peripheral lung. I. Metabolism of benzo[a]pyrene, *Lab. Invest.,* 38, 685, 1978.

535. **Stiehl, A., Gundert-Remy, U., Walker, S., Sieg, A., Czygan, P., Kommerell, B., and Raedsch, K.,** Hepatic secretion of bilirubin and biliary lipids in patients with alcoholic cirrhosis of the liver, *Digestion,* 26, 80, 1982.

536. **Sullivan, J. F., Wolpert, P., Williams, R., and Egan, J. D.,** Serum magnesium in chronic alcoholism, *Ann. N.Y. Acad. Sci.,* 162, 947, 1969.

537. **Svoboda, D. J. and Mannering, R. T.,** Chronic alcoholism with fatty metamorphosis of the liver: mitochondrial alterations in hepatic cells, *Am. J. Pathol.,* 44, 645, 1964.

538. **Svoboda, D. J. and Reddy, J. K.,** Some effects of carcinogens on cell organelles, in *Cancer: A Comprehensive Treatise,* Vol. 1, 2nd ed., Becker, I. F., Ed., Plenum Press, New York, 1983, 411—449.

539. **Swerdlow, M. A. and Chowdhury, L. N.,** IgA deposition in liver in alcoholic liver disease, an index of progressive injury, *Arch. Pathol. Lab. Med.,* 108, 416, 1984.

540. **Taddeini, L., Nordstrom, K. L., and Watson, C. J.,** Hypercholesterolemia in experimental and human hepatic porphyria, *Metabolism,* 13, 691, 1964.

541. **Taddeini, L. and Watson, C. J.,** The clinical porphyrias, *Sem. Hematol.,* 5, 335, 1968.

542. **Takikawa, H., Otsuka, H., Beppu, T., Seyama, Y., and Yamakawa, T.,** Serum concentrations of bile acid glucuronides in hepatobiliary diseases, *Digestion,* 27, 189, 1983.

543. **Tamburro, C. H.,** Relationship of vinyl monomers and liver cancers: angiosarcoma and hepatocellular carcinoma, *Semin. Liver Dis.,* 4, 158, 1984.

544. **Teng, Y. S., Jehan, S., and Lie-Injo, L. E.,** Human alcohol dehydrogenase ADH2 and ADH3 polymorphism in ethnic Chinese and Indians of West Malaysia, *Hum. Genet.,* 53, 87, 1979.

545. **Thomsen, O.,** Mechanism and regulation of hepatic bile production with special reference to the bile acid-independent canalicular bile formation, *Scand. J. Gastroenterol.,* Suppl. 97, 1, 1984.

546. **Thomson, A. D., Baker, H. and Leevy, C. M.,** Patterns of 35S-thiamine hydrochloride absorption in the malnourished alcoholic patient, *J. Lab. Clin. Med.,* 76, 34, 1970.

547. **Thompson, R. A., Carter, R., Stokes, R. P., Geddes, A. M., and Goodall, J. A. D.,** Serum immunoglobulins, component levels and autoantibodies in liver disease, *Clin. Exp. Immunol.,* 14, 335, 1973.

548. **Thurman, R. G., Ji, S., and Lemasters, J. J.,** Alcohol-induced liver injury. The role of oxygen, *Rec. Dev. Alcohol,* 2, 103, 1984.

549. **Thurman, R. G., McKenna, W. R., Brentzel, H. J., and Gesse, S.,** Significant pathways of hepatic ethanol metabolism, *Fed. Proc.,* 34, 2075, 1975.

550. **Trennery, P. N. and Waring, R. H.,** Early changes in thioacetamide-induced liver damage, *Toxicol. Lett.,* 19, 299, 1983.

551. **Trivedi, P., Tanner, M. S., Portmann, B., McClement, J., and Mowat, A. P.,** Hepatic peptidyl prolyl hydroxylase activity and liver fibrosis — a prospective study of 94 infants and children with hepatobiliary disorders, *Hepatology,* 4, 436, 1984.

552. **Truitt, E. J. and Walsh, M. T.,** The role of acetaldehyde in the actions of ethanol, in *The Biology of Alcoholism,* Vol. 1, Kissin, B. and Begleiter, H. B., Eds., Plenum Press, New York, 1971, 161—191.

553. **Trulsch, D., Greim, H., Czygan, P., Hutterer, F., and Popper, H.,** Cytochrome P-450 in 7-alpha-hydroxylation of taurodeoxycholic acid, *Biochemistry,* 12, 76, 1973.

554. **Tschudy, D. P., Welland, F. H., Collins, A., and Hunter, G.,** Aminoacetone in acute intermittent porphyria, *Lancet,* 2, 660, 1963.

555. **Tschudy, D. P., Welland, F. H., Collins, A., and Hunter, G.,** The effect of carbohydrate feeding on the induction of delta-aminolevulinic acid synthetase, *Metabolism,* 13, 396, 1964.

556. **Tuma, D. J., Barak, A. J., Schafer, D. F., and Sorrell, M. F.,** Possible interrelationship of ethanol metabolism and choline oxidation in the liver, *Can. J. Biochem.,* 51, 117, 1973.

557. **Tuma, D. J. and Sorrell, M. F.,** Effect of ethanol on hepatic secretory proteins, *Rec. Dev. Alcohol,* 2, 159, 1984.

558. **Tuyns, A. J., Pequignot, G., and Jensen, O. M.,** Nutrition, alcool et cancer de l'oesophage, *Bull. Cancer,* 65, 58, 1978.

559. **Uchida, T., Kronborg, I., and Peters, R. L.,** Acute viral hepatitis: morphologic and functional correlations in human livers, *Hum. Pathol.,* 15, 267, 1984.

560. **Udagawa, M., Horie, Y., and Hirayama, C.,** Aberrant porphyrin metabolism in hepatocellular carcinoma, *Biochem. Med.,* 31, 131, 1984.

561. **Ugarti, G., Pereda, T., Perez, C., Iturriaga, H., Gattas, V., and Bunout, P.,** Nutritional status of alcoholic patients. Its possible relationship to alcoholic liver damage, *Am. J. Clin. Nutr.,* 38, 469, 1983.

562. **Uhlenbruck, G., Beuth, J., and Weidtman, V.,** Liver lectins; mediators for metastases?, *Experientia,* 39, 1314, 1983.

563. **Ulland, B. M., Weisburger, J. H., Yamamoto, R. S., and Weisburger, E. K.,** Antioxidants and carcinogenesis: butylated hydroxytoluene, but not diphenyl-p-phenylenediamine, inhibits cancer induction by N-2-fluorenylacetamide and by N-hydroxy-N-2-fluroenyl-acetamide in rats, *Food Cosmet. Toxicol.,* 11, 199, 1973.

564. **Vallari, R. C. and Pietruszko, R.,** Interaction of human cytoplasmic aldehyde dehydrogenase E1 with disulfiram, *Pharmacol. Biochem. Behav.,* 18(Suppl. 1), 97, 1983.

565. **Vallee, B. L. and Bazzone, T. J.,** Isozymes of human liver alcohol dehydrogenase, *Isozymes Curr. Top Biol. Med. Res.,* 8, 219, 1983.

566. **Van Thiel, D. H.,** Alcohol and its effect on endocrine functioning, *Alcoholism,* 4, 44, 1980.

567. **Van Waes, L. and Lieber, C. S.,** Early perivenular sclerosis in alcoholic fatty liver: an index of progressive liver injury, *Gastroenterology,* 73, 646, 1977.

568. **Van Waes, L. and Lieber, C. S.,** Glutamate dehydrogenase, a reliable marker of liver cell necrosis in the alcoholic, *Br. Med. J.,* 2, 1508, 1977.

569. **Vaughn, F. L. and Bernstein, I. A.,** Molecular aspects of control in epidermal differentiation, *Mol. Cell. Biochem.,* 12, 171, 1976.

570. **Velebny, V., Kasafirek, E., and Kanta, J.,** Desmosine and isodesmosine contents and elastase activity in normal and cirrhotic rat liver, *Biochem. J.,* 214, 1023, 1983.

571. **Verhamme, M., de Wolf-Peeters, C., and Van Steenbergen, W.,** Hepatic injury due to glafenine. Report of two cases and review of the literature, *Neth. J. Med.,* 27, 35, 1984.

572. **Vessell, E. S. and Penno, M. B.,** A new polymorphism of hepatic drug oxidation in humans: family studies on rates of formation of antipyrine metabolites, *Fed. Proc.,* 43, 2342, 1984.

573. **Victor, M.,** Neurologic changes in liver disease, in *Peripheral Neuropathy,* Dyck, P. J., Thomas, P. K., and Lambert, E. H., Eds., W.B. Saunders, Philadelphia, 1975, 1030.

574. **Videla, L., Bernstein, J., and Israel, Y.,** Metabolic alterations produced in the liver by chronic alcohol administration. Increased oxidative capacity, *Biochem. J.,* 134, 507, 1973.

575. **Videla, L. A., Iturriaga, H., Pino, M. E., Bunuot, D., Valenzuela, A., and Ugarte, G.**, Content of hepatic reduced glutathione in chronic alcoholic patients: influence of the length of abstinence and liver necrosis, *Clin. Sci.*, 66, 283, 1984.

576. **Vierling, J. M.**, Hepatic injury by prescription medication, *Proc. Annu. Meet. Med. Sect. Am. Counc. Life Insur.*, 1983, 79—86.

577. **Vierucci, A., De Martino, M., Graziani, E., Rossi, M. E., London, W. T., and Blumberg, B. S.**, A mechanism of liver cell injury in viral hepatitis: effects of hepatitis B virus on neutrophil function in vitro and in children with chronic active hepatitis, *Pediatr. Res.*, 17, 814, 1983.

578. **Vinores, S. A., Churey, J. J., Haller, J. M., Schnabel, S. J., Custer, R. P., and Sorof, S.**, Normal liver chromatin contains a firmly bound and larger protein related to the principal cytosolic target polypeptide of a hepatic carcinogen, *Proc. Natl. Acad. Sci. U.S.A.*, 81, 2092, 1984.

579. **Vitale, J. J. and Coffey, J.**, Alcoholism and vitamin metabolism, in *The Biology of Alcoholism*, Vol. 1, Kissin, B. and Begleiter, H., Eds., Plenum Press, New York, 1971, 327—352.

580. **von Bahr, C., Groth, C. G., Jansson, H., Lundgren, G., Lind, M., and Glaumann, H.**, Drug metabolism in human liver in vitro: establishment of a human liver bank, *Clin. Pharmacol. Ther.*, 27, 711, 1980.

581. **Vyas, G. N., Dienstag, J. L., and Hoofnagle, J. H.**, Eds., *Viral Hepatitis and Liver Disease*, Grune & Stratton, 1984.

582. **Walsh, M. J., Truitt, E. B., Jr., and Davis, V. E.**, Acetaldehyde mediation in the mechanism of ethanol-induced changes in norepinephrine metabolism, *Mol. Pharmacol.*, 6, 416, 1970.

583. **Watanabe, A., Takei, N., Hayashi, S., and Nagashima, H.**, Serum neutral amino acid concentrations in cirrhotic patients with impaired carbohydrate metabolism, *Acta Med. Okayama*, 37, 381, 1983.

584. **Wattenberg, L. W.**, Inhibition of carcinogenic and toxic effects of polycyclic hydrocarbons by phenolic antioxidants and ethoxyquin, *J. Natl. Cancer Inst.*, 48, 1425, 1972.

585. **Wattenberg, L. W.**, Inhibitors of chemical carcinogenesis, *Adv. Cancer Res.*, 26, 197, 1978.

586. **Weinbren, K. and Billing, B. H.**, Hepatic clearance of bilirubin as index of cellular function in regenerating rat liver, *Br. J. Exp. Pathol.*, 37, 199, 1956.

587. **Weisburger, J. H. and Williams, G. M.**, Chemical carcinogenesis, in *Toxicology, the Basic Science of Poisons*, Casarett, L. J. and Doull, J., Eds., Macmillan, New York, 1975, 84—138.

588. **Weisz, G., Udvardy, M., Dalmi, L., and Kulcsar, A.**, Serum alpha-fetoprotein in chronic liver disease, *Acta Med. Hung.*, 40, 155, 1984.

589. **Welch, W. R., Prat, J., Robboy, S. J., and Herbst, A. L.**, Pathology of prenatal diethylstilbestrol exposure, *Pathobiol. Annu.*, 13(Part 1), 201, 1978.

590. **Werner, S. C., Hanger, F. M., and Kritzler, R. A.**, Jaundice during methyl testosterone therapy, *Am. J. Med.*, 8, 325, 1950.

591. **Westphal, U., Ott, H., and Gedigk, P.**, Azorubin-binding capacity of normal and pathological sera, *Proc. Soc. Exp. Biol. Med.*, 76, 838, 1951.

592. **Saunders, J. B., Wodak, A. D., Morgan-Capner, P., White, Y. S., Portman, B., Davis, M., and Williams, R.**, Importance of markers of hepatitis B in alcoholic liver disease, *Br. Med. J. Clin. Res.*, 286, 1851, 1983.

593. **Whitlock, J. P., Jr., Cooper, H. L., and Gelboin, H. V.**, Aryl hydrocarbon (benzopyrene) hydroxylase is stimulated in human lymphocytes by mitogens and benz(a)anthracene, *Science*, 177, 618, 1972.

594. **Whitmer, D. I., Hauser, S. C., and Gollan, J. L.**, Mechanisms of formation, hepatic transport and metabolism of bile pigments, *Prog. Clin. Biol. Res.*, 152, 29, 1984.

595. **Williams, G. M.**, The pathogenesis of rat liver cancer caused by chemical carcinogens, *Biochem. Biophys. Acta*, 605, 167, 1980.

596. **Williams, R. R. and Horm, J. W.**, Association of cancer sites with tobacco and alcohol consumption and socioeconomic status of patients: interview study from the Third National Cancer Survey, *J. Natl. Cancer Inst.*, 58, 525, 1977.

597. **Wirth, P. J., Bettis, C. J., and Nelson, W. C.**, Microsomal metabolism of furosemide. Evidence for the nature of the reactive intermediate involved in covalent binding, *Mol. Pharmacol.*, 12, 759, 1976.

598. **Wolke, A. M., Schaffner, F., Kapelman, B., and Sacks, H. S.**, Malignancy in primary biliary cirrhosis. High incidence of breast cancer in affected women, *Am. J. Med.*, 76, 1075, 1984.

599. **Woodhouse, K. W., Williams, F. M., Mutch, E., Wright, P., James, O. F., and Rawlins, M. D.**, The effect of alcoholic cirrhosis on the two kinetic components (high and low affinity) of the microsomal O-deethylation of 7-ethoxycoumarin in human liver, *Eur. J. Clin. Pharmacol.*, 26, 61, 1984.

600. World Health Organization, Cancer agents that surround us, *World Health*, 9, 16, 1964.

601. **Worner, T. M. and Lieber, C. S.**, Plasma glutamate dehydrogenase: a marker of alcoholic liver injury, *Pharmacol. Biochem. Behav.*, 13(Suppl. 1), 107, 1980.

602. **Wu, A., Chanarin, I., Slavin, G., and Levi, A. J.**, Folate deficiency in the alcoholic — its relationship to clinical and haematological abnormalities, liver disease and folate stores, *Br. J. Haemat.*, 29, 469, 1975.

603. **Wu, A., Grant, D. E., and Hambley, J.,** Reduced serum somatomedin activity in patients with chronic liver disease, *Clin. Sci. Mol. Med.,* 47, 359, 1974.
604. **Wu, A., Slavin, G., and Levi, A. J.,** Elevated serum gamma-glutamyltransferase (transpeptidase) and histological liver damage in alcoholism, *Am. J. Gastroenterol.,* 65, 318, 1976.
605. **Wynder, E. L.,** The epidemiology of large bowel cancer, *Cancer Res.,* 35, 3388, 1975.
606. **Wynder, E. L., Hultberg, S., Jacobson, F., and Bross, I. J.,** Environmental factors in cancer of the upper alimentary tract: Swedish study with special reference to Plummer-Vinson syndrome, *Cancer,* 10, 470, 1957.
607. **Wynn, V., Landon, J., and Kaweraul, E.,** Studies of hepatic function during methandienone therapy, *Lancet,* 1, 69, 1961.
608. **Yaffe, S. J., Levy, G., Matsuzawa, T., and Baliah, T.,** Enhancement of glucuronide conjugation capacity in a hyperbilirubinemic infant due to apparent enzyme induction by phenobarbital, *N. Engl. J. Med.,* 275, 1461, 1966.
609. **Yamamoto, H., Tanaka, M., Nakabayashi, H., Sato, J., Okochi, T., and Kishimoto, S.,** Intestinal-type alkaline phosphatase produced by human hepatoblastoma cell line HUH-6 clone 5, *Cancer Res.,* 44, 339, 1984.
610. **Yoshida, A.,** Differences in the isozymes involved in alcohol metabolism between caucasians and orientals, *Isozymes Curr. Top. Biol. Med. Res.,* 8, 245, 1983.
611. **Zaki, F. G.,** Ultrastructure of hepatic cholestasis, *Medicine,* 45, 537, 1966.
612. **Zakim, D., Boyer, T. D., Montgomery, C., and Kanas, N.,** Alcoholic liver disease, in *Hepatology — A Textbook of Liver Disease,* Zakim, D. and Boyer, T. D., Eds., W.S. Saunders, Toronto, 1982, 739—778.
613. **Zetterman, R. K. and Leevy, C. M.,** Immunologic reactivity and alcoholic liver disease, *Bull. N.Y. Acad. Med.,* 51, 533, 1975.
614. **Ziemlanski, S. and Wartanowicz, M.,** Effects of ethanol and various dietary fats on the levels of thiamine, riboflavin, niacin, and folic acid in the liver, *Acta Physiol. Pol.,* 33(Suppl. 24), 55, 1982.
615. **Zinneman, H. H. and Levi, D. F.,** Separate autoimmune mechanisms for 7S and 19S globulins in Laennec's cirrhosis, *Arch. Intern. Med.,* 124, 153, 1969.
616. **Borthwick, N. M. and Smellie, R. M. S.,** The effects of oestradiol-17beta on the ribonucleic acid polymerases of immature rabbit uterus, *Biochem. J.,* 147, 91, 1975.
617. **Estabrook, R. W., Hildebrandt, A., Remmer, H., Schenkman, J. B., Rosenthal, O., and Cooper, D. Y.,** Role of cytochrome P-450 in microsomal mixed function oxidation reactions, Biochemic des Sauerstoffs, *19 Colloquium der Gesellschaft fur Biologische Chemie,* Hess, B. and Staudinger, H. J., Eds., Springer-Verlag, Berlin. 1969, 142.
618. **Feuer, G., Miller, D. R., Cooper, S. D., de la Iglesia, F. A., and Lumb, G.,** The influence of methyl groups on toxicity and drug metabolism, *Int. J. Clin. Pharmacol.,* 7, 13, 1973.
619. **Gelboin, H. F.,** Mechanisms of induction of drug metabolism enzymes, in *Handbook of Experimental Pharmacology,* Vol. 2, Brodie, B. B. and Gillette, J. R., Eds., Springer-Verlag, Berlin, 1971, 431.
619a. **Gelboin, H. V. and Wiebel, F. J.,** Studies on the mechanism of aryl-hydrocarbon hydroxylase induction and its role in cytotoxicity and tumorigenicity, *Ann. N.Y. Acad. Sci.,* 179, 529, 1971.
620. **Hildebrandt, A. G., Remmer, H., and Estabrook, R. W.,** Cytochrome P-450 of liver microsomes — one pigment or many, *Biochem. Biophys. Res. Commun.,* 30, 607, 1969.
620a. **Hildebrandt, A. G., Leibman, K. C., and Estabrook, R. W.,** Metyrapone interaction with hepatic microsomal cytochrome P-450 from rats treated with phenobarbital, *Biochem. Biophys. Res. Commun.,* 37, 477, 1696.
621. **Spelsberg, T. C., Thrall, C., Webster, R., and Pikler, G.,** Isolation and characterization of the nuclear acceptor that binds the progesterone-receptor complex in hen oviduct, *J. Toxicol. Environ. Health,* 3, 309, 1977.
622. **Tulkens, P. and Trouet, A.,** *Membranes and Disease,* Bolis, L., Hoffman, J. F., and Lead, A., Eds., Raven Press, New York, 1976, 141.
623. **Tulkens, P. and Trouet, A.,** The uptake and intracellular accumulation of aminoglycoside antibiotics in lysosomes of cultured rat fibroblasts, *Biochem. Pharmacol.,* 27, 415, 1978.
624. **Woollam, D. H. M.,** Principles of teratogenesis: mode of action of thalidomide, *Proc. R. Soc. Med.,* 58, 497, 1965.

FURTHER READINGS

Arias, I. M., Popper, H., Schachter, D., Shafritz, D. A., Eds., *The Liver, Biology and Pathobiology,* Raven Press, New York, 1982.
Cameron, H. M., Linsell, D. A., and Warwick, G. P., Eds., *Liver Cell Cancer,* Elsevier, Amsterdam, 1976.
Cimino, J. A., Ed., *Cancer and the Environment,* Mary Ann Liebert Publishers, New York, 1983.
Farber, E. and Fisher, M. M., Eds., *Toxic Injury of the Liver,* Part A and Part B, Marcel Dekker, New York, 1979.

Gitnick, G., Ed., *Hepatology,* Vol. 6, Year Book Medical Publishers, Chicago, 1986.

Lapis, K. and Johannessen, J. V., Ed., *Liver Carcinogenesis,* Hemisphere Publishing Corporation, Washington, 1979.

Lieber, C. S., *Medical Disorders of Alcoholism, Pathogenesis and Treatment,* W. B. Saunders, Philadelphia, 1982.

Plaa, G. L. and Hewitt, W. R., Eds., *Toxicology of the Liver,* Raven Press, New York, 1982.

Riddell, R. H., *Pathology of Drug-Induced and Toxic Diseases,* Churchill Livingstone, London, 1982.

Schiff, L., Ed., *Diseases of the Liver,* 3rd ed., J. B. Lipincott, Philadelphia, 1969.

Sherlock, S. and Summerfield, J. A., *Color Atlas of Liver Disease,* Year Book Medical Publishers, Chicago, 1978.

Stricker, B. H. Ch. and Spoelstra, P., *Drug-Induced Hepatic Injury,* Elsevier, Amsterdam, 1985.

Zakim, D. and Boyer, T. D., *Hepatology, A Textbook of Liver Disease,* W. B. Saunders, Philadelphia, 1982.

Zimmermann, H. J., *Hepatotoxicity, The Adverse Effects of Drugs and Other Chemicals on the Liver,* Appleton-Century-Crofts, New York, 1978.

Chapter 4

DISEASES OF THE NERVOUS SYSTEM

I. INTRODUCTION

The nervous system shows many more specialized features compared to any other organ. This elaborate system contains complicated anatomical and functional structures and exhibits several unique metabolic processes. The inherent complex structure is one of the major obstacles in advancing our biochemical knowledge in many areas concerning the activity of the central nervous system. Much of this organization has not been established. For instance, information on the basic biochemical processes of different types of neuron or glial cells is still limited. Yet disorders of the human nervous system can be interpreted in terms of disturbed functions of specific anatomical structures or abnormalities of regular biochemical processes.[41,69,83,206]

The response of the nervous system to injury is similar in principle to the rest of the body. In many instances, the cellular reaction of neurons, glia cells, and myelin sheaths to injury shows similarities to other cells. The course of basic processes such as inflammation and repair and degeneration and neoplasia occurs in the brain in the same fashion as in other organs, but the resemblance is obscured by the complexity of the cerebral architecture.[174,588] Further, differences lie in the fact that a number of factors determine whether or not a biochemical lesion or structural damage causes neurologic disfunction.[303,346] In some regions, lesions develop without producing clinical symptoms, such as the frontal lobe. In contrast to these silent areas, smaller changes may produce distressing effects on other parts of the brain. Sometimes the nervous system may be able to adapt to a great extent to a slowly evolving lesion, but the same lesions may elicit a sudden clinical impairment.[309]

The signs of disorder in neurological functions also show variations according to the anatomic level of the nervous system involved. The organization of the basic structural unit, the neuron, and the basic functional unit, the reflex, both become increasingly complex from the peripheral nerve to the spinal cord up the brainstem, diencephalon, and, finally, to the cerebral hemispheres. The consequence of a structural damage or failure of a biochemical reaction is fairly uniform and can be predicted at low anatomic levels. However, as increasing numbers of structural systems, reflexes, and biochemical processes are involved, the result of a lesion at these highest levels shows a great degree of variation and is less predictable.[240,298] Many special conditions are known to be related to neurological diseases such as Leigh disease.[348,480] Creutzfeld-Jakob disease,[571,581] Alzheimer disease,[77,161,260,374,461,469,476,502,554,566] Salla disease,[27,490] Klinefelter's syndrome,[223,434] Parkinson's syndrome,[89,166,222,622] Wernicke-Korsakoff psychosis,[394,395,585] Huntington syndrome,[66] Reye syndrome,[357] and Hartnup disease.[556]

Many disorders of the nervous system originate from metabolic or nutritional disorders,[193,196,276,287,358] related to anoxia or hypoglycemia,[132,170,202,239,402,532,548] or deficiency of some essential factors,[167,180,196] or have a genetic origin, such as inborn errors of metabolism. The clinical manifestation and progress of these conditions may be significantly more complicated and catastrophic as compared to other tissues or organs.[138] Some neurologic disorders are secondary to hepatic, renal, endocrine systemic disease, tumors, and infections.[18,23,25,34,60,100,203,254,308,336,424] Biochemical and physiological mechanisms underlying cerebrovascular disorders, ischemic vascular disease, or intracranial hemorrhage are similar to cardiovascular events and basic changes occuring during the development of atherosclerosis. Some disorders are, however, more pronounced. The effects of infectious diseases on the central nervous system, such as pyogenic bacteria, fungal infections, or viral dis-

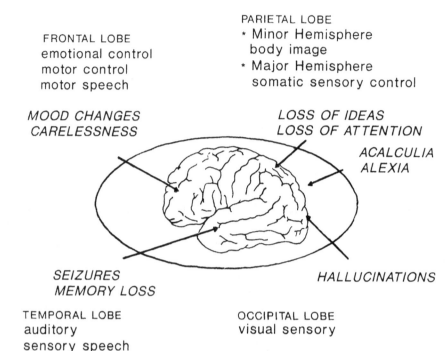

FRONTAL LOBE
emotional control
motor control
motor speech

PARIETAL LOBE
* Minor Hemisphere
body image
* Major Hemisphere
somatic sensory control

MOOD CHANGES
CARELESSNESS

LOSS OF IDEAS
LOSS OF ATTENTION

ACALCULIA
ALEXIA

SEIZURES
MEMORY LOSS

HALLUCINATIONS

TEMPORAL LOBE
auditory
sensory speech

OCCIPITAL LOBE
visual sensory

FIGURE 1.   Examples of neurological disorders associated with focal regions of the cerebral hemispheres.

eases, show variations[187] and can be more intense and deteriorating as compared to their actions on other organs. There are several special disorders, such as degenerative and demyelinating diseases, which are specific to the nervous system. Cerebral lesions have general deleterious effects on many neurologic and mental faculties irrespective of their location and depending in part upon their extent.[164,309]

In addition to the various direct neurological alterations brought about by the lesion of the function and structural system, specific symptoms may be associated with the involvement of focal regions of the cerebral hemispheres (Figure 1). Damage to the frontal lobe causes changes in mood and careless behaviour; parietal lobe damage produces inability to formulate ideas or to carry out actions through the transmission of the motor pathways. This may be associated with sensory inattention. These defects may be due to a hemisphere damage or to localized impairment of biochemical processes. Temporal lobe involvement is often linked with seizures; extensive bilateral changes lead to pronounced memory disturbances. Lesions of the occipital lobe cause vision defects and bring about hallucinations. Diffuse degenerative conditions involving central regions can be associated with generalized hyperreflexia and dysarthria. Lesions of the hypothalamus and pituitary may produce endocrine diseases. Besides these important interrelationships and generalized effects, only some specialized aspects of brain metabolism, which are peculiar to the nervous system, will be discussed in this chapter. Particularly, the role of neurotransmitters, certain amino acids, and neuropeptides will be emphasized.[256,334,340,346,450,451,520,598,602,616] This information is essential for the basic understanding of the interplay of biochemical and associated pathological alterations that underlie the clinical manifestations of neurological disease processes.

II. STRUCTURAL CHANGES

The basic units of the nervous system are the neurons and macroglia.[448] These unique structures have distinctive morphologic and functional characteristics and elicit specific biochemical reactions. The human brain contains approximately 20 billion neurons of somewhat heterogeneous structure and shows significant variations in neurological disease. Each neuron forms and receives about 100 synapses. Specific cortical and brain stem areas and nuclei elicit different susceptibilities to the injurious agent. The localization of function in specific areas also affects the onset and severity of specific disorders. For instance, although etiologic factors determine the progression of the deterioration of biochemical processes and tissue changes are essentially the same in the development of an infant in various brain areas, the frontal region of the hemispheres responds differently to small zones of ischemia and have different clinical consequences than similar lesions in the lateral medulla.

The effects of infarcts or any disease processes in the nervous system are essentially the same, but these are disorders with involvement of a highly selective structural pattern. The effects of most injurious agents acting upon the nerve cell and manifesting in neuronal abnormalities are related basically to cellular metabolism.

The neurons require a continuous supply of oxygen, glucose, and many other metabolites and therefore are very sensitive to changes of the local environment.[607] Similar to other organs, both lethal and nonlethal changes follow injury. However, at birth, humans possess essentially the full final complement of nerve cells; lost neurons are not replaced by regeneration. Mild changes such as swelling of the neurons and dispersal of the endoplasmic reticulum represent equivalent changes to cloudy swelling and loss of basophilia as in damaged liver and other cells. These changes and other abnormalities of various cytoplasmic organelles are highly significant in the interpretation of disease processes of the nervous system. Shrinking of neurons and unit loss are highly convincing proofs of disease.

During necrosis due to infarction, anoxia, hypoglycemia, trauma or viral infection, the nuclei become pycnotic and fragmented, cell bodies are shrunken and more eosinophylic, and the number of neurofibrils and endoplasmic reticulum membranes are reduced. Atrophy of the neuron occurs slowly in progressive degenerative disease and develops as an age-related process. The axons and dendrites become irregular in shape, and part of the axon undergoes fragmentation and lysis. These cells eventually die and are replaced by glial proliferation to some degree. In contrast to axonal fragmentation in cerebral matter, peripheral nerves are able to undergo some regeneration. The functional success of this process is highly variable. If there is a significant gap due to the fragmentation process, many axons will be lost.[333]

Neuronal inclusions characterize a number of inborn errors, virus infections, and other diseases (Plate 1). In disorders of sphingolipid metabolism, the neuronal cytoplasm is significantly distended and contains secondary lysosomes filled with lipids. In virus infections, Parkinson's disease and in idiopathic familial myoclonus epilepsy, characteristic inclusion bodies or large spherical intracytoplasmic structures are found. These structures contain straneous fibrillar material.

Glial cells are also affected by various abnormalities; however, these cells are considerably more resistant to anoxia or ischemia than to necrosis. Destructive lesions cause gliosis or formation of glial scars. During this process, glia cells usually undergo considerable-hypertrophy and are apparently proliferate. This proliferation is usually secondary to destructive lesions of either neurons or myelin. There is an increase of astrocytes in selective areas where myelin is destroyed, but the number of oligodendroglia is reduced. It may be that oligodendroglia are converted to astrocytes and these structures participate in glial scar production.[611]

Changes in myelin sheaths are easily recognizable features in a wide range of disease processes. In destructive lesions following infarcts, myelin sheaths are broken down and dissolved in the destroyed tissue parallel with the loss of neural and glial structures. When axons are lost, the corresponding myelin sheaths are also destroyed in both the central and peripheral nervous systems such as in Wallerian degeneration. Several toxic and metabolic

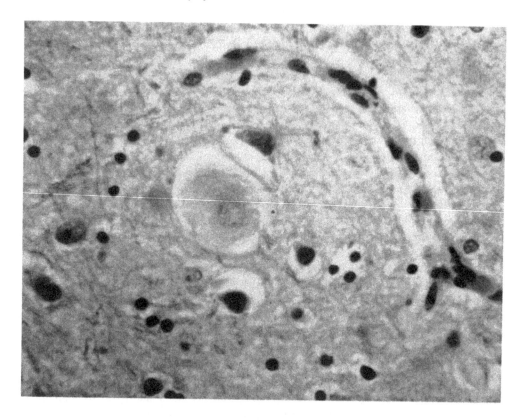

PLATE 1.   Degenerative changes in neurons from a brain with Pick's disease.

changes affect primarily myelin sheaths, mainly Schwann cells; widespread demyelination occurs in areas of chronic cerebral edema and following exposure to carbon monoxide.[59,92,238,252] In these disorders, the demyelinating process is secondary to other factors. Peripheral nerves show multiple foci of demyelination in many toxic and metabolic neuropathies, while axons remain relatively intact and are interspersed between normal myelinated and remyelinated segments. Chronic uremia and diabetes mellitus are connected with primary demyelination of the peripheral nerves. Diphteria toxin also affects primarily the peripheral myelin and Schwann cells. Myelin formation is defective in the developing brain in various inherited diseases of inborn errors of metabolism. In primary demyelinating disease, one or more components of the myelin sheath are selectively destroyed. In the latter groups, there is little or no damage to the neurons or axons and time integrity is maintained.

Independent of cause, the breakdown of myelin follows a similar pattern in the central and in the peripheral nervous systems. First, the sheaths lose regularity, and the lamellae become separated and arranged in abnormal configurations. With the loss of structure, lipoprotein substances coalesce, some of them are metabolized to neutral lipids, and numerous globules are formed which are digested by macrophages. Primary demyelination is accompanied by loss of oligodendroglia and gliosis. In demyelinated peripheral nerves, Schwann cell proliferation and endoneural fibrosis are common. Myelin is generally not replaced in the central nervous system following degeneration. Remyelination takes place more readily in the peripheral nerves.

A. DOWN'S DISEASE

This disease occupies the largest group among disorders of the central nervous system, causing mental retardation. Down's disease is associated with a specific chromosome abnormality and is the most common of all chromosomal disorders in man. It is also known as mongolism or mongolian idiocy. The basis of Down's disease is the aneuploidy; the cells of the affected persons usually show 47 chromosomes with trisomy for number 21. In such cases, one of the patient's parents may be an asymptomatic carrier. Probably an aberration in the oogenesis rather than spermatogenesis is responsible for this disease. The parental chromosomes are normal and the abnormality originates from one of the meiotic cell divisions at conception or from the early cleavage of the zygote. Since increased age of the mother is associated with increased incidence of Down's disease, the abnormality of maternal chromosomes is the probable cause of this disorder. In addition to regular Down's disease with simple trisomy, possible translocation between this and another chromosome may occur, and in some cases, mosaicism of the trisomy and sex chromosome anomaly have also been shown. Current molecular biology studies are aimed at determining the gene responsible for the disease.

The incidence of Down's disease is influenced by environmental and genetic factors which increase the occurence of nondisjunction and trisomy. Oocytes are dormant in the ovaries for a long time before they are completely mature; this and conditions during ovulation and fertilization render them more vulnerable to noxious effects which may interfere with chromosome pairing on union with the sperm cell. Exposure to X-ray irradiation of the mother has also been considered in the pathogenesis.

Many biochemical changes are found in children with Down's disease. These abnormalities are quantitative rather than qualitative. In this disorder, the defective homeostasis is aggravated by the chromosomal anomaly. Serum proteins show some defects, which are age dependent to some extent. Essentially, total serum protein levels are normal, α- and γ-globulins are increased, and albumin is decreased. Abnormalities of protein transport across cell membranes can cause these changes. There are differences in peptide patterns from identical serum-globulin fractions between normal individuals and patients with Down's disease. Serum calcium is reduced and urinary calcium excretion is low. However, serum phosphate levels are essentially normal, and there is defective transport of fat soluble vitamins. The reduced calcium level is in connection with defects of the skeletal and nervous system found in Down's disease and may be associated with the deficiency in the absorption, transport, and utilization of vitamin D. Insufficient parathyroid activity may also be related to the altered calcium metabolism.

Patients with Down's disease show defects in tryptophan metabolism.[520] This may be related to vitamin B_6 deficiency since this coenzyme is more readily depleted from patients than from normal individuals. Particularly, the pathway of tryptophan conversion to serotonin is affected; blood levels of serotonin are low in the trisomic form of the disease compared to healthy cohorts. Patients with Down's disease translocation have intermediate values. The fall of serum serotonin is related to the activity of 5-hydroxytryptophan decarboxylase which is a pyridoxal phosphate dependent enzyme (Figure 2). In the case of Down's disease, blood serotonin levels show further reduction with DL-penicillamine, a vitamin B_6 antagonist, is administered. In newborn babies, blood 5-hydroxytryptamine levels are low due to the functional immaturity of the 5-hydroxytryptophan decarboxylase system. In Down's disease, the inadequate utilization of vitamin B_6 and defective transport of tryptophan and its metabolites are responsible for the continued inadequate serotonin levels. Regional brain 5-hydroxytryptamine levels are reduced in senile Down's syndrome, similarly to Alzheimer disease.[493,621]

III. NARCOSIS AND SLEEP

The study of narcosis and excitation provides a initial tool when we evaluate various disease processes of the nervous system.[195,278,445] The sleep of depressed patients shows

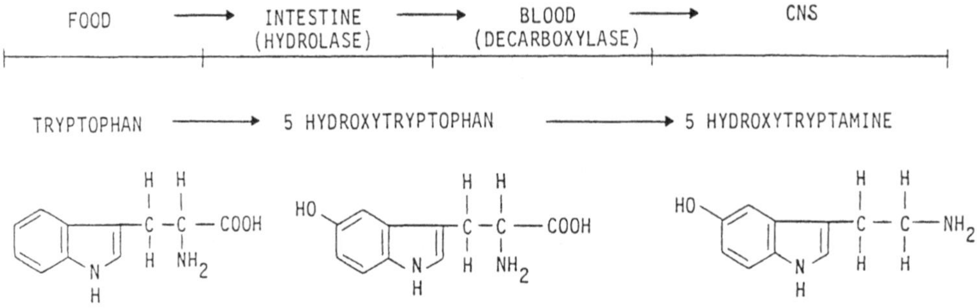

FOOD $\longrightarrow$ INTESTINE $\longrightarrow$ BLOOD $\longrightarrow$ CNS
(HYDROLASE) (DECARBOXYLASE)

TRYPTOPHAN $\longrightarrow$ 5 HYDROXYTRYPTOPHAN $\longrightarrow$ 5 HYDROXYTRYPTAMINE

FIGURE 2. Biosynthesis of serotonin and the role of various tissues.

variations.[261] There are also many disorders of sleep.[318,376,529] It has been reported that various barbiturates are capable of inhibiting the oxygen consumption of brain preparations *in vitro* as well as *in vivo*.[407] This inhibitory action is selective and connected with the mainstream of energy-producing reactions. The oxidation of glucose, lactate, and pyruvate are depressed; glutamate oxidation is also affected, but to a lesser extent, while no changes occur in succinate oxidation.[402]

It is not known whether the narcotic effects of these drugs are the direct outcome of a slowing down of the oxidative metabolism of the brain neurons or whether the reduction of the respiration is the end result of a reduction of other cerebral activities brought about by modulating effects on excitation, conduction, or synaptic transmission. If the primary effect of the drug is to inhibit oxidation, it may be expected that the energy-rich phosphates would be depleted in the narcotized brain. However, during sleep or anaesthesia the levels of adenosine triphosphate, phosphocreatine, and acetylcholine remain normal, whereas lactic acid, inorganic phosphate, and ammonia levels are low. These findings indicate that under the effect of the narcotics, a state of economy occurs; the energy is nonutilized rather than the energy-producing mechanism being blocked. It must be remembered that cell respiration is an integration of complex chained reactions, and it is still possible that at some point in this chain barbiturates or other narcotics may affect the function before any measurable effect can be detected in overall cell respiration rate.

There is experimental evidence that alcohol, ether, and some other anaesthetics also depress cerebral metabolism *in vivo*. Ether anesthesia can cause 10 to 40% reduction of oxygen utilization of the brain. No specific chemical groups are required in the molecule to exert anesthetic action and no chemical reaction takes place between the drugs and the organism. The depressing action is connected with changes on the cell membrane rather than with any structure of the intracellular space. The anaesthetic is probably dissolved in the membrane lipid and interferes with the movement of sodium and potassium across themembrane. This is associated with a depression of higher cortical functions by the inhibition of certain synaptic pathways so the number of neurons firing per unit of time is reduced. This lowers the entry of sodium into neurons, sodium pump activity is decreased, and adenosine triphosphate and, consequently, oxygen consumptions are decreased. In these interrelated reactions, interactions with proteins probably play a major role. Conformational changes have been shown with albumin, myoglobin, and β-lactoglobulin.

The brain has an absolute dependence on the oxidation of carbohydrates. Lack of glucose by any means will depress cerebral metabolism and consequently affecting function. Insulin-induced hypoglycemia can also reduce brain metabolism. The effect is reversible if the hypoglycemia is of short duration and not excessive. There are differences in the events occurring during ischemia and hypoglycemia. During hypoglycemia, metabolic changes are different from those in circulatory failure, and the onset of functional and metabolic changes is slow. The tricarboxylic acid cycle is functioning and the concentration of endogenous substrates is enough to maintain energy metabolism for 20 to 25 min. Hypoglycemia may occur in the brain associated with liver disease, insulin-secreting tumors, and insulin overdose. The clinical signs of hypoglycemia, such as increased perspiration and tachycardia, are due to the release of large amounts of epinephrine. Drowsiness and confusion are apparent when blood glucose is reduced to 30 mg/dl, and coma ensues at 20 mg/dl. Below this level there is loss of neurons. Prolonged hypoglycemia can produce permanent damage, mental and psychological disorders, and death. Infantile hypoglycemia is found to be a significant cause of neonatal brain damage.

Circulatory factors alter the pattern and rate of development of ischemic changes in the brain. Under normal conditions, brain cells absorb oxygen and glucose from the blood. Glucose is the major source of energy and is utilized for many structural requirements although other essential substances are also extracted. Despite the dependence of the brain on glucose, at rest the brain takes up only a fraction of the available glucose from the blood. When oxygen supply is ample, the brain produces small amounts of lactate which is eliminated into the venous blood.

The decline of cerebral blood flow by vascular block or reduction of cardiac output initiates autoregulatory mechanisms. The large brain vessels adjust to this situation and attempt to maintain constant blood flow. Local changes including a mechanical myogenic response to decreased pressure and modification of the metabolism are important factors in this regulation. An increase of tissue pCO_2 and decrease of pO_2 cause vasodilatation. In addition to lower pH, lower affinity of hemoglobin for oxygen raises the level of oxygen retained locally. When this mechanism fails due to inadequate blood supply, major tissue changes result.

Anoxia, hypoglycemia, and generalized cerebral ischemia have similar effects on the brain.[117,607] The central effects of anoxia, however, are linked with extensive removal of major metabolites from the brain such as citrate, hexosephosphates, adenosine triphosphate, and creatine phosphate; in contrast, pyruvate accumulates. If cerebral circulation is stopped completely, within 10 to 15 s, unconsciousness occurs. Most susceptible neurons die within 5 to 10 min, mainly in the cerebral and cerebellar cortex and globus pallidus. If the circulation is restored after several minutes, brain functions may be restored in lower levels, since the loss of cortical neurons brings about dementia with signs of focal or generalized cerebral damage.

There are reports suggesting that various fragments from the pituitary hormone, such as β-lipotropin, elicit sedative action on the central nervous system and may be involved in the process of sleep. Methionine-enkephalin, a tetrapeptide, and leucine-enkephalin, a related pentapeptide, have transient analgesic effects. Larger fragments of the hormone α-endorphin containing 16 and β-endorphin containing 21 amino acids exert potent long-lasting analgesia when injected to various experimental animals. These observations may imply that peptide fragments are important neuromodulators of the central nervous system, and their function is connected with sleep mechanisms. The behavioural action of these peptides shows striking similarity to those of some central nervous system neuropeptides and may be involved in psychopathological conditions which can be controlled by neuroleptic drugs. The changes in neuropeptides may be associated with alterations of the enzyme activity responsible for the production of these peptides from the intact hormone.

IV. EXCITATION AND CONVULSION

Excitation in the central nervous system is associated with events leading to the firing of the neurons and generation of action potentials.[217] Potential differences are related to positive charges on the outside and negative charges on the inside of the nerve membrane. The permeability of the resting membrane to sodium is very limited. Excitation alters this

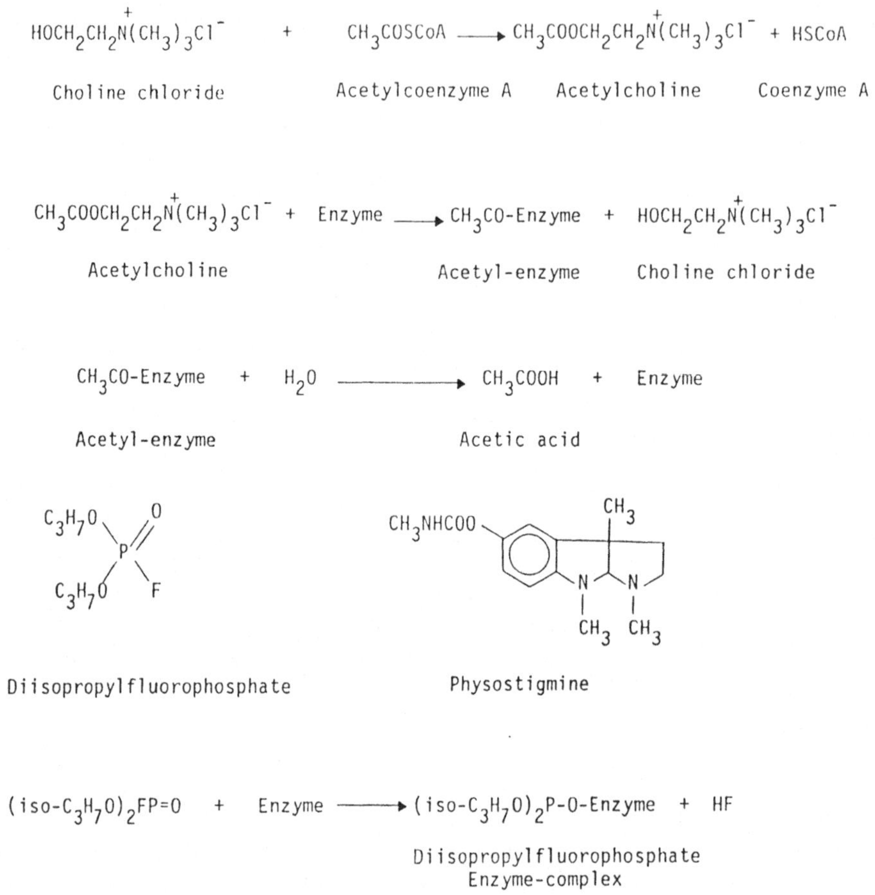

$$HOCH_2CH_2\overset{+}{N}(CH_3)_3Cl^- \quad + \quad CH_3COSCoA \longrightarrow CH_3COOCH_2CH_2\overset{+}{N}(CH_3)_3Cl^- + HSCoA$$

Choline chloride   Acetylcoenzyme A   Acetylcholine   Coenzyme A

$$CH_3COOCH_2CH_2\overset{+}{N}(CH_3)_3Cl^- + Enzyme \longrightarrow CH_3CO-Enzyme + HOCH_2CH_2\overset{+}{N}(CH_3)_3Cl^-$$

Acetylcholine   Acetyl-enzyme   Choline chloride

$$CH_3CO-Enzyme \quad + \quad H_2O \longrightarrow CH_3COOH \quad + \quad Enzyme$$

Acetyl-enzyme   Acetic acid

Diisopropylfluorophosphate   Physostigmine

$$(iso-C_3H_7O)_2FP=O \quad + \quad Enzyme \longrightarrow (iso-C_3H_7O)_2P-O-Enzyme \quad + \quad HF$$

Diisopropylfluorophosphate
Enzyme-complex

FIGURE 3. Biosynthesis and metabolism of acetylcholine, including inhibitors diisopropyfluo-rophosphate and physostigmine.

property resulting in momentary sodium flux and the local depolarization is followed by a reversal of polarity and generation of an action potential. The recovery of the cell to resting state involves a release of sodium and an intake of potassium ions. This mechanism is probably regulated by a membrane-linked complex enzyme system which needs adenosine triphosphate for this function.

In convulsive states, metabolic changes in the brain are generally opposite to changes seen in narcosis. Rapid utilization of energy-rich phosphates, glucose, and oxygen occurs and apparently are necessary to maintain the high levels of activity during convulsions. When oxygen consumption is increased, there is a rise in the brain lactic acid, adenosine diphosphate, inorganic phosphate, and ammonia contents. At the same time, levels of glycogen, glucose, adenosine triphosphate, phosphocreatine, and acetylcholine fall.

Excitation can be caused by some cell products. Neurohormones, such as acetylcholine, mediate the transmission of the nerve impulse across synaptic junctions. At the nerve endings acetylcholine is synthesized according to a simple process (Figure 3) and is present in bound form to acetylcholine receptors.[340] Binding induces conformational changes linked to the discharge of calcium ions from protein carboxyl or sulfhydryl groups (Figure 4). The release of calcium may cause further conformation changes in phospholipids and other membrane components. These chain reactions bring about the movement of 20 to 40,000 ions across the membrane per molecule of acetylcholine released. Thus, the chemical transmission of a nerve impulse is generated by acetylcholine. When acetylcholine is liberated in a free

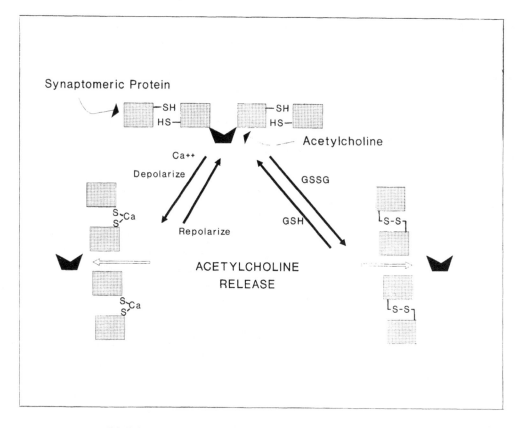

FIGURE 4.   Mechanism of acetylcholine release in presynaptic vesicles.

form, it elicits its action on the postsynaptic membranes, altering membrane permeability and causing changes in ionic concentrations leading to changes in the electric potential. The release is connected with nerve excitation. The free acetylcholine is rapidly removed by hydrolysis due to acetylcholinesterase activity. The removal of this mediatory restores the conformation of the membrane to the preexcitatory state. Numerous chemicals and drugs inhibit this enzyme. Physostigmin is one of the best known reversible competitive inhibitors. Organophosphorus derivatives are important esterase inhibitors. These compounds, such as diisopropylfluorophosphate, elicit an irreversible action by producing a stable enzyme-inhibitor complex (Figure 3).

The release of bound acetylcholine from the synapsis may be linked to the presence of reduced glutathione. Generally, the communication between most nerve cells depends on the transfer of transmitters. According to current concepts, this involves accumulation of vesicles at the presynaptic region, transport to vesicle release sites, rearrangement of these sites, and the discharge of transmitter and its movement across the synaptic membranes. Glutathione participates in the activation of presynaptic vesicles and in the promotion of transmitter release (Figure 4).

A. PEPTIDES AND NERVE EXCITATION

The existence of a peptide, substance P, in nerve tissue has been known for a long time,[290,356,470] but extensive research on the possible functional role of this peptide and of other peptides of neuronal and nonneuronal origin has emerged from recent studies. Until now, several peptides of hypothalamic and anterior pituitary origin have been isolated from neural tissue.[557] They are primarily involved in the regulation of hormone release. However, some of these peptides function as conventional neurotransmitters mediating short-term changes in neuronal excitability.[355] They also participate in long-term regulation of both nerve excitation and efficacy of synaptic transmission.[342] The peptides involved in neural activity include substance P, oxytocin, lysine vasopressin, angiotensin II, thyrotropin releasing factor, luteinizing-hormone releasing factor, and somatostatin (growth hormone-release-inhibiting factor).[209] The structures of these peptides are given in Volume I, Chapter 2, Figures 13, 14, and 10.

Substance P is distributed widely but unevenly across the nervous system. It is present in relatively high amounts in the sensory system, hypothalamus, substantia nigra, and myenteric plexuses and affects neuronal activity causing excitation of motoneurons and other spinal and cortical neurons. This peptide may be a general transmitter mediating sensory input into the central nervous system.[342,343] Substance P is probably released from the spinal cord. Areas of this organ with primary afferent terminals contain high concentrations of this peptide; it accumulates at ligations which are placed on sensory axons.

Similar to substance P, glutamate has also been suggested to mediate sensory input. Both the peptide and the free amino acid are present in the same part of the nervous system. The peptide is transported from the sensory cell toward the spinal cord, whereas there are no apparent changes in glutamate levels. Both glutamate and substance P depolarize spinal cord cells. The onset of the effects of substance P is slow but long lasting; in exciting motoneurons, it is more potent by several orders of magnitude than glutamate. Moreover, glutamate-evoked increased activity is depressed by the peptide. The modulation of the glutamate effect and the long-lasting nature of substance P response indicates that substance P may be a regulator of neuronal excitability rather than an actual transmitter involved in mediating sensory input. Thus, secretion of this peptide may be involved in the long-term regulation of synaptic transmission. Changes in the secretion usually bring about important consequences for synaptic events in cells exposed to substance P. The action of substance P seems to be highly specific and closely related peptides such as physalamin and eledoisin are inactive. The secretion of this peptide may show variations among various states: activity, sleep, conditioning, estrus cycle, or day rhythm. Age also may change the level of peptide secretion, making it more or less easy for incoming excitatory synaptic events to produce threshold effect. The role of substance P in regulating sensory transmission may not be limited to postsynaptic processes which are propagated through the central nervous system; chronic pathological changes may represent the basis of disorders of sensory receptors and transmission.

Beyond the extraneuronal action of the various neurohypophysial peptides, antidiuretic hormone is involved in the physiology of the supraoptic neurosecretory system. Lysine vasopressin, and a wide variety of agents including norepinephrine and acetylcholine depressthese cells, and only a small percentage of cells are excited by the antidiuretic hormone.[43,44] The inhibitory action of the other substances seems to be specific for the supraoptic neurosecretory system, since cortical cells are either unresponsive or excited by the peptide. In the excitation of the paraventricular neurosecretory system, oxytocin is the primary acting peptide.[420] Angiotensin II has well established peripheral effects regulating blood pressure and volume. Its effect on the central nervous system is specific, and it is associated with a pressor response, drinking behaviour, or the release of antidiuretic hormone. Angiotensin II is synthesized centrally and peripherally from the circulating precursor angiotensin I by the action of the converting enzyme. All components of this system are also present in the central nervous system. Angiotensin II occurs mainly in the form of the decapeptide precursor. Its conversion to the active substance is dependent on the availability of the converting enzyme.[620] It has not been revealed whether the centrally mediated pressor effect of this angiotensin II is due to the centrally produced substance or it is related to the peripheral peptide which gains access to various areas of the central nervous system.

Angiotensin II-stimulated drinking behavior is localized primarily to the subfornical organ, although other areas of the central nervous system are also participating, but do not respond uniformly.[209] The regulation of the hypothalamic excitation of subfornical neurons and subsequent initiation of drinking behaviour have not yet been established. The release of antidiuretic hormone by angiotensin II involves the supraoptic neurosecretory system.[432] A structure-activity study revealed that the effect of angiotensin II can be counteracted by [cysteine[8]] angiotensin II and [sarcosine[1]-isoleucine[8]] angiotensin II.[215]

Accumulating evidence shows that several releasing factors are located outside their hypothalamic sites of origin; they are also found in nerve ending fractions of the brain.[459,509] Some of these peptides alter the response of the central nervous system to depressants and stimulants. Thyrotropin releasing factor (thyroliberin) reverses pentobarbital toxicity and reduces the convulsive dose of strychnine. In contrast, somatostatin causes an opposite effect.[458] Thyrotropin releasing hormone, luteinizing hormone releasing factor (gonadoliberin) and somatostatin cause a uniform depression of neuronal activity in the areas of cortex, hypothalamus, brainstem, and cerebellum. Brain norepinephrin metabolism is modified by ovariectomy,[23] and L-dopa stimulates the secretion of human growth hormone.[82] These studies suggest a transmitter function on local feedback regulations.[535] Some releasing factors modulate the behaviour of experimental animals. Although the cellular mechanism underlying the specific behavioural patterns remains to be elucidated, these investigations are suggestive that certain psychological disorders are based on neuroendocrinological factors and may be associated with the production of abnormal quantity or quality of neuronal peptides, or with changes in the control of peptide release, or termination of this action by specific or non-specific peptidases. The regulation of the rate of peptide metabolism and the control of synthesis and conversion of these specific peptides are probably important determinants of mental health.

Some dicarboxylic amino acids also have excitatory effects on spinal neurons, including L-glutamic, N-methylaspartic, and homocysteic acids. The mechanism of action of these amino acids is not known. They probably bind to specific receptor sites and cause membrane depolarization.

B. EPILEPSY

Epilepsy represents a complex of symptoms, associated with periodic transient changes characterized by convulsive movements and alteration of the state of consciousness. The clinical manifestation and pathological conditions of epileptic attacks are very variable.[524] The fundamental cause of idiopathic epilepsy is difficult to assess since it is not related to any characteristic structural change with the exception of focal epilepsy. Due to these variations in epileptic convulsions, less information is available on metabolic changes in the brain than on artifically induced seizures.[233,245] Seizures provide an example on how the abnormality is related to biochemical changes. In these disorders, an alarming episode disturbs the function of the central nervous system, followed usually by a fairly quick restoration of normal functions. The epileptogenic convulsions appear primarily as the manifestation of altered biochemical actions with no detectable underlying structural defects. Both general and specific factors influence the onset of seizures. They occur frequently in association with systemic febrile illnesses or secondary to underlying organic brain disease. Genetic factors provide increased liability. The majority of seizures manifest without any detectable cause, however, and factors such as hyperventilation, hypoglycemia, or specific afferent stimulation can often precipitate the incidence.

One of two functions are impaired in the epileptic brain. Either there is an increased excitation of motor nerve cells or a paralysis of an inhibitory mechanism. The second of these mechanisms is the most likely due to dysfunction. The excitatory and inhibitory neurons are mutually antagonistic. If this antagonism is disrupted, seizures can be seen, resulting from an apparent increase in excitation. One proposed theory involves changes in levels of

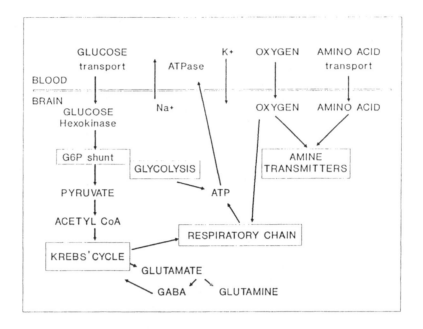

FIGURE 5. Carbohydrate and energy metabolism in the epileptic brain.

the neurotransmitters in the brain.[387,439] Some of the neurotransmitters are inhibitory and some are excitatory. Acetylcholine, one of the major neurotransmitters in the brain has bothexcitatory and inhibitory actions, depending upon receptor that is involved. Excitatory responses have mixed nicotinic and muscarinic properties, whereas those responses for inhibition are exclusively muscarinic.[227] Dopamine, noradrenaline, and serotonin are all inhibitory by hyperpolarizing the membrane of the neurons. The principal pathways of each transmitter originate from the brain stem, the brain's deep central core. This suggests that most generalized seizures originate from discharges in the brain stem which contains the reticular activating system. This area sends efferent fibers throughout the brain, thus resulting in generalized seizures. If acetylcholine increases, the level of dopamine or serotonin decreases, leading to increased excitation and hence seizures.

Discharges usually occur as the result of periodic membrane instability in a group of neurons. This leads to hyperactive and hypersynchronous neuronal firing. The hyperdepolarization leads to excessive neuronal firing which interrupts the normal function of the nervous system leading to clinical seizures. Various excitory and inhibitory chemicals can modify the balance of ions across the membrane causing membrane polarization.

The onset of epilepsy is considered to occur as the consequence of an essentially uncontrolled discharge of cortical neurones. The convulsions are associated with an abnormal acetycholine metabolism. Evidence that epilepsy represents a chronic biochemical defect in the brain is provided when epileptogenic cortical tissue has been studied *in vitro*. From patients suffering epilepsy with focal cortical seizures, cortical tissue has been removed and two biochemical abnormalities have been found: increased acetylcholine and cholinesterase activity and failure to form bound acetylcholine when slices of cortex are incubated in glucose and eserine-containing solutions. Protein[178] and glucose[202] metabolism in the brain is also altered in epilepsy (Figure 5).

The increased cholinesterase activity may be an adaptive response to the increased tendency to release acetylcholine resulting from partial failure in binding. In many instances, an increased concentration of free acetylcholine is associated with increased seizure susceptibility.[227] The injection or acetylcholine into the carotid artery or intraventricular spaces in the brain induces electroencephalogram patterns characteristic of grand mal seizures. The cerebrospinal fluid of epileptic patients contains measureable amounts of acetylcholine, which does not occur in normals. These findings underline the conclusion that abnormal acetylcholine metabolism may be the major biochemical lesion in this disease and may be the causative factor producing a state of excitatory instability particularly in focal areas.

Further evidence for the role of increased free acetylcholine in epilepsy is obtained from animal experiments. Injection of diisopropyl fluorophosphonate to experimental animals resulted in electroencephalographic changes similar to those seen in epilepsy. This compound inactivates the effects of acetylcholinesterase. The inhibition of this enzyme by a variety of chemical agents brings about an accumulation of acetylcholine and a block of nerve conduction. In experimental animals, death caused by the administration of such inhibitors is associated with a complete inhibition of brain acetylcholinesterase.

The failure in the formation of bound acetylcholine has been demonstrated in cerebral cortex slices obtained from animals poisoned with methionine sulphoximine. This compound produces seizures in animals very closely resembling those of human epilepsy. Addition of glutamine or asparagine to the incubation-medium restores the binding of acetylcholine. These amino acids show similar effects on human focal epileptogen tissue and glutamic acid elicits no effect. Several of these amino acids, especially glutamine, glycine, and, partic ularly, large amounts of γ-aminobutyric acid (GABA), are found in brain tissue.[63] These amino acids serve as neurotransmitters in the central nervous system. GABA is the principal inhibitory transmitter in the brain and glutamate is the principal excitatory transmitter. Glycine has inhibitory functions. The local accumulation of glutamine or decrease of GABA can result in excess excitation and induce convulsion.

The effect of these substances is connected with glutamine synthesis and metabolism (Figure 6). Methionine sulphoximine has been shown to inhibit the enzyme glutamine synthetase both *in vitro* and *in vivo* (Figure 7).[519] The inhibition is biphasic: reversible competition with glutamine and irreversible interaction with ATP, to form enzyme-bound methionine sulfoximine phosphate. This compound remains in the brain for long periods, and during that time brain glutamine synthetase activity returns slowly to the normal level.

The enzyme decarboxylase requires pyridoxal phosphate (vitamin B_1) as coenzyme. The effect of GABA has been demonstrated on the brain; it exerts a state of neuronal activity. When applied locally, GABA produces changes in electrical activity. GABA decarboxylase is reduced in the brain when epileptiform convulsions develop.

The treatment of epilepsy by antiepileptic drugs has been primarily based on laboratory trials. The enhancement of the synaptic transmission during repetitive stimulation is the major contributory factor in the continuation of the seizure; this is diminished by anticonvulsant drugs.[242] Most of these compounds promote an efflux of sodium from the neurons. This tends to stabilize the hyperexcitability which is the result of excessive stimulation or changes associated with the reduction of the gradient of membrane sodium concentration. Subsequently, this decreases postsynaptic potentiation and limits the discharge from a cortical focus. The changes in ionic concentration are related to the local concentration of acetylcholine. Although drugs with diverse chemical structures have been effective as anticonvulsants, some structural relationships with acetylcholine may provide support to the nature of biochemical lesion underlying epilepsy.

C. MIGRAINE

Migraine can be regarded as a reaction in the central nervous system which is related to a lowered threshold of cerebral mechanisms in a combination with several precipitating factors.[49,273] The endogenous precipitants include stress, menstruation and oral contraceptives, alcohol, dietary sensitivity, fasting and hunger, and photo stimulation. Heredity is participating in this disease, but the contributing exogenous and endogenous factors are

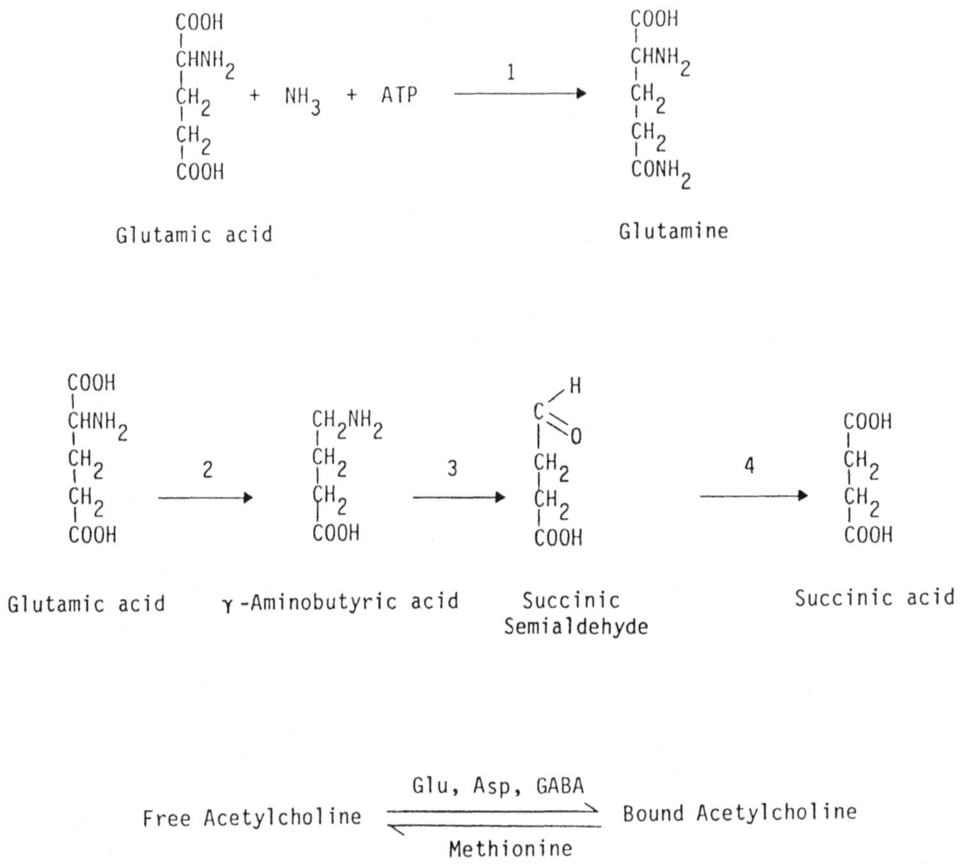

$$
\begin{array}{c}
\text{COOH} \\
| \\
\text{CHNH}_2 \\
| \\
\text{CH}_2 \\
| \\
\text{CH}_2 \\
| \\
\text{COOH}
\end{array}
\;+\; \text{NH}_3 \;+\; \text{ATP} \;\xrightarrow{\;1\;}\;
\begin{array}{c}
\text{COOH} \\
| \\
\text{CHNH}_2 \\
| \\
\text{CH}_2 \\
| \\
\text{CH}_2 \\
| \\
\text{CONH}_2
\end{array}
$$

Glutamic acid   Glutamine

$$
\begin{array}{c}
\text{COOH} \\
| \\
\text{CHNH}_2 \\
| \\
\text{CH}_2 \\
| \\
\text{CH}_2 \\
| \\
\text{COOH}
\end{array}
\xrightarrow{\;2\;}
\begin{array}{c}
\text{CH}_2\text{NH}_2 \\
| \\
\text{CH}_2 \\
| \\
\text{CH}_2 \\
| \\
\text{COOH}
\end{array}
\xrightarrow{\;3\;}
\begin{array}{c}
\text{C}\diagdown\text{H} \\
\diagup\diagdown\text{O} \\
| \\
\text{CH}_2 \\
| \\
\text{CH}_2 \\
| \\
\text{COOH}
\end{array}
\xrightarrow{\;4\;}
\begin{array}{c}
\text{COOH} \\
| \\
\text{CH}_2 \\
| \\
\text{CH}_2 \\
| \\
\text{COOH}
\end{array}
$$

Glutamic acid γ-Aminobutyric acid   Succinic Semialdehyde   Succinic acid

$$
\text{Free Acetylcholine} \;\underset{\text{Methionine}}{\overset{\text{Glu, Asp, GABA}}{\rightleftharpoons}}\; \text{Bound Acetylcholine}
$$

FIGURE 6. Biosynthesis of glutamine and aminobutyric acid and their action on acetylcholine binding.

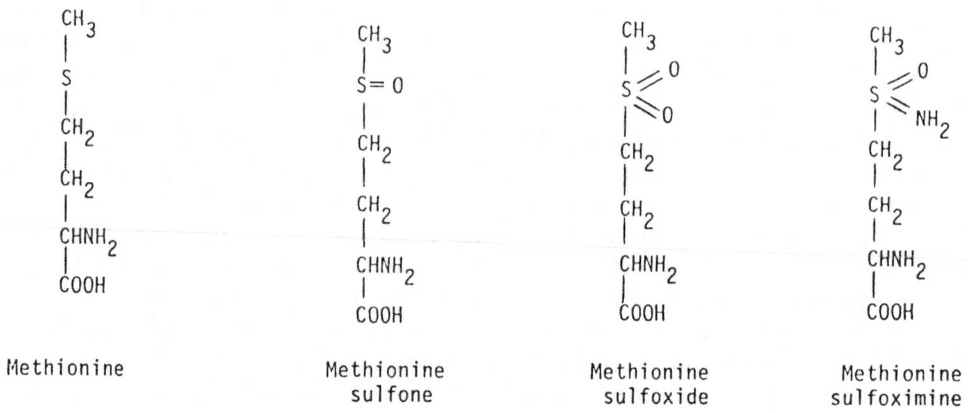

$$
\begin{array}{c}
\text{CH}_3 \\
| \\
\text{S} \\
| \\
\text{CH}_2 \\
| \\
\text{CH}_2 \\
| \\
\text{CHNH}_2 \\
| \\
\text{COOH}
\end{array}
\qquad
\begin{array}{c}
\text{CH}_3 \\
| \\
\text{S}=\text{O} \\
| \\
\text{CH}_2 \\
| \\
\text{CH}_2 \\
| \\
\text{CHNH}_2 \\
| \\
\text{COOH}
\end{array}
\qquad
\begin{array}{c}
\text{CH}_3 \\
| \\
\text{S}\diagup\diagup^{\text{O}}_{\diagdown\text{O}} \\
| \\
\text{CH}_2 \\
| \\
\text{CH}_2 \\
| \\
\text{CHNH}_2 \\
| \\
\text{COOH}
\end{array}
\qquad
\begin{array}{c}
\text{CH}_3 \\
| \\
\text{S}\diagup\diagup^{\text{O}}_{\diagdown\text{NH}_2} \\
| \\
\text{CH}_2 \\
| \\
\text{CH}_2 \\
| \\
\text{CHNH}_2 \\
| \\
\text{COOH}
\end{array}
$$

Methionine   Methionine sulfone   Methionine sulfoxide   Methionine sulfoximine

FIGURE 7. Structures of methionine and methionine analogs.

important in the trigger mechanism. The migraine headache is connected with a period of vasoconstriction of cerebral blood vessels during the stage of premonitory symptoms, followed by a subsequent vasodilatation which is accompanied by pain.

Some abnormalities in migraine reside in carbohydrate metabolism. In comparison to normal subjects, glucose tolerance is impaired in migraine patients. The relative shortage

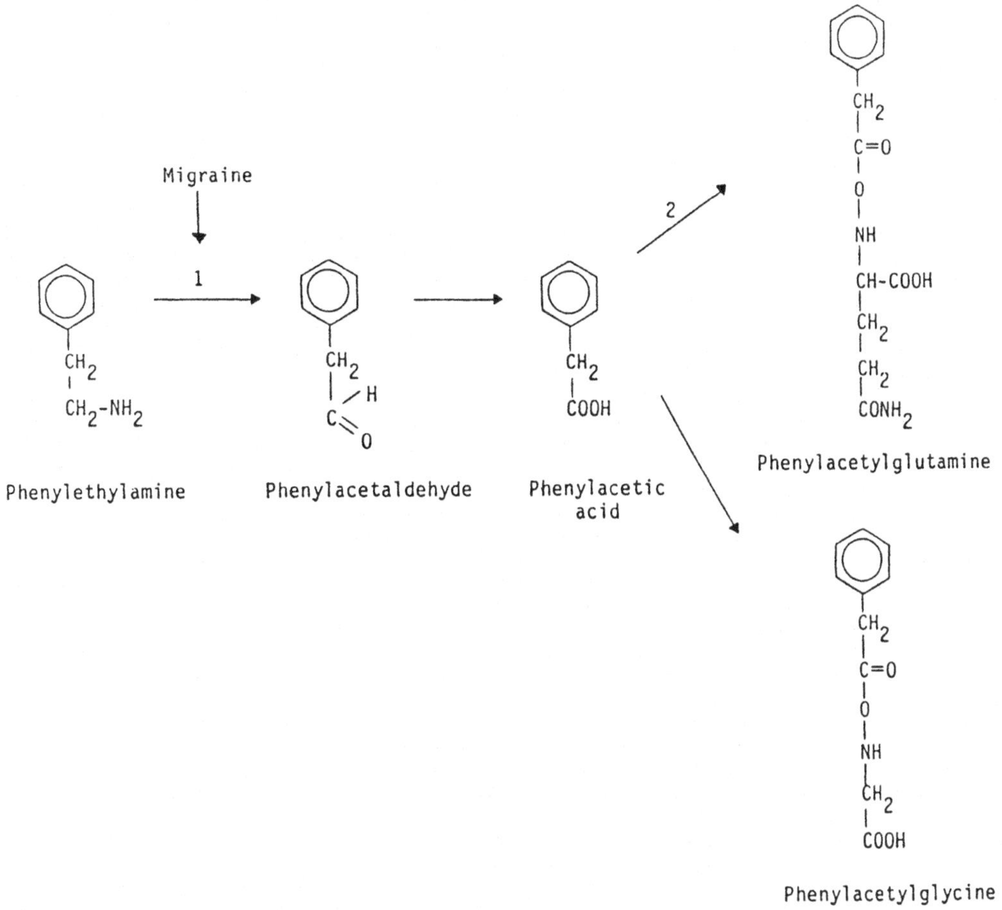

FIGURE 8. Metabolism of phenylethylamine in migraine.

of carbohydrate may be an important factor in the genesis of attacks in susceptible individuals after fasting or strenuous exercise. In the state of relative carbohydrate depletion, the response of the central nervous system may be abnormal in migraine subjects.

In migraine attacks some alterations in tyramine or catecholamine metabolism have been shown.[149] The metabolism of tryptophan is also modified.[145,520] Therefore, these compounds play an important role in the pathogenesis of this disease. A connection between migraine and these amines is found when headaches and hypertensive crises develop in certain individuals being treated with monoamine oxidase inhibitors and eating cheese. Cheese contains large amounts of tyramine and phenylethylamine, and the inhibition of monoamine oxidase in the intestine and liver allows the absorption of these constituents. These amines influence peripheral adrenergic receptors. However, they are inactivated in normal subjects by monoamine oxidase.[232] This evidence suggests that tyramine may be responsible for the migraine attack.[272] Further proof of this conclusion is derived from clinical experience. Tyramine hydrochloride given in 100 mg oral doses regularly precipitated typical attacks of migraine headache in migraine patients.[237] Recent studies have shown that migraine patients have highly reduced phenylethylamine oxidizing ability resulting in lower urinary output of phenylacetic acid (Figure 8). Tyramine oxidation is also diminished, and smaller decreases in dopamine and 5-hydroxytryptamine oxidation have been noted. These enzymes occur in multiple forms in brain and platelets and are subdivided into two major forms, A and B. Type A has a preference for serotonin, epinephrine, and norepinephrine, whereas type B

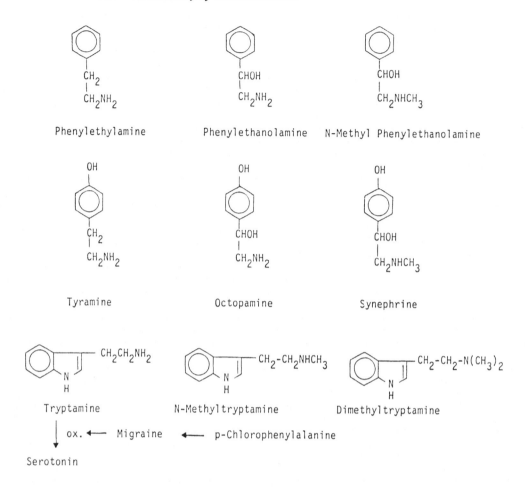

FIGURE 9.   Structure of natural trace amines and their role in migraine.

for phenylethylamine and several other trace amines. Dopamine, tyramine, and tryptamine are oxidized by either type A or B monoamine oxidases.

Certain dietary factors appear to be associated with the onset of the attack in migraine patients; chocolate, cheese, or citrus fruits are most frequently quoted foodstuffs. Oranges are known to contain considerable amounts of octopamine and *N*-methyloctopamine or synephrine (Figure 9). Apart from tyramine, there may be other compounds related to migraine. Patients suffering from dietary migraine excrete significantly less free tyramine and far less conjugated tyramine than control subjects. It has been suggested that dietary factors may precipitate an inborn defect in the metabolism of tyramine and related factors.

Reserpine is also known to produce migraine attacks in susceptible people. It was found that plasma serotonin level falls following reserpine treatment, and a headache can be relieved by intravenous serotonin.[528,541] Normal serotonin turnover is necessary to maintain the painless physiological condition. Under normal conditions the continuous flow of sensations arrives to the brain from the periphery because of an inhibiting system. This inhibition has been suggested to occur at the pain gate located in the thalamus and spinal cord, and 5-hydroxytryptamine is the biochemical mediator (Figure 10). Normally no pain is apparent; however, following peripheral stimulation most sensations will go through the gate, and pain is registered. Spontaneous pain is related to a possible vulnerability of serotonin metabolism,[541] and it may begin when 5-hydroxytryptamine deficiency ensues. Reserpine releases norepinephrine and other amines from stores and reduces the levels of endogenous

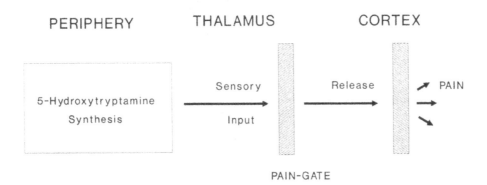

FIGURE 10. Schematic illustration of the pain gate.

5-hydroxytryptamine in brain and peripheral nerves (Figure 11). Administration of *p*-chlorophenylalanine to patients with untreatable migraine provokes a depletion of 5-hydroxytryptamine by selectively inhibiting its synthesis which confirms the role of this amine in pain production (Figure 12).

In migraine headaches, a lowering of the threshold of the vascular and nervous receptors to monoamines and correlated drugs is quite easily recognizable. The exact mechanisms of how serotonin deficiency causes pain in the brain is not clear at present. However, it is possible that similar courses of action happen in the periphery as well as in the central nervous system.[273] Monoamines such as 5-hydroxytryptamine, dopamine, and norepinephrine are mediators of affectivity, body temperature, sleep, water imbalance, nausea, or sex.[109,333,350,426,451,507] All these functions are implicated in migraine attacks, and the correlation between these functions confirms that the abnormal monoamine metabolism is linked with pain at the periphery and originated from the central nervous system (Table 1).

V. DEGENERATIVE DISEASES

Degenerative diseases include chronic slowly progressive disorders of the nervous system. Many diseases in this category are rarely seen, but others are quite common. There are several disorders with unknown or uncertain etiology, and many affect selectively certain groups of neurons and related functional properties (Table 2). Most entities are primarily diseases of the neurons or axons, and structural abnormalities in glial cells and myelin sheaths are secondary. Some diseases begin in infancy or childhood, while others occur in later life. However, the age of onset and progression are roughly similar within one type of impairment.

When a nerve is damaged or cut, characteristic degenerative changes take place. These changes are associated with metabolic lesions of the nerve cell. The high rate of metabolic processes in the brain depends mainly on the utilization of glucose and various components of the vitamin B complex participate. A deficiency of these water-soluble vitamins renders the nervous system particularly sensitive to changes leading to impairment and disease. Nerve degenerative processes also occur in thiamine deficiency. Therefore, these two neurological disorders may originate from a similar basic biochemical disturbance.

A. NERVE DEGENERATION

Lesions of the nerves are associated with characteristic degenerative changes of injured nerve cells.[161] These changes are primary or secondary, depending on the initial integrity of the axon and its interaction with the myelin sheath and the Schwann cell. Severing the axon triggers the degeneration process of the myelin sheath which is completely and irreversibly destroyed so that regeneration cannot be accomplished. Demyelination also occurs

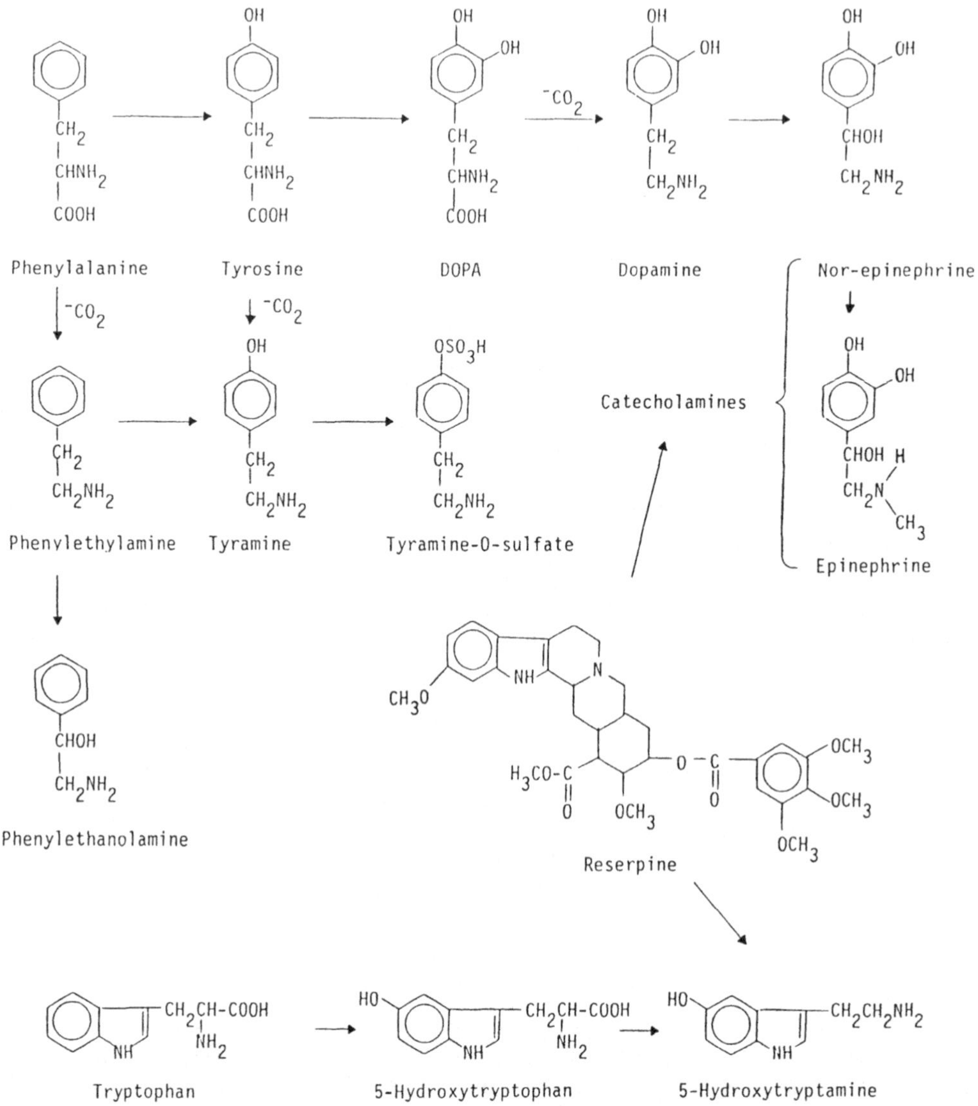

Phenylalanine → Tyrosine → DOPA $\xrightarrow{-CO_2}$ Dopamine → Nor-epinephrine

Phenylalanine: CH_2–$CHNH_2$–$COOH$
Tyrosine (OH): CH_2–$CHNH_2$–$COOH$
DOPA (OH, OH): CH_2–$CHNH_2$–$COOH$
Dopamine (OH, OH): CH_2–CH_2NH_2
Nor-epinephrine (OH, OH): $CHOH$–CH_2NH_2

Phenylalanine $\xrightarrow{-CO_2}$ Phenylethylamine
Tyrosine $\xrightarrow{-CO_2}$ Tyramine → Tyramine-O-sulfate

Phenylethylamine: CH_2–CH_2NH_2
Tyramine (OH): CH_2–CH_2NH_2
Tyramine-O-sulfate (OSO_3H): CH_2–CH_2NH_2

Catecholamines {

Epinephrine (OH, OH): $CHOH$–CH_2N\textlangle$\begin{smallmatrix}H\\CH_3\end{smallmatrix}$

Phenylethanolamine: $CHOH$–CH_2NH_2

Reserpine

Tryptophan: CH_2CH–$COOH$, NH_2 → 5-Hydroxytryptophan (HO): CH_2CH–$COOH$, NH_2 → 5-Hydroxytryptamine (HO): $CH_2CH_2NH_2$

FIGURE 11. Pathways of biosynthesis of important brain amines.

both in the central and the peripheral nervous system as the result of a primary demyelinating disease or secondary degeneration. In degenerative processes the neuron and its myelinsheath undergo structural destruction. Characteristic changes take place in Wallerian degeneration peripheral to the point of damage. Other conditions also produce secondary demyelination, including metabolic disorders, cerebral edema, anoxia, a variety of neuron intoxications, and tract compression.

In contrast to the irreversible changes, milder effects in the peripheral nervous system may allow regeneration to proceed from the proximal stump. The axonal elongation requires protein synthesis which mainly takes place in the neuronal perikaryon. When the normal axon is restored, the myelin sheath is reconstructed around the axon and homeostasis is reestablished. Nerve regeneration follows a typical time course, and the various stages include integrated associations between the restoration of structure and electrical and behavioral activity.

The process of Wallerian degeneration shows similarities in the peripheral and central

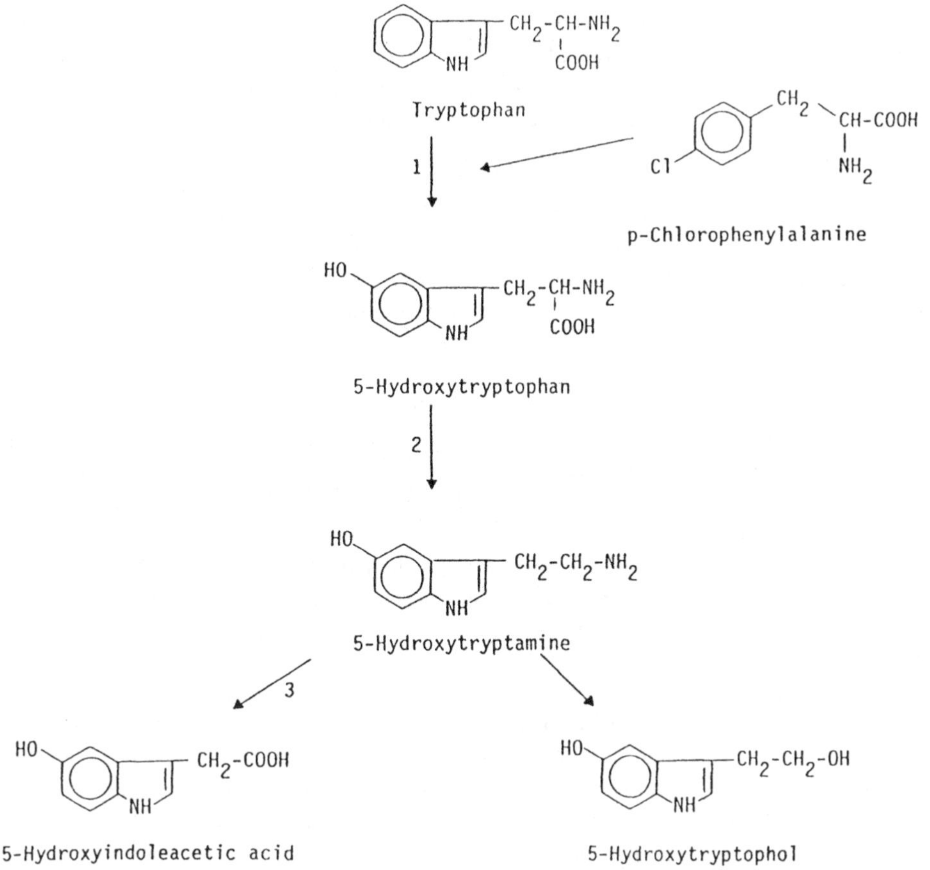

FIGURE 12. Competitive inhibition of serotonin biosynthesis by chlorophenylalanine.

TABLE 1 **Normal Range of Catecholamines** **Excretion in Urine**	
Catecholamine	**24-h Concentrations**
Epinephrine	9—34 μg
Norepinephrine	11—69 μg
Homovanillic acid	3.7—7.5 mg
Vanilmandelic acid	0.7—6.8 mg
Metanephrine	28—110 μg
Normetanephrine	78—370 μg

TABLE 2 **Various Degenerative Diseases and** **Corresponding Anatomical Sites**	
Degeneration	**Disease**
Cerebral cortex	Alzheimer's disease
	Pick's disease
Basal ganglia	Parkinson's disease
	Huntington's chorea
Spinocerebellar system	Friedrich's ataxia
	Cerebellar degeneration
Motor system	Motor neuron disease
Peripheral nerves	Muscular atrophy

nervous system. The fragmentation during the degeneration process in the brain is similar to the degenerating peripheral nerves, but the breakdown of myelin sheaths occurs more slowly in the central than in the peripheral system. After axonal degeneration, the myelin sheath in the peripheral nerve disintegrates with the Schwann cells. However, the myelin sheaths in the central nerve fibers first collapse, become engulfed by phagocytes, and then are digested. A difference may appear in the course of biochemical actions between the two nervous systems.

In the peripheral system, the biochemical changes show three stages. During the first phase of degeneration the axon is physically destructed in 7 to 8 d, and the organized structure of the proteolipid moieties of the myelin sheath loses stability. Early biochemical changes alter the configuration of the individual lipoproteins, initiating the physical fragmentation of the myelin. In this stage there is no apparent change in the main protein classes found in the nerves such as neurokeratin and proteolipid-protein. The physical and chemical changes cause subsequent instability and modification of the lipoprotein structure of the myelin sheath mainly consisting of progressive dissociation of the lipid from the protein portion. The second stage, 8 to 30 d, is connected with cellular proliferation and biochemical processes responsible for the removal of lipids. Active proteolysis also takes place in this stage. Peptidase activity, particularly acidic proteinase found in nerve organelles, is increased in both the proximal and distal stumps of the damaged nerve. The action of neutral proteinase, which is the main constituent of the myelin sheath itself, is raised in the preliminary phase and later, indicating a response to cellular proliferation. In the third stage, collagen is synthesized representing the process of fibrosis. Protein synthesis is quickly reduced after injury in the functionally altered neurons, then it rises above normal levels within 24 h reaching peak at 7 d and decreasing to normal levels at about day 30 from the beginning of the injury. The increased protein synthesis in the altered neurons coincides with the appearance of chromatolysis. Injured neurons lose their normal protein synthesizing capability which is restored rapidly. However, if regeneration does not occur, protein synthesis decreases steadily to below normal levels resulting in the production of collagen rather than in the replacement of original neural proteins.[34]

The time sequence of changes occurring in the proteolipid-protein pattern of degenerating tracts of white matter is different from that of peripheral nerves. The initial decrease of protein synthesis is prolonged up to 140 to 150 d and illustrates the general tendency that nerve cells of the central system show a delayed response to injury. The principal difference between the degenerating peripheral nerve and central white matter is the marked retardation in the removal of various substances in the latter. This may be a reflection of a less intense response of the glia cell in comparison which Schwann cells.

The changes in protein synthesis and degradation associated with proteinase activity and protein synthesis may derive from alteration of the membrane permeability of the various organelles in the neurons from the damaged peripheral nerve.[270] Proteinases contain proteolipids which may be responsible for their enzyme activity. Therefore, the primary modifications of the macromolecular organization of the neuronal structures and denaturation of lipoproteins occuring during early stages of neuron injury are associated with conformational changes of these complex molecules. Reduced enzyme activity may represent unmasking of the enzyme function. Later, increased enzyme activity may be related to changes in membrane permeability due to the injury or release of proteolipid from protein binding through the action of cytolytic substances, such as lysolecithin or lysophosphatidylethanolamine. These phospholipids are normally present in small amounts in the nervous system and exert a direct cytolytic or myelinolytic action on the cell, releasing enzymes from lysosomes of myelin. This step may be the initiator of the demyelinating process, indicating the participation of neural lysosomes in events of Wallerian degeneration. Lysosome-like particles are described in neuronal cells, axon, and glial cells and in the Schwann cell. It may be that lysosomal activity largely of axonal origin is responsible for the degradation and enzyme changes manifesting in the early stage of degeneration.

Early stages of Wallerian degeneration are considered associated with lysosomes, and the degradative process sets in through released enzymes. Lysosomes also contain acid phospholipid hydrolyzing enzymes (phospholipases). Phospholipases catalyze the release of free fatty acids from endogenous lipids. Free fatty acids act as cytolytic substances, they can labilize and disrupt mitochondrial membranes and the release of proteolytic enzymes from damaged mitochondria, as well as from lysosomes and can produce further alterations on membrane structure.

Wallerian degeneration alters lipid composition in a similar fashion both in the peripheral and central nervous system, although these changes take longer in the central tract. During the first stage, changes in lipid concentration of the nerve are slight. The loss of myelin lipids becomes apparent during the second week. The reduction includes a progressive decrease of phospholipids mainly in the distal part of the damaged peripheral nerve. The decrease is first significant in spingomyelin, phosphatidylethanolamine, and phosphatidylserine contents, later in lecithin and ethanolamine plasmalogen, and finally, in phosphatidylinositol. Lysolecithin increases while cholesterol is reduced, particularly after the second phase. At the same time, cholesterol ester increases, unlike in intact nerve which contains no esterified derivative. Triglycerides are also decreased, and mono- and diglycerides are elevated.

Irreversible damage of neurons is linked with initial increases of neuronal RNA and DNA in the first stage, followed by a gradual reduction of these constitutents from the neuron and the distal segment of the injured axon, leading finally to a complete loss.

A number of enzymes also altered in the nerve during Wallerian degeneration. In the degenerating nerve the levels of acetylcholinesterase falls following lesions, butyrylcholinesterase is increased or unaltered at the beginning, and it slowly returns to the normal level. These differences are related to their cellular distribution; acetylcholinesterase is found in the neurons, whereas butyrylcholinesterase is associated with the myelin sheath. Choline acetylase is greatly reduced in association with a decrease of acetylcholine content (Figure 13). These changes may be linked with observed alterations of protein and lipid synthesis, and these cellular components are intrinsic parts of enzyme activity.

B. NERVE REGENERATION

When the peripheral nerve is cut or damaged, the axon is separated from the motoneuron, and a series of adverse reactions set in shortly afterwards. A progressive cellular proliferation begins in both the distal and proximal stumps of the damaged nerve. This proliferation is greater in the proximal part and regenerative processes start if changes in the trophic center are favorable and the retrograde processes normalize within weeks. Progressive reactions become dominant, and successively, the central process of the Schwann cells results in a growing axon tip. This finally leads to a restoration of the structural and functional contact between the damaged parts. If the progression does not take place, the injured cell will be destroyed gradually. Remyelination in the central nervous system is essentially dependent on the activity of reacting glial cells which remyelinate the axons.

Shortly after injury, protein synthesis activity of the injured nerves increases. However, protein concentration decreases in this latency period. During the growth period of the axon and peripheral stem, the cell volume rises and protein synthesis from free amino acids increases. At maturation, when the contact between the nerve cell and periphery is reestablished, cell volume is doubled, and protein content is further elevated. Gradually, the original protein concentration is reached. These changes are associated with the reduction of neutral proteinase activity in both the proximal and distal stumps and with an increase in the rate of protein synthesis mainly in the proximal part. The Schwann cells play an important role in this process. This change is mostly linked with the regenerative activity of the neuron and the axoplasmic flow of newly synthetized proteins.

During the regeneration processes the synthesis of phospholipids is very slow and basically does not differ from intact nerves. There is some transient increase into phosphatidylethanolamine and inositol which may represent a role they play in regeneration. The synthesis of ethanolamine plasmalogens the most abundant constituents of the nervous system remains unaltered.

Enhanced protein synthesis and cytoplasmic swelling are accompanied with high turnover of neuronal RNA. It seems that there is no loss of RNA content during chromatolysis and

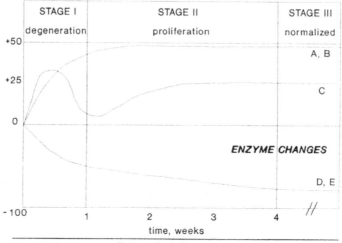

A: acid phosphatase   B: butyril cholinesterase   C: proteinase
D: choline esterase   E: choline acetylase

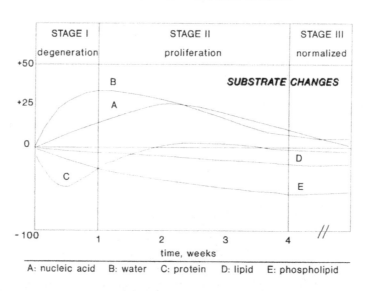

A: nucleic acid   B: water   C: protein   D: lipid   E: phospholipid

FIGURE 13.   Enzyme changes in the nerve during Wallerian degeneration.

is only redistributed in the hypertrophied regenerating neuron. RNA remains constant during the outgrowth, but in the maturation period, there is a doubling of this constituent. In the proximal stump of a regenerating nerve, DNA and RNA both gradually increase due to proliferation. The concentration of RNA is always greater than DNA.

C. DEGENERATION OF THE CEREBRAL CORTEX

1. Alzheimer's Disease

Many forms of degeneration exist in the cerebral cortex.[93,139,223,386] The more common are Alzheimer's disease and Pick's disease. Alzheimer's disease is a general common disorderof middle and late life and the principal cause of presenile and senile dementia.[67,74,77,78,146,155,162,260,374,566] The disease advances imperceptibly and is characterized by generalized deterioration of mental and body functions. The duration of the disease varies from 1 to 10 or more years. The principal lesions are widespread loss of neurons distributed diffusely and symmetrically throughout the cerebral cortex, amyloid plaques, neurofibrillary tangles, and neuroaxonal degeneration (Plate 2).[183,452,478] The involvement of the basal ganglia and other subcortical structures is minimal.

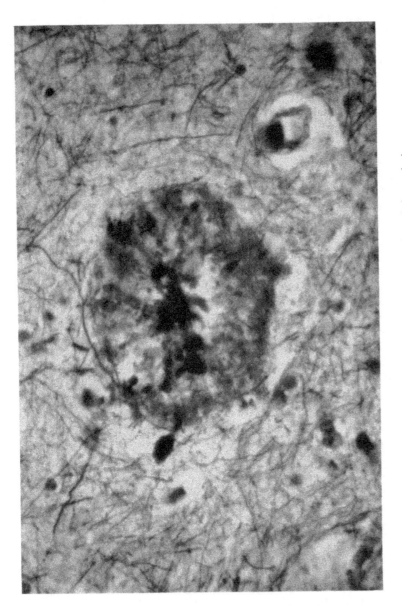

PLATE 2. Microscopic aspect of an Alzheimer plaque in human brain.

In cortical degeneration, the disorder starts with focal alterations of neurites followed by a phagocytic response. Later amyloid protein plaques are deposited and surrounded by few macrophages with swollen neurites containing secondary lysosomes. Amyloid plaques are found in almost all elderly patients, but their number is great only when signs of clinical dementia are apparent and neuronal fallout is detectable. Patchy lesions in the white matter in aging brain and dementia have also been reported.[86] The presence of abnormal proteins characterizes the manifestation of the Alzheimer's disease, although its direct cause is still unknown.[79,80,81,154,383] The deposition of abnormal proteins in the amyloid plaques is found concentrated near old infarcts and their presence probably represents nonspecific degenerative reactions to the causative agent by focal or individual cortical neurons.[38,40] The primary cause may be associated with slowly progressing deterioration of protein synthesis by the endoplasmic reticulum (Nissl substance); its elimination is partly controlled by the production of secondary lysosomes.

Recent publications suggest that various etiological factors are responsible for senile dementia. The neuritic or senile plaques in Alzheimer's disease consist of a dense core of extracellular amyloid surrounded by enlarged neurites containing degenerating mitochondria and lamellar lysosomes with increased hydrolase activity.[554] Neurotransmitter substances,[476,501] such as dopamine and norepinephrine, and the gabanergic system show significant losses with age, but there are no specific changes in Alzheimer dementia. Monoamine oxidase activity is increased in the brain in Alzheimer's disease, and the levels of 5-hydroxytryptamine and 5-hydroxyindoleacetic acid are decreased. Changes in the cholinergic system seem to be related, and choline acetyltransferase activity is reduced and acetylcholine increased in certain cortical areas in Alzheimer's disease and related disorders.[151,218,456,461,469,478,502]

Aluminum concentrations are increased in some brain regions of the brain in Alzheimer's disease 10 to 30 times the normal average concentrations.[135-137,300,569] Since aluminum exhibits cytotoxicity,[468] this metal has been implicated in the pathogenesis of several degenerative processes in the human central nervous system. In some cases, the presence of aluminum in the abnormal tissue may be the consequence of the deteriorated metabolic control. So matotoxin receptors showed reduced numbers in the cerebral cortex in Alzheimer's disease;[53] vasopressin and oxitocin neurons are modified with aging and in senile dementia.[220]

There is a certain relationship between Down's syndrome and Alzheimer's disease. Down's patients as middle-aged adults often become demented and die of a particularly aggressive form of Alzheimer's disease. The onset of this stage is very much a function of age. Since the cause of Down's disease is known due to trisomy of chromsome 21, it is possible that since Alzheimer patients are karyotypically normal individuals, their condition must be due to some sort of disorder in gene expression on that chromosome. Superoxide dismutase, an enzyme coded for by chromosome 21, showed an increase in skin fibroblast in trisomy and in Alzheimer's disease.[627] Regional brain 5-hydroxytryptamine levels are reduced in senile Down's syndrome and in Alzheimer's disease.[493,621]

2. Pick's Disease

In Pick's disease the clinical patterns are loss of memory and progressive dementia. The brain of affected individuals shows diffuse cortical atrophy which is often very severe inone or both frontal or temporal lobes (Plate 3). There is a moderate to extensive loss of neurons in affected areas and usually intense gliosis. Some of the neurons are greatly distended and large cytoplasmic inclusions replace the nuclei. The accumulation of these lipoprotein particles probably represents a metabolic defect related to the disease. There are changes in the presence of trace elements in the impaired neurons.[197]

3. Parkinson's Disease

The symptoms of this disorder are tremor, bradykinesia, and extrapyramidal rigid-

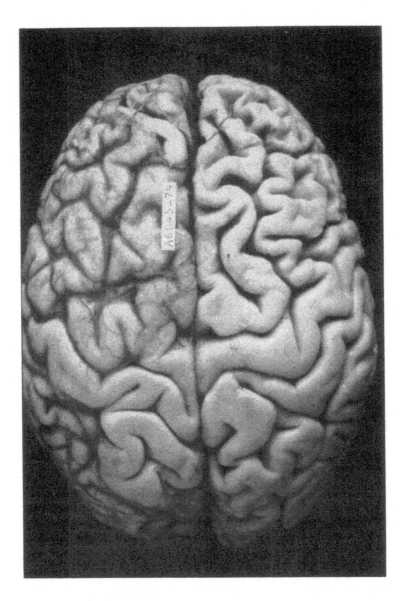

PLATE 3.   Surface aspect of the brain in Pick's disease.

ity.[89,166,222] Certain drugs may produce Parkinson's disease, but that is usually reversible after the withdrawal from the drugs.[295] Essential changes include loss of certain melanin-containing neurons of the brainstem, mainly in the substantia nigra and locus ceruleus.

Parkinson's disease is related to abnormalities of catecholamine metabolism.[30,211,224,441,622] In the normal cerebral tissue, dopamine, noradrenaline, and 5-hydroxytryptamine are found in varying amounts.[109] Neurons of the substantia nigra release catecholamine and mainly dopamine. In Parkinson's disease, the distribution of these transmitters shows changes.[65,66,133,198] There is marked reduction of dopamine in affected areas corresponding to loss of dopamine-producing neurons.[299-301,392] Chemical changes are mainly located in those areas of the brain responsible for the symptoms of the disease, such as the extrapyramidal motor centers. Neuromelanin disappears from the substantia nigra, and dopamine and its metabolites are greatly reduced in the striatum, substantia nigra, and globus pallidus. Enkephalin production is variable in the brain of parkinsonian patients.[559]

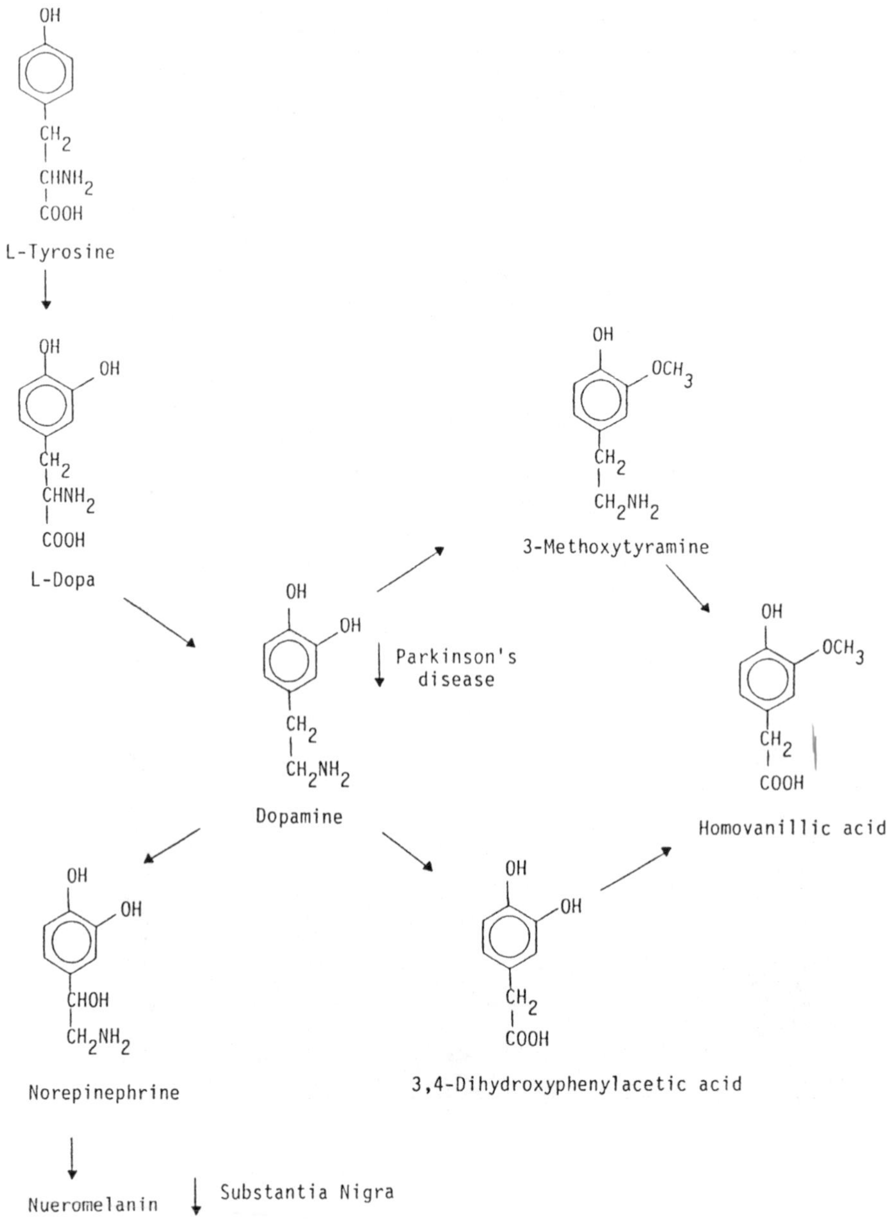

FIGURE 14.   Pathways of biosynthesis and metabolism of catecholamines in Parkinson's disease.

Attempts to replace depleted dopamine have not been successful, because this compound does not penetrate the blood-brain barrier easily.[51] However, cerebral dopamine stores can be replenished by the administration of the precursor L-dopa (dihydroxyphenylalanine) which is carried through the capillary endothelium by a specific mechanism.[377,396] The carboxylase enzyme converts L-dopa to dopamine in the striatum (Figure 14).

There is evidence that the cholinergic system also takes part in this disorder. Acetylcholine is present in the striatum as an excitatory transmitter. Under normal circumstances, some of the inherent activities of this neuroactive compound is inhibited by some pathways. When the disease of the extrapyramidal system becomes manifest, these inhibitory pathways are damaged and the unrelenting inhibition is probably responsible for the clinical symptoms in Parkinson's disease. Improvements achieved in patients with anticholinesterase agents such as tacrine (tetrahydroacridine) and aggravation of the symptoms brought about by cholinergic drugs suggest the role of acetylcholine metabolism in parkinsonism.

Several drugs may cause a Parkinson's syndrome. For example, reserpine depletes the endogenous 5-hydroxytryptamine and dopamine stores of the norepinephrine and other cerebral amines. In large doses, this drug produces depression and other psychic disturbances. Parkinson-like conditions are also produced by this drug. Chlorpromazine and haloperidol elicit similar actions, possibly by inhibiting catecholamine receptors leading to the release of the normal inhibitory effect on the extrapyramidal system. Many drug treatments have been considered to relieve parkinsonian syndromes.[15,377,436]

VI. VITAMIN DEFICIENCY DISORDERS

The brain is distinguished from other tissues because of its relatively high rate of metabolism. It is almost entirely dependent on carbohydrates as source of energy, and it responds rapidly to energy losses when is active and demands are increased by electric excitation of cells. Glucose provides the major source of energy and no alternative substrate has been found to support brain function adequately under normal conditions. The operating pathways of glucose metabolism in the brain are apparently the same as elsewhere in the body. Since the brain has relatively little glucose or glycogen reserves, it is essential to receive them rapidly by the bloodstream to maintain adequate function.

The control mechanism of carbohydrate metabolism in neural tissue is related to the accessibility of glucose to tissues and to the application of this metabolism for ion movements and changes in membrane potentials. The major route of glucose metabolism is glycolysis, and this pathway is regulated by important control points, such as hexokinase and phosphofructokinase enzymes. Moreover, important limiting factors include the amount of substrate and coenzymes present in the tissue, including NAD for dehydrogenase reactions and ADP for kinase reactions such as phosphoglycerate kinase and pyruvate kinase. The activity of pyruvate kinase is dependent on thiamine, and the lack of this exogenous compound in addition to other endogenous factors can considerably influence nervous system function. Pyridoxine, pantothenic acid, and cyanocobalamine deficiencies are also associated with neurological symptoms.[54] Lack of vitamin E exerts deleterious effects on the brain.[196,422]

A. VITAMIN B₁ DEFICIENCY

The lack of endogenous components is involved in the suppression of high enzymatic rates needed for the maintenance of normal function. In particular, thiamine deficiency is associated with various neurological disorders.[101,589,609] Severe and acute thiamine deficiency occurs in many East Asian countries where rice is the main source of food. It has been known for some time that the removal of the rice husks leads to loss of vitamin B_1, yet this complex disease called beri-beri still exists. Three forms of this disease are distinguishable: (1) wet beri-beri is characterized by generalized edema leading to death due to heart failure; (2) dry beri-beri is a chronic nutritional polyneuropathy with degenerative changes in the peripheral nerves leading to muscular degeneration; and (3) infantile beri-beri a chronic disorder often associated with sudden heart failure. The development of these diseases is linked with an alteration of pyruvate metabolism due to lack of thiamine (Figure 15).

Conditions similar to nutritional beri-beri are seen in chronic alcoholics or in patients suffering from chronic cachexia secondary to stomach carcinoma. These diseases respond promptly to thiamine therapy underlying the causal relationship with inadequate thiamine-supply. Chronic alcoholism is commonly associated with thiamine deficiency accounting for one of the most serious central nervous system complications in alcoholics: Wernicke's encephalopathy. This condition is characterized in acute stages by confusion, abnormal

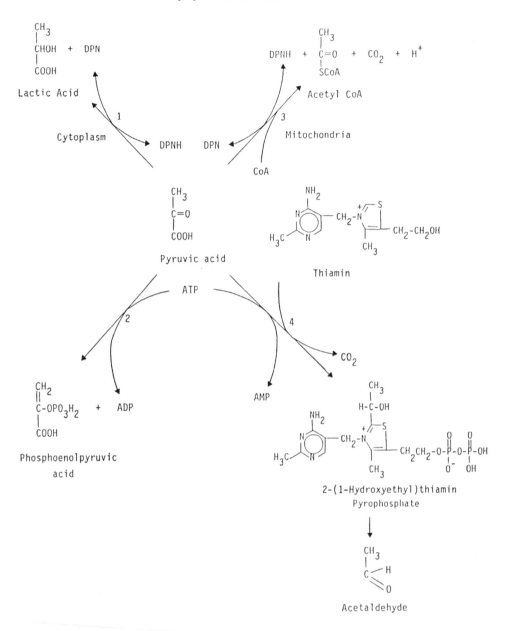

FIGURE 15.   Pathways of pyruvate metabolism and the role of thiamine.

ocular mobility, and ataxia. The pattern of neurologic signs has been reproduced in rhesus monkeys fed a thiamine-deficient diet.[406]

Some well controlled studies carried out on human volunteers have shown that thiamine deficiency brings about mental symptoms such as irritability, depression, defective memory, failure of concentration, subjective and objective changes in peripheral nerves of the lower limbs, impairment of sensations, weakness of the feet and muscles, and tenderness of the calf muscles. Some of these changes, particularly the mental symptoms, improve rapidly with thiamine therapy, whereas the various signs of peripheral neuropathy reverse later. The prolonged response lag after the administration of the coenzyme suggests that some irreversible or slowly reversible structural changes has occurred in these nerve cells deprived of thiamine.

B. VITAMIN B₆ DEFICIENCY

Vitamin B_6 is intimately concerned with the metabolism of the central nervous system.[586] All compounds implicated as neurotransmitters are synthesized and/or metabolized via vitamin B_6-dependent enzymatic reactions. These include dopamine, norepinephrine, serotonin, tyramine, tryptamine, taurine, histamine, γ-aminobutyric acid, and acetylcholine indirectly. Vitamin B_6 deficiency may be involved in the pathological manifestations of many disorders of the central nervous system such as seizure disorders and parkinsonism.

Swines kept on a vitamin B_6-free diet for 9 to 10 weeks exhibit demyelinization of peripheral nerves and degeneration of axons.[116] In rats, brain development, particularly myelination, was affected by deficiency of vitamin B_6 prior to and including the period of rapid myelination. Maternal deficiency of vitamin B_6 in the rat resulted in decreased myelination of the central nervous system in the progeny.[418] Five weeks of pyridoxine deficiency was sufficient to produce a deficit in active avoidance learning in postweaning rats when the brain development had been almost completed. The active avoidance learning was restored to normal within 1 week by reversal of the pyridoxine deficiency.[547]

In humans, the effects of pyridoxine deficiency have been best demonstrated in infants and children. A typical clinical picture observed in a group of infants including abdominal distress, increased irritability, as well as convulsive seizure and unconsciousness was caused by vitamin B_6 deficiency. Supplementation with pyridoxine-containing preparations promptly alleviated the symptoms.

In tuberculosis patients receiving high doses of the tuberculostatic drug isoniazid, a syndrome resembling vitamin B_6 deficiency has been observed.[612,623] These patients develop peripheral neuropathy which initially is sensory and later shows motor involvement. Other manifestations of isoniazid neurotoxicity include generalized seizures, optic neuritis followed by atrophy, muscle twitching, dizziness, ataxia, paresthesias, stupor, and encephalopathy. In addition, mental abnormalities such as euphoria, transient impairment of memory, separation of ideas and reality, loss of self-control, and psychosis have been reported. The incidence of isoniazid-induced neurotoxicity is increased in malnutrition and in situations causing secondary vitamin B_6 deficiency such as pregnancy, administration of contraceptive steroids, hypertyroidism, infections, and malignancy.[52]

Isoniazid may chelate with pyridoxal phosphate to form pyridoxal phosphate hydrazone complex which in turn inhibits pyridoxal kinase, the enzyme that synthesizes the catalytically active coenzyme pyridoxal phosphate. Hence, isoniazid reduces the tissue concentration of pyridoxal phosphate directly and indirectly (Figure 16).

C. VITAMIN B₆ AND γ-AMINOBUTYRIC ACID SYNTHESIS

In connection with the function of pyridoxal as a codecarboxylase for amino acids, there is one pyridoxal-dependent reaction which is specific to the central nervous system. This reaction is the conversion of glutamic acid to γ-aminobutyric acid (GABA) indicated by a pyridoxal phosphate-dependent L-glutamic acid decarboxylase, a soluble enzyme predominantly of synaptosomal origin. The rate of binding of pyridoxal phosphate to the decarboxylase reveals a two-step mechanism (Figure 17). The steady state concentrations of GABA in various brain areas are governed by glutamic acid decarboxylase and not by GABA-transaminase.[430]

Although having millions of neurons capable of firing, the normal brain is relatively resistant to spontaneous seizures due to inhibitory feedback loops that regulate the frequency of firing of individual neurons Synchronization of neuronal firing to the degree necessary to cause self-regenerative neuronal firing and seizure is present. During a seizure, many more neurons than normal in a particular part of the brain fire synchronously. This activity may spread to contiguous areas and leads to generalized neuronal discharge. In contrast to the usual EEG pattern, the pattern seen during a major epileptic attack may show peaked,

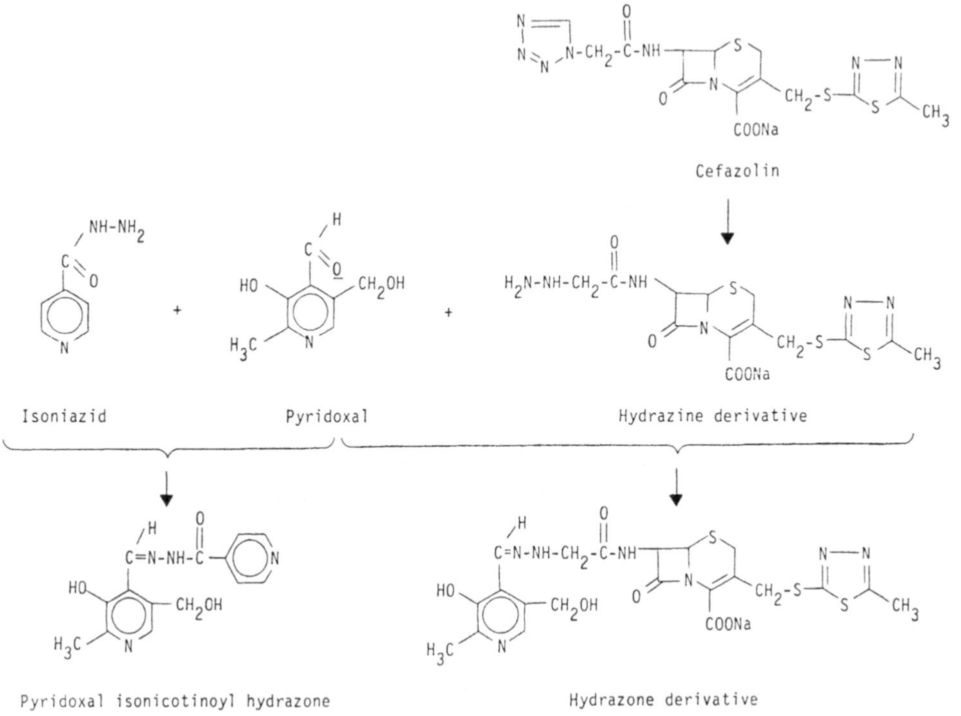

FIGURE 16.   Interaction between pyridoxal phosphate and isoniazid or cefazolin.

high-voltage waves with rapid and repetitive firing, or large, wide, high-voltage slow waves. The fault seems to be due to the lack of normal mechanisms by which neurons inhibit each other and desynchronize their activity. The effects of GABA on peripheral as well as central synaptic activity suggest that this compound functions as a neuronal activity regulator. Although it is most concentrated in brain tissue, traces of GABA are present in nonneural tissues, such as the liver. Also, GABA is not concentrated within synaptic vesicles. This evidence suggests that GABA is always constantly and freshly synthesized and released when needed. The influence of vitamin B_6 on the brain metabolism has been attributed to a GABA shunt, which permits the decarboxylation of glutamic acid to GABA primarily if not exclusively in the brain (Figure 18).

Epileptiform seizures produced by vitamin B_6 deficiency or isoniazid administration may be related to decreased activity of glutamic acid decarboxylase with resultant decreased GABA amounts necessary to regulate neuronal activity in a normal manner. Glutamic acid decarboxylase is more susceptible to vitamin B_6 deficiency in comparison to other vitamin B_6-requiring enzymes such as L-amino acid decarboxylase. Convulsion inhibits oxygen consumption, and GABA is a substrate for cerebral oxidative metabolism. Vitamin B_6 can reverse the inhibition of brain oxygen consumption brought about by vitamin B_6-dependent convulsions in humans. Most anticonvulsants share the property of pyridoxine in protecting against hypoxic convulsion. All of these observations suggested that pyridoxal phosphate controls the activity of glutamic acid decarboxylase, which in turn influences the central nervous system excitability through the synthesis of GABA which has inhibitory activity on the central nervous system.

D. VITAMIN B_6 AND CATECHOLAMINE SYNTHESIS

Amines other than GABA may be involved in the pathogenesis of central nervous system hyperexcitability. For example, raising the concentration of norepinephrine can decrease

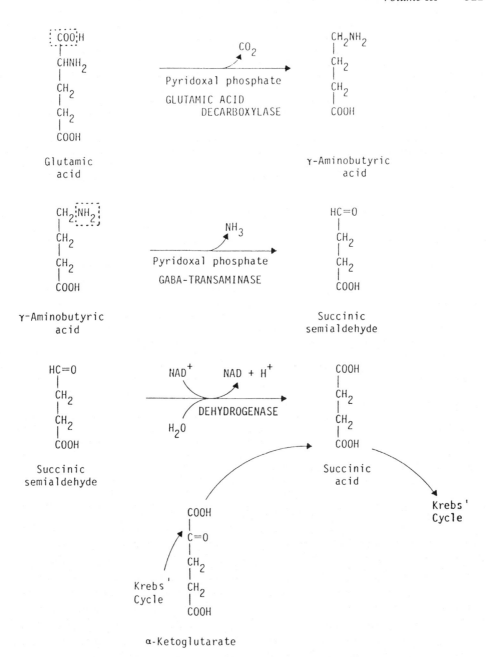

FIGURE 17.   Coenzyme role of pyridoxal phosphate in various steps of aminobutyric acid metabolism.

seizure susceptibility. Dopamine is a neurotransmitter as well as a precursor in the synthesis of norepinephrine.

In the conversion of 3,4-dihydroxyphenylalanine (dopa) to dopamine catalyzed by L-amino acid decarboxylase, pyridoxal phosphate is required as a cofactor. Pyridoxal phosphate and pyridoxal kinase modify dopa decarboxylase activity, which may influence the synthesis of monoamines such as dopamine, norepinephrine, and serotonin. The enzyme L-amino acid decarboxylase is unsaturated at physiological conditions. Its activity and its reaction products can be increased by incubation with pyridoxal phosphate *in vitro*, by administration of pyridoxine *in vivo*, or by agents that elevate the concentration of pyridoxal in the body. The

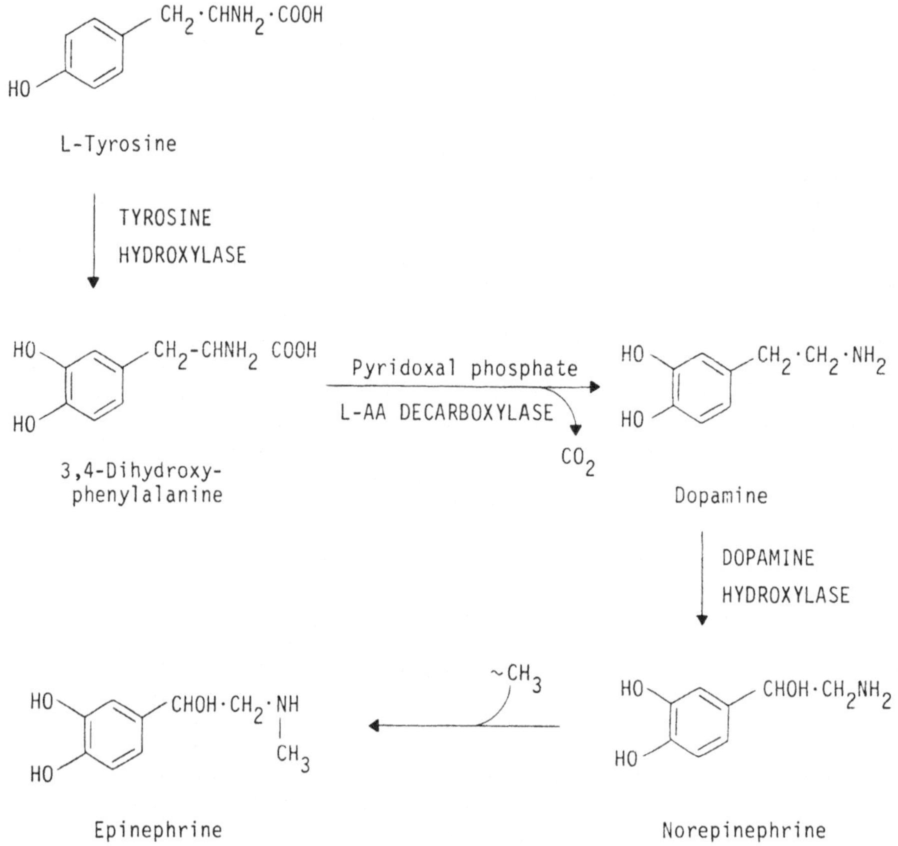

FIGURE 18.   Coenzyme role of pyridoxal phosphate in catecholamine metabolism. L − AA = L-amino acid.

rate of monoamine synthesis varies with the degree of sympathetic nerve activity. There is an inverse relationship between the pyridoxal kinase activity, responsible for the synthesis of the active coenzyme pyridoxal phosphate and the concentrations of brain dopamine, norepinephrine, and serotonin. When the monoamine content of the brain is elevated, the activity of pyridoxal kinase decreases. Conversely, when the concentration of brain mono-amines is lowered, the activity of pyridoxal phosphokinase is elevated. Dopa, dopamine, and norepinephrine inhibit the activity of pyridoxal kinase. This relationship indicates the relationship between brain vitamin B_6 content and metabolism of monoamines, suggesting that monoamines concentration of brain might control the production of pyridoxal phosphate. The brain regulates the concentration of pyridoxal phosphate by modifying the activity of pyridoxal kinase. When the concentration of pyridoxal phosphate is below normal, the kinase becomes activated. Conversely, when the level of the coenzyme rises above normal, the activity of kinase becomes lowered.

Parkinsonism is a disorder characterized by three cardinal symptoms and signs, namely coarse tremor, plastic rigidity, and akinesia. Patients with Parkinson's disease have sub-stantially less striatal dopamine in comparison with normal subjects. Hence, Parkinsonism is considered a striatal dopamine deficiency syndrome, and treatment is orientated toward the normalization of striatal dopamine. This can be achieved by administration of large amounts of L-dopa which is a dopamine precursor.

Since the addition of pyridoxal phosphate increases the activity of dopa decarboxylase, one might expect beneficial effects in administration of pyridoxine to patients with parkin-

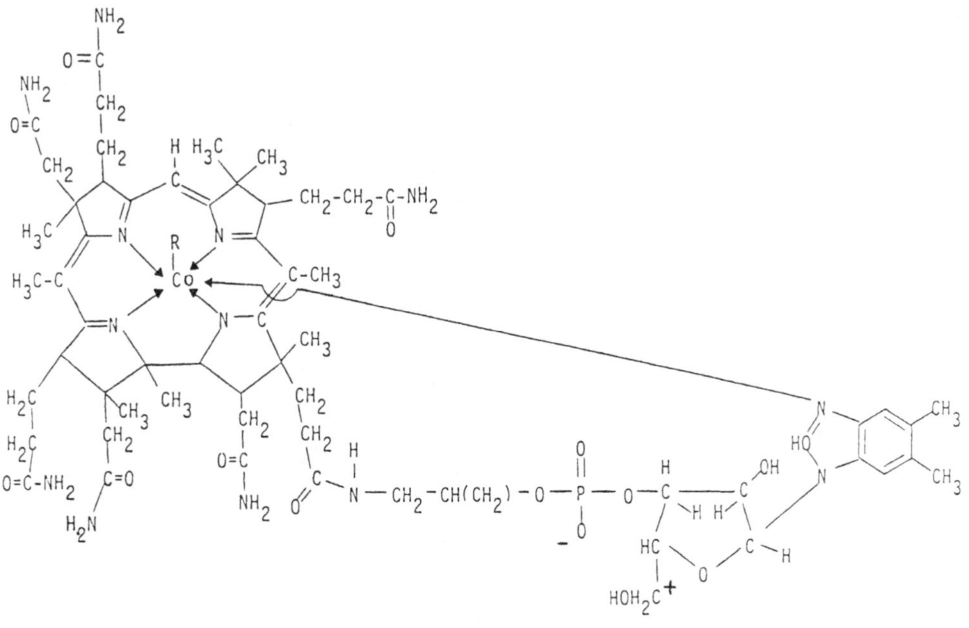

FIGURE 19. Structure of vitamin B₁₂.

sonism who are receiving L-dopa. However, it was found that pyridoxine nullified the beneficial effects of L-dopa, and that adding pyridoxine to L-dopa therapy is of no value. This is due to increased decarboxylation of L-dopa to dopamine peripherally as a result of added pyridoxine, so that there is a consequently decreased availability of L-dopa to the brain. The inhibition of L-dopa central nervous system effects by pyridoxine may result from the formation of a Schiff base between pyridoxine and L-dopa, with subsequent biochemical and pharmacological inactivation of both compounds. Some of the side effects of L-dopa such as the appearance of involuntary movements may be overcome by the use of pyridoxine.

E. VITAMIN B₁₂ DEFICIENCY

Vitamin B_{12} deficiency mainly causes disorders of the hematopoietic system and red cell production. This condition, however, also affects the nervous system connected with patchy, diffuse, and progressive demyelination. The clinical picture resulting from the diffuse, uneven demyelination is one of insidiously progressive neuropathy, often beginning in the peripheral nerves and progressing centrally to involve the posterior and lateral columns of the spinal cord and the brain.

The effect of vitamin B_{12} (Figure 19) is related to folate synthesis and metabolism. A vitamin B_{12}-containing enzyme removes the methyl group from methylfolate, thereby regenerating tetrahydrofolate (THF) from which 5,12-methylene-THF is produced which is required for thymidilate synthesis. Methylfolate is the predominant form of the vitamin in human serum and liver and this compound is stored in the body's folate pool by a vitamin B_{12}-dependent step. In case of vitamin B_{12} deficiency, folate is trapped as methylfolate and thus becomes metabolically useless. The folate trap causes a defect in the DNA synthesis step, responsible for demyelination.

Subacute degeneration of the spinal cord may be due to vitamin B_{12} deficiency. This condition is also connected with pernicious anemia. The relationship between these two diseases has now been clarified. Neurological involvements occur very frequently in the development of anemia and sometimes may even initiate erythrocyte production disorders. The degree of anemia and severity of neurological symptoms does not run parallel. Neurological changes are associated with abnormal metabolism of the nerve cells caused directly by the lack of cyanocobalamin.[42] The mechanism of impairment may be due to the failure of a variety of reactions, particularly methylation reactions which need the participation of vitamin B_{12} coenzyme. It has been shown that this compound is also involved in the reduction of disulphide compounds including glutathione. The disturbance of the ratio between reduced and oxidized glutathione may affect normal regulatory processes of carbohydrate and fat metabolism.

VII. POLYNEURITIS

In this disease the function of peripheral nerves is impaired. The clinical symptoms, therefore, are connected with a widespread disturbance of the nervous system and often the brain is also involved. Because of widespread lesions, this condition is associated with factors affecting the body as a whole.

The main causes of polyneuritis are beri-beri, pellagra, chronic alcoholism, and chemical toxins, including arsenic, other metals, carbon monoxide, and organic compounds such as carbon disulphide, aniline, and nitrobenzene, Metabolic disorders such as diabetes mellitus and porphyria may also cause polyneuritic alterations and cancer or bacterial infections can also produce it.

Generally, thiamine deficiency is considered to be the major biochemical lesion of polyneuritis, but there are other biochemical abnormalities related to other types of polyneuritis. The outstanding defect in thiamine deficiency is the impairment of normal pyruvate metabolism, resulting in increased blood levels.

Alcoholic polyneuritis shows a striking resemblance to dry beri-beri. This condition is due to thiamine deficiency caused by the unbalanced, nutritionally deficient diet of alcoholics. When an adequate diet rich in thiamine was taken, the disease subsided, even though alcohol was also consumed. The existence of thiamine deficiency in alcoholic polyneuritis is supported by the findings of low levels of vitamin B_1 and cocarboxylase and high levels of pyruvate in blood.

Polyneuritis is often caused by metal poisoning, related to the enzyme system responsible for pyruvate oxidation which contains highly reactive sulfhydryl groups. A number of toxic agents can inhibit pyruvate oxidation by interaction with these groups leading to high blood pyruvate levels. Arsenic, mercury, and other heavy metals act in this way and clinical symptoms of neuritis associated with the toxic action of metal ions resemble also dry beri-beri neuritis. Polyneuritis caused by poisoning with heavy metals can be distinguished from thiamine deficiency by using the pyruvate tolerance test (Figure 20).[116]

Polyneuritis is sometimes connected with the intake of organophosphorus compounds. Tri-*o*-cresylphosphate is a neurotoxic organophosphorus compound that causes severe motor neuritis (Figure 21). This effect was discovered in 1930 when the paralysis caused by one constituent of Jamaica ginger extract was used for making some beverages. The "ginger paralysis" was also observed in patients with pulmonary tuberculosis treated with phosphocreosote. The tri-*o*-cresylphosphate is converted in the body to a more reactive compound, a cyclic metabolite, which produces the toxic effects. The metabolite is a potent cholinesterase inhibitor and causes neurotoxic symptoms at low dose levels of 4 mg/kg body weight.

Interstitial neuritis is connected with inflammation of the connective tissue of peripheral nerves causing pain and motor impairment. The cause of the pain is due to the inflammatory exudate exercising a pressure on the nerve fibers, and in later stages the nervous tissue is replaced by connective tissue overgrowth.

Polyneuritis may occur in pregnancy, probably related to nutritional factors. Persistent vomiting, unsuitable diet, and the increased requirements of the fetus may contribute to the nutritional deficiency during pregnancy. Where beri-beri is endemic, pregnancy may predispose this condition.

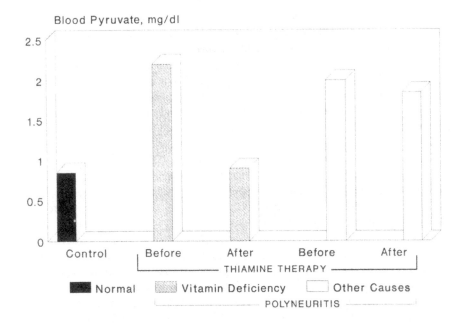

FIGURE 20. Variations in blood pyruvate levels in polyneuritis.

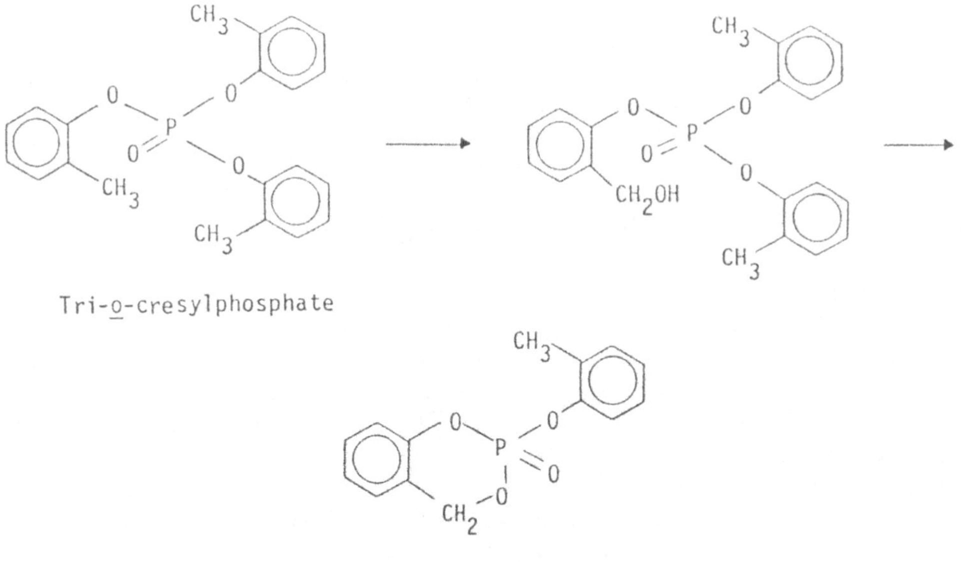

Tri-o-cresylphosphate

Cyclic metabolite

FIGURE 21. Metabolism of tri-*o*-cresylphosphate.

Acute infective polyneuritis is a diffuse infectious disease of the nervous system involving the spinal cord, peripheral nerves, and occasionally, the brain. This is probably one of the most common conditions of polyneuritis. A number of cases were observed among troops during the war. There is an initial febril state with no nervous symptoms followed by a latency period which may last from a few days to several weeks. Symptoms in this stage are usually headache, vomiting, and pains in the back and limbs. At the end of this period paralytic conditions develop very suddenly. The acute onset and associated high fever suggest an infection due to a microorganism. The toxins produced probably affect the lower neurons.

Since most neuritis conditions are associated with thiamine depletion, the determination of blood pyruvate values provide a good indication on the form of the disease. It is considerably elevated in the blood in thiamine-deficiency neuritis, particularly in the acute advanced beri-beri. In subacute or chronic types, pyruvate levels are usually found within the normal range or only slightly raised. The increase of pyruvate is not always apparently related to the degree of thiamine deficiency. In cases of less severe degrees of thiamine deficiency, it is necessary to give a loading dose of glucose. This leads to an abnormal amount of pyruvate formation in the tissues and elevated blood pyruvate levels.

VIII. DISEASES OF DEMYELINATION

Myelin sheaths are highly specialized structures in the central nervous system interfascicular obligodendroglia and in the peripheral system Schwann cells. Myelin is very reactive to ischemia or trauma and disintegrates if the axon is lost by injury. In some disease conditions, myelin-forming cells or myelin sheaths are primary targets and axonal alterations, gliosis, and phagocytosis follow secondarily. A wide variety of injuries can bring about destruction of the myelin sheath. Sometimes the demyelinating disease is secondary to damage of the neurons. Demyelinating diseases are relatively common disorders, but their etiology in most cases is unknown. Characteristic symptoms are scattered and localized areas show myelin breakdown and gliosis. The main locations of the demyelinated areas are the white matter of the brain, spinal cord, and optic nerves. Demyelination is considered to be the reaction of the nervous system to injury and the primary cause of this lesion can be, therefore, very different.

Various demyelinating disorders include multiple sclerosis, encephalomyelitis, several forms of diffuse sclerosis, complications of vaccination or infections, measles, German measles, chicken pox, small pox, mumps, complications of hepatic disease, porphyria, eclampsia, and uremia.[4,23,424,434,571,585] Acquired immune deficiency syndrome (AIDS) is often associated with progressive diffuse leukoencephalopathy.[18,60,336] Many data indicate reduced concentrations of mediators,[205,225,265,302,394,395,555,617] neurohormones,[373,389,412,488,489] various enzymes,[270,333,335,348,414] and changes in immunoregulation.[595,596]

A. MULTIPLE SCLEROSIS

Multiple sclerosis is a chronic and relapsing disorder which usually begins in early adult life. The symptoms and signs indicate multiple locations in the central nervous system.[10] In this disease, scattered plaques of demyelination and glial sclerosis occur throughout the nervous system. The optic nerves, brain stem, cerebral peduncles, and spinal cord are the most commonly affected regions; peripheral nerves are usually unaffected. The size of the plaques varies from microscopic to 1 to 2 cm or even larger. The plaques are clearly distinguishable from the surrounding tissue and show a tendency to occur symmetrically. As a consequence of plaques, myelin undergoes a process of erosion or lysis.

The clinical symptoms of multiple sclerosis depend on the location and size of plaques. Early stages usually point to one or more acute focus, and the symptoms of the lesions usually develop rapidly, but is often markedly improved with little functional deficit remaining. The recovery is usually incomplete and accumulation of the relapses leads to a gradual, permanent disability. The first symptoms of weakness and monocular blindness or double vision indicate spinal cord damage and the involvement of the optic nerves.

Pathogenetic factors of multiple sclerosis have not yet been clearly established. It is suggested that the plaque formation in the case of multiple sclerosis is caused by local anoxia in the brain, resulting form thrombotic occlusion of small blood vessels. Sometimes plaques occur around veins which contradicts their relationship to anoxia. Another theory relates to the deficiency of trace metals.[292] Demyelinating disease occurs naturally in young lambs and is due to a deficiency of copper ions in the pasture. Ewes grazing in this copper-deficient pasture have low levels of copper in blood and milk. The progression of this disease can be inhibited by copper administration. In lambs, copper is required for the normal formation of myelin. The mechanisms by which copper participates in this complex process has not been elucidated.

In contrast to copper ions, the presence of excessive amounts of heavy metal ions in soil or water has been suggested to have a role in the development of multiple sclerosis. High lead content is considered to be a causative factors. Some data indicate that the teeth lead content in multiple sclerotic patients is elevated. Contradictory findings have also been reported.

Lipid changes are more consistent in tissues of multiple sclerosis patients. Alteration of lipid patterns in blood and cerebrospinal fluid and especially changes in polyunsaturated fatty acid residues are important findings in multiple sclerosis. This finding is congruent with the suggestion that high-fat diets and diets relatively deficient in unsaturated long-chain fatty acids may predispose susceptible individuals to multiple sclerosis. The total cholesterol, mainly free cholesterol and total phospholipid, are also elevated in the cerebrospinal fluid. In contrast, cholesteryl ester content, especially cholesteryl linoleate, is reduced in the serum. The levels of linoleic acid, however, remained unaffected in both serum and cerebrospinal fluid.

The white matter from the brain of multiple sclerosis subjects contains less phospholipid than normals, and sphingomyelin and ethanolamine plasmalogen appear to be the lipids involved. The process leading to loss of phospholipid may be similar to the predemyelinating removal of phospholipid in the very early stage of Wallerian degeneration, reflecting damage to mitochondria and axoplasm. Small amounts of cholesterol esters have also been found in such white tissue through these esters are absent from the normal brain.

Virologic and immunologic investigations revealed the function of infection with slow viruses as possible causes of multiple sclerosis lesions.[4,314,385,466] A very long initial period of latency lasting for several months to several years trigger off remissions and exacerbations of the disease condition. The primary event in multiple sclerosis, the myelin damage, results from a viral infection early in life expressed later on as an immune process (Figure 22) associated with an increased immunoglobulin production.[204,568] Multiple sclerosis patients show abnormalities in the relative amounts of fatty acids present in a variety of tissues, particularly unsaturated and polyunsaturated fatty acids, and palmitoleic, oleic, and arachidonic acids show reductions in the lecithin fraction of the white matter. Leukocytes of multiple sclerosis patients also contain less polyunsaturated fatty acids.[10,50,76] Variations in the activity of proteolytic enzymes and loss of basic proteins in and around multiple sclerosis plaques[199] and polypeptides[125] related to viral antibody in the cerebrospinal fluid have been associated with the disease.

It has been suggested that lysosomal acid proteinases of neuronal and glial cells are involved in the pathogenesis of demyelination. These lysosomal enzymes may liberate basic proteins from the myelin sheaths. The basic protein or encephalitogenic fragment of the myelin sheath is very characteristic for adult myelin. It appears gradually and is essential for the maintenance of the proper structure. Both in the peripheral nerve and in the central nervous system this protein is lost in an early step of demyelination. The basic protein is a vulnerable part of the membrane and is released by lysosomal proteolytic enzymes. The lysosomal changes also affect 2',3'-cyclic nucleotide 3-phosphohydrolase, an important enzyme in the active period of myelination. The activity of this enzyme is greatly reduced in multiple sclerosis.

Immunological processes may also play part in the pathogenesis of multiple sclerosis.[588] Patients often elicit cellular responses to nervous tissue antigens and have demonstrated impairment of mixed leukocyte reactions. Typical multiple sclerosis lesions contain a small

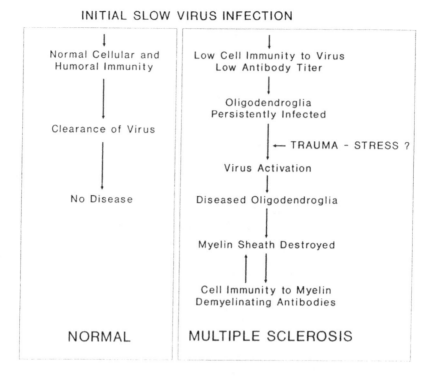

FIGURE 22.   Schematic presentation of the pathogenesis of multiple sclerosis.

number of inflammatory cells in the border-zone of the plaques, which may play a role in the autophagocytic reactions in later stages of the disease. All these findings indicate that the course of multiple sclerosis is a highly complex process.

B. ENCEPHALOMYELITIS

Allergic responses of the central nervous system are also suspected causative factors. Encephalomyelitis or acute infections in childhood may be associated with the progress of the disease, and present evidence suggests the involvement of an infectious agent as well as the immune system. The infectious agent is probably a virus, since it has been found that multiple sclerosis patients usually have higher measles or mumps antibody titers than normal. Some patients have high immunoglobulin levels in the cerebrospinal fluid, suggesting that an infectious agent is associated with the disease. The presence of inclusion bodies and multinucleated giant cells in demyelinated areas implicate further a viral etiology.

The released encephalitogenic proteins are also probably responsible for the immune response associated with multiple sclerosis. These biochemical changes are recognized in the protein levels of cerebrospinal fluid. Multiple sclerosis shows no effects on plasma proteins, but elevated globulin content appears more frequently in the cerebrospinal fluid. This parameter still cannot be used for diagnosis since only 20 to 50% of the cases give positive results. However, a positive correlation has been demonstrated between the concentration of cerebrospinal fluid immunoglobulin G and the increased amount of this immunoglobulin in multiple sclerosis plaques.

IX. METABOLIC DISEASES

Many mental impairments are related to metabolic disorders causing retardation or decreased cognitive function. In these disorders, accumulation of excessive amounts of metabolites or abnormal body constituents in the tissues are observed. Mental defects may be related to inborn or acquired errors of metabolism. The genetic hereditary basis of some conditions has been established, but in many diseases it is still far from clear in spite of extensive studies.[27] Various genetic defects are associated with mental retardation. However, even when the genetic effect is fairly well established, the correlation with functional lesions may be obscure. Moreover, the differentiation between inborn and acquired causes is not always simple. The brain defect in phenylketonuria has genetic origin and the exact nature of the biochemical lesion and its site are known; in hyperglycinemia, however, the error can be either inborn or acquired.

The conditions of metabolic disorders associated with abnormal brain function are numerous, and their number is likely to increase still further, but the overall contribution of the metabolic disorders to the prevalance of mental retardation is not large. Many children with metabolic disorders die in early infancy before the cause of disease can be established, and the true incidence therefore, may be greater than reported. The most frequently occurring diseases are phenylketonuria, lipidosis, galactosemia, hyperglycinemia, homocystinuria, argininosuccinic aciduria, gargoylism, mucopolysaccharidoses, and generalized aminoaciduria. In this chapter, we consider only the most frequently occurring conditions.

A. AMINOACIDURIAS

Many diseases of inborn errors of metabolism are associated with aminoaciduria.[297] The disorder may be primarily related to (1) enzyme defects in the intermediary metabolism or transport of amino acids such as phenylketonuria and Hartnup disease; (2) secondary interference with hepatic or renal metabolism causes by the action of an endogenous or exogenous substance, resulting in overflow and elimination of excess amino acids such as Wilson's disease; or (3) the consequence of heavy metal poisoning. Excess tissue levels of a given amino acid may inhibit the transport of other amino acids into the brain and their utilization for protein synthesis.[46,47] Respiration, synthesis of neurotransmitter substances, and myelination may also be affected. Some amino acids serve as neurotransmitters,[48] implying that altered tissue levels may cause derangement in the neuronal network function.[49] In some cases, the plasma level of an amino acid is elevated, and due to overflow, it appears in theurine. In others, the plasma level is low. In some diseases the anomaly of amino acid metabolism caused by an enzyme defect does not appear as accumulation in the plasma, since there is no renal mechanism for its reabsorption. Such amino acids are normally present within the cell and due to the no-threshold level they are eliminated in the urine, such as cystathionine and argininosuccinic acid. A large number of the genetic disorders of amino acid metabolism are coupled with neurologic symptoms, most commonly with mental retardation.[472]

In most aminoacidurias only a few amino acids are excreted in urine. This selectivity is related to the presence of several enzymatic transport systems in the kidney. Separate mechanisms are associated with the transport of neutral monocarboxylic acids, acidic dicarboxylic acids (glutamic, aspartic), and basic diamino acids (arginine, ornithine, lysine). The imino acids (proline, hydroxyproline) are transported by mechanisms similar to that of glycine. Cystine shares the transport mechanism of basic amino acids, and methionine is probably transported by a separate system operating in the kidney. In several types of aminoaciduria, combinations may exist between the various transport mechanisms. Several amino acids can be elevated in the plasma as the result of lesions in hepatic enzymes with or without participation of renal transport mechanisms. This condition may represent the combination of an overflow and no-threshold aminoaciduria. In some cases, the defective metabolism of an amino acid in the liver and a defect in tubular reabsorption in the kidney results in both overflow and renal aminoaciduria. The various sites of defects can be located by the determination of the amino acid in the serum or plasma and in the urine. Elevated serum levels probably represent pure overflow, other types of aminoacidurias show increased urinary excretion. These screening procedures can be applied for the purpose of detection of the metabolic disorder in question. It is important to note that although aminoacidurias are primarily connected with enzyme defects in various organs, such as liver or kidney, mental retardation is very frequent in many of these disorders.

1. Phenylketonuria

The symptoms of the disease develop soon after birth and can be diagnosed within weeks thereafter by the presence of increased plasma phenylalanine sometimes up to 30 times above normal levels.[194] At the same time, large amounts of phenylpyruvate are excreted in the urine. If not treated, signs of mental retardation can be observed after 6 months. Seizures and various other neurological abnormalities occur including tremors, microcephaly, electroencephalogram abnormalities, eczema, and reduced pigmentation of hair and skin. Usual stages of motor development are delayed, such as sitting, walking, and talking. The neurological changes run parallel with the degree of mental defect and in general, they are worse in severely affected individuals. Epileptic seizures and muscular toxicity often accompany the disease at an early stage. In older children and adults the process establishes a stationary level, but life expectancy is reduced. The incidence of phenylketonuria is about 1 in 10,000 to 25,000 births. Most of these patients are in mental institutions.

Phenylketonuria is an autosomal recessive disease and is characterized by the absence or defect of an enzyme, phenylalanine hydroxylase.[221] The enzyme represents the most effective pathway of phenylalanine metabolism and the highest activity is normally found in the liver. Biopsy studies have confirmed that phenylalanine hydroxylase is almost completely inactive or absent in phenylketonuria and that there is an adaptive increase in enzymes catalyzing the conversion of phenylalanine along other pathways, such as the production of phenylacetylglutamine. In the degradation of this amino acid, tyrosine is an intermediate which is further metabolized via p-hydroxyphenylpyruvic and homogentisic acid to carbon dioxide and water. Quantitatively less important pathways produce thyroxine, adrenaline, noradrenaline, and melanine (Figure 23). The accumulation of phenylalanine in body fluids such as blood, cerebrospinal fluid, and duodenal juice, and the diversion of phenylalanine metabolism into pathways which have minor importance in normal individuals are the results of the metabolic block in phenylketonuria. Therefore, in the diseased state alternate routes become dominant and as a consequence, o-tyrosine, o-hydroxyphenyl-lactic, pyruvic, and acetic acids are formed. The quantitative increase of these compounds is characteristic to this disease. In normal blood, phenylalanine levels are between 1 and 2 mg/dl. During the first days of life before the hepatic hydroxylase system is fully developed, phenylalanine levels rise up to 6 mg/dl or even higher, particularly in babies with low birth weight. This increase is transient and returns to normal shortly after birth in the postnatal period. In untreated phenylketonuric patients, however, phenylalanine is further increased and may reach 50 to 100 mg/dl. Part of this elevated phenylalanine is excreted in the urine mainly as phenylpyruvic acid. Some related diseases such as alkaptonuria and albinism are also associated with the abnormal metabolism of phenylalanine or tyrosine (Figure 23). Animal experiments established that phenyl acetate causes neurotoxicity in experimental phenylketonuria.[369]

The metabolism of tryptophan is also altered. High phenylalanine content of tissue fluids inhibits the interstitial absorption of this amino acid. Additional abnormalities are associated with the bacterial action of the intestinal flora on the excess amount of tryptophan.

The exact mechanism determining how metabolic abnormalities of these aromatic amino acids lead to the impairment of intelligence in phenylketonuria has not been firmly agreed upon. One or more of the related substances elicit toxic action on the developing brain. The overall increase of phenylalanine in the extracellular space competes with the transport of

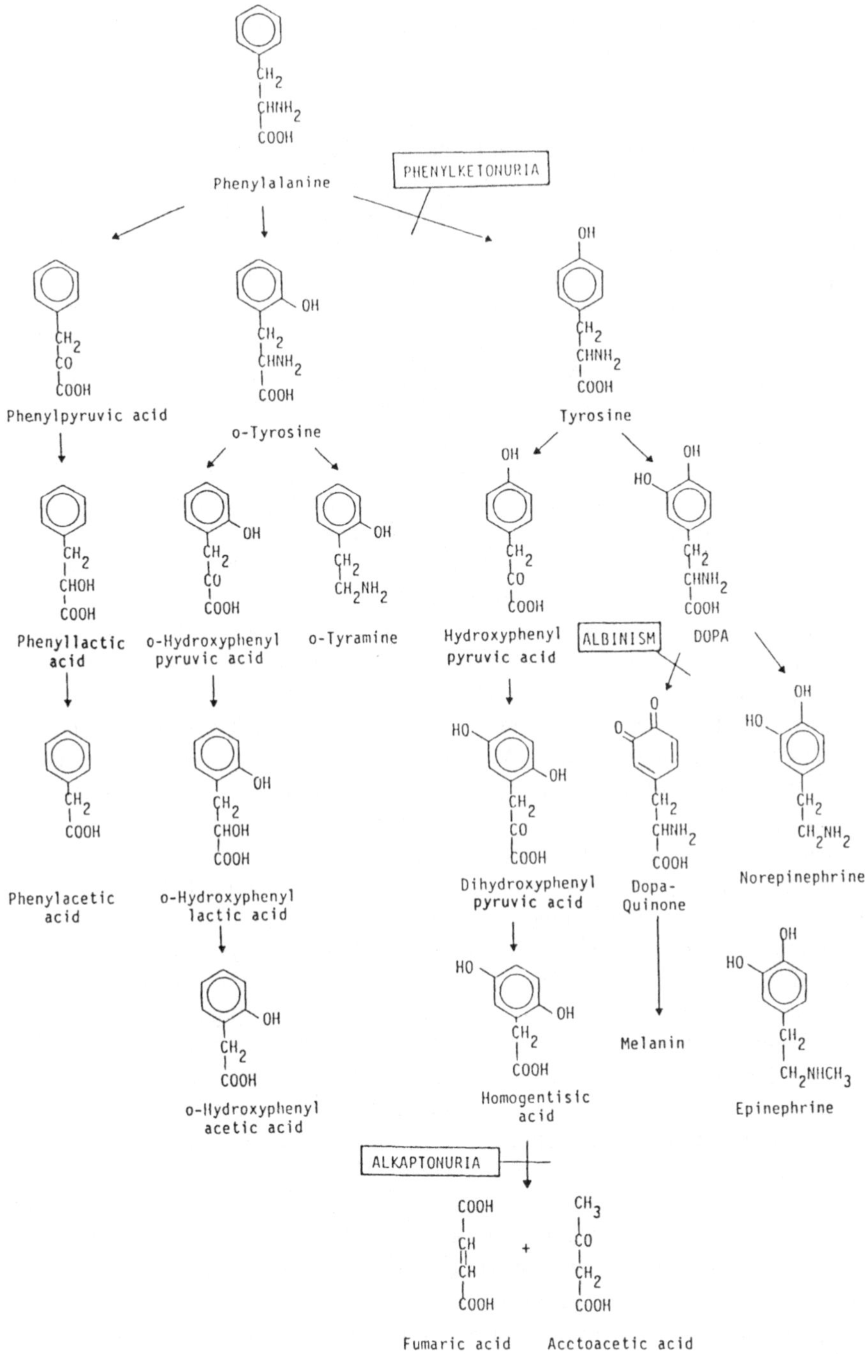

FIGURE 23.   Schematic presentation of the pathogenesis of phenylketonuria, albinism and alkaptonuria.

other amino acids across the blood-brain barrier, and the lack of essential amino acids causes the impairment of protein synthesis, with subsequently abnormal cognitive brain function. This is congruent with the abnormalities in the composition of cerebral proteins. Several metabolites obtained in the serum and urine of phenylketonurics inhibit important enzymes of tyrosine and tryptophan metabolism *in vitro*, such as aromatic amino acid decarboxylase. *o*-Hydroxyphenylacetic acid inhibits cerebral glutamic acid decarboxylase and the formation of glutamic and γ-aminobutyric acid may be impaired. Depletion of glutamine may potentiate the brain damage seen in phenylketonuria, and phenylpyruvic acid blocks the conversion of dihydroxyphenylalanine to epinephrine.

Phenylalanine inhibits tryptophan hydroxylase by reducing the transfer of tryptophan across the nerve ending membranes. Subsequently, the transformation of tryptophan to serotonin becomes deficient. Serotonin plays a role in the synaptic transmission of certain areas of the brain, and therefore, the decrease of serotonin synthesis may be another plausible cause of mental retardation. The administration of serotonin can counteract the toxic action of high phenylalanine levels in the brain. Phenylethylamine can be an immediate causative factor also. This compound is formed in phenylketonurics when the concentration of phenylalanine is high, and particularly when further oxidation is inhibited. Amine oxidase inhibitors bring about an aggravation of neurological symptoms. It may be that an interaction between the mechanisms responsible for the mental effects depends on the degree of maturation of the nervous system.

Lipid abnormalities also accompany phenylketonuria. Cholesterol and cerebroside contents in the white matter are decreased. Hydroxy fatty acid content and unsaturated:saturated fatty acid ratios in cerebroside and sulfate fractions are reduced. The lowered amount of cerebroside and cholesterol in the cells reflects the reduced proportion of myelin relative to other lipid-containing membranes in impaired areas.

Phenylketonuric babies are presumed to be normal at birth due to the protective action of the maternal phenylalanine hydroxylase system *in utero*. However, due to the enzyme defect, high phenylalanine levels induce antenatal brain damage. This can be prevented by the reduction of dietary phenylalanine intake.[87] Since phenylalanine is an essential amino acid, it cannot be completely excluded. Morphologic changes are related to the interference with normal maturation. Myelination is generally defective, or localized in areas of white matter where postnatal myelin deposition has failed to occur. There is impaired cortical layering, persistence of heterotopic gray matter, and cystic degeneration of the white matter.

The therapy of phenylketonuric patients consists of phenylalanine limitation in the diet by replacing the protein with an amino acid mixture free of phenylalanine. In patients kept on this diet, the major biochemical abnormalities are reversed. Phenylalanine and metabolites are decreased in the tissue and extracellular spaces to normal values, and abnormal protein components disappear in the plasma with the treatment. Skin and pigment changes are also cleared, and pigmentation is increased during therapy. The treatment ameliorates most neurological signs of phenylketonuria, with the exception of structural changes if the start of treatment has been delayed. Muscular hypertoxicity also decreases. Longer periods of treatment are necessary for normalization; however, when phenylanine is readministered all abnormalities promptly return.

Sometimes it is adequate to place patients on a low phenylalanine-containing diet for 2 to 3 years and discontinue the strict diet afterwards. Presumably, after this period, the brain structure is sufficiently formed and various enzyme activities are established so that the enzyme deficiency characteristic of phenylketonuria will no longer influence the function of the brain. In adulthood, however, returning to the normal diet may have serious implications. Female phenylketonurics raised on low phenylalanine diet during childhood may show normal development, and they can switch to a more palatable, normal diet. However, if they remain on normal diet during pregnancy, the baby may be born with phenylketonuria and likely be mentally retarded.

2. Histidinemia

Neurological impairments in this condition include speech defects, convulsions, and ataxia. There are, however, normal individuals who do not exhibit severe abnormality of mental function. This inborn error is related to an anomaly in histidine metabolism.[54] Nor-

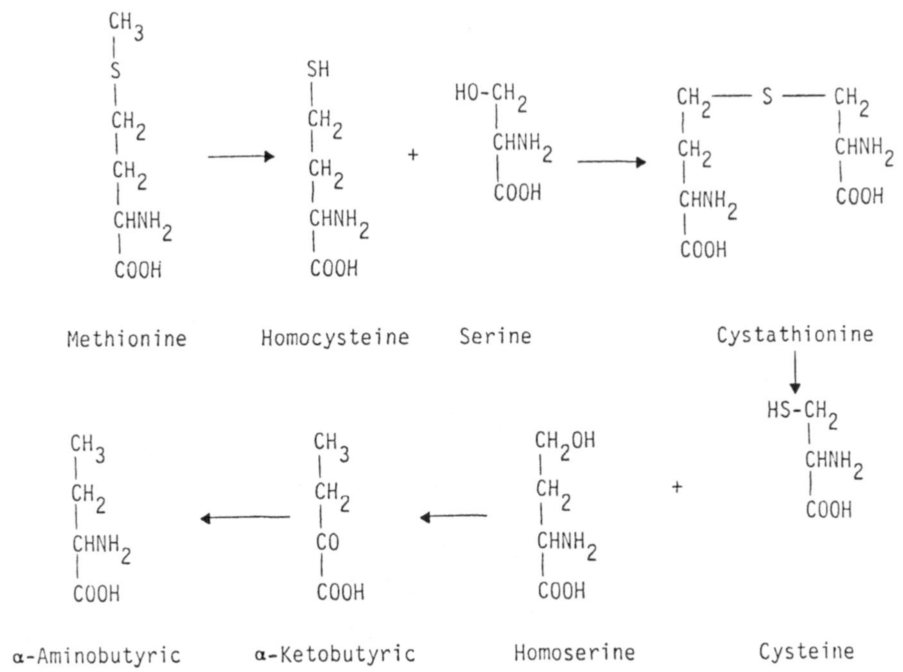

FIGURE 24.   Sequential metabolic steps in homocystinuria and cystathionuria.

mally, the most important pathways in the conversion of this amino acid are the formation of formiminoglutamic acid and glutamic acid via urocanic acid (Figure 24). In patients with histidinemia, the transformation of histidine to urocanic acid is interrupted. In consequence, histidine accumulates in blood and cerebrospinal fluid. The urinary excretion of histidine and its metabolites is elevated, and as expected from the location of the enzyme, urocanic acid is absent from the perspiration of the affected subjects.

The biochemical lesion in histidinemia shows some resemblance to phenylketonuria. In this disease, metabolic pathways which are normally negligible become dominant. In histidinemia imidazole-pyruvic, -lactic, and -acetic acids are eliminated in the urine. The normal urinary clearance of histidine is several times greater than that of phenylalanine and tends to limit the importance of secondary pathways in histidinemia as compared with phenylketonuria. The excretion of these substances is therefore intermittent depending on histidine intake.

There are striking differences in the consequences of lesions due to histidinemia or phenylketonuria. The lower incidence of severe subnormality in histidinemia may be related to the higher renal clearance of histidine as compared to phenylalanine. Histidinemic children have about 10 times higher histidine levels in the blood than normal adults or children, whereas serum phanylalanine rises 20 or 50 times above normal levels. Furthermore, the accumulated tissue histidine and its metabolites may exert less cytotoxic action or inhibition of enzymes in related metabolic pathways.

3. Branched Chain Ketoaciduria

This condition is a rare degenerative disorder of the nervous system transmitted as an autosomal recessive trait. It is also called maple syrup disease, due to the distinctive peculiar odor of the urine and perspiration, reminiscent of the natural maple syrup. Branched chain ketoaciduria manifests during the first week of life with varying severity and causes early death. The symptoms show progressive involvement of the nervous system and prominent features include seizures, irregular respiration, and muscular rigidity alternating with opisthotonus and flaccidity. Some untreated children develop spasticity and survive for several years with severe mental retardation.

The disease is associated with a failure of oxidative decarboxylation of branched chain amino acids. Three keto acids — α-ketoisovaleric, α-ketoisocaproic and α-keto-β-methylvaleric acids — metabolites of valine, leucine and isoleucine, respectively, are accumulated in the serum and cerebrospinal fluid and excreted in the urine in great amounts. These keto acids are also present in tissues in large concentrations, and secondarily, the plasma levels of valine, leucine, and isoleucine are also increased. Alloisoleucine is also present in serum, formed probably by transamination from α-keto-β-methylvaleric acid. The impaired decarboxylation brings about an increased production of α-ketobutyric acid responsible for the odor. The enzyme systems responsible for the oxidative decarboxylation of α-keto acids arefound in hepatic mitochondria and leukocytes. The reaction requires coenzyme A as a cofactor. Patients with maple syrup disease cannot combine keto acids with coenzyme A during oxidative decarboxylation and in some cases, conversion of the coenzyme A complex is blocked.

If untreated infants survive, pathological changes develop in the cerebral white matter similar to the alterations caused by phenylketonuria, and these effects may be more pronounced. The cortex shows generalized immaturity, and the number of cortical layers is reduced. Central myelination is significantly diminished, and the lipid content is greatly decreased. Cerebrosides, sulfatides, and proteolipid protein concentrations are negligible in affected areas. These structural and biochemical changes and some of the neurological symptoms can be prevented if the dietary intake of branch chained amino acids is restricted. It is probable that the increased concentration of these amino acids and the accumulation of their metabolites are responsible for the development of mental retardation, rather than the enzyme block. The presence of β-hydroxy-β-methylglutaric aciduria indicates neurological changes and connected with the pathological symptoms in Reye disease.[357]

4. Homocystinuria and Cystathionuria

These diseases are inborn errors of methionine metabolism, associated with metabolic blocks in the transformation of these compounds to various derivatives[110] (Figure 24). The frequency of these conditions is second to that of phenylketonuria. They are transmitted by an autosomal recessive gene, affecting the nervous system, and most patients are mentally subnormal or retarded. Some homocystinuric infants suffer from fits. Generalized dysrhythmia, skeletal deformities, ectopia lentis accompanied by tremor of the iris are major symptoms. In cystathionuria, the psychiatric symptoms resemble those of paranoid psychosis.

The basic metabolic lesion in homocystinuria is the deficiency of cystathione synthetase normally present in the liver and brain. In some patients, this enzyme has been detected in the optic lens. The lack of this enzyme causes accumulation of homocystine and methionine in the blood and excretion of homocystine in the urine in excessive quantities. Several other metabolic products including *S*-adenosyl-L-methionine are also present in the urine. Levels of cystathionine are low in the brain and other tissues of homocystinuric patients, whereas homocysteine is present in greater amounts. Some homocysteine is methylated to methionine and some is oxidized to homocystine. Folic acid content of the serum is decreased, probably due to increased demands for its metabolite *N*-5-methyltetrahydrofolic acid, needed in the methyl transfer reactions between homocysteine and methionine. In homocystinuria, cysteine cannot be synthetized from methionine, this is why supplementation of this amino acid becomes essential in these patients.

In cystathionuria, the biochemical lesion occurs at the cystathionase level and consequently, cystathione accumulates in tissues. The amount of this amino acid in blood is apparently normal due to rapid renal clearance and large quantities are eliminated in urine.

Cystathione synthetase and cystathionase both function with pyridoxal phosphate as coenzyme. A deficiency of this factor, or reduced affinity of the enzyme to the coenzyme in cystathionuric patients influences the biochemical responsiveness. This may also alter pathways of amino acid metabolism where pyridoxal phosphate is required.

Multiple infarcted areas are seen in the brain of homocystinuric patients. Cystathionine, present normally in high concentrations, is absent, indicating the local involvement of the missing enzyme. Primary structural changes are found in blood vessels independent of their diameter. Intimal thickening and fibrosis are mostly characteristic and major branches with fraying elastic fibers are also found in the aorta. Arterial and venous thomboses occur in many organs. It may be that homocysteine is responsible for the vascular lesion although the mechanism has not been revealed. The mental defect can be associated with cystine or cystathionine deficiency or excess methionine. The way how brain damage develops is still obscure since it is not yet clear what the role of cystathionine is, other than as intermediate in cysteine synthesis.

5. Hyperglycinemia

This condition occurs in two forms: idiopathic or ketotic hyperglycinemia and hyperglycemia with hypooxaluria or nonketotic hyperglycemia. Both forms are characterized by elevated blood glycine levels. The symptoms of this metabolic disorder appear soon after birth and death follows very quickly. The severity of the neonatal manifestations of the disease suggests that some cases die *in utero*. The clinical symptoms are vomiting, lethargy, metabolic and respiratory acidosis, and acetonuria. In some cases, extreme hypotonia and abnormal electrocardiogram have found. Infants surviving the first few months developed thrombocytopenia, neutropenia, and osteoporosis. Protein feeding or the administration of some amino acids, such as valine, leucine, isoleucine, methionine, or threonine, provoke acute attacks. It is curious that glycine elicits no adverse symptoms although hyperglycinemia is the major sign of the disease. During attacks the urinary excretion of several ketones is highly elevated, such as acetoacetic acid, acetone, methyl ethyl ketone, methyl isopropyl ketone, 2-pentanone, 3-pentanone, which intermittently disappear and reappear.

The underlying biochemical lesion is probably the defective function of the conversion of glycine to serine. The incorporation of glycine into the porphyrin skeleton is also faulty. It may be, however, that that anomaly of glycine metabolism and the elevation of blood glycine levels are secondary consequences of a more basic metabolic disturbance. Neuropathological changes are similar to those caused by branched-chain ketonuria, such as delayed myelination and severe degeneration of the white matter.

In the nonketotic hyperglycinemia the increased blood glycine levels are not parallelled by changes in other amino acids. There is no associated ketoacidosis nor hematologic abnormalities. The excretion of oxalic acid in the urine is diminished. Brain damage is severe in this condition. A deficiency in glycine oxidase has been suggested as the cause of this biochemical lesion, but recent studies show defects in the transformation of glycine to hydroxymethyltetrahydrofolic acid.

6. Disorders of Urea Synthesis

Several metabolic defects are linked with the urea cycle which are in most cases associated with mental abnormality. These disorders include argininosuccinic aciduria, citrullinuria, hyperammonemia, hyperornithinemia, hyperlysinemia, homocitrullinemia, and congenital lysine intolerance. These biochemical lesions probably are derived from an autosomal recessive transmission. Many features are common, such as moderate to severe mental retardation, convulsions, vomiting, and intermittent stupor attacks.

The enzyme defect in all conditions is only partial since complete inhibition of urea production is incompatible with life and may be capable of inducing additional quantities of the deficient enzyme. When protein intake is normal, urea is synthesized at normal or subnormal rates and blood urea concentrations are within normal range. The reduced binding capacity of the mutant enzyme is partly corrected by the mass effect of substrate accumulation. Protein loading increases blood ammonia concentration, and the neurological symptoms may be attributed to ammonia intoxication.

In argininosuccinic aciduria, the defect is in the enzyme argininosuccinase localized in the liver, brain, and blood cells where only traces of argininosuccinase activity have been demonstrated. Large amounts of argininosuccinic acid accumulates in body fluids as a consequence of this lesion. The highest quantity is found in the cerebrospinal fluid and higher than in plasma. Massive amounts are excreted in the urine daily, comparable to the glomerular filtration rate. Beside the general neurological symptoms, this disease is characterized by ataxia, hepatomegaly, and brittle hair. An interesting observation indicates that thyroid hormones may be capable of inducing additional quantities of the deficient enzyme.

The major feature of citrullinuria is the presence of large amounts of citrullin in body fluids. In this condition, the plasma level is higher than that in the cerebrospinal fluid. Argininosuccinic acid synthetase activity is defective and, consequently, great amounts of citrullin are excreted in the urine. The production and elimination of citrullin is related to dietary protein intake.

In hyperammonemia, the only established biochemical defect is the elevated blood ammonia level. This even may be associated with the deficiency of ornithine transcarbamylase or carbamyl phosphate synthetase. These enzymes are located in the liver and both types of disorders have been demonstrated. Consumption of a low-protein-containing diet reduces blood ammonia.

Hyperlysinemia probably contains more than one disease form. In this condition, normal or high protein intake brings about increased lysine levels in cerebrospinal fluid and plasma. Ammonia and arginine are also raised. On the other hand, the urinary amino acid excretion is normal. Low lysine containing diets prevent the changes from the normal amino acid pattern. The enzymes of the urea cycle are present, however, lysine metabolism is impaired and the increased lysine is a potent inhibitor of arginase. The inhibition of arginase activity affects the urea cycle and decreases detoxication by ammonia. In hyperlysinemia, defects exist in the incorporation of lysine into proteins, because the clinical symptoms of seizures and the appearance of weakness of the muscles and anemia in patients are similar to the actions of lysine deficient diets.

Congenital dietary lysine intolerance elicits different symptoms from hyperlysinemia. Lethargy, episodes of vomiting, and hepatic coma occur intermittently, associated with increased quantities of ammonia, lysine, and arginine in blood. These symptoms disappear on low protein diet, but can be provoked by the administration of lysine. A partial reduction of hepatic lysine dehydrogenase activity is probably responsible for the metabolic error.

B. LIPIDOSES

In these disorders abnormal amounts of lipids are accumulated in neural tissue causing progressive degeneration.[84,490,437] The storage and degenerative processes primarily involvethe neurons. The brain contains normally 50 to 70% lipids in the dried white matter, and 30 to 45% in the grey, showing the importance of these constituents in neurological diseases. The abnormal metabolism of lipids is associated with neurological symptoms in infants suffering from conditions such as Gaucher's disease, Hurler's disease, Niemann-Pick disease, Tay-Sachs disease, Fabry's disease, and generalized gangliosidosis. There are several variations among these inborn errors of metabolism, and lipids are not the only substances that accumulate in lipidosis. Sometimes abnormal amounts of polysaccharides are also accumulated, such as in Hurler's disease, referred also as mucopolysaccharidosis. All lipidoses are fairly rare, the commonest being Hurler's disease.

TABLE 3
Enzyme Defects in Lipidoses Affecting the Central Nervous System

Defective enzyme	Disease	Lipid accumulation
Sphyngomyelinase	Niemann-Pick	Sphyngomyeline
β-Glucosidase	Gaucher	Glucocerebroside
α-Galactosidase	Fabry	Ceramide trihexoside
β-Galactosidase	Krabbe	Ceramide galactoside
Sulfatidase	Metachromatic leukodistrophy	Ceramide galactose-3-sulfatide
β-Galactosidase	Ceramide lactoside lipidosis	Ceramide lactoside
Hexosaminidase A	Tay-Sachs	Ganglioside GM_2
Hexosaminidase A and B	Tay-Sachs variant (Sandhoff)	Globoside and ganglioside GM_2
β-Galactosidase	Generalized gangliosidosis	Ganglioside GM_1
α-Fucosidase	Fucosidosis	H-isoantigen

Neuronal storage of lipids is a common parameter in these disorders. The accumulation of the abnormal material sooner or later destroys the neurons and atrophy and sclerosis of the tissue develop following all loss. There is wide variation in the extent, intensity, and regional distribution of lesions. Early onset of the disease is usually accompanied by more diffuse neuronal involvement and a more rapid deterioration process. The reticuloendothelial system is often involved and may be minimal, affecting only a few cells in the spleen, lymph gland, or liver, or may be extensive and dominate the clinical symptoms of the disease. In some cases, the visceral involvement determines the course, and the nervous system shows minor changes or even may be entirely unaffected.

These diseases have a common genetic background. The frequency of familial incidence of lipidoses shows Mendelian recessive transmission, suggesting that the causes are probably inherited enzyme lesions. The precise site of the biochemical lesions is in some cases controversial, but a common feature that these metabolic diseases are characterized by is the inability to degrade various sphingolipids (Table 3).

1. Niemann-Pick Disease

This hereditary lipid storage disease is also called sphingomyelin lipidosis and occurs as consequence of a genetic defect which follows the distribution of an autosomal recessive characteristic pattern. It often starts in early infancy and symptoms are lack of mental development, epilepsy, blindness, and failure to thrive. Clinical observations reveal enlargement of the liver, spleen, and sometimes the lymph glands. The disease has been subdivided into three forms: cerebral infantile, cerebral juvenile, and noncerebral forms. In the noncerebral variant, the disorder appears later and the course is milder than the two other ones.

The profound damage in the central nervous system is associated with increased sphingomyelin, gangliosides, several ganglioside derivatives, and cholesterol in the grey matter. In the brain, sphingomyelin is not confined to the grey matter, but is also found in the white matter, although its turnover is more rapid in the grey matter. The major compounds accumulating in this condition are sphingomyelin, ceramide phosphorylcholine, and the metabolic defect is linked with the drastic reduction of sphingomyelinase enzyme which catalyzes the hydrolysis of sphingomyelin. The sphingomyelin stored in tissues of patients with Niemann-Pick disease originates in part from erythrocyte stroma, which contains high quantities, besides phosphatidylcholine and -ethanolamine. It is not surprising, therefore that the reticuloendothelial system, where erythrocytes are normally destroyed is one of the places of sphingomyelin storage. Sphingomyelin is also the major lipid component of the plasma membrane of all cells and is an important constituent of subcellular organelles. Thus a large amount of sphingomyelin could continuously arise during the course of cellular turnover of a variety of tissues.[319] There is no increase of sphingomyelin in the blood.

In Niemann-Pick disease, the accumulation of sphingomyelin is greater in the liver and spleen than in the brain. In some patients, cerebral sphingomyelin is not enhanced at all. In the white matter, sphingomyelin with 24 carbon fatty acids dominate, and in the grey matter, it is composed of 18 carbon fatty acids. In the case of the Niemann-Pick disorder, sphingomyelin containing 18 carbon fatty acids is raised in the stored lipid. The increased $C18:C24$-sphingomyelin ratio occurs without an absolute rise of sphingomyelin in many cases of dysmyelination as a nonspecific characteristic parameter. It is associated with many inherited and acquired degenerative disorders of the nervous system and is not confined to Niemann-Pick disease.

2. Gaucher's Disease

This disease exists in three forms. The adult form is characterized by enlargement of the liver and spleen, erosion of the long bones, and accompanying fractures. The bone marrow contains large reticulated cells loaded with lipid and acid phosphatase is elevated in the serum. This enzyme presumably derives from the lysosomes of the so-called Gaucher cells. The infantile form shows the same symptoms, but in addition, pathological changes occur in the central nervous system, resulting in severe subnormality. In the juvenile form, the systemic manifestations progress very rapidly, but the central nervous system is not damaged or only weakly affected.

In Gaucher's disease, the neural changes are frequently severe, and the brain involvement shows marked but patchy loss of nerve cells and neuronophagia. Some neurons store glycolipid, and this substance accumulates also in the liver, spleen, bone marrow, lymph glands, and occasionally the brain, with Gaucher cells. The reticuloendothelial cells accumulate ceramide glucoside or glucocerebroside, and in the spleen it may increase from the normal 0.1 to 0.2% up to 4% in Gaucher's disease.[319] The affected neurons also contain cerebrosides. The metabolic defect comprises the deficiency of glucocerebrosidase which catalyzes the hydrolytic breakdown of glucocerebroside to glucose and N-acylsphingosine (Table 3). This enzyme is also present in normal human brain, and in Gaucher's disease it is reduced to minimum levels or completely absent. The loss of this enzyme activity is the probable cause of the neuropathological manifestations. Gangliosides are the source of glucocerebroside in peripheral tissues of patients suffering from Gaucher's disease and are likely the principal substances of glucocerebroside accumulating in the brain.[85]

One precursor of glucocerebrosides is globoside, N-acetyl-galactosaminyl-galactosyl-galactosyl-ceramide which occurs in great amounts in the stroma of erythrocytes. Leukocytesare other likely sources of glucocerebroside; they contain glycolipids and the precursor or intermediate ceramide lactoside and glucocerebroside occur as predominant lipid constituents. Leukocyte breakdown provides probably most glycolipids. The turnover of gangliosides is fairly rapid in infancy and slows down later in life. In the adult type of Gaucher's disease, there is probably some glucocerebrosidase activity in the brain which metabolizes the glucocerebroside arising from leukocyte gangliosides during the neonatal period. Thus, the residual enzyme activity prevents the development of abnormalities in the central nervous system.

3. Fabry's Disease

Signs and symptoms of this disease are the striking involvement of the skin, kidneys, and brain (Plate 4). The most frequent cause of death is renal failure. The heart may be affected and conduction abnormalities occur in peripheral nerves. The etiology of this disease is not clear at this time. It mainly occurs in males, the genetic defect is linked to the sex chromosome (X) with occasional and variable penetrance in the heterozygous female. In Fabry's disease, excessive amounts of ceramide trihexoside and galactosyl-galactosyl-glucosyl-ceramide accumulate in the kidney, intestine, and lymph nodes. The biochemical

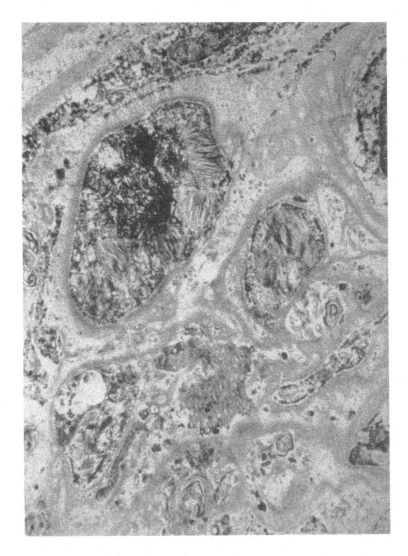

PLATE 4.   Typical inclusion bodies in Fabry's disease.

lesion due to the complete absence of the ceramide trihexosidase which catalyzes the hydrolysis of the terminal sugar molecular from ceramide trihexoside (Table 3). The major site of the enzyme defect is probably the liver, where the quantity of ceramide trihexoside increases tenfold over normal, but other tissues also have this enzyme activity. Serum trihexoside levels are elevated, but there is no evidence of considerable accumulation of the lipid in brain or kidney. Hemizygous males with the full syndrome have no ceramide trihexosidase activity at all in their tissues. In female carriers of the Fabry trait, the enzyme activity is reduced. The source of the stored ganglioside is probably the globoside of the erythrocyte stroma. The trihexoside is considerably water soluble and is transported from the tissues involved into the kidney via the bloodstream. Digalactosylceramide is stored to some extent in the kidney.

4. Tay-Sachs Disease

Tay-Sachs disease is the most common of lipidosis, generally manifested in early infancy and characterized by the onset of severe cerebral impairment and blindness. According to the age of occurrence, several forms can be distinguished, such as congenital, infantile, late infantile, juvenile, and adult form. Some of these forms are referred to as amaurotic disease. There are histological and clinical differences between these forms, and neurochemical changes are often inconclusive. Neuronal lipid storage is the common phenomenon, but the amount of lipid stored increases with age.

The clinical picture of Tay-Sachs disease includes progressive apathy, loss of vision and mental deterioration, seizures, progressive motor weakness, spasticity, paralysis, and exaggerated motor response to noise. Death usually occurs before the age of 2 years. If the course of the disease is slower, the life span is extended.

The major biochemical change in this disease is the accumulation of a glycolipid in the brain (Table 3). Gangliosides are a class of sialic acid containing glycolipids, normally found at highest concentration in the ganglion-cell-rich fraction of the brain. In the normal brain, GM_1 and GM_{1ax} are the predominant gangliosides, GM_2 is present only in minute quantities. In the Tay-Sachs brain, GM_2 ganglioside is accumulated and there is a relative decrease of other gangliosides. GM_2 has been named Tay-Sachs ganglioside. This is the monosialosylceramide trihexoside, N-acetylgalactosaminyl(N-acetylneuraminosyl)-galactosyl-glucosyl ceramide. The corresponding asialo compound, N-acetylgalactosaminylgalactosyl-glucosyl ceramide, is also present, but to a smaller extent. The biochemical defect in this disorder is the deficiency of a specific hexosaminidase. In the peripheral tissue, N-acetylneuraminic acid must be cleared from the Tay-Sachs ganglioside and the sialidase enzyme responsible for this process is present in patients with Tay-Sachs disease, with faulty degradation of N-acetylneuraminic acid molecule. Due to the lack of the hexosaminidase component, Tay-Sachs ganglioside and its asialo-derivatives are accumulated. These compounds inhibit the activity of brain sialidase. The inhibition of this reaction is apparently the rate-limiting step in ganglioside catabolism in Tay-Sachs disease, and as a consequence, ceramide lactoside and glucocerebroside are also stored in moderate amounts in cerebral tissue in late stages of the disease.

Generalized gangliosidosis or GM_1-gangliosidosis is rare and shows rapid and progressive cerebral degeneration. Infants die generally before the second year of life. Skeletal deformities and liver enlargement are frequent, unlike in Tay-Sachs disease. In other forms of amaurotic family idiocy, the increase of ganglioside content could not be always confirmed by chemical analysis. In some cases, the ganglioside pattern is normal; in several juvenile and adult cases, the concentration of brain lipids is reduced, but GM_2 ganglioside is raised. This resembles that of proper Tay-Sachs disease, although the increase was less marked. In the late infancy form, there is an increase of GM_1 ganglioside and a relative decrease of the other gangliosides. There is sometimes no evidence of lipid overproduction or of structural abnormalities in the brain gangliosides. The fault may be associated with some enzyme deficiency of ganglioside metabolism, or due to an abnormal binding of the brain ganglioside to a protein, thus preventing degradation. Low concentration of free amino acids in the brain may reflect the protein interference. Membraneous cytoplasmic bodies are found in Tay-Sachs disease and related disorders. These are formed from the aggregation of excess ganglioside with other lipids, proteins, and amino acids by physicochemical processes or by the formation of lysosome-like structures (Plate 5). The accumulation of these secondary lysosomes and derived structures is probably a nonspecific response to prevent cytoplasmic accumulation of endogenous lipid or may represent an acceleration of accentuated aging processes. The formation of abnormal cellular organelles may also be connected with the breakdown of previously formed structures such as lysosomes. It is difficult to establish whether these membranous structures are lysosomes which have incorporated the excessive amount of lipids, or if they are myelin-like aggregates which show lysosome-like structure and characteristics. The association with lysosomal activity is reflected in their biochemical characteristics. The membranous bodies in Tay-Sachs disease, Niemann-Pick disease, late infantile amaurotic idiocy, and in acid mucopolysaccharidoses show acid phosphatase and thiolacetate esterase activity.

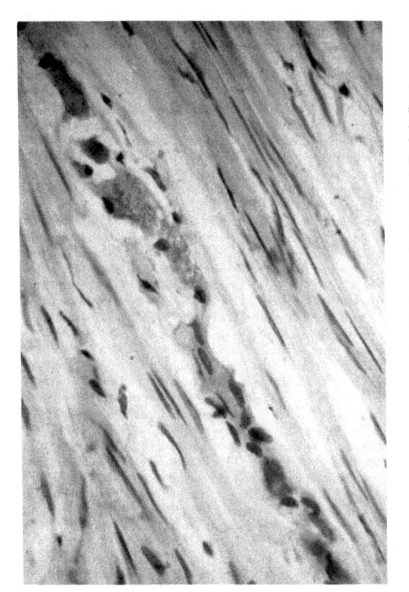

PLATE 5.   Lipid inclusion in neurons from the plexus in an intestinal biopsy in Tay-Sachs disease.

C. LEUKODYSTROPHIES

These are associated with abnormalities of myelin formation and metabolism. The combination of lipids and proteins to form the myelin sheath is involved in these disorders. Myelin formation takes place on the surface of Schwann cells or oligodendrocytes, where lipid molecules are linked spontaneously to produce multimolecular aggregates. Protein and polysaccharide units are then attached to the lipid particles. The myelin sheath is formed by a spiral winding of these layers around the axis giving rise to the characteristic lamellar structure. The synthesis of adequate lipids and proteins, and the proper aggregation of protein and lipid molecules in order and proportion are important during myelination and remyelination. Myelin sheath proteins are denatured, consequently, the metabolism of the lipid moieties of this membrane is very slow. Only small components, such as phosphatidylinositol, show rapid turnover associated with the control of impermeability of certain areas in the nerve membrane.

The maintenance of this process depends on the viability of metabolically active oligodendrocytes, and any factor which causes a reduction of activity provokes the disintegration of the associated myelin sheath. Interference with the synthesis of myelin proteins or lipids due to a deficiency of essential enzymes, cofactors or metabolites results in structurally imperfect myelin sheaths and dysmyelination takes place. Such sheaths are very fragile and prematurely degenerate, particularly when a toxic metabolite, such as in phenylketonuria or histidinemia, interferes with brain metabolism.

Myelin formation is abnormal in leukodistrophies and degeneration occurs mainly in the white matter of the cerebrum and less frequently in the cerebellum and other structures. The grey matter is only secondarily involved. The neurological manifestations include epilepsy, paralysis, blindness, and progressive dementia. Some congenital cases show marked mental retardation, but they do not progress. Many cases are familial and the transmission is autosomal recessive. The nonfamilial disease is probably associated with inflammatory changes, demyelination, and loss of axis cylinders in the affected white matter areas.

In Krabbe's disease or globoid leukodystrophy, the brain shows a very extensive lack of myelin in the cerebral hemisphere, cerebellum, and brain stem. Glial cells grow over the affected demyelinated areas and the accumulation of globoid cells is seen. There is some reduction in the total amounts of cerebrosides in the brain, although the cerebroside:sulfatide ratio is increased. Krabbe's disease is considered to be a galactocerebroside lipidosis of the white matter (Table 3). The activity of several enzymes involved in sphingolipid metabolism of the brain and other tissues is altered. In particular, in Krabbe's disease, galactocerebrosidase the activity is decreased by 10% of the normal brain.

In metachromatic leukodystrophy or sulfatide lipidoses there is evidence of destruction of axons and the myelin sheaths with variable degrees and gliosis. Metachromatic deposits are present in affected areas usually as coarse homogenous globules in the brain, kidney, and bile ducts associated with dysfunction of these organs (Plate 6). There are two forms of this disease. The late infantile form begins between the ages of 3 and 5 months with death ensuing after about 10 months, preceded by weakness, ataxia, and hypotonus. The adult form shows initially psychological disturbances followed by progressive dementia. The biochemical lesion comprises the sulfatide, galactocerebroside-3-*O*-sulfate ester in both central and peripheral nerve tissues, resulting in a reduction in conduction of affected nerves. The defect is caused by a deficiency sulfuric acid esterase or sulfatase involved in sulfatidecatabolism. There are three distinct enzymes in normal tissue which differ in their subcellular localization, substrate affinity, and optimum pH. These are arylsulfatase A, B, and C. Arylsulfatase A is located predominantly in lysosomes. It is diminished in metachromatic leukodystrophy, and it is probable that ceramide-galactose-3-sulfate is the natural substrate of this enzyme. Other lysosomal enzymes show normal activity.

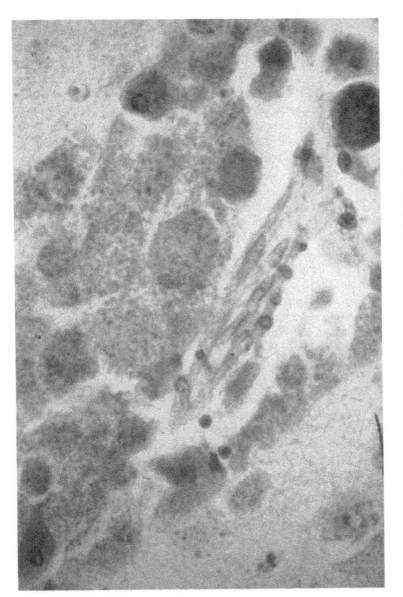

PLATE 6. Neuronal changes in metachromatic leukodistrophy.

D. DISORDERS OF SACCHARIDE METABOLISM

1. Glycogen Storage Diseases

Disorders of glycogen and related macromolecules in the nervous system are linked to the deposition of different polysaccharides. In reactive astrocytosis, glycogen particles are found in areas lacking filaments. Astrocytes proliferating around degenerating axon terminals also show accumulated glycogen. The accumulation of glycogen is associated with an increase of phosphorylase and branching enzyme. However, the mechanism whereby this polysaccharide is retained has not yet been established. Normal astrocytes contain substantial amounts of enzyme which synthetise and catabolize glycogen and sometimes the pathological changes occurring in astrocytes are connected with severe acute or chronic liver disease.

2. Mucopolysaccharidoses

These inherited disorders cause an abnormal accumulation of mucopolysaccharides or glycoproteins in the body.[437] Some aspects of these disorders are also associated with abnormal lipids. The interrelationship between mucopolysaccharide and lipid metabolism is important in the analysis of these disorders. The composition of gangliosides containing lipids with oligosaccharide chains also show variations in these diseases.

3. Hurler's Disease

Gargoylism or Hurler's disease is a common form of lipidosis. Its manifestations are variable, usually associated with enlargement of the liver and spleen, deafness, cardiac defects, corneal clouding, and occasional by mental retardation. The genetic and biochemical heterogeneity of the disease indicates that it may be transmitted as an autosomal recessive defect or the transmission is sex linked.

The biochemical changes are related to the accumulation of different mucopolysaccharides. These are important constituents of connective tissue, particularly cartilage, blood vessels, and corneae, where these substances form the amorphous ground substance. Many clinical features of Hurler's disease are linked with defects of connective tissue metabolism. The properties of the connective tissue depend partly on the interaction between mucopolysaccharides and other proteins, particularly collagen. If the binding in the complex structure between the protein and polysaccharide is weak, the mucopolysaccharide may diffuse out of the tissue. This is due to abnormal protein structure or advanced local hydrolysis. In gargoylism, the primary defect is associated with an abnormal protein-mucopolysaccharide interaction, and abnormal amino acid metabolism, particularly of serine, has been reported. In order to correct the interaction anomaly interaction, an overproduction of mucopolysaccharides takes place from normal protein mucopolysaccharide complexes, leading to increased synthesis of mucopolysaccharides of less importance. This is confirmed by the reports of the urinary excretion of excessive amounts of chondroitin sulfate B and heparitin sulfate in gargoylism, in contrast to normal urine where chondroitin sulfate A is predominant, and only small amounts of the C form and heparitin sulfate are present.

The abnormal biochemical findings include lipid disorders and high levels of glycolipids containing gangliosides occur in the brain. This may be a direct effect due to derangement of the metabolism of nerve cells or indirectly through changes in the connective tissue of the blood vessels or meninges. The molecular distribution of brain glycosides is also abnormal in Hurler's syndrome. Increased amounts of monosialogangliosides, GM_1, GM_2, and GM_3 are found, particularly the normally minor component GM_2, Tay-Sachs ganglioside, GM_3, and hematoside are enhanced. Slight increases of these monosialogangliosides are common in many degenerative neurological disorders, but they are less prominent than those in Hurler's disease. Lysosomal acid β-galactosidase activity is markedly reduced in the brain, liver, spleen, and skin.

4. Galactosemia

The symptoms of this condition usually start immediately after birth, and the infant dies soon if the disease is not controlled. The disorder, however, may occur in a milder form causing mental retardation, hepatic cirrhosis, and cataracts. The biochemical defect comprises an inhibition of galactose 1-phosphate uridyl transferase activity.

Uridine diphosphoglucose is one of the precursors of cerebrosides and mucopolysaccharides, and the failure of enzyme activity blocks the formation of these essential molecules. The loss results in increased blood galactose levels and galactose 1-phosphate accumulation in various tissues. In particular, the elevated saccharides initiate multiple defects in kidney tubules impairing the reabsorption of amino acids, glucose, and protein. The proteinuria is, however, usually mild.

Galactosemia is often accompanied by hypoglycemia and may be involved in the onset of the mental symptoms. Galactose 1-phosphate, when formed in excess amounts, cannot be easily eliminated. It may be that this compound is directly or indirectly responsible for toxic manifestations. There is some evidence that the fetal brain may be damaged as a consequence of galactose accumulation. Treatment with a lactose-free diet brings about dramatic improvements to the galactosemic patient.

E. ABNORMAL COPPER METABOLISM
1. Wilson's Disease

The usual consequence of Wilson's disease or hepatolenticular degeneration is dementia.[606] People suffering from this disorder exhibit extrapyramidal neurological signs such as muscular rigidity, tremor, and uncoordination. The lesion causes damage in the basal ganglia, resulting in paralysis and increasing dementia, and nodular cirrhosis in the liver. Wilson's disease usually starts in late childhood or adolescence and sometimes remains unrecognized, but liver failure and cirrhosis appear before the neurological involvement becomes apparent.

Wilson's disease is a metabolic disorder associated with abnormal accumulation of copper in most tissues.[70,143,442,592,531] The absorption of copper from the alimentary tract and urinary excretion is high, while elimination in the bile is low. Plasma copper levels of these patients are somewhat reduced. The distribution of copper is widespread in various parts of the brain, liver, and kidney. Analyses of the various tissues of patients suffering from Wilson's disease demonstrated four- to tenfold increases over control values. The biochemical lesion is linked with a fundamental fault in the synthesis of the copper-carrying protein ceruloplasmin. Normally, copper is firmly bound to protein, and 40 to 60% of the total blood copper is attached to globulin, 35 to 55% to albumin and other proteins, and less than 5% of the total is loosely bound. In the cells, copper is combined with proteins such as ceruloplasmin, cerobrocupreine, hepatocupreine, and tyrosinase. Some of the copper complexes possess enzyme activity. In Wilson's disease, significantly greater amounts of copper react directly with copper reagents, indicating that less copper is firmly bound. Moreover, more copper is retained in the tissue, and larger amounts are excreted although copper levels and ceruloplasmin are low. These differences suggest that the biochemical lesion may be a failure of the ceruloplasmin synthesis. The excessive deposition of the metal leads ultimately to liver cirrhosis and proximal tubule damage in the kidney. The renal defect upsets the reabsorption of amino acids, peptides, proteins, and many other body constituents such as glucose, uric acid, calcium, and phosphate. Aminoaciduria and proteinuria are common symptoms in the late stages of the disease. Loss of calcium and phosphate may induce fractures, osteomalacia, and rickets. Copper accumulates in the brain in hepatolenticular degeneration and its action is similar to the relation of copper deficiency to demyelination in newborn lambs. Pathological amounts of copper are found in various brain proteins which are normally copper-free. The therapy of this condition is connected with the possible removal of copper from the brain. Dimercaptol (BAL) and penicillamine (β,β'-dimethylcysteine) have been used successfully.[250] These drugs reduce the neurological symptoms to a minimum, but there are indications that cirrhosis persists in the liver.

2. Menkes' Disease

Menkes' disease is characterized by peculiar hair (kinky-hair syndrome), neurological impairment, and severe mental retardation. The cerebral cortex and white matter are extensively degenerated. Copper levels are low in the liver and brain, and high in other tissues. It is likely that the disease is due to defects in the homeostatic control of copper metabolism. There is a relative deficiency of copper-dependent enzymes related to abnormal and metallothionein gene regulation in response to copper.[358] In Menkes' disease, metallothionein synthesis is defective, which binds copper, and other metallothionein binding metals (mercury, cadmium, zinc) are increased. Abnormalities include increased levels of serum lipids.[72]

X. NEUROTOXICITY OF CHEMICAL AGENTS

A. BLOOD-BRAIN BARRIER

The entry of various substances into the central nervous system is protected by the blood-brain barrier. This barrier represents certain cellular structures in glial cells (astrocytes)[611] that are less permeable to chemicals than most other areas of the body. The capillary endothelial cells of the central nervous system are also tightly joined and only few pores, if any, are left between cells. Protein concentration in the interstitial fluid is much less than elsewhere in the body, therefore, transport processes connected with protein carriers are very much reduced. These three factors act together as a preventative mechanism and inhibit the free diffusion of many chemicals and toxicants into the brain in appreciable amounts and thus decrease their toxicity or hinders their contact with sensitive sites.

Basically, the entry of toxicants into the brain is similar to their transfer across any other cells in the body. Only free toxicants which are not bound to plasma protein are free to go into the brain tissue. The passage of large molecules, such as proteins, and large peptides does not usually happen or it is greatly retarded. Ingestion of protein toxins will, therefore, only cause peripheral toxicity, unless via very large concentrations some fragment quantities may defect the effectivity of the blood-brain barrier.

The blood-brain barrier is a highly lipophilic membrane and lipid solubility plays a major role in determining the rate of entry of various toxicants into the central nervous system. Nonpolar, lipid soluble substances are transported into the brain fairly quickly, whereas if a substance is ionized, it will not penetrate the central nervous system because it is not lipid soluble. If a substances is nonionized, it enters the brain with a rate proportional to its lipid solubility. A highly lipid-soluble compound readily goes through the blood-brain barrier. The entry of a less lipid-soluble substance is inhibited.

Methylmercury, which is a lipid-soluble toxicant, enters the brain with relative ease as compared to inorganic mercury which does not pass through the blood-brain barrier easily. The conversion of inorganic mercury to methylmercury by plankton and microbial action (bioactivation) and the subsequent uptake of methylmercury by fish in the food chain and its accumulation in fish tissue (biomagnification) resulted in the Minamata disease, connected with extreme brain disfunction and permanent neurological damage.

Since many nutrients, including amino acids and carbohydrates, are polar compounds, the brain has a mechanism to obtain these essential molecules. Although the entry of polar molecules into the brain is reduced or totally prevented, the adequate transport of nutrient molecules is dependent on specific blood-brain barrier mechanisms. Such systems have been described for amino acids (separate for neutral, basic, and acidic amino acids), carboxylic acids, hexoses, and inorganic ions.[68,282,450] These systems are highly specific, however, potential toxicants with structures similar to physiological substrates may enter the brain by bypassing the blood-brain barrier.

The protective action of the blood-brain barrier varies in the different brain areas. The cortex, pineal body, posterior pituitary, and the lateral nuclei of the hypothalamus are more permeable than any other parts of the brain. The function of the choroid plexus is parallel with the blood-brain barrier. It separates the blood from the cerebrospinal fluid. Besides the role of astrocytes, an extra blood-brain barrier structure has been considered known as supraependymal structures. These are bathed in the cerebrospinal fluid and are exposed to molecules which do not pass into deep brain tissue. Possibly these structures monitor neuroendocrine functions, and specific pores in the barrier in this region allow the transport of specific endogenous molecules into the brain. However, other molecules, including putative neurotoxicants, may go through these openings, although they do not pass through other parts of the blood-brain barrier. The functions of these supraependymal sites are particularly affected by toxic chemicals.

Many factors can modify the permeability of the blood-brain barrier. Embryonic and fetal brain have greater accessibility to toxic chemicals, and even immediately after birth, there is a great passage of xenobiotics. The blood-brain barrier is not developed completely at birth and this is the reason why some substances are more toxic to newborns than to adults. For example, morphin is three to ten times more toxic to the newborn than in the adult because of the higher permeability of the blood-brain barrier. In phenylketonuric babies, excess amounts of phenylalamine can cause brain damage after birth, but exert no neurological symptoms in children about 4 years old or older.

Many toxicants can alter the function of the blood-brain barrier. Organic solvents, including alcohol and sodium desoxycholate, can disrupt the blood-brain barrier. Destruction of the membrane lipid in astrocytes by cobra venom containing phospholipase increases the permeability of the blood-brain barrier. Heavy metals, including lead, also alter blood-brain barrier function, the consequence being encephalomyelopathy in newborns and less brain damage in adults due to differences in the development of this barrier. The changes caused by various toxicants on the blood-brain barrier may be reversible or irreversible, but in any case, they influence the toxicity of other xenobiotics at subsequent exposure.

B. DRUG-INDUCED NEUROTOXICITY

Several drugs cause side effects in the nervous system. These include drugs affecting mood and consciousness, several antibiotics, antiparasitics, and other drugs.[40,42,151,189,242,375,492,513,536,546] Among the mood modifying drugs, major tranquilizers exert actions on the extrapyramidal motor system and evoke behavioral and autonomic effects often blending with their therapeutic properties.[541] Especially in elderly patients, the side effects of phenothiazines, thioxanthenes, and butyrophenones are associated with hallucinations, impaired autonomic reflexes, and extrapyramidal syndromes including parkinsonism, tardive dyskinesia, and acute dystonic reactions.[15] Acute dystonic reactioins occur shortly after initiating treatment. Parkinsonian syndromes develop gradually after prolonged treatment and can be reversed by reducing the antipsychotic agent or by using an anti-parkinsonian drug.

These side effects, and particularly the symptoms of the tardive dyskinesia, are connected with chronic dopamine receptor blockade resulting in functional excess of brain dopamine and supersensitivity. The symptoms of dyskinesia are particularly likely to develop after discontinuation of drug treatment.[134,339]

Tricyclic antidepressants often produce toxic side effects related to two major actions: blockade of amine metabolism and the central-peripheral cholinergic system.[177] Tricyclics block the amine reuptake mechanism in the presynaptic area, and therefore the synaptic transmitter remains in a functionally active state for longer periods. These drugs show

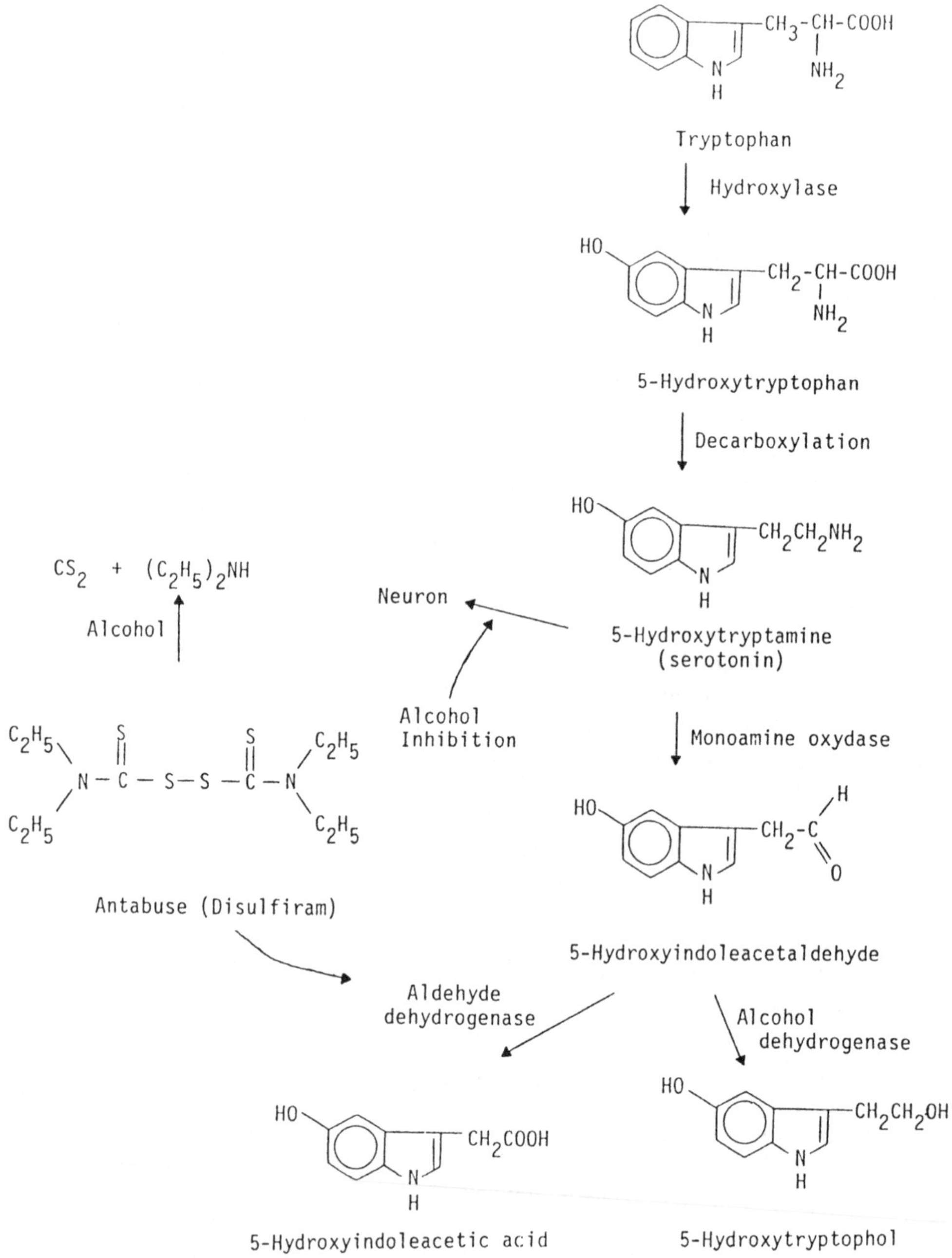

FIGURE 25.   Behaviural effect of alcohol due to interference with serotonin metabolism.

selective activity. Tricyclics with teritary amine groups block more strongly the amino pump for serotonin than for nonepinephrine.[537] Acute intoxication is followed by a central nervous system anticholinergic syndrome, with confusion and delirious state, followed by sedation and central anticholinergic effects causing coma. Severe complications may also occur, particularly in aged patients.[576]

Acute and chronic alcohol abuse has many neurological consequences due to interference with serotonin metabolism (Figure 25).[147,184,185,191,307,354,362,464] The disorders of the nervous

TABLE 4
Frequent Reactions to Alcohol According to Anatomical Region of the Brain

Frontal lobe:
  Loss of inhibition, self control, will power, aprosexia, euphoria, excitation, logorrhea, and maljudgement
Psychomotor areas:
  Aproxia, ataxia, dyslalia, dyslexia
Parietal lobe:
  Diplopia, stereovision altered, color confusion, hallucinations
Basal nuclei:
  Tremors, neurovegetative alterations, stupor, apathy, athetosis, spasms
Cerebellum:
  Altered gait, loss of equilibrium
Pons-medulla:
  Hypothermia, hypoventilation, hypotension, emesis

system related to alcoholism can be grouped in four categories: (1) direct toxic actions; (2) effects related to the withdrawal of alcohol; (3) indirect effects, probably connected with associated malnutrition such as peripheral neuropathy, cerebellar degeneration, or Wernicke's disease; and (4) neurological symptoms associated with hepatic dysfunction.[308]

Direct effects of acute alcohol intoxication or drunkeness include euphoria, an apparent decrease of the anxiety levels, nausea, dizziness, unsteady gait, and slurred speech[287] (Table 4). The initial state can further progress to stupor and coma with respiratory depression. The degree of intoxication is largely dependent on the amount of alcohol consumed and the rate of alcohol metabolism. The metabolism is relatively constant, but modified by previous alcohol consumption and actual dietary intake. Interactions occur between alcohol and barbiturate or diazepam on the hypothalamus-pituitary-adrenal function in chronic alcoholics.[405] The consumption of large amounts of alcohol during pregnancy may cause damage to the embryo and abnormal fetal development.[463] Chronic alcoholic mothers may give birth to children with dysmorphic features and mentally deficient children.[274,550]

Alcohol withdrawal syndrome occurs in a predictable manner in chronic alcoholics and is related to the degree of preceeding alcohol intake.[247,604] The withdrawal symptoms are connected with irregular tremors, severe tremulousness, disordered perception, and frank visual and auditory hallucinations. In a small percentage of patients, generalized seizures occur and alcoholic polyneuropathy develops.[316] Delirium tremens constitutes a major withdrawal syndrome. Patients display confusion and extreme agitation, restlessness, and excess motor activity. In fatal cases, hyperthermia or circulatory collapse may lead to death.[584].

The peripheral axonal neuropathy associated with chronic alcoholism may be connected with nutritional deficiency rather than with a direct effect of alcohol.[210,570,590] Most studies of alcoholic neuropathy include patients with nutritional deficiency,[150] but the controversy still exists. A recent study suggests that the condition is not caused by vitamin deficiency since only about 66% of the patients had low blood thiamine levels[61] and in another report, 86% of the alcoholics were deficient in thiamine, with concomitant reductions of one or more additional vitamins including pyridoxine, nicotinic acid, or pantothenic acid.[210]

Among many drugs causing neurological side effects, thalidomide should be mentioned. This drug was introduced as a sedative-hypnotic and became widely used due to its favorable therapeutic index. Chronic therapeutic doses of thalidomide caused pain in the feet and muscle cramps and sensory loss. In later stages, motor involvements occurred, suggesting widespread loss of fibers in peripheral nerves and posterior columns of the spinal cord. Participation of central nervous system components in this disease has also been suggested.[230]

C. NEUROTOXICITY OF CHEMICALS

Many   chemicals   exert   adverse   effect   on   the   nervous   system.[33,35,56,94,113,114,128,152,163,175,181,229,236,255,313,349,400,427,429,438,440,511,513,561] In this section, only

TABLE 5
Cellular Targets of Neurotoxicants

Neural target	Examples of toxicant
Neuron	Doxorubicin
	Aluminum
	Cadmium
	Mercury
	Lead
	Phenothiazine
Axon, proximal,	B,β¹-iminodiproprionitrile
distal	Acrylamide, carbon disulfide, hexacarbons
Schwann cell	Actinomycin D
	Ethidium bromide
	Cuprizone
	Hexachlorophene
	Triethyltin
Glia	Nortiptyline
	Bilirubin
	CCl_4

the most important ones are discussed, including cyanide, methyl alcohol, methyl chloride, methyl bromide, toluene, trichloroethylene, tetrachlorobiphenyl, and other industrial solvents.[12,13,36,257,280,293,296,328,332,337,366,371,372,431,498,543,544,564,576] Exposure to any of these chemicals causes nervous system dysfunction. Toxic symptoms often include staggering gait, tremors, weakness, paresthesia, blurred vision, and impairment of short-term memory. Neurological abnormalities persist for various periods of time. The acute effects of some chemicals may extend for as long as 10 weeks after exposure. Occupational contact with various chemicals can lead to carbon monoxide,[55,92,112,129,214,235,238,246,252,367,368,532,548] peripheral neuropathy, and other nervous disorders (Table 5).[16,28,55]

Carbon monoxide is an odorless, colorless, and tasteless gas and very toxic. Exposure to carbon dioxide can cause headaches, dizziness, weakness, nausea, vomiting, loss of muscle control, and dimness of vision.[129,532,548] Gasoline-powered vehicles, kerosene or coal stoves, wood burned in a fireplace or stoves, and charcoal grills produce some carbon monoxide. Tobacco smoking also contributes to carbon monoxide content of the air, but only in very small amounts.[246]

Carbon monoxide poisoning causes changes in regional blood flow connected with shunt of the perfusion to more critical organs. Carbon monoxide can decrease the capability of the blood to transport oxygen and produce anoxia.[92] It binds hemoglobin to form carboxyhemoglobin.[112] The presence of carboxyhemoglobin results in a significant reduction of blood oxygen content, but the ambient concentration of carbon monoxide is rarely high enough to result in a detectable reduction of the arterial p_{O_2}. The slowly developing hypoxia causes a compensatory response by increasing cardiac output and peripheral vasodilation. In acute carbon monoxide poisoning, fainting and unconsciousness are very common a long time before death occurs. Tachycardia and ECG changes indicating hypoxia manifest at 30% carboxyhemoglobin saturation. Unconsciousness, convulsions, coma, and death are associated with 50 to 80% saturation.[532] The early effects of carbon monoxide are reversible, the carboxyhemoglobin is fully dissociable and reverses to oxyhemoglobin. Carbon monoxide is excreted through the lungs.

Nonsmoking adults do not have normally more than 1% carboxyhemoglobin of the total circulating heme pigments in their blood, but heavy smokers may have much higher values up to 5 to 10% saturation. Combustion of fossil fuels and motor vehicle exhaust contain 4 to 7% carbon monoxide. The basic carboxyhemoglobin level in the blood is not caused by environmental exposure to carbon monoxide. It is generated endogenously mainly from the catabolism of hemoglobin. The breakdown of cytochromes and catalase provide small amounts of carbon monoxide. The methylene bridge of the heme molecules is metabolized to carbon monoxide in equivalent amounts with bilirubin. In hemolytic disease, carbon monoxide production is enhanced due to increased heme catabolism.

Chronic exposure to carbon monoxide exerts an effect on the cerebral function, leading to neuropathological changes.[55,92,235,238,548] Carbon monoxide affects pregnant women, causes some reduction of fetal development, and reduces the weight and height of the newborn. Cigarette smoking, probably carbon monoxide, however, stimulates the production of lung surfactants in premature babies born from smoking mothers.[367,368] The major consequences of carbon monoxide damage to neural structure is encephalopathy.[214,252,352] Cerebral and prolonged anoxia produces capillary injury with edema and small hemorrhages most frequently in the central nervous system, heart, and lungs. Death may result from respiratory failure, broncho-pneumonia, pulmonary edema, cardiac failure, or cerebral damage. Permanent damage to the nervous system or heart may remain after recovery from acute poisoning.

Cyanide salts are employed in metallurgy, electroplating, and in the manufacture of mirrors. Hydrogen cyanide is applied as a fumigant in the production of synthetic fibers. Chronic cyanide poisoning from occupational hazard is very infrequent. Environmental exposure may occur from the consumption of fruit such as peaches, apricots, cherries, bitter almonds, and cassava (*Manihot esculenta*). Consumption of cassava in large quantities is associated with a neurological condition prevalent in Nigeria. The ingestion of cyanogenic plants is linked with other tropical neurological disorders.[586]

Cyanide is a fast-acting and extraordinary potent toxic compound. Inhalation of hydrogen cyanide or digestion of inorganic cyanide salts can cause acute cyanide poisoning and as little as 300 mg potassium cyanide can be lethal. Hydrogen cyanide may cause death within 1 minute; death occurs within 4 hours after swallowing cyanide salts. Hydrogen cyanide and inorganic cyanide salts are rapidly absorbed from the lung and gastrointestinal tract. The toxicity is associated with its reaction with the three-valent iron in cytochrome oxidase. The formation of cytochrome oxidase-cyanide complex inhibits oxygen utilization, and the cells die from hypoxia. Cyanide does not interfere with the oxygen saturation of hemoglobin. However, the pink color of the venous blood shows that the tissue utilization of oxygen is inadequate. Patients develop headaches, hyperventilation, convulsion, and death. Acute cyanide poisoning only displays a few changes in the brain, mainly swelling and small subarachnoid hemorrhages. However, surviving individuals have residual damage to the central nervous system resulting from anoxic injury.

Chronic exposure to dietary cyanide is considered the cause of the development of an ataxic neuropathy syndrome frequent in Nigeria.[361,443] The main staples of the region are cassava and other plants which contain cyanogenic glycides. This diet significantly elevates plasma thiocyanate levels. Many individuals also show riboflavin deficiency. The neuropathy is slowly progressive, starting with parasthesia of the feet and numbness of the hands. Diminished hearing, visual loss, and weakness of the legs and ataxic gait develop with the progress of the disease. Nerve conduction is abnormal in the lower extremities. Chronic exposure to cyanide in cigarette smoke has been suggested to cause visual loss in the tobacco-alcohol amblyopia syndrome. The large ethanol consumption and undernourishment may be more important factors in this condition than cyanide.

Acute toxicity of methanol is connected with headache, acidosis, circulatory collapse, respiratory failure, and blindness.[380,521] Chronic toxicity starts with a decrease of the pupillary light reflex followed by pupil dilatation.[399] Subsequently, a loss of acuity occurs. The optic disc and surrounding retina become edematous. Experimentation with monkeys showed accumulation of mitochondria in optic nerve axons. Intracranial pressure is increased in relation to stasis of axonal transport. The ocular action of methanol is associated with its metabolism to formic acid.[380,381] When formate is administered to monkeys, gross and microscopic changes in the visual system showed the same changes as seen in human cases of methanol poisoning.

It has been suggested that the general neurotoxicity of methanol is also due to its biotransformation to formic acid, which causes a decrease of cytochrome oxidase activity in affected cells.[433] Subsequently, adenosine triphosphate (ATP) levels are reduced. The consequences of ATP reduction are (1) a decrease in Na^+K^+-ATP-ase activity which impairs electrolyte balance and causes a decrease in electrical activity and visual dysfunction; (2) water and sodium penetrate into the cells, contributing to swelling of oligodendrocytes and inner mesaxons, axonal compression with stasis of axonal transport, and swelling of axons and optic disc edema; and (3) the energy requiring axonal transport becomes static.[532]

Methyl chloride and methyl bromide also exert some toxicity on the nervous system.[12,321,419] Methyl chloride is an odorless gas at room temperature and applied in the production of synthetic rubber and plastic. Some cases of methyl chloride-induced neurotoxicity has been reported in workers exposed to this compound. The toxic symptoms include staggering gait, weakness, tremors, blurred vision, and impairment of short-term memory. These abnormalities persist for over 10 weeks after exposure. Long-term exposure to dichloromethane exerts irreversible effects on the brain.[500]

Methyl bromide is a colorless gas at room temperature and has been used as insecticide fumigant, refrigerant, and in fire extinguishers. Acute exposure to methyl bromide causes visual and speech disturbances, convulsions, and delirium. Chronic toxicity is associated with peripheral neuropathy, as well as cerebellar and pyramidal dysfunctions. In chronic conditions, the first signs are paresthesia of the limbs and deep reflexes which become sluggish or absent. Markedly altered gait and staggering are also found. Mental status and pyramidal signs remain normal. The recovery from these abnormalities is slow, sometimes between 2 to 8 months after onset of symptoms. Methyl bromide is toxic to the lungs and kidney also.

Trichloroethylene is a multipurpose solvent and applied in paint and rubber industry as a degreasing agent and in dry cleaning. It acts predominantly on the nervous system.[102,208] Acute exposure produces dysfunction of the facial and optic cranial nerves. Recovery is slow and occurs over a period of months. The pathological mechanism of the cranial neuropathy is not established, but probably is connected with demyelination. Chronic exposure results in trigeminal neuropathy, visual disturbances, tremors, and impaired memory. The major effect of hexachlorobenzene is porphyria with neurological impairment.[462] Hexachlorophene is neurotoxic.[467,471]

Entry of polychlorinated (PCB) and polybrominated biphenyls (PBB) into the human body results in neurological symptoms.[121] Polychloro or polybromobiphenyls are very stable, highly fat soluble compounds and stay in living organisms for a long time. In 1968, an outbreak of PCB toxicity occurred in Japan (Yoshu disease) caused by PCB-contaminated rice oil used for cooking. Affected individuals developed peripheral neuropathy, acne-form skin eruptions, and pain and numbness in the limbs.[423]

PBB is used as fire-retardant chemicals and basically considered nontoxic compounds. In 1973 in Michigan, a mixture of PBB was accidentally used in animal feed substituting magnesium oxide. This resulted in contamination of a wide area and thousands of people who consumed milk and food containing PBB and developed abnormal liver function, hair loss, chloracne, and a decreased number of effective T cells. In addition, loss of appetite, stomach pain, irritability, fatigue, and numbness of the extremities occurred in some individuals. Prolonged sural nerve latencies, fatigue, poor coordination, and depression may represent neurotoxic symptoms.[281]

Toluene is a widely used solvent in the paint industry and in the manufacture of dyes and explosives. Acute exposure to this compound produces narcosis and depression of the nervous system.[317] Low levels cause fatigue, nausea, and uncoordination. Chronic exposure is associated with ataxic gait, unsteadiness, bizarre behavior, and emotional instability.[75,326,338] Benzene is more toxic than toluene; workers exposed to this solvent showed abnormal electroencephalogram patterns.[328]

D. INTOXICATIONS WITH TRACE METALS

Prolonged exposure to trace amounts of heavy metals can produce degenerative changes in the central nervous system and in peripheral nerves.[503] Chelating therapy can reduce the toxic actions of these metals.[279] These include lead, mercury, manganese, aluminum, bismuth, lithium, thallium, and organic tin.[94,159,188,304,331,345,359,360,487,542,591] Some of these effects on the nervous system are iatrogenic, connected with industrial exposure at the workplace, or caused by environmental contamination. Acute toxic encephalopathy developed in patients taking bismuth subnitrate orally for the treatment of gastrointestinal disorders.[382,552]

Occasionally, lithium causes neurological manifestations. This drug is applied for the treatment of periodic depression and can give rise to severe intoxication associated with confusion, tremors, occasional fits, and rarely, acute generalized polyneuropathy.[94,274] Another example is diethyl tin iodide which is used to treat boils, but contained triethyl tin impurity which causes acute cerebral edema, headaches, drowsiness, and even epilepsy.[6,360,542]

1. Lead Poisoning

Chronic lead poisoning causes neurological symptoms.[103,123,416] Industrial lead intoxication was once quite common, but has been greatly decreased by restrictions on the use of lead and the development of adequate preventive measures at the workplace. Lead poisoning still occurs among plumbers, painters, and battery-makers.[56,111,169,304,344,360,517] Sucking or licking furniture or walls covered with lead paint causes poisoning in children with subsequent brain dysfunction.[46,47,269,526] Tetraethyl lead is a highly toxic compound used in gasoline as an antiknocking agent.[517] Vehicle exhaust fumes contain lead that causes serious environmental contamination and when inhaled chronically, lead to neurological disorders.[468] Due to this potentially dangerous action, many countries are now introducing legislation to decrease or even eliminate the tetraethyl lead content of motor fuel.

The principal route of lead absorption is the digestive tract and some enters the body through the lungs. About 90% of the ingested lead is not absorbed. The part which is absorbed from the gut goes first into the red blood cells, then is stored primarily in the liver, kidney, and bone, and a small fraction is concentrated in the brain or skeletal muscle. There is a gradual transfer of lead from various tissue depots into bone. In chronic lead intoxication, about 95% of the lead is stored in the bones as phosphate. The transfer and storage of lead in the bone is facilitated by calcium salts. Lead is accumulated in the bone over a person's lifetime; its metabolism and excretion are very slow. It is mobilized by acidosis and released into the blood stream and eliminated in feces and urine.[249,327]

Rapid mobilization due to acidosis may lead to an attack of encephalopathy.[601] Toxic demyelination is the usual consequence of chronic low level lead exposure.[56,107,179]

Acute encephalopathy is common in children below 2 years old; it is rare in adults.[14,249] It is characterized by convulsions, irritability, delirium, and coma. The cerebrospinal fluid is often abnormal, lead is present, and glucose content is increased together with an excess of lymphocytes and globulin. Lead intoxication interferes with various processes of heme synthesis. Patients with lead poisoning excrete increased amounts of coproporphyrin III and δ-aminolevulinic acid in the urine.[249,286,408] The synthesis of the δ- and β-chains in hemoglobin is also defective in lead poisoning.[600] Convulsions and defects of cognition and memory occur in chronic encephalopathy.[153,190] Raised blood lead levels are associated with impaired cognitive and behavioral functioning,[506] related to an interference with brain energy metabolism,[97] or cyclic AMP synthesis.[429] Lead neuropathy affects usually the muscles of the fingers and wrist first and the muscles of the upper arm later. The lower limbs are occasionally affected. Lead neuropathy is characteristically a predominant motor neuron disease, and sensory signs and symptoms are usually slight.[108]

2. Mercury Poisoning

Acute poisoning produces neurological symptoms.[118,126,127,256] Chronic exposure occurs in industry, and one form is entitled Minamata disease.[120,491,530,538,567] Chronic intoxication leads to a syndrome of tremors, limb weakness and ataxia, and personality changes characterized by irritability, insomnia, and fatigability. Often, selective damage occurs to the granular cell layer in the cerebellum. Both organic and inorganic mercury poisoning may cause this condition.

A special case of chronic mercury intoxication characterizes the Minamata disease.[388,558,567] This was noted in villages near Minamata Bay in Japan. This disorder is manifested by symptoms of peripheral neuropathy, cerebellar ataxia, loss of hearing and sight, and occasionally, development of progressive encephalopathy. In fatal cases, neuronal damage was found in the cerebral cortex and in the granular cell layer of the cerebellum. The cause of this condition was the ingestion of fish contaminated with methylmercury salts[378,534] derived from effluent of a fertilizer factory containing inorganic mercury. The inorganic mercury is converted to methylmercury by planktons and this way the toxic hazard became biomagnified. Plankton is taken up up by fish and through the food chain eating methylmercury contaminated fish, toxicity is manifested in man representing the epidemic outbreak of Minamata disease.[1,234] A similar syndrome has been reported among Canadian Indians whose main staple was fish.[599]

Chronic mercury poisoning is found under some working conditions such as inhalation of mercury vapor in thermometer workers,[7,587] or in workers exposed to volatile inorganic mercury compounds in chlor-alkali plants.[351] Excessive use of mercurous chloride laxatives resultes in neurological symptoms.[160] Occasionally, contamination of food with mercury compounds is responsible for motor-sensory polyneuropathy, such as eating bread made from wheat treated with methylmercury as occurred in an epidemy in Iraq.[505] Poisoned Iraqi children showed motor weakness and ataxia, many with visual loss remained permanently blind and only a few recovered partial vision, and some cases improved. Children born to mothers exposed to methylmercury exhibited marked psychomotor retardation. Accidental ethylmercury poisoning resulted from the consumption of the meat from a pig which had eaten seeds treated with a fungicide containing ethylmercury chloride. Children who died of poisoning showed severe damage to the brain, spinal cord, peripheral nerves, skeletal muscle, and myocardium.[124]

3. Manganese Poisoning

This condition is due to the inhalation of manganese dust and occurs among manganese miners in Chile and in Central Europe. The clinical symptoms include extrapyramidal Parkinson-like effects, slurred speech, and slowness. Irritability, variable euphoria, and emotional instability sometimes is followed by fatigue, somnolence, and lethargy.[468]

4. Aluminum Poisoning

This disease was noted in patients undergoing renal dialysis. Due to a high concentration of aluminium in water supply, this trace element is deposited in the brain and results in the onset of encephalopathy, leading to progressive dementia and death. In some areas in Great Britain (Glasgow, Newcastle upon Tyne) or the U.S. (Denver), renal and bone diseases also occur in high incidence.[39,99,353,391,398,453]

E. BIOLOGICAL NEUROTOXINS

Many biological toxins cause neurotoxicity. These include botulism, diphtheria and tetanus toxin, snake and bee venom, mushroom poisoning, and lathyrism.[57,58,96,130,324,533,551,594] Botulism is associated with generalized weakness and bulbar dysfunction brought about by the ingestion of spoiled food due to *Clostridium botulinum* contamination.[533] *C. botulinum* is a ubiquitous soil organism and its spores are very resistant. Botulinus toxin A is among the most lethal substances known, as little as 10^{-5} μg will kill a 20 g mouse. The toxin is synthesized under anaerobic conditions by *C. botulinum*.[341] The protoxin is only slightly toxic; toxic residues are formed when proteolytic enzymes cleave certain amino acids from this molecule.[171]

Botulinum toxin is the most potent biological poisonous substance known today, in nanogram amounts, it causes fatal neuromuscular paralysis.[525] Seven different neurotoxins have been identified: toxins A through G. In most human cases, types A and B were identified. After ingestion, the toxin reaches the blood stream and leaks out of intramuscular capillaries into neuromuscular junctions where it interferes with synaptic transmission. Botulinum toxin blocks neuromuscular transmissions at cholinergic synapses and inhibits acetylcholine release.[323,481] The results are blurred vision and diplopia, followed by weakness of the bulbar muscle, areflexia, and general paralysis leading to respiratory failure.

Several strains of *C. botulinum* exist, and the action of the various toxins is indistinguishable. Types A, B, and E are the most common, causing the disease in North America, Europe, and Japan, respectively.[115] The effects of botulinum poisoning in man varies from a mild subclinical disease to a fulminating condition leading to death within a day. Gastrointestinal symptoms usually begin 12 to 36 h after ingestion, predominant in the early stages and include nausea, vomiting, and diarrhea. Neurologic manifestations may occur simultaneously or after a 1 to 3 h delay, and consist of signs of cranial nerve dysfunction followed by systemic weakness. Respiratory paralysis is frequent, usually abrupt, and this is the main cause of death. Botulinum toxin binds to peripheral cholinergic presynaptic axon terminals and blocks the release of acetylcholine.[533] The toxin exerts apparently no effects on the central nervous system, possibly because the molecule is too large to traverse the blood-brain barrier.[615]

Diphtheria is a disease caused by the lysogenic strains of *Corynebacterium diphtheriae*.[393,597] During active infection, prophage genomes are incorporated into DNA. The disease is now rare in most countries due to the fact that children are immunized at an early age. Absorption occurs at the local site of bacillar infection and most intensely following pharyngeal and bronchial infections.[248] Diphtheria toxin is extremely potent, 10^{-4} mg will kill a guinea pig.[130,248,449] It exerts a profound action of the peripheral nervous system causing extensive proximal demyelination in the ganglia and adjacent nerve roots, mainly in places where the blood-brain barrier is incomplete. Cardiac effects are also very frequent, mainly connected with abnormalities of carnitine metabolism leading to decreased oxidation of long chain fatty acids and accumulation of triglycerides.[610]

Tetanus is brought about by infections with the Gram-positive anaerobe microorganism *Clostridium tetani*.[288,289,384] The spores of this anaerobe microbe are found in soils throughout the world. Locally produced toxin penetrates into the central nervous system through motor nerves. The toxin tetanospasmin is bound to presynaptic nerve endings in muscle and then transported to the perikarya of anterior horn cells.[475] The toxin blocks the release of the inhibitory neurotransmitter, glycine.[447]

Tetanus is characterized by generalized rigidity and convulsive spasms. From deep wounds in anaerobic conditions the toxin is absorbed and shows a relatively long incubation period which may last for 8 weeks. Irritability, headaches, and stiffness of the jaw may occur within 2 weeks of infection.[8,57] Neonatal tetanus is very severe and occurs during the first 2 weeks of life due to umbilical cord infection by *C. tetani*.

Snake venoms contain a complex mixture of toxic proteins which act on several organs with ensuing neurotoxicity or hemolysis.[589] Snake neurotoxins are rapidly absorbed from subcutaneous tissues and distributed throughout the body, with high concentration at the motor end plates, where the primary action manifests. Scorpion venoms or scorpamines are lethal neurotoxins. They contain small basic proteins and hyaluronidase which increase capillary permeability. The mechanism of action of these toxins resides in the presence of disulfide bridges and lysine residues.[71,168,411] Certain spider's bites cause a variety of signs, ranging from local pain and necrosis to systemic hemolysis and nervous system dysfunction. Tarantulas secrete occasionally toxic venom, but the most toxic is the black widow spider, *Lactrodectus mactans,* which causes frequent and severe neurologic dysfunction.,[71,589] Bee stings can exert nervous system actions. Severe anaphylactic reactions are accompanied by cerebral edema and vascular congestion. Widespread demyelination can exert effects on the peripheral and central nervous system. A relationship has been reported between the action of bee stings and local mononeuropathies.[508]

Mushroom poisoning or mycetism is connected with widely varying classes of neurotoxins.[364] These include *Amanita muscaria,* which produces ibotenic acid, muscimol and muscazone, and Inocybes and Clitocybes mushrooms, which produce muscarine. *Amanita phalloides* is the most toxic mushroom; they synthesize amatoxins: cyclic octapeptides and phallotoxins:cyclic heptapeptides.[90,165,268] The principal amatoxin is amanitin, and the most important phallotoxin is phalloidin. The action of various mushroom toxins resides in the effects on several nerve functions such as GABA-like action inhibiting central neurons, inhibition of RNA polymease II, depletion of nuclear RNA preventing protein synthesis, and disruption or dissolution of cell membranes and membranes of lysosomes, endoplasmic reticulum, and Golgi bodies.[176,231,268]

1. Effects of Neurotoxins

Neurotoxic compounds cause a wide variety of effects on the nervous system. Many neurotoxins affect specific regions of the brain stem and produce toxic injury to specific cell functions or specific cell types. The site of action of several biological toxins on motor neurons has been established.[473] The neuronal impairment can be selective producing an inhibition of protein synthesis, altering maintenance of the myelin structure, and blocking synaptic transmission, axonal transport, or conduction of action potentials.

There are certain toxins which block protein synthesis, such as diphtheria and polio virus infection-produced toxins. The neuronal perikaryon is the principal site of macromolecular synthesis. Proteins and glycoproteins are produced on perikaryal ribosomes attached to the Nissl bodies which represent the endoplasmic reticulum in the nervous cell. Polio virus infection blocks protein synthesis in the neuronal cell body, resulting in complete stoppage, death of the motor neuron, and paralysis. Diphtheria toxin, a highly neurotoxic protein occurs in some strains of *Corynebacterium diphtheriae.*[449] The diphtheria toxin impairs protein synthesis and its action is localized to the Schwann cells responsible for the maintenance of myelin. The result of diphtheria toxemia is demyelination, failure of conduction, and paralysis.[277,449,466] These effects result in neuropathy by demyelinating peripheral nerves. Palatal weakness and blurring of vision occur at early stages, followed by involvement of other cranial nerves and generalized motor sensory neuropathy.

Some neurotoxins block the conduction of the axonal transport, such as β,β'-iminodipropionitrile. The axon is not only responsible for generating and propagating bioelectric currents, but functions as a conductor for a highly complex delivery system which works in two directions. β,β'-Iminodipropionitrile affects proximal axons, the site where proteins enter transport. This toxin impairs slow transport mechanisms along the axons and causes proximal neurofilamentous swelling, distal axonal atrophy, and weakness.[262,263]

Other toxins block the conduction of axon potentials at nodes of Ranvier, such as tetrodotoxin. Tetrodotoxin is produced by a variety of species including the puffer fish (*Tetraodontidae*), blue-ringed octopus, and California newt.

This toxin is concentrated in the ovaries of the puffer fish which is carefully prepared and consumed as a delicacy in Japan. People digesting the toxin develop circumoral paresthesia, numbness of the limbs and tongue, rapidly deteriorating to progressive paralysis. Tetrodotoxin blocks sodium channels resulting in a failure of neuronal transmission. Saxitoxin is the toxic principle found in the Alaskan butter clam *Saxidomas giganteus*. It is produced by the marine plankton *Gonyaulax catenella* and *G. tamarensis*. It has similar action to tetrodotoxin,[322,510,523] and impairs impulse conduction. Blockade of the sodium channels prevents the development of inward currents leading to conduction failure.[105,294,495]

Tetanus and botulinum toxins alter synaptic transmission. A neurotoxic protein is produced in wounds contaminated by *Clostridium tetani* tetanospasmin, which when it reaches the central nervous system, results in tetanus. This condition represents an interference of inhibitory synaptic inputs on spinal motor neurons.[474] Tetanospasmin causes functional disturbances of the balance between excitation and inhibition.[578] The active toxin reaches the central nervous system by retrograde axonal transport. It is defected first within the perikaryon on motor neurons and causes tetanus when the toxin reaches the inhibitory synapses of the spinal cord.[144] Clinical manifestations include muscle spasms, rigidity, and tetanic seizures.[267]

XI. PSYCHE DISORDERS

Affective disorders and functional psychoses can be viewed primarily as psychological reactions rather than disease conditions.[485] However, the relevance of somatic factors indicate that these can be considered disorders of normal cellular processes as much as atherosclerosis or hepatic diseases,[158] or severe dietary restrictions.[496] There are wide variations in the symptoms of these psychological disorders. The major symptoms of depression and mania are exaggerations of moods, whereas schizophrenia is characterized by disturbance of emotional or affective responses to the environment, withdrawal from the society, peculiar thinking, and secondary hallucinations. Evidence is accumulating that there are biochemical links between some forms of affective disorders and abnormal functions of certain neurotransmitters.[29,32,243]

A. TRACE AMINES AND BEHAVIOUR

Several transmitters of nervous impulses operate such as acetylcholine, serotonin, norepinephrine, and dopamine in central synaptic junctions.[30,32,426,515] The development of affective disorders is linked with some abnormalities of these biogenic amines.[512] Interference with the central effects of acetylcholine causes severe mental disturbances, but the action on behaviour is diffuse and very general.[310] On the other hand, brain levels of catecholamines and serotonin show more specific alterations.[265,311,528] The catecholamines affect the function of the sympathetic nervous system and regulate the body adaption to environment changes.[29,514] Relative or absolute changes of brain catecholamines are correlated with increased motor activity and improved performance and alertness, whereas changes in serotonin content are associated with disorientation and sedation, high doses of serotonin cause agitation, and excitation and seizures.

Conditions of severe stress decrease norepinephrine levels in the brain independent of whether the stress is induced by emotional, physical, or pharmacological stimulation.[40,516] In contrast, brain serotonin levels remained unchanged or sometimes are even elevated.[397] Animals with an emotional response show depressed norepinephrine levels. Since stress usually causes increased excretion of catecholamines and their metabolites, the reduction of norepinephrine levels in stress is probably due to increased discharge. Increased norepinephrine turnover in the brain and other tissues has been observed in cold stress, stress due to electric shock, ethanol intoxication, exercise, and in crowding situations. Sedation on the other hand diminishes the turnover of catecholamines. The effect of stress on brain norepinephrine levels may be abolished by sedatives such as chlorpromazine.

Stress also raises the turnover of serotonin in the brain, although there is no changes in the amount. In the brain of cold-stressed animals, the activity of the rate-limiting enzyme in serotonin biosynthesis, tryptophan 5-hydroxylase is increased. Electric shock increases serotonin synthesis in the rat brain. The turnover of serotonin in the brain is less in isolated animals than in group-living animals exposed to more stress. These findings show that stress-induced acceleration of nonepinephrine turnover is linked with defensive-aggressive functions, and that increased turnover of serotonin is associated with fear.

Catecholamines and serotonin do not cross the blood-brain barrier in appreciable amounts, but the parent compounds 3,4-dihydroxy-L-phenylalanine (dopa) and 5-hydroxy-L-tryptophan do so. These amino acids affect some brain functions. The concentrations of catecholamines and serotonin are raised by dopa and 5-hydroxytryptophan, respectively. Dopa exerts alerting effects on animals and improves the performance of conditioned response tests probably after being converted to catecholamine in tissues. These actions represent direct effects on the central nervous system since they are potentiated by the administration of monoamine oxidase inhibitors. In contrast to dopa, 5-hydroxytryptophan has deteriorating effects on test performance, and this action is enhanced by monoamine oxidase inhibitors. In low doses, 5-hydroxytryptophan produces drowsiness, sedation, and lethargy, and at high doses excitement, agitated behavior suggestive of fear and rage, and/or an increased emotional tension. Dopa and 5-hydroxytryptophan elicit contrasting actions on electroencephalogram; dopa shows arousal patterns, and 5-hydroxytryptophan induces changes observed in sleep.

Specific inhibitors of serotonin and catecholamine synthesis can also provide evidence for the opposite effects of these biogenic amines (Figure 11). Methyl-*p*-tyrosine, an inhibitor of tyrosine hydroxylase, brings about low brain catecholamine levels, but no effects on serotonin. This compound impairs performance and diminishes motor activity of animals, effects which are reversed by dopa or a monoamine oxidase inhibitor. Reduction of serotonin levels of *p*-chlorophenylalanine, a tryptophan hydroxylase inhibitor, causes no sedation (Figure 12).[435] Recent analysis of the ventricular fluid for catecholamine derivatives revealed interesting differences in various illnesses of the central nervous system.

Emotional behaviour is linked to the activity of the endocrine system,[320,454] and the hypothalamus plays an important regulatory role.[131] The regulation is mediated by excitatory and inhibitory impulses it receives from higher and lower brain centers and the release of pituitary hormones via nervous pathways and through the hypophyseal portal system. Genetically selectively bred animals responding to mild stress situations with fearful behaviourdisplay reduced thyroid, adrenocortical, and gonadal activities (Figure 26).[291] These changes have been modulated by regulatory peptides. Gonadotropin affects hypothalamic catecholamines,[131] and progesterone influences mood and behavior.[271,320]

Many hormones produced by the pituitary and other endocrine glands influence the electrical activity of the brain.[45] Some hypothalamic releasing factors which regulate the secretion of hormones from the anterior pituitary gland have a similar influence on the central nervous system.

Three hypothalamic-adenohypophyseal peptides, thyrotropin-releasing hormone, growth-hormone-release inhibiting factor, and somatostatin and luteinizing hormone releasing factor are localized in the extrahypothalamic region of the central nervous system and in certain extraneuronal regions such as the pineal gland,[82,379,420,608,619] brain synaptosomes, and nerve terminals. These peptides affect behaviour by direct action on the brain. Administration of thyrotropin-releasing hormone induces behavioural effects in rats, luteinizing hormone releasing factor induces mating behavior, and somatostatin potentiates the behavior action of

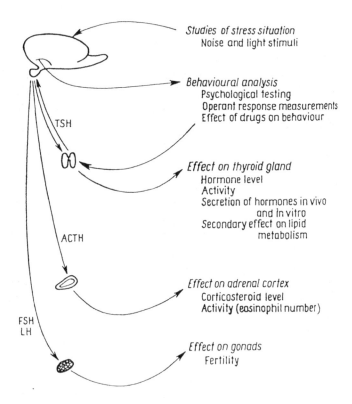

Studies of stress situation
Noise and light stimuli

Behavioural analysis
Psychological testing
Operant response measurements
Effect of drugs on behaviour

TSH

Effect on thyroid gland
Hormone level
Activity
Secretion of hormones in vivo
and in vitro
Secondary effect on lipid
metabolism

ACTH

Effect on adrenal cortex
Corticosteroid level
Activity (eosinophil number)

FSH
LH

Effect on gonads
Fertility

FIGURE 26.   Variations in hormone levels due to emotional differences. Albino rats were selectively bred for different emotional behavior using light and noise stimulation exerting minor stress situation.[628-631] This selection resulted in animals with courageous and active behavior associated with elevated blood levels of thyroid and adrenal hormones and increased sexual activity and fertility as compared with animals showing fearful and timid behavior. TSH, thyrotrophic hormone; ACTH, adrenocorticotrophic hormone; FSH, follicle stimulating hormone; LH, luteinizing hormone.

D,L-dihydroxyphenylalanine. These findings together with neural localization and the existence of high affinity binding sites in extrahypothalamic tissues suggest the role of these peptides in neuronal function.[80] It is possible that hypothalamic releasing or release-inhibiting peptides are liberated simultaneously, both at median eminence terminals and at central synapses, and hence act as neurohormones and as neurotransmitters. The neurotransmitter function of the releasing factors in addition to their classical hormonal role may provide a possible mechanism for the coordination of different aspects of hypothalamic activities.[311] Neurons in the hypothalamus which secrete releasing factors can influence the secretion of pituitary hormones as well as affect behavior.[31,333]

Observations indicate that lithium attenuates motor hyperactivity of experimental animals by blocking the release of transmitters or by enhancing intraneuronal amine concentration. These effects are congruent with the involvement of a neurotransmitter with the action of lithium, however, the underlying biochemical mechanism responsible for this effect remains to be clarified.

B. TRACE AMINES AND DISEASE

Abnormal metabolism of catecholamines and serotonin has been implicated in various mental diseases, and various amines present in minute quantities may play a role in brain function. The chemical structure of these compounds is similar to some neurotransmitters and they can interfere with the metabolism of the latter substances (Figure 9). They may take part in neuronal activity and may act as neurotransmitters themselves. The biogenic amines are oxidatively deaminated by monoamine oxidase. This enzyme is found in almost all tissues with the exception of skeletal muscle, blood plasma, and erythrocytes. Major sources of monoamine oxidase enzymes are the nervous tissue and blood platelets.

In the human brain, there are several amines in relatively smaller amounts, such as octopamine, phenylethylamine, phenylethanolamine, tyramine, and their methyl derivatives.[86] These trace amines may be involved in various neurological activities and related diseases. Administration of phenylalanine to experimental animals alone has no effect on brain concentration, but together with a monoamine oxidase inhibitor, it raises octopamine content. Tyrosine elicits no effects, and tyramine causes a 40-fold increase, suggesting that tyramine is the probable precursor of octopamine and its metabolite synephrine (Figure 27). Octopamine is highly and specifically localized in noradrenergic and sympathetic nerves. Stimulation of the sympathetic nerves causes the release of octopamine, indicating that this compound possesses neurotransmitter properties.

Other trace amines, phenylethylamine and phenylethanolamine, are also found in the brain. It is probable that phenylalanine is the precursor of phenylethylamine which is further converted to phenylethanolamine (Figure 11). In the fetal rat, the levels of octopamine and phenylethanolamine are very high at 16 d after gestation, whereas catecholamines are low. There is a sharp fall at about 17 d coinciding with a rise in monoamine oxidase. This observation indicates that these trace amines play an important role in brain development.

Tryptamine, methyltryptamine, and dimethyl tryptamine are also present in brain. The level of these amines is increased after the administration of L-tryptophan, particularly when a monoamine oxidase inhibitor is given simultaneously. The formation of tryptamine and methyltryptamines represents a minor route in tryptophan metabolism (Figure 28).

5-Methoxytryptamine is also present in trace amounts in the central nervous system, and it appears to have a biological significance since it alters behavior and modifies the brain chemical composition. It is probably derived from the neurotransmitter 5-hydroxytryptamine and S-adenosylmethionine by methylation (Figure 29). Deacetylation of 5-methoxy-N-acetyltryptamine also occurs in the brain, but this is probably a relatively minor pathway. 5-Methoxytryptamine is a potential precursor in the biosynthesis of 5-methoxymonomethyl or dimethyltryptamine. These N-methylated indoles may play a role in some psychiatric disorders (Figure 30).

The function of these trace amines is related to the monoaminergic system. The mode of action of these compounds involves the process of neurotransmission acting directly or indirectly. They are synthetized in the cytoplasm of the neuron, interact with synaptic membranes, and produce continuous activation. This activation creates a synaptic potential responsible for the synapsic transmission. Any imbalance in the amount of trace amines caused by enzyme defects, altered membrane permeability, presence of drugs or toxic compounds, or dietary changes may be involved in the onset of some neurological and psychiatric illnesses. Some of these amines are behaviorally active with abnormal amounts excreted in parkinsonism, affective disorders, schizophrenia, migraine, and hepatic and renal coma.[148,232,265,334,501] The administration of phenylalanine and a phenylalanine hydroxylase inhibitor to pregnant rats increased the octopamine/noradrenaline ratio in the fetal brain from 2:1 to 13:1. Octopamine is elevated in hepatic failure, which may be linked to neurological symptoms. The hypothalamic levels of octopamine are 12 times higher in children who died of acute hepatic encephalopathy or Reye's syndrome.[357] Octopamine may act as a false neurotransmitter in these liver diseases. The enzyme responsible for the methylation of these amines is present in platelets; the activity of the platelet enzyme shows differences in various mental disorders. There is a significant increase in schizophrenic patients both in acute and chronic conditions, and it is also elevated in affective disorders or slightly reduced in alcoholics.

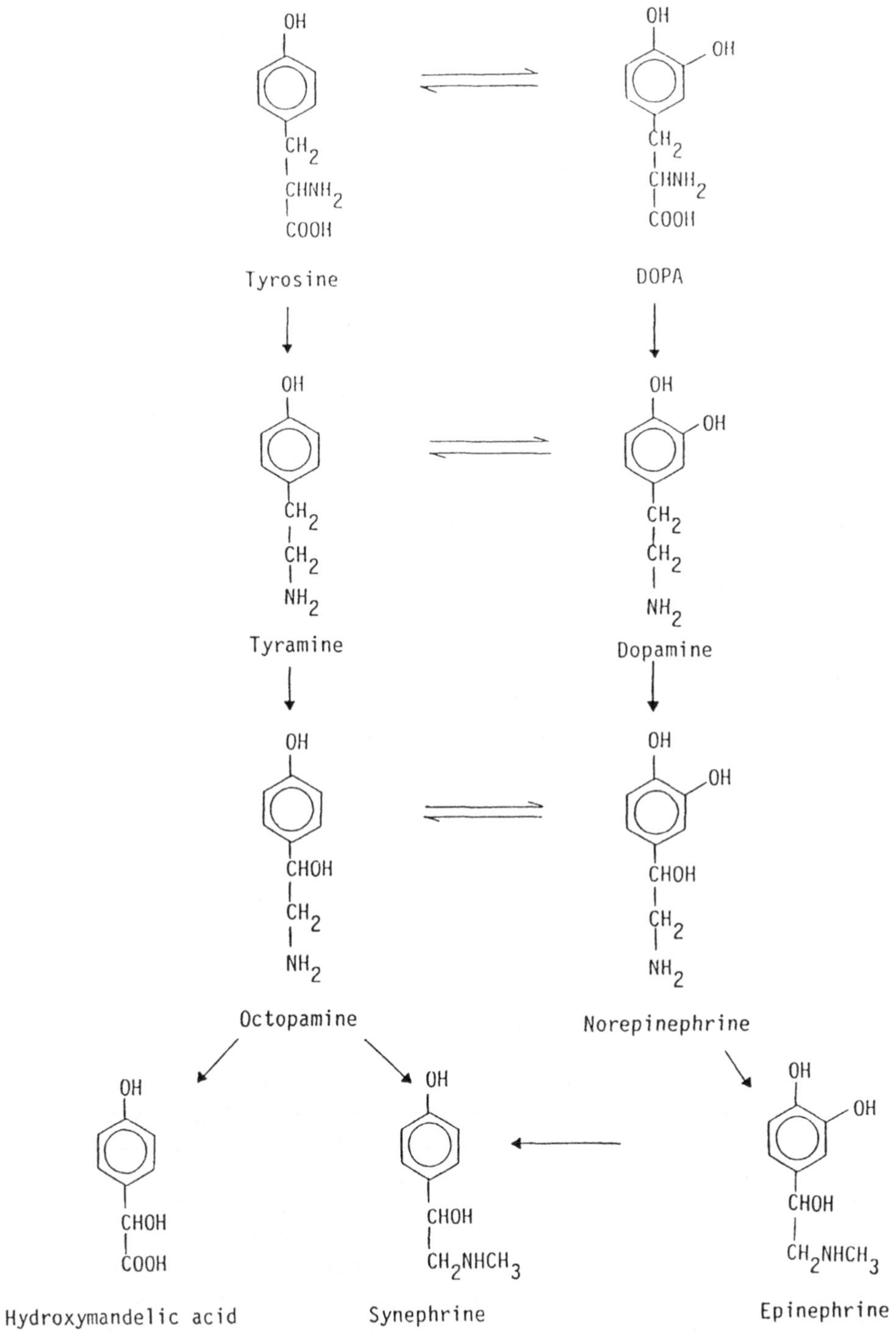

FIGURE 27. Schematic representation of tyrosine metabolism leading to the formation of various trace amines.

C. TRACE AMINES AND AFFECTIVE DISORDERS

Clinical experience also supports the role of catecholamine metabolism in affective disorder. Severe physical or psychological stress reduces the brain catecholamine level and precipitates attacks of depression. Electroconvulsive treatment of depression causes a massive discharge of adrenergic neurons in the central and peripheral nervous systems indicated by

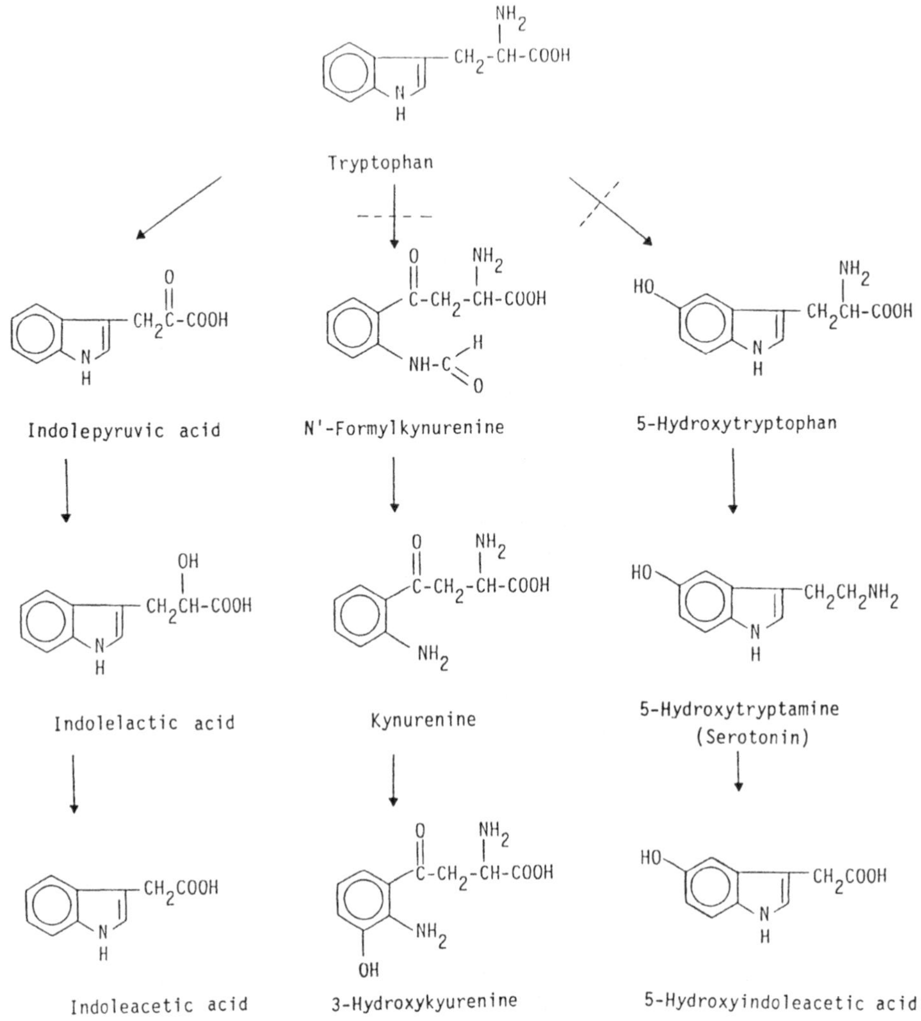

FIGURE 28.   Metabolic transformation of tryptophan.

decreased of cerebral norepinephrine levels and increased conversion to normetanephrine. These changes are reflected by elevated plasma catecholamine levels. Patients with depressive illness show significant decreases in the urinary output of conjugated tyramine, probably to an *O*-sulfate; free tyramine excretion is also reduced.

The amount of catecholamines and metabolites excreted in the urine show differences in metabolism and release rates in various affective disorders.[265,616] In cyclic manic-depressive psychosis, patients excrete high amounts during the manic phase and low amounts in the depressive phase. The excretion of norepinephrine is normal in patients suffering from reactive neurotic depression, whereas in psychotic depression, the excreted norepinephrine is extremely variable. The excretion of vanillylmandelic acid, one of the major metabolites of catecholamines, is enhanced during the manic phase in patients with cyclic affective psychosis. Some of these levels are influenced by variations of diuresis and may reflect changes in peripheral nerves. However, the activities of the central and peripheral sympathetic systems may be parallel.

Several reports indicate that serotonin metabolism may also be implicated in affective illnesses.[528,541] A decrease of 5-hydroxyindole acetic acid, the major metabolite of serotonin,

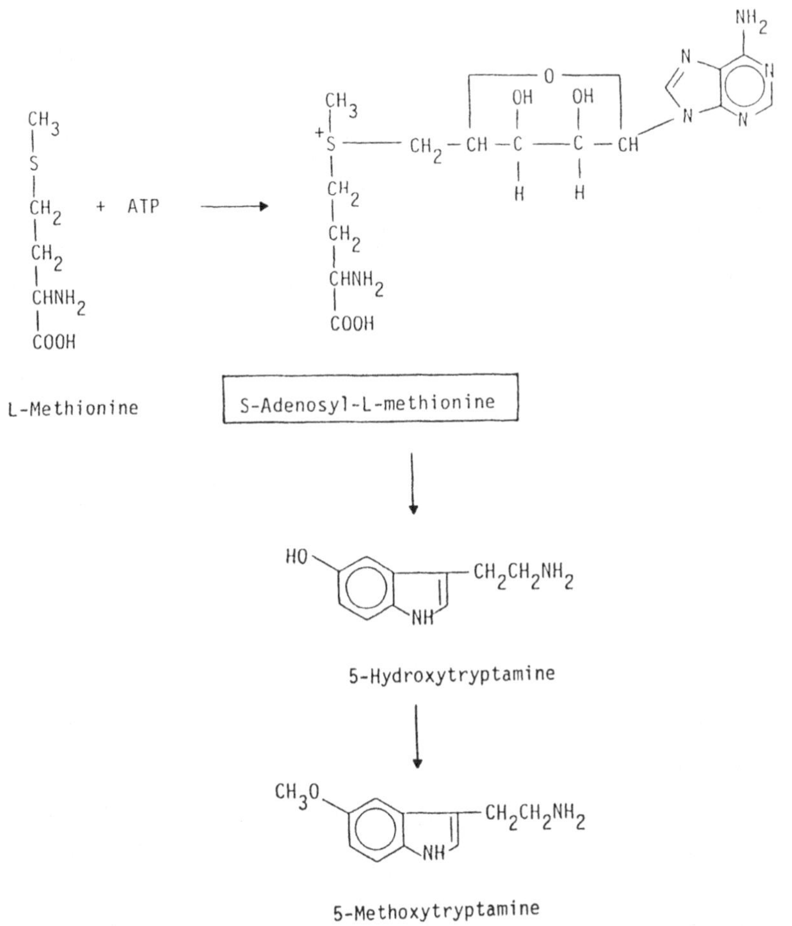

FIGURE 29.   Methylation of 5-hydroxytryptamine via the methyl donor S-adenosylmethionine.

is found in the cerebrospinal fluid of depressed patients. However, the level of this compound is not restored to normal upon clinical recovery. Further, 5-hydroxyindole acetic acid is reduced in early mania, but some studies revealed no differences in 5-hydroxyindole levels in the cerebrospinal fluid between depressed and schizophrenic patients. The urinary excretion of 5-hydroxyindole acetic acid is significantly greater during the manic than the depressed state. Patients suffering from retarded depression with apathy excrete more of this metabolite than patients with agitated depression and anxiety.

Large doses of tryptophan potentiate the antidepressant action of monoamine oxidase inhibitors; it may be effective alone. This action is likely the result of increased levels of tryptamine caused by the inhibition of monoamine oxidase activity. Tryptamine produces central excitation and seizures probably by displacing serotonin in serotonergic neurones. The successes of tryptophan therapy is probably due to the correction of tryptamine deficiency in the brain. Depression is also linked with an increase of tryptophan pyrrolase activity related to an increased adrenocortical activity. The metabolism of indoles and tryptophan may be involved in the course of affective diseases, the correlation with one phase of mood or the other is, however, apparent.

D. DEPRESSION AND MANIA

Changes in water and mineral metabolism occur in affective disorders, particularly in the cyclic form of manic depressive illness.[401,580] The output of water and sodium is reduced

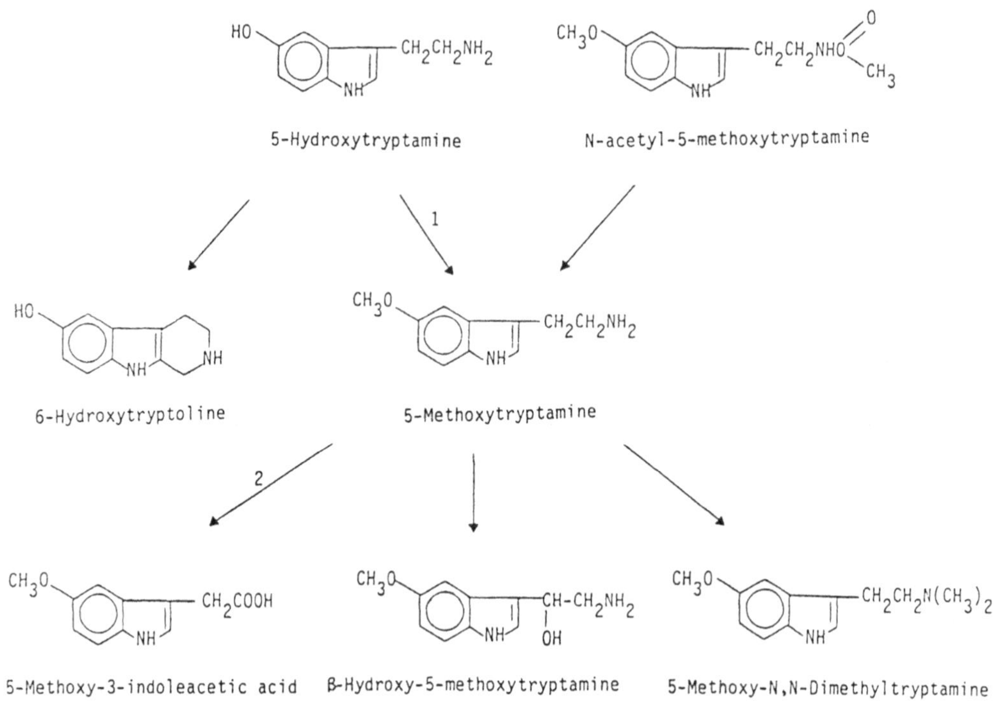

FIGURE 30.   Schematic representation of metabolic intermediates derived from 5-methoxytryptamine.

during the depressed phase and elevated during the manic phase. The retention of exchangeable sodium increased in depressed patients may be due to sodium retention in the extra- or intracellular fluid. After recovery, exchangeable sodium decreases, which corroborates the role of water and sodium changes in this disease. The increase of intracellular sodium and possible decrease of potassium indicates reduced efficiency of the sodium pump and increased in membrane permeability.[347] However, the maintenance of selective distribution of sodium and potassium ions is essential for membrane potential and for nerve excitability. The observed changes of ion distribution in depression probably represent an overall lowered resting and action potential in the central and peripheral nervous systems in depression.

Lithium therapy of manic patients cautions the association of water changes with the disease process.[94] Total body water and intracellular water are increased by lithium. Total body potassium is elevated in manic patients and reduced in depressed patients during lithium therapy. Electrolyte shifts occur in adrenocortical insufficiency as well as in hyperactivity; therefore, the changes in water and mineral metabolism in affective disorders may represent changes of adrenocortical activity in these diseases. This relationship has been further confirmed by the investigations of 17-hydroxycorticosteroid excretion in depressed patients. Several patients who attempted or committed suicide showed significantly higher corticoid excretion than other depressed patients, particularly during the last week before suicide. Patients with psychotic depression produce increased quantities of cortisol during illness; these high levels return to normal during recovery. Psychotic depression is associated with increased serum and urine levels of 17-hydroxycorticosteroids, whereas these are normal in reactive depression. The role of a depressor substance was suggested a long time ago,[205] and the participating of the acetylcholine system was also raised.[310] Mineral metabolism is controlled by the regulatory action of hormones from the adrenal cortex and posterior pituitary and with the autonomic centers in the diencephalon. This suggests that changes in mineral metabolism are linked with neurotransmitter amines. Norepinephrine is also associated with depressive reactions.[98]

XII. SCHIZOPHRENIA

Some forms of this disorder have genetic determinants. The fundamental symptoms include disturbances of emotional or affective responses to the envrionment, bizarre thought disorders, and withdrawal from societal interactions. Secondary symptoms include many dramatic manifestations of schizophrenia such as hallucinations and delusions.

Biochemical studies revealed diverse abnormalities in electrolyte, carbohydrate, protein, amino acid, and lipid metabolism.[62,64,104,497] However, the major successes in establishing the mechanism of schizophrenic abnormality stems from studies of central nervous system stimulants. Amphetamine and related compounds have two effects on the brain processes in schizophrenics. At large doses, psychosis with symptoms very similar to acute paranoid schizophrenia are elicited. At small doses, amphetamine exacerbates schizophrenic symptoms. The extension of these observations suggests that catecholamines are involved in the etiology of this illness. Among the various derivatives, dopamine plays a primary role in amphetamine psychosis and aggravation of schizophrenia. This is supported by highly significant reductions in the activity of monoamine oxidase (MAO) found in platelets of both chronic and acute schizophrenic patients. As the result of reduced enzyme activity an excess dopamine-like activity is evoked in the brain. Lower dopamine β-hydroxylase activity in the brain in schizophrenia is also found.[24] However, another comparative analysis of the activity of this enzyme in six different regions of the brain from schizophrenic patients revealed no abnormality.[141,142] Further studies on the properties of MAO in schizophrenia and other mental diseases have shown two types of this enzyme A and B. The activity of MAO type A is blocked by low concentrations of clorgyline; noradrenaline and serotonin are specific substrates for this enzyme. MAO type B can only be inhibited by high concentrations of clorgyline and deprenyl, which is a selective inhibitor of this enzymes. Specific substrates are benzylamine, 2-phenylethylamine and N-methylhistamine.

Abnormalities in turnover or function of dopamine metabolism, has been also considered as a major factor in the etiology of schizophrenia. This hypothesis is based on the view that the dopamine system in schizophrenic patients is hyperactive. Various findings indicate that many chemicals (amphetamine, apomorphine, methylphenidate, and L-dopa) elevate dopamine concentrations in the brain and at the same time induce mental states analogous to acute paranoid schizophrenia. It was also observed that most antipsychotic drugs (e.g., phenothiazines and butyrophenones) appreciably reduce the activity of dopamine-dependent system in the body.[226,581] An increase in the density of dopamine receptors in the striatrum and nucleus accumbens correlates mainly with positive symptoms of schizophrenia.[370,446,447]

A more detailed analysis showed that D_2 receptors are increased and D_1 receptors are unchanged in the striatum isolated after death from the brains of untreated patients. It is likely that the increase of D_2 receptors is linked with the pathogenesis of this disease.[140] Schizophrenia, therefore, may develop from the hyperactivity of dopaminergic transmission or genetically determined metabolic errors, leading to increased production of dopamine metabolites. Failure of the local dopamine elimination due to impaired flow or through a fault in methyl transfer reaction catalyzed by N-5-methyltetrahydrofolate-dopamine methyl transferase, may be the direct biochemical defect.[519] This, however, can be an indirect consequence of a deficiency in 5,10-methyltetrahydrofolate reductase enzyme responsible for the supply of the methyl donor methyltetrahydrofolate.

The isolation of trace amines raises the possibility of their involvement in schizophrenia. Phenylethylamine has also been suggested to play a possible role in the pathogenesis of this illness. Phenylethylamine possesses the pharmacological properties of amphetamine when it is protected from degradation, but it is sensitive to monoamine oxidase action. In amphetamine, the presence of the methyl group prevents it from acting as a substrate for monoamine oxidase. It is probable that the chronic form of schizophrenia arises from ex-

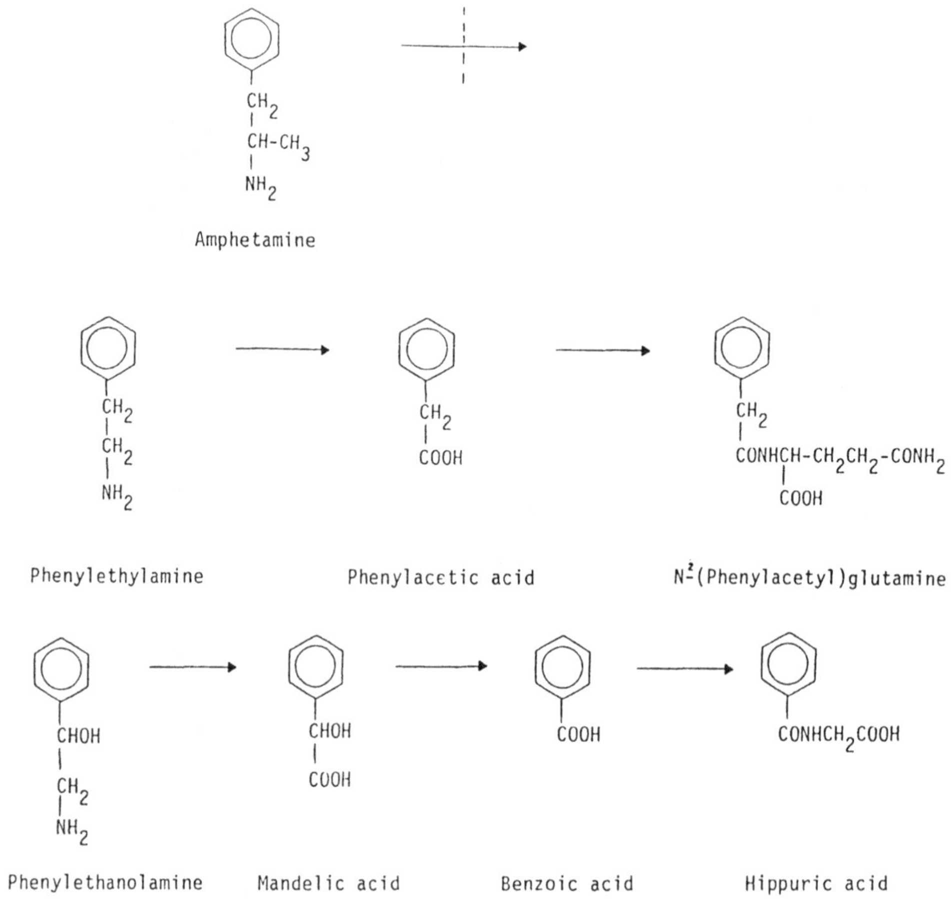

Amphetamine

Phenylethylamine   Phenylacetic acid N^2(Phenylacetyl)glutamine

Phenylethanolamine   Mandelic acid   Benzoic acid   Hippuric acid

FIGURE 31. Metabolism of amphetamine and phenylethylamine in schizophrenia.

aggerated response by overproduction of this amine, or from the deficiency of phenylamine-specific monoamine oxidase B localized in the platelet.[90] Indeed, during acute exacerbation of this disease platelet monoamine oxidase activity is decreased. No apparent decrease of activity is noted in the brain of schizophrenics.

Phenylethylamine is metabolized to phenylacetic acid which is partly excreted in conjugated form. This compound may contribute to the action of phenylethylamine in the central nervous system. This observation is supported by the finding that the conjugation of benzoic acid to hippuric acid is deficient in some patients with catatonic schizophrenia (Figure 31).[91]

A methylating process participates in the synthesis of phenylethylamine.[519] The brain contains an enzyme system which can N-methylate indoleamines and phenylethylamine. All these methylations use S-adenosylmethionine as methyl donor, which derives from methionine by activation. It has been found that when various amino acids are given to schizophrenic patients, only methionine worsened the actual symptoms. The methionine effect is associated with the methylation reaction, although in the brain, it shows a relatively weak enzyme activity. 5-Methyltetrahydrofolic acid can also serve as methyl donor in the methylation of several amines. Enzyme activity accelerated, more with this cofactor than with S-adenosylmethionine, suggesting a more important role of this pathway in the brain. Some methylated products are active substrates such as bufotenin or very potent psychomimetic substances such as 5-methoxy-N,N-dimethyltryptamine. The recent importance of trace amines may suggest that failure in their production by methylation process is relevant to schizophrenia.[92] Variations in the activity of the amine-methylating enzyme may be responsible for the development of abnormal mental function and for the onset of mental disturbances such as schizophrenia. The action of methylation of these amines does not exclude the possibility that other neurotransmitters such as acetylcholine and GABA also play some role.

An integral approach explains the disturbances of biochemical homeostasis of the brain found in schizophrenia.[285] It was suggested that at least three basic systems of the brain are involved in the development of the schizophrenic process: the reticular formation of the forebrain and the midbrain, the limbic system of the forebrain, and the corpus striatum.[301] Combination of disturbances of the noradrenergic and dopaminergic systems become manifested in the disease and other neurotransmitters are involved in the pathophysiological process such as serotonin, acetylcholine, GABA, and noradrenalin. In the acute phase of the illness, noradrenaline is significantly elevated in the cerebrospinal fluid.[330] In untreated schizophrenia, this catecholamine is also increased in the tissue.[251] It seems that there is a relationship between the hyperactive state of the noradrenergic system of patients with schizophrenia and factors inducing anxiety. Reports are contradictory on the role of serotonin.[213,251,479,545]

Some abnormalities of sulfur-containing amino acid metabolism are found in schizophrenia. These may be due to the action of methionine as methyl donor, causing a shift in methyl transferase activity and, consequently, an abnormal metabolism of related compounds (Figure 29). Patients with schizophrenia also have higher taurine and lower cystine levels in plasma.[93] Immunological responses showed elevations as reflected in increased IgA levels.[549]

XIII. PSYCHE AND ADRENOCORTICAL STEROIDS

The clinical manifestations of adrenocortical insufficiency indicate that adrenocortical hormones exert a great influence on the central nervous system.[518] Patients suffering from Addison's disease exhibit neurological and psychological symptoms including apathy, irritability, depression, and mental aberrations. The psyche is influenced profoundly, and psychological derangements appear to form an integral part of this disease syndrome. Occasionally, frank psychosis develops in Addison's disease as the result of adrenocortical steroid deficiency. Many changes can be reversed by therapy with a combination of cortisone and deoxycorticosterone.

Adrenal cortical hyperfunction is also connected with mental disturbances. Such changes have been found in patients with Cushing syndrome and in patients being treated with adrenocortical steroids or adrenocorticotropin. In Cushing disease, the psychiatric disorders and underlying mental symptoms represent wide variations. Nevertheless, the psyche alterations induced by adrenocorticotrophic hormone and 17-hydroxysteroids are similar to those observed in association with adrenal cortical hyperfunction. The overall view of both disorders suggests that mental derangements and psychological symptoms are linked with the corticosteroids metabolism.

Analysis of the human brain reveals the presence of cortisol, tetrahydrocortisol and $11\beta,17\alpha,20\beta,21$-tetrahydroxy-pregn-4-ene-3-one. The concentration of cortisol in the brain is about 25 to 30 times higher than that in the blood, indicating that cortisol readily enters the organ. Blood levels of this steroid are about 15 to 40 times higher than in the cerebrospinal fluid. Intrathecally administered cortisol also disappears very quickly. These data indicate that the steroid is removed from the cerebrospinal fluid by a process of bulk flow in order to maintain a balance between the low and high level in the cerebrospinal fluid and blood respectively. The increased concentration of cortisol and corticosterone in the brain as compared to plasma is probably the result of active transport and subsequent selective bindingto proteins in nuclear and cytoplasmic fractions of brain cells. The nervous tissue contains various enzyme systems which metabolize steroids. Cortisol is converted to cortisone to a marked extent, but only minimal amounts of tetrahydrocortisol and tetrahydrocortisone are produced. NADP-dependent oxidation reactions are common. These enzymes are bound to subcellular particles and the activity of some of them changes with maturation suggesting some roles of these processes in the maturation process.

It is interesting to speculate what are the underlying biochemical processes characterize the symptoms of abnormal behaviour and affective disorders. Adrenal hypofunction affects plasma and brain electrolyte distribution and excitability. Adrenalectomy reduces plasma sodium and raises potassium, the intracellular concentration of sodium in the brain is increased and the turnover of sodium is decreased. Total brain potassium is unchanged, but the ratio of intracellular to extracellular potassium is decreased. These changes indicate that adrenal insufficiency decreases the active transport of sodium out from brain cells. This change is not mediated through the sodium/potassium activated adenosine triphosphatase. It is probably associated with reduction of the oxidative metabolism in the brain which supplies energy to this process. The reduction of active transport of sodium into the cerebrospinal fluid and potassium removal across the choroid plexus alters the electrolyte composition in the cerebrospinal fluid following adrenal hypofunction. The decreased sodium/potassium pump of the brain cell, the increase in the cerebrospinal fluid and extracellular potassium concentration together depolarize the nerve and increase susceptibility to seizures.

The effect of adrenal hyperfunction on brain electrolytes has been studied by the administration of deoxycorticosterone. This treatment does not alter total brain sodium and potassium concentration, but intracellular concentration is markedly decreased, potassium concentration remains unchanged, and the intracellular to extracellular ratio of potassium distribution is increased. The decreased intracellular sodium is associated with decreased brain excitability.

Various corticosteroids such as cortisol, cortisone, and dexamethasone can be applied effectively in man for the treatment of cerebral edema. The probable mechanism of how steroids act in this case is related to the reduction of the abnormal permeability of the structurally intact cerebral vessels. Glucocorticosteroids also decrease the permeability of glial cells to sodium and chloride and decrease their swelling resulted by rapid penetration of these ions during the edema formation.

In experimental animals adrenalectomy causes a significant reduction in cephalic blood flow with concomitantly decreased oxygen consumption. The administration of corticosteroids restores these changes to normal. Some cases of adrenal hypofunction revealed that cerebral blood flow and oxygen utilization are essentially unchanged. The effect of adrenal hyperfunction on blood flow has been studied in man by the administration of cortisone and adrenocorticotrophic hormone. These treatments resulted in a decreased cerebral flow, associated with an increased vascular resistance and with a slight increase of arterial blood pressure. No change was found in the metabolic utilization of oxygen or glucose. However, negative findings have been reported on patients with Cushing's syndrome.

Effects of carbohydrate metabolism on adrenal hypofunction or hyperfunction have not been widely studied. Adrenocorticotrophic hormone and corticosteroids inhibit the oxidation of glucose in tissue and increase glycogen accumulation in the brain. The effect of cortisone on glycogen concentration may be attributed to a dual effect of this compound, such as inhibition of glucose utilization and acceleration of gluconeogenesis. It is probable that the increase in storage of glycogen is derived from increased gluconeogenesis by modifying protein and amino acid metabolism.

In conditions of adrenal hypofunction, the synthesis of protein in the brain is accelerated, and the total free amino acid concentration is markedly decreased with the exception of cysteic acid and glutathione which are increased. Adrenalectomy brings about reductions of glutamic acid, glutamine, GABA, taurine, valine, and cystine, whereas aspartic acid is unaltered. The decrease of GABA is important since this substance is an inhibitory mediator in the cortex and cerebellum. In contrast to hypofunction, it is expected that adrenal hyperfunction, administration of corticosteroids, and adrenocorticotrophic hormone decrease protein synthesis and increase breakdown. In particular, the conversion of glutamic acid to glutamine in human brain is prevented or reversed by deoxycorticosterone. Adrenocortical hormones elicit marked decreasing effects on GABA associated with reduced brain excitability. The effect of these conditions on lipid metabolism is not clear. Adrenocorticotrophic hormone and cortisol enhance brain phospholipid synthesis, and injection of cortisol or estradiol accelerates myelination and cerebroside content in various areas of the brain. The increased myelination and phospholipid production is associated with an enhanced functional development.

It is evident that either the deficiency or excess of adrenocortical hormones bring about marked effects on the function of the nervous system correlated with significant changes in several biochemical constituents. In particular, the ratios of both sodium and potassium concentrations in the brain and cerebrospinal fluid, protein synthesis, carbohydrate utilization, and the concentration of the inhibitory transmitter GABA have been altered. The changes in the GABA concentrations in the cerebral cortex may be one of the main contributing causes to changes of brain excitability. Cortisol and corticosterone are distributed into the brain unchanged where they are selectively bound to the nucleus and cytoplasm. It is possible that neurophysiological effects are mediated through enzyme reactions and through regulation of protein synthesis in brain cells. These investigations are incomplete at present, but hopefully, in time, the neurological and psychological symptoms exhibited by patients with Addison disease and Cushing syndrome can be explained by alterations of the normal biochemical processes which may lead to parallel advances of therapy.

XIV. THE ACTION OF PSYCHOTROPIC DRUGS

Recent studies show that the maintenance of normal personality structure is dependent upon an orderly and highly integrated response of the organism to the endless number of stimuli provided by normal life. However, hallucinations and various degrees of disintegration of personality can be readily produced by many different kinds of substances and procedures. This illustrates how easily the integration of our organism can be disturbed, at times irreversibly.

Psychotropic drugs interfere with response to the normal stimuli and normal biochemical processes of the brain. Apathy and loss of interest in work and life are some of the many consequences. Obviously, low doses elicit no drastic effect, but repeated abuse can bring about grave and often lasting changes, similar in some respects to the disintegration of personality which occurs in certain mental diseases.

In certain individuals, high doses of amphetamine, gives rise to a clinical state closely resembling acute paranoid schizophrenia. Small doses of amphetamine produce exacerbations in schizophrenic patients. Methylphenidate, an amphetamine analog, produces a florid aggravation of schizophrenic symptoms even when taken in extremely low doses and as quickly as 2 min after an intravenous injection. People receiving other psychotomimetic drugs such as lysergide develop psychosis which only differ qualitatively from spontaneous mental disturbances. LSD and related psychedelic drugs such as mescaline and dimethyltryptamine evoke psychotic states. Visual and auditory hallucinations and disturbances of thought processes cause depersonalization and panic states leading to irrational actions and sometimes suicide or homicide. Moreover, LSD induces an increased frequency of chromosomal abnormalities.[104]

XV. PEPTIDES AND NEURAL FUNCTIONS

A. PEPTIDES AND MEMORY

Work on the molecular aspects of memory represents a further extention of the biochemical principles into our understanding of normal neural function and conditions leading to disease.[48] The existence of a molecular code of memory has been established in animal experiments related to hypothalamic and pituitary peptide hormones. Adenocorticotropic hormone and some of its fragments, α- and β-melanocyte-stimulating hormones and vasopressin elicit general effects consolidating memory and delaying its extinction. This effect is independent of the hormone action of these peptides. Desglycinamide derivative of lysin vasopressin isolated from the posterior pituitary brings about a full effect on learning activity. Specific peptides have been identified which are connected with memory transfer processes in the brain of learning animals. Comparatively small peptides containing about 6 to 25 amino acid residues have been formed in the brain of animals learning a new behavior.[119,241,499,573,625] One of these peptides, a pentadecapeptide, has been identified and named scotophobin,[95,266,574] has been isolated from the brain of rats trained to reverse their natural dark preference and to avoid darkness. The peptide is produced in the rat brain only during the training of dark avoidance, and it reaches maximum levels of about 200 ng/g of brain on the sixth day of training. After this peak, it decreases to undetectable amounts by 15 d. Scotophobin is widely distributed in all parts of the brain, but its localization is predominantly in the cortex. When scotophobin is injected intraperitoneally, about 1% is found in the brain 4 h after injection and by 48 h, the time of its maximum behavioural effect, no detectable amounts are found. It is possible that the peptide is incorporated into some cellular structures, perhaps into synaptic membranes. Some synthetic derivatives of scotophobin show full behavioral effect.

When rats were exposed to acoustic stimuli, another peptide, amelebin has been isolated from the brain.[482] This is a hexapeptide and its amino acid sequence has been established: Pyro–Glu–Lys–Gly–Tyr–Ser–Lys. When given to unexposed rats this hexapeptide caused marked reduction in startle responses to sound stimulation. This peptide has also been synthetized, but the synthetic product did not show the full range of action of the natural peptide. This may be due to possible cyclization of the lysine sidegroups. Other conditioning-induced peptides have been demonstrated in the brain of animals trained for shock avoidance, maze running, and avoidance of red and green colors.[119,241,482,499] Peptides resposible for color discrimination have been obtained from the brain of goldfish trained for avoidance-behaviour.[575] Differences were found in these purified peptides between goldfish trained to blue or green avoidance. Another peptide has been isolated from the brain of these fish which are trained to reproduce a swimming behaviour.[625]

So far no peptides identical to the components of animal brain have been isolated from human brain. Many observations, however, suggest that these peptides are not species specific. Scotophobin, ameletin, and other peptides involved in the process of learning in experimental animals share a dipeptide sequence Gly–Tyr and most have Lys as carboxy terminal. The common chemical characteristics found in the structure of specific behavior-inducing peptides support the assumption that closely related molecules are involved in these processes in man. It is, therefore, likely that the biochemical basis of memory is similar between man and that of experimental animals. Differences in color perception, deterioration of mental ability, and senility which progressively set in at old age are probably associated with similar biochemical changes as those established in these representative animal models. These experiments have shown that memory transfer is associated with processes of special peptide synthesis and their incorporation into proteins of the nervous system. Peptide fragments from the hypothalamus and pituitary or from any other peptide hormone-producing gland may serve as appropriate precursors.[91]

It is likely that in the human brain biochemical changes can be correlated with the acquisition and storage of information, and these changes represent an actual neural information. The various peptides found so far related to learned adaptation have different molecular sizes and their utilization for protein synthesis is associated with different enzyme specificities. This suggests that each type of learned behaviour may be accompanied by a distinct peptide sequence. It has been postulated that this information is related specifically to a specific RNA sequence which induces the corresponding protein.[244,305,306] Qualitative and quantitative changes in RNA were found in neurons isolated from the brain of animals in behavioral training. RNA and protein metabolism in the whole brain or in selected areas show some correlation with learning. The application of inhibitors of RNA and protein metabolism confirm these findings, these substances cause an impairment of learning suggesting that an increased RNA and particularly protein synthesis are necessary for the consolidation of acquired information. No specific information can be established so far on the role of the newly synthetized proteins and the participation of the special peptides which have been isolated. Nevertheless, these studies document the possibility that a peptide or protein molecule can record and store a specific memory within its structure.

Besides the hypothalamic peptides a large variety of brain peptides have been identified. These are mostly small peptides such as *N*-acetylaspartylglutamic acid, glutamyl di- and tripeptides, tryptophanyl peptides, and lysyl peptides. These may occur in considerate quantities probably in peptide secreting cells. Peptides released at the synaptic junction are possible neurotransmitters and modulate neuronal activity which governs the performance of the nervous system. They may influence peptide and protein synthesis and control the type of protein being synthetized by the nerve cell. In particular, modulators may act on the presynaptic neurons by influencing the amount of available transmitters, the amount of transmitter released, and the rate and time course of release. They may also act on the postsynaptic neurons regulating the quantity of available receptors and their affinity for the transmitters.

Many recognized neurotransmitters are amines derived from amino acids by decarboxylation. Decarboxylation processes are associated with important cofactors and their presence may influence the production of these biogenic amines. Sometimes the decarboxylated compounds may be further modified chemically. Some unchanged amino acids can also function as transmitters such as glycine and glutamic acid. Amino acids may represent a basic coding system in the nervous system and by constructing the peptide chains with increasing complexity, they form the foundation of many brain functions.

B. PEPTIDES AND DISEASE

Minor or major alterations in the basic coding system involved in amino acid metabolism and peptide and protein synthesis are not only related to learning and memory, but associated with many mental illness such as aminoacidurias, vitamin deficiency polyneuritis, and other disorders linked to these body constituents directly or indirectly. Neuropeptides are present in neurological tumors.[11]

Study of neuropeptides introduced a new and promising trend in biological psychiatry in the mid 1970s. Endogenous morphine may play a role in the development of mental disorders including schizophrenia. Typical representatives of this group are α-, β-, and γ-endorphins, methionine-endorphin, and leucine-endorphin; from a structure point of view, they are fragments of the β-lipotropin molecule. Two competing hypotheses link endogenous opiates to the development of schizophrenia. One of them postulates a decrease in the concentrations of endogenous opiates in the body; the other suggests a connection with increased levels.[157,172,200,421,425,494,565,577] Positive therapeutic effects of des-tyrosine-γ-endorphin in the treatment of schizophrenia support the involvement of the endogenous endorphin family in the clinical manifestation of neurological disorders.[201,582] In spite of this controversy, endogenous opiates undoubtedly play an important role in the formation of an individual mental status, but the role of these compounds in the development of various mental diseases has not yet been established.

XVI. CEREBROSPINAL FLUID

The cerebrospinal fluid (CSF) provides physical support for the brain, acting as a cushion and protecting it from shocks. It takes part in regulating the intracranial pressure. The fluid possesses an excretory function by removing various products of cerebral metabolism such as carbon dioxide, hydrogen, and lactate ions. Through intracerebral transport, the CSF contributes biologically active substances within the central nervous system. It also participates in the functions of the blood-brain barrier by regulating extracellular fluid composition of the brain, both in normal circumstances and in disease.

The CSF is mainly secreted by the choroid plexus in the cerebral ventricles. The fluid is largely formed by active secretion and transport. The total volume of the CSF varies between 70 and 120 ml, the rate of formation is about 0.35 ml/min, and it is replaced several times daily. The CSF constantly undergoes a process of dialysis where various chemical constituents from the blood are exchanged. Cerebral metabolites are also present in the CSF representing biochemical parameters of brain function.[415]

Clinical and experimental observations have established that the CSF shows variations in pathological conditions. These include abnormalities in pressure and in cytological and biochemical composition.

The normal CSF pressure in adults in a horizontal position is 60 to 150 mm of water. It is often lower in children, where the normal pressure level is between 45 and 90 mm. Significant changes occur with postural alterations, physical exertion, arterial hypertension, and coughing.[605] Abnormally high pressure is found in cases of hemorrhage, benign intracranial hypertension, intracranial tumor, hypervitaminosis A, and in various forms of encephalitis, encephalopathy, and meningitis. A subnormal pressure occurs in head injury and dehydration.

The CSF is normally clear and colorless. Any visible discoloration is due to the presence of pigments and this condition is pathological. The fluid becomes turbid when it contains about 400 cells/mm^3. Turbidity of the CSF is due to excess polymorphonuclear cells, present in acute meningitis in great numbers, and the supernatant fluid may turn to yellow. Excess of cells in the CSF called pleocytosis indicates meningeal irritation, but not necessarily represents infection. Blood may be present in the CSF as a result of head injury or product of hemorrhage in the subarachnoid space.

The composition of normal lumbar CSF is fairly constant and there is close similarity with that of serum, except for glucose, protein, and total lipid content, which are lower. The CSF contains some substances also present in variable amounts in the serum, such as cyclic AMP, cyclic GMP, homovanillic acid, 5-hydroxyindoleacetic acid, norepinephrine, acetylcholine, choline, prostaglandin PGF$_2$, β-endorphin, cholecystokinin, and gastrin. Homovanillic acid is derived from dopamine; hydroxyindoleacetic acid is a metabolite of serotonin. Some patients with parkinsonism with high CSF homovanillic acid levels do not respond well to levodopa treatment as well as those with low levels.[537] Down's syndrome patients show low blood serotonin, but the CSF 5-hydroxyindoleacetic acid level is normal.[173] These studies, however, indicate that the biochemical basis of nervous system disorders are connected with abnormalities of biogenic amines, including depression and schizophrenia,[415,504] although several neurotransmitters do not cross the blood-brain barrier.[613]

A. Biochemical Changes in Cerebrospinal Fluids

Severe diseases of the central nervous system alter the structural organization, resulting in generalized or localized increase in permeability of the blood-brain barrier. Some changes accompany normal functions of the nervous tissue such as shifts of ions through membranes

TABLE 6
Status of Cerebrospinal Fluid in
Conditions Affecting the Brain Stem

Normal:[a]
  Alzheimer's disease
  Wernicke encephalopathy
  Epilepsy
  Parkinson's disease
  Migraine
  Beri beri
  Pellagra
Abnormal:[b]
  Neoplasia
  Multiple sclerosis
  Polyneuritis
  Cerebrovascular accident
  Meningitis
  Krabbe's disease (protein ↑)
  Metachromatic leukodystrophy (protein ↑)

[a] Clear, 70 to 180 mmH$_2$O pressure, 15 to 45 mg/dl
    protein, 0 to 10 WBC/mm^3, 45 to 80 mg/dl glucose.
[b] Xanthochromic, increased pressure, protein and
    WBC's color appearance usually accompanies
    changes in protein concentration or WBC counts.

of neurons and glial cells. However, gross changes in barrier permeability are associated with pathological conditions. Although the hematoencephalic barrier is still a hypothetical structure, it has a considerable importance. If the integrity of this barrier is damaged, the CSF shows increased substances of low molecular weight, passage of macromolecules which can be either endogenous or exogeneous. A number of pathological factors influence the severity of lesions related to the derangement of permeability and determine the number and types of molecules appearing in the cerebrospinal fluid (Table 6).

Many generalized disease conditions affect the permeability of the blood-brain barrier,[282] such as cerebral edema due to trauma, toxic chemicals, inflammation, cerebral anoxia, brain injury, and brain tumors. The effects are ranging from relatively mild and transient interference to severe and widespread destruction, influencing the number and quantity of substances that are present in the cerebrospinal fluid. The modifications in its composition may occur in pathological cases.[292,560] Analysis of the cerebrospinal fluid may therefore provide an indication of a disease process manifest in the central nervous system.

The total protein content of normal CSF is 0.15 to 0.45 g/l, mainly in an albumin to globulin ratio of 8:1. The protein concentration increases until age 30, and between ages 20 and 50, it is higher in men than in women. Total protein levels remain normal in many neurological disorders such as arteriosclerosis, multiple sclerosis, and presenile dementia. Elevated protein levels in the CSF are very common. A moderate increase is associated with inflammatory diseases of the brain and meninges, such as in various forms of meningitis, encephalitis, poliomyelitis, and even in multiple sclerosis.[186] The presence of an intracranial tumor or cerebral hemorrhage may also moderately elevate CSF protein content. It is also increased in some degenerative diseases, such as familial spastic paraplegia, and Refsum's disease, or decreased after strokes or epileptic seizures. Qualitative differences may characterize some diseases such as brain tumors and metastases.[11]

Most proteins found in serum are present in the cerebrospinal fluid; high molecular weight fractions are associated with modification of the blood-brain barrier. These are apparent in the majority of multiple sclerosis patients and in brain or medullary tumors. The presence of fibrinogen represents pathological damage since this protein is absent from normal CSF. In inflammatory diseases, bacterial and viral infections bring about a rise in the globulin fraction;[365] this increase mainly manifests in the IgG fraction and sometimes in IgA.[216] Terminal component of complement (Cg) is present in CSF of patients with multiple sclerosis.[417]

Various enzymes in the CSF show correlations with neurological disorders. Acid and alkaline phosphatase activity is increased in psychiatric diseases, β-glucuronidase in demyelination, creatine phosphokinase in cerebral tumors, epilepsy, and intracranial hypertension.[37] α_1-Antitrypsin is present in variable amounts in the CSF of patients with various neurological diseases.[457] Ferritin content of the CSF and serum shows changes indicating clinical relevance to neurological disorders.[207,527]

Some hypothalamic and pituitary hormones show abnormalities in depression, related to control mechanisms and adrenal actions regulating ACTH release.[460] In animal experiments, very sensitive immunohistochemical techniques have established the localization of these hormones in various regions of the anterior pituitary.[458,459] Thyrotropic releasing hormone levels show variations in the CSF in several neurological diseases.[412] CSF vasopressin, oxytocin, somatostatin, and β-endorphin levels are abnormal in Alzheimer's disease.[483] CSF vasopressin is increased in many neurological and psychiatric disorders,[530] and variations occurring in plasma and CSF vasopressin concentrations are characteristic of dementia.[540] In schizophrenia, CSF contains endorphins.[494] Lactic acid content is elevated in the CSF of patients with infections of the central nervous system.[88] Lactic acidosis manifests in certain myelopathies.[413,480] Acid-base changes also occur in the CSF concurrent with brain disease.[106]

Amino acid levels of the cerebrospinal fluid are different from the levels in blood and show greater vaiations.[284] The quantity of total amino acids is enhanced in meningitis, normal, in tumors, and reduced in multiple sclerotic children. In Parkinson's disease glutamic acid is reduced and other amino acids are increased.[264] In aminoacidopathies, the detection of the amino acids in the cerebrospinal fluid provides a key for the diagnosis such as phenylketonuria, homocystinuria, and argininosuccinic aciduria (Table 5).[583] 5-Hydroxyindole derivatives are present in CSF of patients with psychiatric or neurological disease[26] and in acute delirium.[312]

The concentration of lipids in the cerebrospinal fluid may be useful for diagnostic purposes. In Tay-Sachs disease and in metachromatic leukodistrophy, all lipids are increased, including phospholipids, gangliosides, cerebrosides, fatty acids, neutral fats, cholesterol, and cholesteryl esters. Fatty acid levels are raised in schizophrenia and manic-depression states, but normal in multiple sclerosis. In schizophrenia, the presence of an abnormal lipoprotein has also been reported. Menkes' disease is also connected with abnormal lipid changes in the CSF and serum.[72]

Total phospholipid content of the CSF may be increased in several neurological diseases, particularly connected with demyelinating processes.[624] Cholesterol and cholesteryl ester content is also increased in some neurological diseases, especially in multiple sclerosis.[259] Among various enzymes, the activity of aspartate aminotransferase is raised in multiple sclerosis.[156,257,325] Angiotensin-converting enzyme is enhanced in Alzheimer's disease and Parkinson's disease as in progressive supranuclear palsy.[626] Some of these enzymes may have derived from the serum.[603] Creatine kinase activity is enhanced in muscular distrophy and isoenzyme studies confirmed that this enzyme is derived from the brain.[522] Abnormality of this enzyme, together with aldolase, often manifest in acute psychoses.[404] Brain diseases are often associated with elevated levels of certain enzymes in the serum. Nonspecific esterases and various acid and alkaline proteinases are increased in some cerebral disorders, 2',3'-cyclic nucleotide 3'-phosphohydrolase may be raised in demyelinating diseases.[38] The specificity of the enzyme tests is questionable, and therefore, their usefulness for routine diagnosis has been doubted.[219] Ascorbic acid levels are decreased in the serum of chronic psychiatric patients.[410]

REFERENCES

1. **Aberg, B., Ekman, L., Falk, R., Greitz, U., Persson, G., and Smiths, J. O.**, Metabolism of methylmercury (203Hg) compounds in man, *Arch. Environ. Health*, 91, 478, 1969.
2. **Acker, W., Aps, E. J., Majumdar, S. K., Shaw, G. K., and Thomson, A. D.**, The relationship between brain and liver damage in chronic alcoholic patients, *J. Neurol. Neurosurg. Psychiatry*, 45, 984, 1982.
3. **Adams, C. W. M., Orton, C. C., and Zilkha, K. J.**, Arterial catecholamine and enzyme histochemistry in migraine, *J. Neurol. Neurosurg. Psychiatry*, 2, 237, 1968.
4. **Adams, J. M.**, Measles antibodies in patients with multiple sclerosis, *Neurology*, 17, 707, 1967.
5. **Agamonolis, D. P., Potter, J. L., Kerrick, M. K., and Sternberger, N. H.**, The neuropathology of glycine encephalopathy: a report of five cases with immunohistochemical and ultrastructural observations, *Neurology (Minneapolis)*, 32, 975, 1982.
6. **Alajouanine, T., Derobert, L., and Thieffry, S.**, Etude clinique d'ensemble de 210 cas d'intoxication par les sels organiques d'etain, *Rev. Neurol.*, 98, 85, 1958.
7. **Albers, J. W., Cavender, G. D., Levine, S. P., and Langolf, G. D.**, Asymptomatic sensorimotor polyneuropathy in workers exposed to elemental mercury, *Neurology*, 32, 1168, 1982.
8. **Alender, C. B.**, Isolation and characterization of sea urchin toxin, *Toxicon*, 3, 9, 1965.
9. **Ali, M. M., Murthy, R. C., Mandal, S. K., and Chandra, S. V.**, Effect of low protein diet on manganese neurotoxicity III: brain neurotransmitter levels, *Neurobehav. Toxicol. Teratol.*, 7, 427, 1985.
10. **Allen, I. V.**, The pathology of multiple sclerosis — fact, fiction and hypothesis, *Neuropathol. Appl. Neurobiol.*, 7, 169, 1981.
11. **Allen, J. M., Hoyle, N. R., Yeats, J. C., Ghatei, M. A., Thomas, D. G., and Bloom, S. R.**, Neuropeptides in neurological tumors, *J. Neurooncol.*, 3, 197, 1985.
12. **Allen, N.**, Solvents and other organic compounds, in *Handbook of Clinical Neurology, Intoxications of the Nervous System*, Vol. 36, Part I, Vinken, P. J. and Bruyn, G. W., Eds., North Holland, Amsterdam, 1979, 361—376.
13. **Allen, N., Mendell, J. R., Billmaier, D. J., Fontaine, R. E., and O'Neill, J.**, Toxic polyneuropathy due to methyl-n-butylketone, *Arch. Neurol. Chicago*, 32, 209, 1975.
14. **Alvares, A. P., Kapelner, S., Sassa, S., and Kappas, A.**, Drug metabolism in normal children, lead-poisoned children and normal adults, *Clin. Pharmacol. Ther.*, 17, 179, 1975.
15. American College of Neuropsychopharmacology — Food and Drug Administration Task Force, Neurologic syndromes associated with antipsychotic-drug use, *N. Engl. J. Med.*, 289, 20, 1973.
16. **Aminoff, M. J.**, Electrophysiologic recognition of certain occupation-related neurotoxic disorders, *Neurol. Clin.*, 3, 687, 1985.
17. **Amin-Zaki, L., Majeed, M. A., Clarkson, T. W., and Greenwood, M. R.**, Methylmercury poisoning in Iraqi children: clinical observations over two years, *Br. Med. J.*, 1, 597, 1978.
18. **Anders, K., Steinsapir, K. D., Iverson, D. J., Glasgow, B. J., Layfield, L. J., Brown, W. J., Cancilla, P. A., Verity, M. A., and Vinters, H. V.**, Neuropathologic findings in the acquired immunodeficiency syndrome (AIDS), *Clin. Neuropathol.*, 5, 1, 1986.
19. **Andersen, O.**, Clinical evidence and therapeutic indications in neurotoxicology, exemplified by thallotoxicosis, *Acta Neurol. Scand. Suppl.*, 100, 185, 1984.
20. **Anthony, M., Hinterberger, H., and Lance, J. W.**, The possible relationship of serotonin to the migraine syndrome, *Res. Clin. Stud. Headache*, 2, 29, 1969.
21. **Anthony, M. and Lance, J. W.**, Monoamine oxidase inhibition in the treatment of migraine, *Arch. Neurol. Chicago*, 21, 263, 1969.
22. **Anton-Tay, F., Anton, S. M., and Wurtman, R. J.**, Mechanism of changes in brain norepinephrine metabolism after ovariectomy, *Neuroendocrinology*, 6, 265, 1970.
23. **Anzil, A. P. and Dosic, S.**, Peripheral nerve changes in porphyric neuropathy, *Acta Neuropathol.*, 42, 12, 1978.
24. **Arato, M., Bagdy, G., Blumel, F., Perenyi, A., and Rihmer, Z.**, Csokkent szerum dopamin-B-hidroxilaz aktivitas paranoid schizopreniaban, *Ideggyogyaszati Szemle*, 35, 355, 1982.
25. **Armstrong, D.**, Central nervous system infections in the immunocompromised host, *Infection*, 12(Suppl. 1), 558, 1984.
26. **Ashcroft, G. W., Crawford, T. B. B., and Eccleston, D.**, 5-Hydroxyindole compounds in the cerebrospinal fluid of patients with psychiatric or neurological diseases, *Lancet*, 2, 1049, 1966.
27. **Aula, P., Autio, S., Raivio, K. O., Rapola, J., Thoden, C.-J., Koskela, S.-L., and Yamashina, I.**, ''Salla disease'': a new lysosomal storage disorder, *Arch. Neurol. Chicago*, 36, 88, 1979.
28. **Auld, R. B. and Bedwell, S. F.**, Peripheral neuropathy with sympathetic overactivity from industrial contact with acrylamide, *Can. Med. Assoc. J.*, 96, 652, 1967.
29. **Axelrod, J.**, Brain monoamines: biosynthesis and fate, *Neurosci. Res. Program Bull.*, 9, 188, 1971.
30. **Axelrod, J.**, Methylation reactions in the formation and metabolism of catecholamines and other biogenic amines, *Pharmacol. Rev.*, 18, 95, 1966.

31. **Axelrod, J.,** The pineal gland, *Endeavour,* 29, 4, 1970.

32. **Axelrod, J. and Winshilboum, R.,** Catecholamines, *N. Engl. J. Med.,* 287, 237, 1972.

33. **Azmitia, E. C.,** Reengineering the brain serotonin system: localized application of specific neurotoxins and fetal serotonergic neurons into the adult CNS, *Adv. Neurol.,* 43, 493, 1986.

34. **Bahemuka, M.,** Malignant hypertension: a review of the neurological features in 34 consecutive patients, *East Afr. Med. J.,* 62, 560, 1985.

35. **Baker, E. L.,** Epidemiologic issues in neurotoxicity research, *Neurobehav. Toxicol. Teratol.,* 7, 293, 1985.

36. **Baker, E. L., Jr., Smith, J. J., and Landrigan, P. J.,** The neurotoxicity of industrial solvents: a review of the literature, *Am. J. Ind. Med.,* 8, 207, 1985.

37. **Banerji, A. P., Jayam, A. V., and Desai, A. D.,** Creatine phosphokinase activity of cerebrospinal fluid in muscular dystrophy and other neurological disorders, *Neurol. Bombay,* 17, 123, 1969.

38. **Banik, N. L., Mauldin, L. B., and Hogan, E. L.,** Activity of $2',3'$-cyclic nucleotide $3'$-phosphohydrolase in human cerebrospinal fluid, *Ann. Neurol.,* 5, 539, 1979.

39. **Banks, W. A. and Kastin, A. J.,** Aluminium increases permeability of the blood-brain barrier to labelled DSIP and β-endorphin: possible implications for senile and dialysis dementia, *Lancet,* 2, 1227, 1983.

40. **Barbeau, A.,** Dopamine and blood pressure regulation, *Clin. Res.,* 17, 634, 1969.

41. **Barbeau, A.,** Dopamine and disease, *Can. Med. Assoc.,* 103, 824, 1970.

42. **Barbeau, A. and Giroux, J-M.,** Levodopa and psoriasis, *Lancet,* 1, 204, 1972.

43. **Barker, J. L., Crayton, J. W., and Nicoll, R. A.,** Supraoptic neurosecretory cells: adrenergic and cholinergic sensitivity, *Science,* 171, 208, 1971.

44. **Barker, J. L., Crayton, J. W., and Nicoll, R. A.,** Supraoptic neurosecretory cells: autonomic modulation, *Science,* 171, 206, 1971.

45. **Barker, J. L., Ifshin, M., and Gainer, H.,** Studies on bursting pacemaker potential activity in molluscan neurons. III. Effects of hormones, *Brain Res.,* 84, 501,1975.

46. **Barltrop, D.,** Environmental lead and its paediatric significance, *Postgrad. Med. J.,* 45, 129, 1969.

47. **Barltrop, D.,** Lead poisoning in childhood, *Postgrad. Med. J.,* 44, 537, 1968.

48. **Bartus, R. T., Dean, R. L., Beer, B., and Lippa, A. S.,** The cholinergic hypothesis of geriatric memory dysfunction, *Science,* 217, 408, 1982.

49. **Basser, L.,** The relation of migraine and epilepsy, *Brain,* 92, 285, 1969.

50. **Bates, D., Fawcett, P. R. W., Shaw, D. A., and Weightman, D.,** Polyunsaturated fatty acids in treatment of acute remitting multiple sclerosis, *Br. Med. J.,* 2, 1390, 1978.

51. **Bauer, R. B. and McHenry, J. T.,** Comparison of amantadine, placebo, and levodopa in Parkinson's disease, *Neurol. Minneapolis,* 24, 715, 1974.

52. **Baumblatt, M. J. and Winston, F.,** Pyridoxine and the pill, *Lancet,* 1, 832, 1970.

53. **Beal, M. F., Mazurek, M. F., Tran, V. T., Chattha, G., Bird, E. D., and Martin, J. B.,** Reduced numbers of somatostatin receptors in the cerebral cortex in Alzheimer's disease, *Science,* 229, 289, 1985.

54. **Bean, W. B., Hodges, R. E., and Daum, K.,** Pantothenic acid deficiency induced in human beings, *J. Clin. Invest.,* 34, 1073, 1955.

55. **Beard, R. R. and Grandstaff, N.,** Carbon monoxide exposure and cerebral function, *Ann. N.Y. Acad. Sci.,* 174, 385, 1970.

56. **Beattie, A. D., Moore, M. R., Goldberg, A., Finlayson, M. J. W., Graham, J. F., Mackie, E. M., Main, J. C., McLaren, D. A., Murdoch, R. M., and Stewart, G. T.,** Role of chronic low-level lead exposure in the aetiology of mental retardation, *Lancet,* 1, 589, 1975.

57. **Beaty, H. N.,** Tetanus, in *Harrison's Principles of Internal Medicine,* Thorn, G. W., Adams, R. D., Braunwald, E., Isselbacher, K. I., and Petersdorf, R. G., Eds., McGraw-Hill, New York, 1977, 886—890.

58. **Beaty, H. N. and Graebner, R. W.,** Botulism, in *Harrison's Principles of Internal Medicine,* Thorn, G. W., Adams, R. D., Braunwald, E., Isselbacher, K. I., and Petersdorf, R. G., Eds., McGraw-Hill, New York, 1977, 890—892.

59. **Beckett, W. S., Moore, J. L., Keogh, J. P., and Bleecker, M. L.,** Acute encephalopathy due to occupational exposure to arsenic, *Br. J. Ind. Med.,* 43, 66, 1986.

60. **Beckham, M. M. and Rudy, E. B.,** Acquired immunodeficiency syndrome: impact and implication for the neurological system, *J. Neurosci. Nurs.,* 18, 5, 1986.

61. **Behse, F. and Buchthal, F.,** Alcoholic neuropathy: clinical, electrophysiological and biopsy findings, *Ann. Neurol.,* 2, 95,1977.

62. **Berger, P.,** Biochemistry and the schizophrenias: old concepts and hypotheses, *J. Nerv. Ment. Dis.,* 169, 90, 1981.

63. **Berl, S., Lajtha, A., and Waelsch, H.,** Studies of glutamic acid metabolism in the central nervous system, in *Chemical Pathology of the Nervous System,* Folch-Pi, J., Ed., Pergamon Press, Oxford, 1961.

64. **Berlet, H. H., Matsumoto, K., Pscheidt, G. R., Spaide, J., Bull, C., and Himwich, H. E.,** Biochemical correlates of behavior in schizophrenic patients, *Arch. Gen. Psychiatry,* 13, 521, 1965.

65. **Bernheimer, H.,** Distribution of homovanillic acid in the human brain, *Nature (London),* 204, 587, 1964.

66. **Bernheimer, H., Birkmayer, W., and Hornykiewicz, O.,** Brain dopamine and the syndromes of Parkinson and Huntington, *J. Neurol. Sci.,* 20, 415, 1973.
67. **Besson, J.,** Dementia: biological solution still a long way off, *Br. Med. J.,* 287, 926, 1983.
68. **Betz, A. L.,** Transport of ions across the blood-brain barrier, *Fed. Proc.,* 45, 2050, 1986.
69. **Bice, A. N., Wagner, H. N., Frost, J. J., Natarajan, T. K., Lee, M. C., Wong, D. F., and Links, J. M.,** Simplified detection system for neuroreceptor studies in the human brain, *J. Nucl. Med.,* 27, 184, 1986.
70. **Bickel, H., Neale, F. C., and Hall, G.,** A clinical and biochemical study of hepatolenticular degeneration (Wilson's disease), *Quart. J. Med.,* 26, 527,1957.
71. **Biery, T. L.,** *Venomous Arthropod Handbook,* United States Government Printing Office, Washington, D.C., 1978.
72. **Blackett, P. R., Lee, D. M., Donaldson, D. L., Fesmire, J. D., Chan, W. Y., Holcombe, J. H., and Rennert, O. M.,** Studies of lipids, lipoproteins, and apolipoproteins in Menkes' disease, *Pediatr. Res.,* 18, 864, 1984.
73. **Boegman, R. J. and Bates, L. A.,** Neurotoxicity of aluminum, *Can.J. Physiol. Pharmacol.,* 62, 1010, 1984.
74. **Bondareff, W.,** Age and Alzheimer disease, *Lancet,* 1, 1447, 1983.
75. **Boor, J. W. and Hurtig, H. I.,** Persistent cerebellar exposure to toluene, *Ann. Neurol.,* 2, 440, 1977.
76. **Bornstein, M. B., Miller, A. I., Teitelbaum, D., Arnon, R., and Sela, M.,** Multiple sclerosis: trial of a synthetic polypeptide, *Ann. Neurol.,* 11, 317, 1982.
77. **Bowen, D. M.,** Biochemical assessment of neurotransmitter and metabolic dysfunction and cerebral atrophy in Alzheimer's disease, in *Biological Aspects of Alzheimer's Disease,* Katzman, R., Ed., Albert Einstein College of Medicine, New York, 1983, 219.
78. **Bowen, D. M. and Davison, A. N.,** Dementia in the elderly: biochemical aspects, *J. R. Coll. Physicians London,* 18, 25, 1984.
79. **Bowen, D. M., Smith, C. B., White, P., and Davison, A. N.,** Neurotransmitter-related enzymes and indices of hypoxia in senile dementia and other abiotrophies, *Brain,* 99, 459, 1976.
80. **Bowen, D. M., Smith, C. B., White, P., Flack, R. H. A., Carrasco, L. H., Gedye, J. L., and Davison, A. N.,** Chemical pathology of the organic dementias. II. Quantitative estimation of cellular changes in postmortem brains, *Brain,* 100, 427, 1977.
81. **Bowen, D. M., Smith, C. B., White, P., Goodhardt, M. J., Spillane, J. A., Flack, R. H. A., and Davison, A. N.,** Chemical pathology of the organic dementias. I. Validity of biochemical measurements on human post-mortem brain specimens, *Brain,* 100, 397, 1977.
82. **Boyd, A. E., III, Lebovitz, H. E., and Pfeiffer, J. B.,** Stimulation of human-growth-hormone secretion by L-dopa, *Lancet,* 2, 1425, 1970.
83. **Bradshaw, J., Geffen, G., and Nettleton, N.,** Our two brains, *New Sci.,* 59, 628, 1972.
84. **Brady, R. O.,** Hereditary fat-metabolism diseases, *Sci. Am.,* 229, 88, 1973.
85. **Brady, R. O., Kanfer, J. N., Bradley, R. M., and Shapiro, D.,** Demonstration of a deficiency of glucocerebroside-cleaving enzyme in Gaucher's disease, *J. Clin. Invest.,* 45, 1112, 1966.
86. **Brant-Zawadski, M., Fein, G., Van Dyke, C., Kiernan, R., Davenport, L., and deGroot, J.,** MR imaging of the aging brain: patchy white-matter lesions and dementia, *Am. J. Nucl. Res.,* 6, 675, 1985.
87. **Brimblecombe, F. S. W., Blainey, J. D., Stoneman, M. E. R., and Wood, B. S. B.,** Dietary and biochemical control of phenylketonuria, *Br. Med. J.,* 2, 793, 1961.
88. **Brook, I., Bricknell, K. S., and Overturf, G. D.,** Measurement of lactic acid in cerebrospinal fluid of patients with infections of the central nervous system, *J. Infect. Dis.,* 137, 384, 1978.
89. **Brown, E. L. and Knox, E. G.,** Epidemiologic approach to Parkinson's disease, *Lancet,* 1, 974, 1972.
90. **Brown, J. H.,** *Toxicology and Pharmacology of Venoms from Poisonous Snakes,* Charles C Thomas, Springfield, IL, 1973.
91. **Brown, M. and Vale, W.,** Central nervous system effects of hypothalamic peptides, *Endocrinology,* 96, 1333, 1975.
92. **Brucher, J. M.,** Neuropathological problems posed by carbon monoxide poisoning and anoxia, *Prog. Brain Res.,* 24, 75, 1967.
93. **Brust, J. C. M.,** Dementia and cerebrovascular disease, in *The Dementias,* Mayeux, R. and Rosen, W. G., Eds., Raven Press, New York, 1983, 131.
94. **Brust, J. C. M., Hammer, J. S., Challenor, Y., Healton, E. B., and Lesser, R. P.,** Acute generalized polyneuropathy accompanying lithium poisoning, *Ann. Neurol.,* 6, 360, 1979.
95. **Bryant, R. C., Santos, N. N., and Byrne, W. L.,** Synthetic scotophobin in goldfish: specificity and effect on learning, *Science,* 177, 635, 1972.
96. **Buck, R. W.,** Mushroom toxins-a brief review of the literature, *N. Engl. J. Med.,* 285, 681, 1961.
97. **Bull, R. J., Stanaszek, P. M., O'Neill, J. J., and Lutkenhoff, S. D.,** Specificity of the effects of lead on brain energy metabolism for substrates donating a cytoplasmic reducing equivalent, *Environ. Health Persp.,* 12, 89, 1975.

98. **Bunney, W. E., Jr. and Davis, J. M.,** Norepinephrine in depressive reactions, *Arch. Gen. Psychiatry*, 13, 483, 1965.

99. **Burks, J. S., Alfrey, A. C., Huddlestone, J., Novenberg, M. D., and Lewis, E.,** A fatal encephalopathy in chronic haemodialysis patients, *Lancet*, 1, 764, 1976.

100. **Busard, B. L., Renier, W. O., Gabreels, F. J., Jasper, H. H., van Haelst, U. J., and Sloff, J. L.,** Lafora's disease. Comparison of inclusion bodies in skin and in brain, *Arch. Neurol.*, 43, 296, 1986.

101. **Butterworth, R. F., Giguere, J. F., and Besnard, A. M.,** Activities of thiamine-dependent enzymes in two experimental models of thiamine-deficiency encephalopathy: 1. The pyruvate dehydrogenase system, *Neurochem. Res.*, 10, 1417, 1985.

102. **Buxton, P. H., Hayward, M.,** Polyneuritis cranialis associated with industrial trichloroethylene poisoning, *J. Neurol. Neurosurg. Psychiatry*, 30, 511, 1967.

103. **Byers, R. K.,** Lead poisoning. Review of literature and report on 45 cases, *Pediatrics*, 23, 585, 1959.

104. **Cade, J. F. J.,** A significant elevation of plasma magnesium levels in schizophrenia and depressive states, *Med. J. Aust*, 1, 195, 1964.

105. **Cahalan, M.,** Voltage clamp studies on the node of Ranvier, in *Physiology and Pathobiology of Axons*, Waxman, S. G., Ed., Raven Press, New York, 1978, 155—168.

106. **Cameron, I. R.,** Acid-base changes in cerebrospinal fluid, *Br. J. Anaesthiol.*, 41, 213, 1969.

107. **Cammer, W.,** Toxic demyelination: biochemical studies and hypothetical mechanisms, in *Experimental and Clinical Neurotoxicology*, Spencer, P. S. and Schaumburg, H. H., Eds., Williams & Wilkins, Baltimore, 1980, chap. 17.

108. **Campbell, A. M. G., Williams, E. R., and Barltrop, D.,** Motor neurone disease and exposure to lead, *J. Neurol. Neurosurg. Psychiatry*, 33, 877, 1970.

109. **Carman, J. S.,** Hyperdopaminergic states, a continuum, *Lancet*, 1, 1249, 1972.

110. **Carson, N. A. J. and Raine, D. N.,** *Inherited Disorders of Sulphur Metabolism*, Williams & Wilkins, Edinburgh, 1971.

111. **Catton, M. J., Harrison, M. J. G., Fullerton, P. M., and Kazantzis, B.,** Subclinical neuropathy in lead workers, *Br. Med. J.*, 2, 80, 1970.

112. **Caughey, W. S.,** Carbon monoxide bonding in hemeproteins, *Ann. N.Y. Acad. Sci.*, 174, 148, 1970.

113. **Cavanagh, J. B.,** Organo-phosphorus neurotoxicity, a model "dying-back" process comparable to certain human neurological disorders, *Guy's Hosp. Rep.*, 112, 303, 1963.

114. **Cavanagh, J. B.,** The significance of the "dying-back" process in experimental and human neurological disease, *Int. Rev. Exp. Pathol.*, 3, 219, 1964.

115. Center for Disease Control, Botulism in the United States, 1899—1973, United States Department of Health, Education and Welfare Publication, Washington, DC, 74-8279, 1974.

116. **(Anonymous),** Central nervous system changes in deficiency of vitamin B-6 and other B-complex vitamins, *Nutr. Rev.*, 33, 21, 1975.

117. **Chan, P. H., Fishman, R. A., Longar, S., Chen, S., and Yu, A.,** Cellular and molecular effects of polyunsaturated fatty acids in brain ischemia and injury, *Prog. Brain Res.*, 63, 227, 1985.

118. **Chang, L. W.,** Neurotoxic effects of mercury — a review, *Environ. Res.*, 14, 329, 777.

119. **Chapouthier, G. and Ungerer, A.,** Effet de l'injection d'extraits de cerveau conditionne sur l'apprentissage, *C. R. Acad. Sci. Ser. D*, 267, 769, 1968.

120. **Chen, R. W., Ganther, H. E., Hoekstra, W. G.,** Studies on the binding of methylmercury by thionein, *Biochem. Biophys. Res. Commun.*, 51, 383, 1973.

121. **Chia, L. G. and Chu, F. L.,** A clinical and electrophysiological study of patients with polychlorinated biphenyl poisoning, *J. Neurol. Neurosurg. Psychiatry*, 48, 894, 1985.

122. **Chicheportiche, R., Balerna, M., Lombet, A., Romey, G., and Lazdunski, M.,** Synthesis and mode of action on axonal membranes of photoactivable derivatives of tetrodotoxin, *J. Biol. Chem.*, 254, 1522, 1979.

123. **Chisolm, J. J.,** Lead poisoning, *Sci. Am.*, 221, 15, 1971.

124. **Cinca, I., Dumitrescu, I., Onaca, P., Serbanescu, A., and Nestorescu, B.,** Accidental ethyl mercury poisoning with nervous system, skeletal muscle, and myocardium injury, *J. Neurol Neurosurg. Psychiatry*, 43, 143, 1980.

125. **Clarke, J. K., Dane, D. S., and Dick, G. W. A.,** Viral antibody in the cerebrospinal fluid and serum of multiple sclerosis patients, *Brain*, 88, 953, 1965.

126. **Clarkson, T. W.,** Epidemiological and experimental aspects of lead and mercury contamination of food, *Food Cosmet. Toxicol.*, 9, 229, 1971.

127. **Clarkson, T. W.,** The pharmacology of mercury compounds, *Annu. Rev. Pharmacol.*, 12, 375, 1972.

128. **Clifford, R. F. and Gawel, M.,** Clioquinol neurotoxicity: an overview, *Acta Neurol. Scand.*, 100, 137, 1984.

129. **Coburn, R. F.,** Biological effects of carbon monoxide, *Ann. N.Y. Acad. Sci.*, 174, 1, 1970.

130. **Collier, R. J.,** Diphtheria toxin — mode of action and structure, *Bacteriol. Rev.*, 39, 54, 1975.

131. **Coppola, J. A.**, Turnover of hypothalamic catecholamines during various states of gonadotropic secretion, *Neuroendocrinology*, 5, 75, 1969.
132. **Cotzias, G. C.**, Metabolic modification of some neurologic disorders, *JAMA*, 210, 1255, 1969.
133. **Cotzias, G. C., Von Woert, M. H., and Schiffer, L. M.**, Aromatic amino acids and the modification of Parkinsonism, *N. Engl. J. Med.*, 276, 374, 1967.
134. **Crane, G. E.**, The prevention of tardive dyskinesia, *Am. J. Psychiatry*, 134, 756, 1977.
135. **Crapper, D. R. and De Boni, U.**, Aluminum and the genetic apparatus in Alzheimer's disease, *The Aging Brain and Senile Dementia*, Nandy, K., Ed., Plenum Press, New York, 1977, 229.
136. **Crapper, D. R., Karlik, S., and De Boni, U.**, Aluminum and other metals in senile (Alzheimer) dementia, in *Alzheimer's Disease: Senile Dementia and Related Disorders*, Vol. 7, Katzman, R., Terry, R. D., and Bick, K. L., Eds., Raven Press, New York, 1978, 472.
137. **Crapper, D. R., Krishnan, S. S., and Quittkat, S.**, Aluminum, neurofibrillary degeneration and Alzheimer's disease, *Brain*, 99, 67, 1976.
138. **Crome, L. C. and Stern, J.**, *Pathology of Mental Retardation*, Churchill Livingstone, London, 1972.
139. **Cross, A. J., Crow, T. J., Johnson, J. A., Dawson, J. M., and Peters, T. J.**, Loss of endoplasmic reticulum — associated enzymes in affected brain regions in Huntington's disease and Alzheimer-type dementia, *J. Neurol. Sci.*, 71, 137, 1985.
140. **Cross, A. J., Crow, T. J., and Owen, F.**, ^{3}H-Flupenthixol binding in postmortem brains of schizophrenics: evidence for a selective increase in dopamine D_2 receptors, *Psychopharmacology*, 74, 122, 1981.
141. **Crow, T. J.**, Catecholamine reward pathways and schizophrenia: the mechanism of the antipsychotic effect and the site of the primary disturbance, *Fed. Proc.*, 38, 2462, 1979.
142. **Crow, T. J.**, Is schizophrenia an infectious disease?, *Lancet*, 1, 173, 1983.
143. **Cumings, J. N.**, The copper and iron content in the brain and liver in the normal and in hepatolenticular degeneration, *Brain*, 71, 410, 1948.
144. **Curtis, D. R.**, Tetanus toxin as a neuropharmacological tool, in *Neuropoisons — Their Pathophysiological Actions*, Vol. 1, Simpson, L. L., Ed., Plenum Press, New York, 1971, 263—282.
145. **Curzon, G., Theaker, P., and Phillips, B.**, Excretion of 5-hydroxyindoly acetic acid (5 HIAA) in migraine, *J. Neurol. Neurosurg. Psychiatry*, 29, 85, 1966.
146. **Cutler, N. R., Haxby, J. V., Duara, R., Grady, C. L., Kay, A. D., Kessler, R. M., and Rapoport, S. I.**, Clinical history, brain metabolism, and neuropsychological function in Alzheimer's disease, *Ann. Neurol.*, 18, 298, 1985.
147. **Cutting, J.**, Neuropsychiatric complications of alcoholism, *Br. J. Hosp. Med.*, 28, 335, 1982.
148. **Dahlstrom, A. and Fuxe, K.**, Evidence for the existence of monoamine-containing neurons in the central nervous system, *Acta Physiol. Scand.*, 62(Suppl. 232), 1, 1964.
149. **Damasio, H. and Beck, D.**, Migraine, thrombocytopenia and serotonin metabolism, *Lancet*, 1, 240, 1978.
150. **Dastur, D. K., Manghani, D. K., Osuntokun, B. O., Sourander, P., and Kondo, K.**, Neuromuscular and related changes in malnutrition: a review, *J. Neurol. Sci.*, 55, 207, 1982.
151. **Davadatta, S.**, Isoniazid-induced encephalopathy, *Lancet*, 2, 440, 1965.
152. **Davenport, J. G., Farrell, D. F., and Sumi, S. M.**, 'Giant axonal neuropathy' caused by industrial chemicals: neurofilamentous axonal masses in man, *Neurology*, 26, 919, 1976.
153. **David, O. J.**, Blood lead levels, behavior and intelligence, *Lancet*, 1, 866, 1974.
154. **Davies, P., Katzinan, R. D., and Terry, R. D.**, Reduced somatostatin-like immunoreactivity in cerebral cortex from cases of Alzheimer disease and Alzheimer senile dementia, *Nature (London)*, 288, 279, 1980.
155. **Davies, P. and Maloney, A. J. F.**, Selective loss of central cholinergic neurons in Alzheimer's disease, *Lancet*, 2, 1403, 1976.
156. **Davies-Jones, G. A. B.**, Lactate dehydrogenase and glutamic oxalacetic transaminase of the cerebrospinal fluid in neurological disease, *J. Neurol. Sci.*, 11, 583, 1970.
157. **Davis, G., Buchsbaum, M. S., and Bunney, W. E., Jr.**, Research in endorphins and schizophrenia, *Schizophr. Bull.*, 5, 244, 1979.
158. **Davis, J. M.**, Theories of biological etiology of affective disorders, *Int. Rev. Neurobiol.*, 12, 145, 1970.
159. **Davis, L. E., Standefer, J. C., Kornfeld, M., Abercrombie, D. M., and Butler, C.**, Acute thallium poisoning: toxicological and morphological studies of the nervous system, *Ann Neurol.*, 10, 38, 1981.
160. **Davis, L. E., Wands, J. R., Weiss, S. A., Price, D. L., and Girling, E. F.**, Central nervous system intoxication from mercurous chloride laxatives, *Arch. Neurol.*, 30, 428, 1974.
161. **Davison, A. N. and Cuzner, M. L.**, Immunochemistry and biochemistry of myelin, *Br. Med. Bull.*, 33, 60, 1977.
162. **Deakin, J. F. W.**, Alzheimer's disease: recent advances and future prospects, *Br. Med. J.*, 287, 1323, 1983.
163. **De Jager, A. E. J., Van Weerden, T. W., Houthoff, H. J., and De Monchy, J. G. R.**, Polyneuropathy after massive exposure to parathion, *Neurology*, 31, 603, 1981.
164. **DeWied, D.**, Peptides and behavior, in *Memory and Transfer of Information*, Zippel, H. P., Ed., Plenum Press, New York, 1973, 373.

165. **De Wolff, F. A.,** Neurologic aspects of mushroom intoxications, in *Handbook of Clinical Neurology, Chemical Intoxication of the Nervous System,* Part I, Vol. 36, Vinken, P. J. and Bruyn, G. W., Eds., North-Holland, Amsterdam, 1979, 259—546.

166. **de Yebenes, J. G., Gervas, J. J., Iglesias, J., Mena, M. A., Martin del Rio, R., and Somoza, E.,** Biochemical findings in a case of Parkinsonism secondary to brain tumor, *Ann. Neurol.,* 11, 313, 1982.

167. **DiDonato, S., Rimoldi, M., Moise, A., Bertagnoglio, B., and Uziel, G.,** Fatal ataxic encephalopathy and carnitine acetyltransferase deficiency: a functional defect of pyruvate oxidation?, *Neurology,* 29, 1578, 1979.

168. **Diniz, C. R. and Corrado, A. P.,** Venoms of insects and arachnids, in *International Encyclopedia of Pharmacology and Therapeutics,* Sect. 71, Vol. 2, Raskova, H., Ed., Pergamon Press, Oxford, 1971, 117—140.

169. **Dolcourt, J. L., Hamrick, H., O'Tauma, L., Wooten, J., and Baker, E.,** Increased lead burden in children of battery workers, *Pediatrics,* 62, 563, 1978.

170. **Dougherty, J. H., Jr., Rawlinson, D. G., Levy, D. E., and Plum, F.,** Hypoxic-ischemic brain injury and vegetative state: clinical and neuropathologic correlation, *Neurology,* 31, 991, 1981.

171. **Drachman, D. B.,** Botulinum toxin as a tool for research on the nervous system, in *Neuropoisons: Their Pathophysiological Actions* Simpson, L. L. and Curtis, D. R., Eds., Plenum Press, New York, 1971, 325—347.

172. **Drysdale, A., Deacon, R., Lewis, P., Olley, J., Electricwala, A., and Sherwood, R.,** A peptide-containing fraction of plasma from schizophrenic patients which binds to opiate receptors and induces hyperreactivity in rats, *Neuroscience,* 7, 1567, 1982.

173. **Dubowitz, V. and Rogers, K. J.,** 5-Hydroxyindoles in the cerebrospinal fluid of infants with Down's syndrome and muscle hypotonia, *Dev. Med. Child Neurol.,* 11, 730, 1969.

174. **Duffner, P. K., Cohen, M. E., and Freeman, A. I.,** Pediatric brain tumors: an overview, *CA: A Cancer Journal for Clinicians,* 35, 287, 1985.

175. **Duffy, F. H., Burchfield, J. L., Bartels, P. H., Gaon, M., and Sim, V. M.,** Long-term effects of an organophosphate upon the human electroencephalogram, *Toxicol. Appl. Pharmacol.,* 47, 161, 1979.

176. **Duffy, T. J.,** Pharmacology of mushroom poisoning, *N. Engl. J. Med.,* 289, 379, 1973.

177. **Dunleavy, D. L. F., Brezinova, V., and Oswald, I.,** Changes during weeks in effects of tricyclic drugs on the human sleeping brain, *Br. J. Psychiatry,* 120, 663, 1972.

178. **Dwyer, B. E., Wasterlain, C. G., Fujikawa, D. G., and Yamada, L.,** Brain protein metabolism in epilepsy, *Adv. Neurol.,* 44, 903, 1986.

179. **Dyck, P. J., O'Brien, P. C., and Ohnishi, A.,** Lead neuropathy II. Random distribution of segmental demyelination among "old internodes" of myelinated fibres, *J. Neuropathol. Exp. Neurol.,* 36, 570, 1977.

180. **Dyck, P. J., Yao, J. K., Knickerbocker, E., Holman, R. T., Gomez, M. R., Hayles, A. B., and Lambert, E. H.,** Multisystem neuronal degeneration, hepatosplenomegaly and adrenocortical deficiency associated with reduced tissue arachidonic acid, *Neurology,* 31, 925, 1981.

181. **Dyball, R. E. J., Dyer, R. G., and Drewett, R. F.,** Chemical sensitivity of preoptic neurons which project to the medial basal hypothalamus, *Brain Res.,* 71, 140, 1974.

182. **Dyer, R. G. and Dyball, R. E.,** Evidence for a direct effect of LRF and TRF on single unit activity in the rostral hypothalamus, *Nature (London),* 252, 486, 1974.

183. **Ebner, K., Liss, L., Couri, D., and Chou, M.,** Relationship between the neurofibrillary tangle, neuraxonal degeneration, aluminum level and clinical symptomology, *Fed. Proc.,* 34, 3564a, 1975.

184. Editorial, Alcohol and the brain, *Br. Med. J.,* 1, 1168, 1976.

185. Editorial, Alcoholism, an inherited disease?, *Br. Med. J.,* 281, 1301, 1980.

186. Editorial, CSF protein in psychiatric disorders, *Br. Med. J.,* 1, 582, 1970.

187. Editorial, Herpes virus and psychiatric disorders, *Br. Med. J.,* 1, 418, 1971.

188. Editorial, Idiosyncratic neurotoxicity: clioquinol and bismuth, *Lancet,* 1, 857, 1980.

189. Editorial, Interactions of drugs and amines in the brain, *N. Engl. J. Med.,* 286, 542, 1972.

190. Editorial, Lead and mental handicap, *Lancet,* 1, 365, 1978.

191. Editorial, Minor brain damage and alcoholism, *Br. Med. J.,* 1, 283, 455, 1981.

192. Editorial, Neurological complications of influenza, *Br. Med. J.,* 1, 248, 1970.

193. Editorial, Nutrition and the developing brain, *Lancet,* 2, 1349, 1972.

194. Editorial, Problems of phenylketonuria, *Br. Med. J.,* 4, 695, 1971.

195. Editorial, Sleep and metabolism, *Br. Med. J.,* 2, 650, 1973.

196. Editorial, Vitamin E deficiency, *Lancet,* 1, 423, 1986.

197. **Ehmann, W. D., Alauddin, M., Hossain, T. I. M., and Markesbery, W. R.,** Brain trace elements in Pick's disease, *Ann. Neurol.,* 15, 102, 1984.

198. **Ehringer, H. and Hornykiewicz, O.,** Verteilung von Noradrenalin und Dopamin (3-Hydroxy-tyramin) in Gehirn des Menschen under Verhalten beim Erkrankungen des extrapyramidalen Systems, *Klin. Wochenschr.,* 38, 1236, 1960.

199. **Einstein, E. R., Csejtey, J., Dalal, K. B., Adams, C. W. M., Bayliss, O. B., and Hallpike, J.,** Proteolytic activity and basic protein loss in and around multiple sclerosis plaques: combined biochemical and histochemical observations, *J. Neurochem.,* 19, 653, 1972.

200. **Emrich, H., Holit, V., Kissling, W., Fischer, M., Lasfe, H., Heinemann, H., von Zerssen, D., and Herz, A.,** Endorphin-like immunoreactivity in cerebrospinal fluid and plasma of patients with schizophrenia and other neuropsychiatric disorders, *Pharmacopsychiatria,* 12, 269, 1979.

201. **Emrich, H., Zandig, M., Kissling, W., Dirlich, G., von Zerssen, D., and Herz, A.,** D-β-glycyl-endorphin in schizophrenia: a double blind trial in 13 patients, *Pharmakopsychiatrie,* 13, 290, 1980.

202. **Engle, J., Kuhl, D. E., Phelps, M. E., and Mazzioatta, J. C.,** Interictal cerebral glucose metabolism in partial epilepsy and its relation to EEG changes, *Ann. Neurol.,* 12, 510, 1982.

203. **Epstein, B. S., Epstein, J. A., and Postel, D. M.,** Tumors of spinal cord simulating psychiatric disorders, *Dis. Nerv. Syst.,* 32, 741, 1971.

204. **Esiri, M. M.,** Multiple sclerosis: a quantitative and qualitative study of immunoglobulin-containing cells in the central nervous system, *Neuropathol. Appl. Neurobiol.,* 6, 9, 1980.

205. **von Euler, U.S. and Gaddum, J. H.,** Unidentified depressor substance in certain tissue extracts, *J. Physiol.,* 72,74, 1931.

206. **Fastbom, J., Pazos, A., Probst, A., and Palacios, J. M.,** Adenosine A1 receptors in human brain: characterization and autoradiographic visualization, *Neurosci. Lett.,* 65, 127, 1986.

207. **Fehling, C. and Qvist, I.,** Ferritin concentration in cerebrospinal fluid, *Acta Neurol. Scand.,* 71, 510, 1985.

208. **Feldman, R. G.,** Trichloroethylene, in *Handbook of Clinical Neurology, Intoxications of the Nervous System,* Vol. 36, Part I, Vinken, P. J. and Bruyn, G. W., eds., North-Holland, Amsterdam, 1979, 457—476.

209. **Felix, D. and Akert, K.,** The effect of angiotensin II on neurones of subfornical origin, *Brain Res.,* 76, 350, 1974.

210. **Fennelly, J., Frank, O., Baker, H., and Levy, C. M.,** Peripheral neuropathy of the alcoholic: I. Aetiological role of aneurin and other B-complex vitamins, *Br. Med. J.,* 1290, 1964.

211. **Fibiger, H. C.,** The neurobiological substrates of depression in Parkinson's disease: a hypothesis, *Can. J. Neurol. Sci.,* 11, 105, 1984.

212. **Filla, A., DeMichele, G., Brescia Morra, V., Palma, V., DiLauro, A., DiGeronimo, G., and Campanella, G.,** Glutamate dehydrogenase in human brain: regional distribution and properties, *J. Neurochem.,* 46, 422, 1986.

213. **Fillon, G. and Fillon, M.,** Modulation of affinity of postsynaptic serotonin receptors by antidepressant drugs, *Nature (London),* 292, 349, 1981.

214. **Finck, P. A.,** Exposure to carbon monoxide: review of the literature and 567 autopsies, *Mil. Med.,* 131, 1513, 1966.

215. **Fischer-Ferraro, C., Nahmod, V. E., Goldstein, D. J., and Finkelman, S.,** Angiotensin and renin in rat and dog brain, *J. Exp. Med.,* 133, 353, 1971.

216. **Fischer-Williams, M. and Roberts, R. C.,** Cerebrospinal fluid proteins and serum immunoglobulins. Occurrence in multiple sclerosis and other neurological diseases: comparative measurement of globulin and the IgG class, *Arch. Neurol.,* 25, 526, 1971.

217. **Fisher, A. E.,** Chemical stimulation of the brain, *Sci. Am.,* 210, 60, 1964.

218. **Fishman, E. B., Siek, G. C., MacCallum, R. D., Bird, E. D., Volicer, L., and Marquis, J. K.,** Distribution of the molecular forms of acetylcholinesterase in human brain: alterations in dementia of the Alzheimer type, *Ann. Neurol.,* 19, 246, 1986.

219. **Fishman, R. A.,** *Cerebrospinal Fluid in Diseases of the Nervous System,* W. B. Saunders, Philadelphia, 1980.

220. **Fliers, E., Swaab, D. T., Pool, C. W., and Verwer, R. W.,** The vasopressin and oxytocin neurons in the human supraoptic and paraventicular nucleus; changes with aging and in senile dementia, *Brain Res.,* 342, 45, 1985.

221. **Ford, R. C. and Berman, J. L.,** Phenylalanine metabolism and intellectual functioning among carriers of phenylketonuria and hyperphenylalaninaemia, *Lancet,* 1, 767, 1977.

222. **Forno, L. S.,** Pathology of Parkinson's disease, in *Movement Disorders,* Marsden, C. D. and Fahn, S., Eds., Butterworths, London, 1982, 25.

223. **Forssman, H. and Hambert, G.,** Incidence of Klinefelter's syndrome among mental patients, *Lancet,* 1, 1327, 1963.

224. **Foster, N. L., Newman, R. P., LeWitt, P. A., Gillespie, M. M., Larsen, T. A., and Chase, T. N.,** Peripheral beta-adrenergic blockade treatment of Parkinsonian tremor, *Ann. Neurol.,* 16, 505, 1984.

225. **Fox, R. H., Davies, T. W., Marsh, F. P., and Urich, H.,** Hypothermia in a young man with an anterior hypothalamic lesion, *Lancet,* 1, 185, 1970.

226. **Fredrickson, P. and Richelson, E.,** Dopamine and schizophrenia — a review, *J. Clin. Psychiatry,* 40, 399, 1979.

227. **Friedlander, W. J., Ed.,** Current reviews, the role of the neurotransmitters in the epilepsies, *Adv. Neurol.,* 13, 85, 115, 124, 1975.
228. **Frohman, L. A.,** Clinical neuropharmacology of hypothalamic releasing factors, *N. Engl. J. Med.,* 286, 1391, 1972.
229. **Fullerton, P. M.,** Toxic chemicals and peripheral neuropathy: clinical and epidemiological features, *Proc. R. Soc. Med.,* 62, 201, 1969.
230. **Fullerton, P. M. and Kramer, M.,** Neuropathy after intake of thalidomide, *Br. Med. J.,* 2, 855, 1961.
231. **Fume, L.,** Mechanism of action of phalloidin, *Lancet,* 1, 1284, 1965.
232. **Fuxe, K.,** Evidence for the existence of monoamine neurons in the central nervous system IV. The distribution of monoamine nerve terminals in the central nervous system, *Acta Physiol. Scand. Suppl.,* 247, 37, 1965.
233. **Gallhofer, B., Trimble, M. R., Frackowiak, R., Gibbs, J., and Jones, T.,** A study of cerebral blood flow and metabolism in epileptic psychosis, *J. Neurol. Neurosurg, Psychiatry,* 48, 201, 1985.
234. **Ganther, H. E.,** Modification of methylmercury toxicity and metabolism by selenium and vitamin E possible mechanisms, *Environ. Health Perspect.,* 25, 71, 1978.
235. **Garland, H. and Pearce, J.,** Neurological complications of carbon monoxide poisoning, *Q. J. Med.,* 36, 445, 1967.
236. **Garland, T. O. and Patterson, M. W. H.,** Six cases of acrylamide poisoning, *Br. Med. J.,* 4, 134, 1967.
237. **Ghose, K., Coppen, A., and Carroll, D.,** Intravenous tyramine response in migraine before and during treatment with indoramin, *Br. Med. J.,* 1, 1191, 1977.
238. **Ginsberg, M. D.,** Carbon monoxide intoxication: clinical features, neuropathology and mechanisms of injury, *J. Toxicol. Clin. Toxicol.,* 23, 281, 1985.
239. **Ginsberg, M. D.,** Delayed neurological deterioration following hypoxia, in *Cerebral Hypoxia and its Consequences, Advances in Neurology,* Fahn, S., Davis, J. N., and Rowland, L. P., Eds., Raven Press, New York, 1979, 21.
240. **Giulian, D., Allen, R. L., Baker, T. J., and Tomozawa, Y.,** Brain peptides and glial growth I. Glia-promoting factors as regulators of gliogenesis in the developing and injured central nervous system, *J. Cell Biol.,* 102, 803, 1986.
241. **Giurgea, C., Daliers, J., and Rigaux, M. L.,** Pharmacological studies on an elementary model of learning — the fixation of an experience at spinal level. II Specific shortening of the spinal cord fixation time (SFT) by a brain extract, *Arch. Int. Pharmacodyn. Ther.,* 191, 292, 1971.
242. **Glaser, G. H.,** Antiepileptic drugs: mechanisms of action, in *Advances in Neurology,* Vol. 27, Penry, J. K. and Woodbury, D. M., Eds., Raven Press, New York, 1980.
243. **Glassman, A.,** Indoleamines and affective disorders, *Psychosom. Med.,* 31, 107, 1969.
244. **Glassman, E.,** The biochemistry of learning: an evaluation of the role of RNA and protein, *Annu. Rev. Biochem.,* 39, 605, 1969.
245. **Glover, V., Sandler, M., Grant, E., Rose, F. C., Orton, D., Wilkinson, M., and Stevens, D.,** Transitory decrease in platelet monoaminooxidase activity during migraine attacks, *Lancet,* 1, 391, 1977.
246. **Goldsmith, J. R.,** Contribution of motor vehicle exhaust, industry and cigarette smoking to community carbon monoxide exposures, *Ann. N.Y. Acad. Sci.,* 174, 122, 1970.
247. **Goldstein, D. B.,** The alcohol withdrawal syndrome. A view from the laboratory, *Rec. Dev. Alcohol,* 4, 231, 1986.
248. **Goldstein, E. and Hoeprich, P. D.,** Diphtheria, in *Infectious Diseases,* Hoeprich, P. D., Ed., Harper & Row, New York, 1977, 247—255.
249. **Goldstein, G. W. and Diamond, I.,** Metabolic basis of lead encephalopathy, in *Brain Dysfunction in Metabolic Disorders,* Vol. 53, Plum, F., Ed., Williams & Wilkins, New York, 1974.
250. **Goldstein, N. P., Tauxe, W. N., McCall, J. T., Randall, R. V., and Gross, J. B.,** Wilson's disease (hepatolenticular degeneration). Treatment with penicillamine and changes in hepatic trapping of radioactive copper, *Arch. Neurol.,* 24, 391, 1971.
251. **Gomes, V. C. R., Shanley, B. C., Potgieter, L., and Roux, J. T.,** Noradrenergic over-activity in chronic schizophrenia: evidence based on cerebrospinal fluid noradrenaline and cyclic nucleotide concentrations, *Br. J. Psychiatry,* 137, 346, 1980.
252. **Gordon, E. B.,** Carbon-monoxide encephalopathy, *Br. Med. J.* 1, 1232, 1965.
253. **Gordon, R. D., Wolfe, L. K., Island, D. P., and Liddle, G. W.,** A diurnal rhythm in plasma renin activity in man, *J. Clin. Invest.,* 45, 1587, 1966.
254. **Gosling, R., Kerry, R. J., and Orme, J. E.,** Creatine phosphokinase activity in newly admitted psychiatric patients, *Br. J. Psychiatry,* 121, 351, 1972.
255. **Goto, I., Matsumura, M., Inoue, N., Murai, Y., Shida, K., Santa, T., and Kuroiwa, Y.,** Toxic polyneuropathy due to glue sniffing, *J. Neurol. Neurosurg. Psychiatry,* 37, 848, 1974.
256. **Grant, C. A.,** Pathology of experimental methylmercury intoxication: some problems of exposure and response, in *Mercury, Mercurials and Mercaptans,* Miller, M. W. and Clarkson, T. W., Eds., Charles C Thomas, Springfield, IL, 1973.

257. **Grasso, P., Sharratt, M., Davies, D. M., and Irvine, D.,** Neurophysiological and psychological disorders and occupational exposure to organic solvents, *Food Chem. Toxicol.,* 22, 819, 1984.

258. **Green, J. B., Oldewurtel, H., O'Doherty, D. S., Foster, F. M., and Sanchez-Longo, L. P.,** Cerebrospinal fluid glutamic oxalacetic transaminase activity in neurologic disease, *Neurology,* 7, 313, 1957.

259. **Green, J. B., Papadopoulos, N., Cevallos, W., Foster, F. M., and Hess, W. C.,** The cholesterol and cholesterol ester content of cerebrospinal fluid in patients with multiple sclerosis and other neurological diseases, *J. Neurol. Neurosurg. Psychiatry,* 22, 117, 1959.

260. **Greenwald, B. S. and Davis, K. L.,** Experimental pharmacology of Alzheimer disease, in *The Dementias,* Mayeux, R. and Rosen, W. G., Eds., Raven Press, New York, 1983, 87.

261. **Gresham, S. C., Agnew, H. W., and Williams, H. L.,** The sleep of depressed patients, *Arch. Gen. Psychiatry,* 13, 503, 1965.

262. **Griffin, J. W., Hoffman, R. M., Clark, A. W., Carroll, P. T., and Price, D. L.,** Slow axonal transport of neurofilament proteins: impairment by '-imino-dipropionitrile, *Science,* 202, 633, 1978.

263. **Griffin, J. W., Price, D. L., Engel, W. K., and Drachman, D.,** The pathogenesis of reactive axonal swellings: role of axonal transport, *J. Neuropathol. Exp. Neurol.,* 36, 214, 1977.

264. **Gumpert, J., Sharpe, D., and Curzon, G.,** Amine metabolites in the cerebrospinal fluid in Parkinson's disease and the response to levodopa, *J. Neurol. Sci.,* 19, 1, 1973.

265. **Gutman, Y. and Weil-Malherbe, H.,** The intracellular distribution of brain catecholamines, *J. Neurochem.,* 14, 619, 1967.

266. **Guttman, H. N., Matwyshyn, G., and Warriner, G. H.,** Synthetic scotophobin-mediated passive transfer of dark avoidance, *Nature (London) New Biol.,* 235, 26, 1972.

267. **Habermann, E.,** Tetanus, Infections of the nervous system, in *Handbook of Clinical Neurology,* Vol. 33, Part I, Vinken, P. J. and Bruyn, G. W., Eds., North-Holland, Amsterdam, 1978, 491—547.

268. **Habermann, E. and Cheng-Raude, D.,** Central neurotoxicity of apamin, crotamin, phospholipase A and L-amanitin, *Toxicon,* 13, 465, 1975.

269. **Haley, T. J.,** Saturnism, pediatric and adult lead poisoning, *Clin. Toxicol.,* 4, 11, 1971.

270. **Hallpike, J. F. and Adams, C. W. M.,** Proteolysis and myelin breakdown: a review of recent histochemical and biochemical studies, *Histochem. J.,* 1, 559, 1969.

271. **Hamburg, D. A.,** Effects of progesterone on behavior, *Res. Pub. Assoc. Res. Ment. Dis.,* 43, 215, 1966.

272. **Hanington, E.,** The effect of tyramine in inducing migrainous headache, in *Background to Migraine, Second Migraine Symposium,* Cochran, A. L., Eds., Heinemann, London, 1967, 113—19.

273. **Hanington, E., Jones, R. J., Amess, J. A. L., and Wachowicz, B.,** Migraine: a platelet disorder, *Lancet,* 2, 720, 1981.

274. **Hansen, H. E. and Amdisen, A.,** Lithium intoxication (report of 23 cases and review of 100 cases from the literature), *Q. J. Med.,* 47, 123, 1978.

275. **Hanson, J. W., Streissguth, A. P., and Smith, D. W.,** The effect of moderate alcohol consumption during pregnancy on fetal growth and morphogenesis, *J. Pediatr.,* 92, 457, 1978.

276. **Harding, A. E., Muller, D. P. R., Thomas, P. K., and Willison, H. J.,** Spinocerebellar degeneration secondary to chronic intestinal malabsorption: a vitamin E deficiency syndrome, *Ann. Neurol.,* 12, 419, 1982.

277. **Harrison, B. N., McDonald, W. I., and Ochoa, J.,** Remyelination in the central diphtheria toxin lesion, *J. Neurol. Sci.,* 17, 293, 1972.

278. **Hartmann, E. L.,** The sleep-dream cycle and brain serotonin, *Psychom. Sci.,* 8, 479, 1967.

279. **Hartvig, P.,** Chemical principles of chelate therapy in neurotoxicology, *Acta Neurol. Scand.,* 100, 199, 1984.

280. **Hashimoto, K. and Aldridge, W. N.,** Biochemical studies on acrylamide, a neurotoxic agent, *Biochem. Pharmacol.,* 19, 2591, 1970.

281. **Hass, J. R., McConnell, E. E., and Harvan, D. J.,** Chemical and toxicologic evaluation of Fire Master BP-6, *J. Agr. Food Chem.,* 26, 94, 1978.

282. **Hawkins, R. A.,** Transport of essential nutrients across the blood brain barrier of individual structures, *Fed. Proc.,* 45, 2055, 1986.

283. **Hayreh, M. S., Hayreh, S. S., Baumbach, G.L., Cancilla, P., Martin-Amat, G., Tephly, T. R., Martin, K. E., and Makar, A. B.,** Methyl alcohol poisoning III. Ocular toxicity, *Arch. Ophthalmol.,* 95, 1851, 1977.

284. **Heiblim, D. I., Evans, H. E., Glass, L., and Agbayani, M. M.,** Amino acid concentrations in cerebrospinal fluid, *Arch. Neurol.,* 35, 765, 1978.

285. **Heimann, H.,** Biologie der Schizophrenie, *Arch. Neurol. Psychiatry,* 132, 193, 1983.

286. **Heinberg, S. and Nikkanen, J.,** Enzyme inhibition by lead under normal urban conditions, *Lancet,* 1, 63, 1970.

287. **Hellstrand, E.,** Brain metabolism and human gait-a PET study, *Acta Physiol. Scand.,* 125, 555, 1985.

288. **Helting, T. B. and Zwisler, O.,** Structure of tetanus toxin. I. Breakdown of the toxin molecule and discrimination between polypeptide fragments, *J. Biol. Chem.,* 252, 187, 1977.

289. **Helting, T. B. and Zwisler, O.,** Structure of tetanus toxin. II. Toxin binding to ganglioside, *J. Biol. Chem.*, 252, 194, 1977.

290. **Henry, J. L., Krnjevic, K., and Morris, M. E.,** Substance P and spinal neurones, *Can. J. Physiol. Pharmacol.*, 53, 423, 1975.

291. **Henry, J. P., Stephens, P. M., Axelrod, J., and Meuller, R. A.,** Effect of psychosocial stimulation on the enzymes involved in the biosynthesis and metabolism of noradrenaline and adrenaline, *Psychosom. Med.*, 33, 227, 1971.

292. **Hershey, C. O., Hershey, L. A., Varnes, A., Vibhakar, S. D., Lavin, P., and Strain, W. H.,** Cerebrospinal fluid trace element content in dementia: clinical, radiologic and pathologic correlations, *Neurology*, 33, 1350, 1983.

293. **Herskowitz, A., Ishii, N., and Schaumburg, H.,** n-Hexane neuropathy, *N. Engl. J. Med.*, 285, 82, 1971.

294. **Hille, B.,** Ionic basis of resting and action potentials, in *Handbook of Physiology, The Nervous System*, Vol. 1, Section 1, Kandel, E. R., Ed., The American Physiological Society, Bethesda, MD, 1977.

295. **Hillarp, N. A., Fuxe, K., and Dahlstrom, A.,** Demonstration and mapping of central neurons containing dopamine, noradrenaline, and 5-hydroxytryptamine and their reactions to psychopharmaca, *Pharmacol. Rev.*, 18, 727, 1966.

296. **Hogstedt, C. and Axelson, O.,** Long-term health effects of industrial solvents — a critical review of the epidemiological research, *Med. Lav.*, 77, 11, 1986.

297. **Hommes, F. A.,** Amino acidaemias and brain maturation: interference with sulphate activation and myelin metabolism, *J. Inherit. Metab. Dis.* 8(Suppl. 1), 121, 1985.

298. **Hope, K., Philip, A. E., and Loughran, J. M.,** Psychological characteristics associated with XYZ sex-chromosome complement in a state mental hospital, *Br. J. Psychiatry*, 113, 495, 1967.

299. **Hornykiewicz, O.,** Die topische Lokalisation und das Verhalten von Noradrenalin und Dopamin im der Substantia der normalen und Parkinson kranken Menschen, *Wien. Klin. Wochenschr.*, 75, 309, 1963.

300. **Hornykiewicz, O.,** Dopamine (5-hydroxytyramine) and brain function, *Pharmacol. Rev.*, 18, 925, 1966.

301. **Hornykiewicz, O.,** Psychopharmacological implications of dopamine antagonists: a critical evaluation of current evidence, *Neuroscience*, 3, 773, 1978.

302. **Hornykiewicz, O., Lisch, H.-J., and Springer, A.,** Homovanillic acid in different regions of the human brain: attempt at localizing central dopamine fibres, *Brain Res.*, 11, 662, 1968.

303. **Humphrey, J. H.,** The value of immunological concepts in medicine, *J.R. Coll. Physicians*, 16, 141, 1982.

304. **Hunter, D.,** *The Diseases of Occupations*, 6th ed., London University Press, London, 1978.

305. **Hyden, H.,** *Biochemistry of the Central Nervous System*, Fourth Int. Congr., Biochem., Pergamon Press, New York, 1959, 64.

306. **Hyden, H. and Egyhazi, E.,** Nuclear RNA changes of nerve cells during a learning experiment in rats, *Proc. Natl. Acad. Sci. U.S.A.*, 48, 1366, 1962.

307. **Ishii, N. and Nishihara, Y.,** Pellagra among chronic alcoholics: clinical and pathological study of 20 necropsy cases, *J. Neurol. Neurosurg. Psychiatry*, 44, 209, 1981.

308. **Ishikawa, A., Ishiyama, H., Enomoto, T., Ozaki, A., Fukao, K., Okamura, T., Isawaki, Y., and Yamamoto, H.,** Hepatic coma and amino acids in the nerve endings of the central nervous system, *Life Sci.*, 37, 2129, 1985.

309. **Jacobson, M. and Hunt, R. K.,** The origins of nerve-cell specificity, *Sci. Am.*, 228, 26, 1973.

310. **Janowsky, D. S., Davis, J. M., El-Yousef, M. K., and Sekerke, H. J.,** Acetylcholine and depression, *Psychosom. Med.*, 35, 459, 1973.

311. **Jenkins, J. S.,** The hypothalamus, *Br. Med. J.*, 99, 1972.

312. **Johansson, B., Roos, B.-E., and Walinder, J.,** 5-HIAA and HVA in cerebrospinal fluid during delirium acutum, *N. Engl. J. Med.*, 286, 1160, 1972.

313. **Johnson, M. K.,** Organophosphorus esters causing delayed neurotoxic effects, *Arch. Toxicol.*, 34, 259, 1975.

314. **Johnson, R. T.,** The possible viral etiology of multiple sclerosis, *Adv. Neurol.*, 13, 1—46, 1975.

315. **Juan, H. and Lembeck, F.,** Influence of prostaglandin E₁, indomethacin, calcium and potassium on the action of nociceptive substances, *Naunyn-Schmiedeberg's Arch. Pharmacol.*, 283, 151, 1974.

316. **Juntunen, J.,** Alcoholic polyneuropathy, *Acta Med. Scand.*, 703, 265, 1985.

317. **Juntunen, J., Matikainen, E., Antti-Poika, M., Suoranta, S., and Valle, M.,** Nervous system effects of long-term occupational exposure to toluene, *Acta Neurol. Scand.*, 72, 512, 1985.

318. **Kales, A. and Kales, J. D.,** Sleep disorders, *N. Engl. J. Med.*, 290, 487, 1974.

319. **Kampine, J. P., Brady, R. O., Kanfer, J. N., Feld, M., and Shapiro, D.,** Diagnosis of Gaucher's disease and Niemann-Pick disease with small samples of venous blood, *Science*, 155, 82, 1967.

320. **Kane, F. J., Daly, R. J., Ewing, J. A., and Keeler, M. H.,** Mood and behavioural changes with progestational agents, *Br. J. Psychiatry*, 113, 265, 1967.

321. **Kantarjian, A. D. and Shaheen, A. S.,** Methyl bromide poisoning with nervous system manifestations resembling polyneuropathy, *Neurology*, 13, 1054, 1963.

322. **Kao, C. Y.,** Tetrodotoxin, saxitoxin and their significance in the study of excitation phenomena, *Pharmacol. Rev.,* 18, 997, 1966.

323. **Kao, I., Drachman, D., and Price, D. L.,** Botulinum toxin: mechanism of presynaptic blockade, *Science,* 193, 1256, 1976.

324. **Kaplan, J. G.,** Neurotoxicity of selected biological toxins, in *Experimental and Clinical Neurotoxicology,* Spencer, P. S. and Schaumburg, H. H., Eds., Williams & Wilkins, Baltimore, 1980, 631—648.

325. **Katzman, R., Fishman, R. A., and Goldensohn, E. S.,** Glutamic-oxaloacetic transaminase activity in spinal fluid, *Neurology,* 853, 1957.

326. **Keane, J. R.,** Toluene optic neuropathy, *Ann. Neurol.,* 4, 390, 1978.

327. **Kehoe, R. A.,** The metabolism of lead in man in health and disease. 2. Metabolism under abnormal conditions, *J. R. Inst. Public Health,* 24, 101, 1961.

328. **Kellerova, V.,** Electroencephalographic findings in workers exposed to benzene, *J. Hyg. Epidemiol. Microbiol. Immunol.,* 29, 337, 1985.

329. **Kelly, J. J., Dreifuss, J. J., and Krnjevic, K.,** Cortical inhibition and gamma-aminobutyric acid, *Exp. Brain Res.,* 9, 137, 1969.

330. **Kemali, D., Del Vecchio, M., and Maj, M.,** Increased noradrenaline levels in CSF and plasma of schizophrenic patients, *Biol. Psychiatry,* 17, 711, 1982.

331. **Kennedy, P. and Cavanagh, J. B.,** Spinal changes in the neuropathy of thallium poisoning, *J. Neurol. Sci.,* 29, 295, 1976.

332. **Kesson, C. M., Baird, A. W., and Lawson, D. H.,** Acrylamide poisoning, *Postgrad. Med. J.,* 53, 16, 1977.

333. **Killifer, F. A. and Stern, W. E.,** Chronic effects of hypothalamic injury, *Arch. Neurol.,* 22, 419, 1970.

334. **Kirshner, N.,** The function of the catecholamines in brain, *J. Neurosurg.,* 24, 165, 1966.

335. **Kish, S. J., Morito, C. L., and Hornykiewicz, O.,** Brain glutathione peroxidase in neurodegenerative disorders, *Neurochem. Pathol.,* 4, 23, 1986.

336. **Kleihures, P., Lang, W., Burger, P. C., Budka, H., Vogt, M., Maurer, R., Luthy, R., and Siegenthaler, W.,** Progressive diffuse leukoencephalopathy in patients with acquired immune deficiency syndrome (AIDS), *Acta Neuropathol. (Berlin),* 68, 333, 1985.

337. **Knave, B., Kolmodin-Hedman, B., Persson, H. E., and Goldberg, J. M.,** Chronic exposure to carbon disulfide: effects on occupationally exposed workers with special reference to the nervous system, *Work Environ. Health,* 11, 49, 1974.

338. **Knox, J. W. and Nelson, J. R.,** Permanent encephalopathy from toluene inhalation, *N. Engl. J. Med.,* 294, 948, 1976.

339. **Kobayashi, R. M.,** Drug therapy of tardive dyskinesia, *N. Engl. J. Med.,* 296, 257, 1977.

340. **Koelle, G. B.,** Acetylcholine — current status in physiology, pharmacology and medicine, *N. Engl. J. Med.,* 286, 1086, 1972.

341. **Koenig, M. G.,** The clinical aspects of botulism, in *Neuropoisons: Their Pathophysiological Actions,* Simpson, L. L. and Curtis, D. R., Eds., Plenum Press, New York, 1971, 283—302.

342. **Konishi, S. and Otsuka, M.,** The effects of substance P and other peptides on spinal neurons of the frog, *Brain Res.,* 65, 397, 1974.

343. **Konishi, S. and Otsuka, M.,** Excitatory action of hypothalamic substance P on spinal motoneurons of newborn rats, *Nature (London),* 252, 734, 1974.

344. **Krigman, M. R., Bouldin, T. W., and Mushak, P.,** Lead, in *Experimental and Clinical Neurotoxicology,* Spencer, P. S. and Schaumburg, H. H., Eds., Williams & Wilkins, New York, 1980, chap. 34.

345. **Krigman, M. R., Bouldin, T. W., and Mushak, P.,** Metal toxicity in the nervous system, *Monogr. Pathol.,* 26, 58, 1985.

346. **Krnjevic, K.,** Chemical signals in the brain, *Image,* 26, 3, 1968.

347. **Krnjevic, K. and Morris, M. E.,** Extracellular accumulation of K⁻ evoked activity of afferent fibers in the cuneate nucleus and dorsal horn of cats, *Can. J. Physiol. Pharmacol.,* 52, 852, 1974.

348. **Kustermann-Kuhn, B., Harzer, K., Schroder, R., Permanetter, W., and Peiffer, J.,** Pyruvate dehydrogenase activity is not deficient in the brain of three autopsied cases with Leigh disease (subacute necrotizing encephalomyelopathy, SNE), *Hum. Genet.,* 4, 68, 1984.

349. **Kuzuhara, S., Kanazawa, I., Nakanishi, T., and Egashira, T.,** Ethylene oxide polyneuropathy, *Neurology,* 33, 377, 1983.

350. **Ladosky, W. and Gaziri, L. C. J.,** Brain serotonin and sexual differentiation of the nervous system, *Neuroendocrinology,* 6, 168, 1970.

351. **Lamm, O. and Pratt, H.,** Subclinical effects of exposure to inorganic mercury revealed by somatosensory-evoked potentials, *Eur. Neurol.,* 24, 237, 1985.

352. **Lapresle, J. and Fardeau, M.,** The central nervous system and carbon monoxide poisoning. II. Anatomical study of brain lesions following intoxication with carbon monoxide (22 cases), *Prog. Brain Res.,* 24, 31, 1967.

353. **Ledermann, R. J. and Henry, C. E.,** Progressive dialysis encephalopathy, *Ann. Neurol.,* 4, 199, 1978.

354. **Lee, K., Moller, L., Hardt, F., Haubek, A., and Jensen, E.,** Alcohol-induced brain damage and liver damage in young males, *Lancet,* 2, 759, 1979.
355. **Leeman, S. E. and Mroz, E. A.,** Substance P, *Life Sci.,* 15, 2033, 1974.
356. **LeGreves, P., Nyberg, F., Terenius, L., and Hokfelt, T.,** Calciton in gene-related peptide is a potent inhibitor of substance P degradation, *Eur. J. Pharmacol.,* 115, 309, 1985.
357. **Leonard, J. V., Seakins, J. W. T., and Griffin, N. K.,** Beta-hydroxy-beta-methylglutaric-aciduria presenting as Reye's syndrome, *Lancet,* 1, 680.
358. **Leone, A., Pavlakis, G. N., and Hamer, D. H.,** Menkes' disease: abnormal metallothionein gene regulation in response to copper, *Cell,* 40, 301, 1985.
359. **LeQuesne, P. M.,** Commentary on contemporary neurotoxicity. Toxic substances and the nervous system: the role of clinical observations, *J. Neurol. Neurosurg. Psychiatry,* 44, 1, 1981.
360. **LeQuesne, P. M.,** Metal-induced diseases of the nervous system, *Br. J. Hosp. Med.,* 28, 534, 1982.
361. **Levine, S.,** Experimental cyanide encephalopathy: gradients of susceptibility in the corpus callosum, *J. Neuropath. Exp. Neurol.,* 26, 214, 1967.
362. **Lewis, P. D.,** Neuropathological effects of alcohol on the developing nervous system, *Alcohol Alcohol,* 20, 195, 1985.
363. **Liddle, G. W. and Hardman, J. G.,** Cyclic adenosine monophosphate as a mediator of hormone action, *N. Engl. J. Med.,* 285, 560, 1971.
364. **Lincoff, G. and Mitchell, D. H.,** *Toxic and Hallucinogenic Mushroom Poisoning,* Van Nostrand Reinhold, New York, 1977.
365. **Link, H.,** Immunoglobulin G and low molecular weight proteins in human cerebrospinal fluid, *Acta Neurol. Scand.,* 43, 28, 1967.
366. **Linz, D. H., de Garmo, P. L., Morton, W. E., Wiens, A. N., Coull, B. M., and Maricle, R. A.,** Organic solvent-induced encephalopathy in industrial painters, *J. Occup. Med.,* 28, 119, 1986.
367. **Longo, L. D.,** The biological effects of carbon monoxide on the pregnant woman, fetus, and newborn infant, *Am. J. Obstetr. Gynecol.,* 129, 69, 1977.
368. **Longo, L. D.,** Carbon monoxide: effects on oxygenation of the fetus in utero, *Science,* 194, 523, 1976.
369. **Loo, Y. H., Potempska, A., and Wisniewski, H. M.,** A biochemical explanation of phenyl acetate neurotoxicity in experimental phenylketonuria, *J. Neurochem.,* 45, 1596, 1985.
370. **Mackay, A. V. P., Iversen, L. L., Rossoz, M., Spokes, E., Bird, E., Arregui, A., Creese, I., and Snyder, S. H.,** Increased brain dopamine and dopamine receptors in schizophrenia, *Arch. Gen. Psychiatry,* 39, 991, 1982.
371. **Magos, L.,** The clinical and experimental aspects of carbon disulfide intoxication, *Rev. Environ. Health,* 2, 65, 1975.
372. **Magos, L. and Jarvis, J. A. E.,** The effects of carbon disulfide exposure on brain catecholamines in rats, *Br. J. Pharmacol.,* 39, 26, 1970.
373. **Mair, R. G., Langlais, P. J., Mazurek, M. F., Beal, M. F., Martin, J. B., and McEntee, W. J.,** Reduced concentrations of arginine vasopressin and MHPG in lumbar CSF of patients with Korsakoff's psychosis, *Life Sci.,* 38, 2301, 1986.
374. **Mann, D. M.,** The neuropathology of Alzheimer's disease: a review with pathogenetic, aetiological and therapeutic considerations, *Mech. Ageing Dev.,* 31, 213, 1985.
375. **Mark, L. C.,** Metabolism of barbiturates in man, *Clin. Pharmacol. Ther.,* 4, 504, 1963.
376. **Markowitsch, H. J. and Pritzel, M.,** The neuropathology of amnesia, *Prog. Neurobiol.,* 25, 189, 1985.
377. **Marsden, C. D., Barry, P. E., Parkes, J. D., and Zilkha, K. J.,** Treatment of Parkinson's disease with levodopa combined with L-alpha-methyldopa-hydrazine, an inhibitor of extracerebral dopa decarboxylase, *J. Neurol. Neurosurg. Psychiatry,* 36, 10, 1973.
378. **Marsh, D. O., Myers, G. J., Clarkson, T. W., Amin-Zaki, L., Tikriti, S., and Majeed, M. A.,** Fatal methylmercury poisoning: clinical and toxicological data on 29 cases, *Ann. Neurol.,* 7, 348, 1980.
379. **Martin, J. B.,** Neural regulation of growth hormone secretion, *N. Engl. J. Med.,* 288, 1384, 1973.
380. **Martin-Amat, G., McMartin, K. E., Hayreh, S. S., Hayreh, M. S., and Tephly, T. R.,** Methanol poisoning: ocular toxicity produced by formate, *Toxicol. Appl. Pharmacol.,* 45, 201, 1978.
381. **Martin-Amat, G., Tephly, T. R., McMartin, K. E., Maker, A. B., Hayreh, M. S., Hayreh, S. S., Baumbach, G., and Cancilla, P.,** Methyl alcohol poisoning. II. Development of a model for ocular toxicity in methyl alcohol poisoning using the Rhesus monkey, *Arch. Ophthalmol.,* 95, 1847, 1977.
382. **Martin Boyer, G.,** Intoxications par les sels de bismuth administre' par voie orale, *Gastroenterol. Clin. Biol.,* 2, 349, 1978.
383. **Martins, R. N., Harper, C. G., Stokes, G. B., and Masters, C. L.,** Increased cerebral glucose-6-phosphate dehydrogenase activity in Alzheimer's disease may reflect oxidative stress, *J. Neurochem.,* 46, 1042, 1986.
384. **Matsuda, M. and Yoneda, M.,** Isolation and purification of two antigenically active "complementary" polypeptide fragments of tetanus neurotoxin, *Infec. Immun.,* 12, 1147, 1975.
385. **Maugh, T. H.,** Multiple sclerosis: genetic link, viruses suspected, *Science,* 195, 667, 1977.

386. **Mayeux, R. and Rosen, W. G., Eds.,** *The Dementias,* Raven Press, New York, 1983.
387. **Maynert, E. W., Marczynski, T. J., and Browning, R. A.,** The role of neurotransmitters in the epilepsies, *Adv. Neurol.,* 13, 79—148, 1975.
388. **McAlpine, D. and Araki, S.,** Minamata disease, *Lancet,* 2, 629, 1958.
389. **McCann, S. M. and Porter, J. C.,** Hypothalamic pituitary stimulating and inhibiting hormones, *Physiol. Rev.,* 49, 240, 1969.
390. **McDermott, J. R., Smith, A. I., Iqbal, K., Wisniewski, H. M.,** Aluminium and Alzheimer's disease, *Lancet,* 2, 710, 1977.
391. **McDermott, J. R., Smith, A. I., Ward, M. K., Parkinson, I. S., and Kerr, D. N. S.,** Brain-aluminium concentration in dialysis encephalopathy, *Lancet,* 1, 907, 1978.
392. **McDonald, R. H., Goldberg, L. I., and McNay, J. L.,** Effects of dopamine in man: augmentation of sodium excretion, glomerular filtration rate and renal plasma flow, *J. Clin. Invest.,* 43, 1116, 1964.
393. **McDonald, W. I. and Kocen, R. S.,** Diphtheritic neuropathy, in *Peripheral Neuropathy,* Vol. 2, Dyck, P., Thomas, P. K., and Lambert, E. H., Eds., W.B. Saunders, Philadelphia, 1984, 2010—17.
394. **McEntee, W. J. and Mair, R. G.,** Memory impairment in Korsakoff's psychosis: a correlation with brain noradrenergic activity, *Science,* 202, 905, 1978.
395. **McEntee, W. J., Mair, R. G., and Langlais, P. J.,** Neurochemical pathology in Korsakoff psychosis: implications for other cognitive disorders, *Neurology,* 34, 648, 1984.
396. **McGoodall, C. and Alton, H.,** Metabolism of 3-hydroxytyramine (dopamine) in human subjects, *Biochem. Pharmacol.,* 17, 905, 1968.
397. **McGreer, P. L.,** The chemistry of the mind, *Am. Sci.,* 59, 221, 1972.
398. **McLachlan, D. R., Kruck, T. P., and Van Berkum, M. F.,** Aluminum and neurodegenerative disease: therapeutic implications, *Am. J. Kidney Dis.,* 6, 322, 1985.
399. **McLean, D. R., Jacobs, H., and Mielke, B. W.,** Methanol poisoning: a clinical and pathological study, *Ann. Neurol.,* 8, 161, 1980.
400. **McMillan, D. E. and Wenger, G. R.,** Neurobehavioral toxicology of trialkyltins, *Pharmacol. Rev.,* 37, 365, 1985.
401. **McNeal, E. T. and Cimbolic, P.,** Antidepressants and biochemical theories of depression, *Psychol. Bull.,* 99, 361, 1986.
402. **Meldrum, B. S.,** Excitatory amino acids and anoxic-ischemic brain damage, *Trends Neurosci.,* 8, 47, 1985.
403. **Meldrum, B. S.,** Neuropathological consequences of chemically and electrically induced seizures, *Ann. N.Y. Acad. Sci.,* 462, 186, 1986.
404. **Meltzer, H. Y.,** Creatinine kinase and aldolase in serum: abnormality common to acute psychoses, *Science,* 159, 1368, 1968.
405. **Merry, J. and Marks, V.,** The effect of alcohol, barbiturate and diazepam on hypothalamic/pituitary/adrenal function in chronic alcoholics, *Lancet,* 2, 960, 1972.
406. **Mesulam, M. M., Van Hoesen, G. W., and Bullers, N.,** Clinical manifestations of chronic B_1 deficiency in the Rhesus monkey, *Neurol. (Minneapolis),* 27, 239, 1977.
407. **Michenfelder, J. D.,** A valid demonstration of barbiturate-induced brain protection in man — at last, *Anaesthesiology,* 64, 140, 1986.
408. **Millar, J. A., Battistini, V., Cumming, R. L. C., Carswell, F., and Goldberg, A.,** Lead and delta-aminolaevulinic acid dehydratase levels in mentally retarded children and in lead-poisoned suckling rats, *Lancet,* 2, 695, 1970.
409. **Miller, F., Menninger, J., and Whitcup, S. M.,** Lithium-neuroleptic neurotoxicity in the elderly bipolar patient, *J. Clin. Psychopharmacol.,* 6, 176, 1986.
410. **Milner, G.,** Ascorbic acid in chronic psychiatric patients, *Br. J. Psychiatry,* 109, 294, 1963.
411. **Minton, S. A.,** *Venom Diseases,* Charles C Thomas, Springfield, IL, 1974.
412. **Mitsuma, T., Nogimovi, T., Sahaski, K., Adachi, K., Kihara, M., and Murakami, K.,** Thyrotropin releasing hormone levels in human cerebrospinal fluid in various neurologic diseases, *Am. J. Med. Sci.,* 29, 164, 1986.
413. **Miyabashi, S., Ito, T., Narisawa, K., Iinuma, K., and Tada, K.,** Biochemical study in 28 children with lactic acidosis in relation to Leigh's encephalomyelopathy, *Eur. J. Pediatr.,* 143, 278, 1985.
414. **Miyatake, T., Atsumi, T., Obayashi, T., Mizuno, Y., Ando, S., Ariga, T., Matsui-Nakamura, K., and Yamada, T.,** Adult type neuronal storage disease with neuraminidase deficiency, *Ann. Neurol.,* 6, 232, 1979.
415. **Moir, A. T. B., Ashcroft, G. W., Crawford, T. B. B., Eccleston, D., and Guldberg, H. C.,** Cerebral metabolites in cerebrospinal fluid as a biochemical approach to the brain, *Brain,* 93, 357, 1970.
416. **Moore, M. R. and Meredith, A.,** The carcinogenicity of lead, *Arch. Toxicol.,* 42, 87, 1979.
417. **Morgan, B. P., Campbell, A. K., and Compston, D. A. S.,** Terminal component of complement (C9) in cerebrospinal fluid of patients with multiple sclerosis, *Lancet,* 2, 251, 1984.

418. **Morre, D. M., Kirksey, A., and Das, G. D.,** Effects of vitamin B-6 deficiency on the developing central nervous system of the rat: myelination, *J. Nutr.,* 108, 1260, 1978.
419. **Moses, H. and Klawans, H. L.,** Bromide intoxication, in *Handbook of Clinical Neurology, Intoxications of the Nervous System,* Vol. 36, Vinken, P. J. and Bruyn, G. W., Eds., North-Holland, Amsterdam, 1979, 291—310.
420. **Moss, R. L., Dyball, R. E. J., and Cross, B. A.,** Excitation of antidromically identified neurosecretory cells of the paraventricular nucleus by oxitocin applied iontophoretically, *Exp. Neurol.,* 34, 95, 1972.
421. **Mueser, K. and Dysken, M.,** Narcotic antagonists in schizophrenia: a methological review, *Schizophr. Bulletin,* 9, 213, 1983.
422. **Muller, D. P. R., Lloyd, J. K., and Wolff, P. H.,** Vitamin E and neurological function, *Lancet,* 1, 225, 1983.
423. **Murai, Y. and Kuroiwa, Y.,** Peripheral neuropathy in chlorobiphenyl poisoning, *Neurology,* 21, 1173, 1971.
424. **Mustajoki, P. and Seppalainen, A. M.,** Neuropathy in latent hereditary hepatic porphyria, *Br. Med. J.,* 2, 310, 1975.
425. **Naber, D., Pickas, D., Post, R., Van Kammen, D., Waters, R., Ballenger, J., Goodwin, F., and Bunney, W. E., Jr.,** Endogenous opioid activity and β-endorphin immunoreactivity in CSF of psychiatric patients and normal volunteers, *Am. J. Psychiatry,* 138, 1457, 1981.
426. **Nagatsu, T., Levitt, M., and Udenfriend, S.,** Tyrosine hydroxylase. The initial step in norepinephrine biosynthesis, *J. Biol. Chem.,* 239, 2910, 1964.
427. **Namba, T., Greenfield, M., and Grob, D.,** Poisoning due to organophosphate insecticides, *Am. J. Med.,* 50, 475, 1971.
428. **Narabashi, T.,** Nerve membrane as a target for environmental toxicants, in *Experimental and Clinical Neurotoxicology,* chap. 16, Spencer, P. S. and Schaumburg, H.H., Eds., Williams & Wilkins, New York, 1980, 225—238.
429. **Nathanson, J. A. and Bloom, F. E.,** Heavy metals and adenosine cyclic 3′,5′-monophosphate metabolism: possible relevance to heavy metal toxicity, *Mol. Pharmacol.,* 12, 390, 1976.
430. National Research Council, Human vitamin B-6 requirements, *N.A.S.N.R.C. Publ.,* 129, 1978.
431. Neurofilamentous axonopathies. The neurotoxicology of acrylamides, hexacarbons, IDPN and carbon disulfide. Proc. 2nd Int. Conf. Neurotoxicology of Selected Chemicals, *Neurotoxicology,* 6, 1—98, 1985.
432. **Nicoll, R. A. and Barker, J. L.,** The pharmacology of recurrent inhibition in the supraoptic neurosecretory system, *Brain Res.,* 35, 501, 1971.
433. **Nicholls, P.,** Formate as an inhibitor of cytochrome oxidase, *Biochem. Biophys. Res. Commun.,* 67, 610, 1975.
434. **Nielson, J.,** Prevalence of Klinefelter's syndrome in patients with mental disorders, *Lancet,* 1, 1109, 1964.
435. **Nies, A., Robinson, D. S., and Ravaris, C. L.,** Amines and monoamine oxidase in relation to aging and depression in man, *Psychosom. Med.,* 33, 470, 1971.
436. **Nutt, J., Williams, A., Plotkin, C., Eng, N., Ziegler, M., and Calne, D. B.,** Treatment of Parkinson's disease with sodium valproate: clinical, pharmacological, and biochemical observations, *Can. J. Neurol. Sci.,* 6, 337, 1979.
437. **O'Brien, J. S.,** The cherry-red spot myoclonus syndrome: a newly recognized inherited lysosomal storage disease due to acid neuraminidase-deficiency, *Clin. Genet.,* 14, 55, 1978.
438. **Ochoa, J.,** Isoniazid neuropathy in man: quantitative electron microscope study, *Brain,* 93, 831, 1970.
439. **Olney, J. W.,** Excitatory transmitters and epilepsy-related brain damage, *Int. Rev. Neurobiol.,* 27, 337, 1985.
440. **Olney, J. W.,** Excitotoxic food additives — relevance of animal studies to human safety, *Neurobehav. Toxicol. Teratol.,* 6, 455, 1984.
441. **Olson, L., Blacklund, E. O., Freed, W., Hoffer, B., Seiger, A., and Shomberg, I.,** Transplantation of monoamine-producing cell systems in oculo and intracranially: experiments in search of a treatment for Parkinson's disease, *Ann. N.Y. Acad. Sci.,* 457, 105, 1985.
442. **O'Reilly, S., Strickland, G. T., Weber, P. M., Beckner, W. M., and Shipley, L.,** Abnormalities of the physiology of copper in Wilson's disease. I. The whole-body turnover of copper, *Arch. Neurol.,* 24, 385, 1971a.
443. **Osuntokun, B. O.,** An ataxic neuropathy in Nigeria, *Brain,* 91, 215, 1968.
444. **Osuntokun, B. O., Montecasso, G. L., and Wilson, J.,** Cassava diet and chronic degenerative neuropathy: an epidemiologic study, *Niger. J. Sci.,* 3, 3, 1969.
445. **Oswald, I., Ashcroft, G. W., and Berger, R. J.,** Some experiments in the chemistry of normal sleep, *Br. J. Psychiatry,* 112, 391, 1966.
446. **Owen, F., Cross, A. J., Crow, T. J., Poulter, M., and Waddington, J. L.,** Increased dopamine receptors in schizophrenia: specificity and relationship to drugs and symptomatology, in *Biological Psychiatry,* Perris, C., Struve, G., and Jansson, B., Eds., Elsevier/North-Holland, 1981, 699—706.

447. **Owen, F., Crow, T. J., Poulter, M., Cross, A. J., Longden, A., and Riley, G. J.,** Increased dopamine receptor sensitivity in schizophrenia, *Lancet,* 2, 223, 1978.

448. **Palay, S. L.,** The role of neuroglia in the organization of the central nervous system, in *Nerve as a Tissue,* Radahl, K. and Issekutz, B., Eds., Hoeber, New York, 1966.

449. **Pappenheimer, A. M., Jr.,** Diphtheria toxin, *Annu. Rev. Biochem.,* 46, 69, 1977.

450. **Pardridge, W. M. and Choi, T. B.,** Neutral amino acid transport at the human blood-brain barrier, *Fed. Proc.,* 45, 2073, 1986.

451. **Parent, A., Saint-Jacques, C., and Poirier, L. J.,** Effect of interrupting the hypothalamic nervous connections on the norepinephrine and serotonin content of the hypothalamus, *Exp. Neurol.,* 23, 67, 1969.

452. **Parker, J. C., Jr. and Philpot, J.,** Postmortem evaluation of Alzheimer's disease, *South Med. J.,* 78, 1411, 1985.

453. **Parkinson, I. S., Ward, M. K., Feest, T. G., Fawcett, P. R. W., and Kerr, D. N. S.,** Fracturing dialysis osteodystrophy and dialysis encephalopathy: an epidemiological survey, *Lancet,* 1, 406, 1979.

454. **Parlatore, A. A.,** Neuroendocrine aspects of psychiatric disorders, *N. Engl. J. Med.,* 289, 808, 1973.

455. **Pastan, I.,** Cyclic AMP, *Sci. Am.,* 14, 97, 1972.

456. **Patocka, J.,** The influence of Al^{+++} on cholinesterase and acetylcholinesterase activity, *Acta Biol. Med. Ger.,* 26, 845, 1971.

457. **Pearl, G. S. and Mullins, R. E.,** Alpha 1-antitrypsin in cerebrospinal fluid of patients with neurologic diseases, *Arch. Neurol.,* 42, 775, 1985.

458. **Pelletier, G., Labrie, F., Arimura, A., and Schally, A. V.,** Electron microscopic immunochemical localization of growth hormone-release inhibiting hormone (somatostatin) in the rat median eminence, *Am. J. Anat.,* 140, 445, 1974.

459. **Pelletier, G., Labrie, F., Puviana, R., Arimura, A., and Schally, A. V.,** Immunohistochemical localization of luteinizing-releasing hormone in the rat median eminence, *Endocrinology,* 95, 314, 1974.

460. **Pepper, G. M. and Krieger, D. T.,** Hypothalamic-pituitary-adrenal abnormalities in depression: their possible relation to central mechanisms regulating ACTH release, in *Neurobiology of Mood Disorders,* Post, R. M. and Ballenger, J. C., Eds., Williams & Wilkins, Baltimore, 1984, 245.

461. **Perry, E. K., Perry, R. H., Blessed, G., and Tomlinson, B. E.,** Changes in brain cholinesterases in senile dementia of Alzheimer's type, *Neuropathol. Appl. Neurobiol.,* 4, 273, 1978.

462. **Peters, H. A., Gocmen, A., Cripps, D. J., Bryan, G. T., and Dogramaci, I.,** Epidemiology of hex-achlorobenzene-induced porphyria in turkey: clinical and laboratory follow-up after 25 years, *Arch. Neurol. Chicago,* 39, 744, 1982.

463. **Pfeiffer, J., Majewski, F., Fischbach, H., Bierich, J. R., and Volk, B.,** Alcohol embryo and fetopathy, *J. Neurol. Sci.,* 41, 125, 1979.

464. **Phillips, S. C.,** Does ethanol damage the blood-brain barrier?, *J. Neurol. Sci.,* 50, 81, 1981.

465. **Phillis, J. W. and Limacher, J. J.,** Substance P excitation of cerebral cortical Betz cells, *Brain Res.,* 69, 158, 1974.

466. **Pleasure, D. B., Feldman, B., and Prockop, D. J.,** Diphtheria toxin inhibits the synthesis of myelin proteolipid and basic proteins by peripheral nerve in vitro, *J. Neurochem.,* 20, 81, 1973.

467. **Pleasure, D. E., Towfight, J., Silberberg, D., and Parris, J.,** The pathogenesis of hexachlorophene neuropathy: in vivo and in vitro studies, *Neurology,* 24, 1068, 1974.

468. **Politis, M. J., Schaumburg, H. H., and Spencer, P. S.,** Neurotoxicity of selected chemicals, in *Experimental and Clinical Neurotoxicology,* Spencer, P. S. and Schaumburg, H. H., Eds., Williams & Wilkins, New York, 1980, chap. 42.

469. **Pomara, N. and Stanley, M.,** The cholinergic hypothesis of memory dysfunction in Alzheimer's disease — revisited, *Psychopharm. Bull.,* 22, 110, 1986.

470. **Powell, D., Leeman, S. E., Treager, G. W., Niall, H. D., and Potts, J. T., Jr.,** Radioimmunoassay for substance P, *Nature (London) New Biol.,* 241, 252, 1973.

471. **Powell, H. C. and Lampert, P. W.,** Hexachlorophene neurotoxicity, in *Neurotoxicity,* Vol. 1, Roizin, L., Shiraki, H., and Grcevic, N., Eds., Raven Press, New York, 1977, 381—402.

472. **Prensky, A. L., Carr, S., and Moser, H. W.,** Development of myelin in inherited disorders of amino acid metabolism, *Arch. Neurol.,* 19, 552, 1968.

473. **Price, D. L. and Griffin, J. W.,** Neurons and ensheathing cells as targets of disease processes, in *Experimental and Clinical Neurotoxicology,* Spencer, P. S. and Schaumburg, H. H., Eds., Williams & Wilkins, Baltimore, 1980, 2.

474. **Price, D. L. and Griffin, J. W.,** Tetanus toxin: retrograde axonal transport of systemically administered toxin, *Neurosc. Lett.,* 4, 61, 1977.

475. **Price, D. L., Griffin, J. W., and Peck, K.,** Tetanus toxin: evidence for binding at presynaptic nerve endings, *Brain Res.,* 121, 379, 1977.

476. **Price, D. L., Kitt, C. A., Struble, R. G., Whitehouse, P. J., Cork, L. C., and Walker, L. C.,** Neurobiological studies of transmitter systems in aging and in Alzheimer type dementia, *Ann. N.Y. Acad. Sci.,* 457, 35, 1985.

477. **Price, D. L., Stocks, A., Griffin, J. W., Young, A., and Peck, K.,** Glycine-specific synapses in rat spinal cord, *J. Cell Biol.,* 68, 389, 1976.
478. **Price, D. L., Whitehouse, P. J., Struble, R. G., et al.,** Basal forebrain cholinergic systems in Alzheimer's disease and related dementias, *Neurosci. Comment.,* 1, 84, 1982.
479. **Prilipko, L. L.,** Biological studies of schizophrenia in Europe, *Schizophr. Bull.,* 12, 83, 1986.
480. **Pronicka, E. and Halikowski, B.,** Metabolic acidosis versus a compensation of respiratory alkalosis in four children with Leigh's disease, *J. Inher. Metab. Dis.,* 7(Suppl. 2), 113, 1984.
481. **Pumplin, D. W. and Reese, T. S.,** Action of brown widow spider venom and botulinum toxin on the frog neuromuscular junction examined with the freeze-fracture technique, *J. Physiol.,* 273, 443, 1977.
482. **Radcliffe, G. J., Jr., and Shelton, J. W.,** Specific facilitation of maze learning by a peptide extracted from trained mouse brain, *Fed. Proc.,* 32, 818, 1973.
483. **Raskind, M. A., Peskind, E. R., Lampe, T. H., Risse, S. C., Taborsky, G. J., and Dorsa, D.,** Cerebrospinal fluid vasopressin, oxytocin, somatostatin, and B-endorphin in Alzheimer's disease, *Arch. Gen. Psychiatry,* 43, 382, 1986.
484. **Rasmussen, H. and Tenehouse, A.,** Cyclic adenosine monophosphate, Ca + + and membranes, *Proc. Natl. Acad. Sci. U.S.A.,* 59, 1364, 1968.
485. **Rawnsley, K.,** Epidemiology of affective disorders. Recent developments in affective disorders, *Br. J. Psychiatry,* (Special Publication) 2, 27, 1968.
486. **Reis, D. J. and Wurtman, R. J.,** Diurnal changes in brain noradrenaline, *Life Sci.,* 7, 91, 1968.
487. **Reiter, L. W. and Ruppert, P. H.,** Behavioral toxicity of trialkyltin compounds: a review, *Neurotoxicology,* 5, 177, 1984.
488. **Renaud, L. P. and Martin, J. B.,** Thyrotropin releasing hormone (TRH): depressant action on central neuronal activity, *Brain Res.,* 86, 150, 1975.
489. **Renaud, L. P., Martin, J. B., and Brazeau, P.,** Depressant action of TRH, LH-RH and somatostatin on activity of central neurones, *Nature (London),* 255, 233, 1975.
490. **Renlund, M., Aula, P., Raivio, K. O., Autio, S., Sainio, K., Rapola, J., and Koskela, S.-L.,** Salla disease: a new lysosomal storage disorder with disturbed sialic acid metabolism, *Neurology,* 33, 57, 1983.
491. **Reuhl, K. R. and Chang, L. W.,** Effects of methylmercury on the development of the nervous system — a review, *Neurotoxicology,* 1, 21, 1979.
492. **Reynolds, E. H. and Trimble, M. R.,** Adverse neuropsychiatric effects of anticonvulsant drugs, *Drugs,* 29, 570, 1985.
493. **Reynolds, G. P. and Godridge, H.,** Alzheimer-like brain monoamine deficits in adults with Down's syndrome, *Lancet,* 2, 1368, 1985.
494. **Rimon, R., Terenius, L., and Kampman, R.,** Cerebrospinal fluid endophins in schizophrenia, *Acta Psychiatry Scand.,* 61, 395, 1980.
495. **Ritchie, J. M. and Rogart, R. B.,** The binding of saxitoxin and tetrodotoxin to excitable tissue, *Rev. Physiol. Biochem. Pharmacol.,* 79, 1, 1977.
496. **Robinson, S.,** Severe psychotic disturbance following crash diet weight loss, *Arch. Gen. Psychiatry,* 29, 559, 1973.
497. **Rodnight, R.,** Schizophrenia: some current neurochemical approaches, *J. Neurochem.,* 41, 12, 1983.
498. **Rosen, I.,** Neurophysiological aspects of organic solvent toxicity, *Acta Neurol. Scand.,* 100, 101, 1984.
499. **Rosenblatt, F., Farrow, J. T., and Rhine, S.,** The transfer of learned behavior from trained to untrained rats by means of brain extracts, *Proc. Natl. Acad. Sci. U.S.A.,* 55, 548, 1966.
500. **Rosengren, L. E., Kjellstrand, P., Aurell, A., and Haglid, K. G.,** Irreversible effects of dichloromethane on the brain after long-term exposure, *Br. J. Ind. Med.,* 43, 291, 1986.
501. **Rossor, M. N.,** Neurotransmitters and CNS disease: dementia, *Lancet,* 2, 1200, 1982.
502. **Rossor, M. N., Svendsen, C., Hunt, S. P., Mountjoy, C. Q., Roth, M., and Iversen, L. L.,** The substantia innominata in Alzheimer's disease: a histochemical and biochemical study of cholinergic marker enzymes, *Neurosci. Lett.,* 28, 217, 1982.
503. **Rothstein, A.,** Cell membrane as site of action of heavy metals, *Fed. Proc.,* 18, 1026, 1959.
504. **Roy, A., Pickar, D., Linnoila, M., Doran, A. R., and Paul, S. M.,** Cerebrospinal fluid monoamine and monoamine metabolite levels and the dexamethasone suppression test in depression, *Arch. Gen. Psychiatry,* 43, 356, 1986.
505. **Rustam, H. and Hamdi, T.,** Methyl mercury poisoning in Iraq — a neurological study, *Brain,* 97, 499, 1974.
506. **Rutter, M.,** Raised lead levels and impaired cognitive/behavioural functioning: a review of the evidence, *Dev. Med. Child Neurol.,* 22, 42, 1980.
507. **Ryba, M., Johansson, K., and Cybulska, A.,** Brain metabolism in deep controlled hypotension in neurosurgical patients, *Eur. J. Neurol.,* 24, 392, 1985.
508. **Saida, K., Mendell, J. R., and Sahenk, Z.,** Peripheral nerve changes induced by bee venom, *J. Neuropathol. Exp. Biol.,* 36, 783, 1977.

509. **Sakai, K. K., Marks, B. H., George, J., and Koestner, A.**, Specific angiotensin II receptors in organ-cultured canine supra-optic nucleus cells, *Life Sci.*, 14, 1337, 1974.

510. **Schantz, E. J., Lynch, J. M., Vayvada, G., Matsumoto, K., and Rapoport, H.**, The purification and characterization of the poison produced by Gonyaulax catenella in axemic culture, *Biochemistry*, 5, 1191, 1966.

511. **Schaumberg, H. H., Aresso, J., Otto, D. A., and Eckerman, D. A.**, Neurotoxic chemical exposure scenarios and suggested solutions, *Neurobehav. Toxicol. Teratol.*, 7, 351, 1985.

512. **Schildkraut, J. J. and Kety, S. S.**, Biogenic amines and emotion, *Science*, 156, 21, 1967.

513. **Schilling, R. F.**, Is nitrous oxide a dangerous anaesthetic for vitamin B-12 deficient subjects?, *JAMA*, 255, 1605, 1986.

514. **Schulsinger, F.**, Psychopathy: heredity and environment, *Int. J. Mental Health*, 1, 190, 1972.

515. **Schute, C. C. D. and Lewis, P. R.**, Comparison of distribution of cholinergic and monoaminergic systems of brain, *Nature (London)*, 212, 710, 1966.

516. **Scott, M.**, Transitory psychotic behavior following operation for tumors of the cerebello-pontine angle, *Psychiatr. Neurol. Neurochir.*, 73, 37, 1970.

517. **Seawright, A. A., Brown, A. W., Aldridge, W. N., Verschoyle, R. D., and Street, B. W.**, *Mechanisms of Toxicity and Hazard Evaluation*, Holmstedt, B., Mercier, R., and Roberfroid, M., Eds., Elsevier/North-Holland, Amsterdam, 1980.

518. **Segraves, R. T.**, Personality, body build and adrenocortical activity, *Br. J. Psych.*, 117, 405, 1970.

519. **Sellinger, O. Z., Schatz, R. A., and Gregor, P.**, Cerebral methylations in epileptogenesis, *Adv. Neurol.*, 44, 465, 1986.

520. **Sharman, D. F.**, Metabolism of tryptamine and related compounds in the central nervous system, *Br. Med. Bull.*, 21, 62, 1965.

521. **Sharpe, J. A., Mostovsky, M., Bilbao, J. M., and Rewcastle, N. B.**, Methanol optic neuropathy: a histopathological study, *Neurology*, 32, 1093, 1982.

522. **Sherwin, A. L., Norris, J. W., and Bulcke, J. A.**, Spinal fluid creatine kinase in neurologic disease, *Neurology*, 19, 993, 1969.

523. **Shimizu, Y.**, Developments in the study of paralytic shellfish toxins, in *Toxic Dinoflagellate Blooms*, Proc. 2nd Int. Conf. Toxic Dinoflagellate Blooms, Taylor, D. L. and Seliger, H. H., Eds., Elsevier North-Holland, New York, 1979, 321.

524. **Siesjo, B. K., Mgvar, M., and Wieloch, T.**, Epileptic grain damage: pathophysiology and neurochemical pathology, *Adv. Neurol.*, 44, 813, 1986.

525. **Simpson, L. L.**, The neuroparalytic and hemagglutinating activities of botulinum toxin, in *Neuropoisons — Their Pathophysiological Actions*, Vol. 1, Simpson, L. L., Ed., Plenum Press, New York, 1971.

526. **Sinder, C., Garten, L. L., and Lewis, P. D.**, The morphological effects of lead on the developing central nervous system, *Neuropathol. Appl. Biol.*, 9, 87, 1983.

527. **Sindic, C. J. M., Collet-Cassart, D., Cambiaso, C. L., Masson, P. L., and Laterre, E. C.**, The clinical relevance of ferritin concentration in the cerebrospinal fluid, *J. Neurol. Neurosurg. Psychiatry*, 44, 329, 1981.

528. **Sirek, A. and Sirek, O. V.**, Serotonin: a review, *Can. Med. Assoc. J.*, 102, 846, 1970.

529. **Sitaram, N. and Gillin, J. C.**, Acetylcholine: possible involvement in sleep and analgesia, in *Brain Acetylcholine and Neuropsychiatric Diseae*, Berger, P. and Davis, K., Eds., Plenum Press, New York, 1979, 311.

530. **Skerfving, S.**, Interaction between selenium and methylmercury, *Environ. Health Perspect.*, 26, 57, 1978.

531. **Smallwood, R. A., Williams, H. A., Rosenoer, V. M., and Sherlock, S.**, Liver-copper levels in liver disease. Studies using neutron activation analysis, *Lancet*, 2, 1310, 1968.

532. **Smith, J. S. and Brandon, S.**, Acute carbon monoxide poisoning — 3 years experience in a defined population, *Postgrad. Med. J.*, 46, 65, 1970.

533. **Smith, L.**, *Botulism, the Organism, its Toxins, the Disease*, Charles C Thomas, Springfield, IL, 1977.

534. **Snyder, R. D. and Seelinger, D. F.**, Methylmercury poisoning: clinical follow-up and sensory nerve conduction studies, *J. Neurol. Neurosurg. Psychiatry*, 39, 701, 1976.

535. **Snyder, S. H.**, Brain enzymes as receptors: angiotension-converting enzyme and enkephalin convertase, *Ann. N.Y. Acad. Sci.*, 463, 21, 1986.

536. **Snyder, S. H.**, Putative neurotransmittes in the brain: selective neuronal uptake, subcellular localization, and interactions with centrally acting drugs, *Biol. Psychiatry*, 2, 367, 1970.

537. **Snyder, S. H. and Yamamura, H. I.**, Antidepressant and the muscarinic acetylcholine receptor, *Arch. Gen. Psychiatry*, 34, 236, 1977.

538. **Somjen, G. G., Herman, S. P., Klein, R., Brubaker, P. E., Briner, W. H., Goodrich, J. K., Krigman, M. R. and Maseman, J. K.**, The uptake of methylmercury in different tissues related to its neurotoxic effects, *J. Pharmacol. Exp. Ther.*, 187, 602, 1973.

539. **Sorensen, P. S., Gjerris, A., and Hammer, M.**, Cerebrospinal fluid vasopressin in neurological and psychiatric disorders, *J. Neurol. Neurosurg. Psychiatry*, 48, 50, 1985.

540. **Sorensen, P. S., Hammer, M., Vorstrup, S., and Gjerris, F.,** CSF and plasma vasopressin concentrations in dementia, *J. Neurol. Neurosurg. Psychiatry,* 46, 911, 1983.

541. **Sourkes, T. L. and Poirier, L. J.,** Serotonin and dopamine in the extrapyramidal system, *Adv. Pharmacol.,* 6, 335, 1968.

542. **Spencer, P. S. and Schaumburg, H. H., Eds.,** *Experimental and Clinical Neurotoxicology,* Williams & Wilkins, New York, 1980.

543. **Spencer, P. S. and Schaumburg, H. H.,** A review of acrylamide neurotoxicity. I. Properties, uses and human exposure, *Can. J. Neurol. Sci.,* 1, 143, 1974.

544. **Spencer, P. S. and Schaumburg, H. H.,** A review of acrylamide neurotoxicity. II. Experimental animal neurotoxicity and pathologic mechanisms, *Can. J. Neurol. Sci.,* 1, 152, 1974.

545. **Stahl, S., Woo, D., Wefford, I., Berger, P., and Ciaranello, R.,** Hyperserotonemia and platelet serotonin uptake and release in schizophrenia and affective disorders, *Am. J. Psychiatry,* 140, 26, 1983.

546. **Sterman, A. B. and Schaumburg, H. H.,** Neurotoxicity of selected drugs, in *Experimental and Clinical Neurotoxicity,* Spencer, P. S. and Schaumburg, H. H., Eds., Williams & Wilkins, Baltimore, 1980, 593—612.

547. **Stewart, C. N., Coursin, D. B., and Bhagavan, H. N.,** Avoidance behavior in vitamin B-6 deficient rats, *J. Nutr.,* 105, 1363, 1975.

548. **Stewart, R. D.,** The effect of carbon monoxide on humans, *J. Occup. Med.,* 18, 304, 1976.

549. **Strahilevitz, M. and Starkey, D. D.,** Increased IgA in schizophrenic patients, *Lancet,* 1, 370, 1970.

550. **Streissguth, A. P., Herman, C. S., and Smith, D. W.,** Intelligence, behavior, and dysmorphogenesis in the fetal alcohol syndrome: a report on 20 patients, *J. Pediatr.,* 92, 363, 1978.

551. **Striefler, M., Cohn, D., Hirano, A., and Schujman, E.,** The central nervous system in a case of neurolathyrism, *Neurology,* 27, 1176, 1977.

552. **Supino-Viterbo, V., Sicard, C., Risvegliato, M., Rancurel, G., and Buge, A.,** Toxic encephalopathy due to ingestion of bismuth salts: clinical and EEG studies of 45 patients, *J. Neurol. Neurosurg. Psychiatry,* 40, 748, 1977.

553. **Sutherland, E. W. and Robison, G. A.,** The role of cyclic 3′,5′-AMP in response to catecholamines and other hormones, *Pharmacol. Rev.,* 18, 145, 1966.

554. **Suzuki, K., Katzman, R., and Korey, S. R.,** Chemical studies on Alzheimer's disease, *J. Neuropathol. Exp. Neurol.,* 24, 211, 1965.

555. **Sweeney, V. P., Perry, T. L., Price, J. D. E., Reeve, C. E., Godolphin, W. J., and Kish, S. J.,** Brain aminobutyric acid deficiency in dialysis encephalopathy, *Neurology,* 35, 180, 1985.

556. **Tahmoush, A. J., Alpers, D. H., Feigin, R. D., Armbrustmacher, V., and Prensky, A. L.,** Hartnup disease: clinical, pathological and biochemical observations, *Arch. Neurol.,* 33, 797, 1976.

557. **Takahasi, T., Konishi, S., Powell, D., Leeman, S. E., and Otsuka, M.,** Identification of the motoneuron-depolarizing peptide in bovine dorsal root as hypothalamic substance, *Brain Res.,* 73, 59, 1974.

558. **Takeuchi, T.,** Neuropathology of Minamata disease in Kumamoto: especially at the chronic state, in *Neurotoxicology,* Roizin, L., Shiraki, H., and Grcevic, N., Eds., Raven Press, New York, 1977.

559. **Taquet, H., Javoy-Agid, F., Giraud, P., Legrand, J. C., Agid, Y., and Cesselin, F.,** Dynorphin levels in parkinsonian patients: Leu-5-enkephalin production from either proenkephalin A or prodynorphin in human brain, *Brain Res.,* 341, 390, 1985.

560. **Taylor, G. R., Grow, T. J., Carter, F. I., and Gamble, S. I.,** Cytopathogenic cerebrospinal fluid from neurological and psychiatric patients, *Exp. Mol. Pathol.,* 42, 271, 1985.

561. **Taylor, J. R.,** Neurological manifestations in humans exposed to chlordecone: follow-up results, *Neurotoxicology,* 6, 231, 1985.

562. **Taylor, J. R.,** Neurotoxicity of certain environmental substances, *Clin. Lab. Med.,* 4, 489, 1984.

563. **Taylor, J. R., Selhorst, J. B., Houff, S. A., and Martines, A. J.,** Chlordecone intoxication in man, I, clinical observations, *Neurology,* 28, 626, 1978.

564. **Teisinger, J.,** New advances in the toxicology of carbon disulfide, *Am. Ind. Hyg. Assoc. J.,* 35, 55, 1974.

565. **Terenius, L., Wahlstrom, A., Lindstrom, L., and Widerloo, E.,** Increased CSF levels of endorphins in chronic psychosis, *Neurosci. Lett.,* 3, 157, 1976.

566. **Terry, R. D. and Katzman, R.,** Senile dementia of the Alzheimer type, *Ann. Neurol.,* 14, 497, 1983.

567. **Tokuomi, H., Uchino, M., Imamura, S., Yamanaga, H., Nakanishi, R., and Ideta, T.,** Minamata disease: (organic mercury poisoning) neuroradiologic and electrophysiologic studies, *Neurology,* 32, 1369, 1982.

568. **Tourtellotte, W. W. and Ma, B. I.,** Multiple sclerosis: the blood-brain-barrier and the measurement of de novo central nervous system IgG synthesis, *Neurology,* 28, 76, 1978.

569. **Trapp, G. A., Miner, G. D., Zimmerman, R. L., Mastri, A. R., and Heston, L. L.,** Aluminum levels in brain in Alzheimer's disease, *Biol. Psychiatry,* 13, 709, 1978.

570. **Tredici, G. and Minassi, M.,** Alcoholic neuropathy — an electron-microscopic study, *J. Neurol. Sci.,* 25, 333, 1975.

571. **Ueda, N., Miyazaki, K., Imai, S., and Fukunishi, R.,** Creutzfeldt-Jakob disease. An autopsy case of the panencephalopathic type and a review of the literature, *Acta Pathol. Jpn.*, 35, 1483, 1985.

572. **Ungar, G.,** Chemical transfer of learned behavior, *Agents Actions*, 1, 155, 1970.

573. **Ungar, G.,** Molecular coding of information in the nervous system, *Naturwissenschaften*, 60, 307, 1973.

574. **Ungar, G., Desiderio, D. M., and Parr, W.,** Isolation, identification and synthesis of a specific-behavior-inducing brain peptide, *Nature (London)*, 238, 198, 1972.

575. **Ungar, G., Galvan, L., and Chapouthier, G.,** Evidence for chemical coding of color discrimination in goldfish brain, *Experientia*, 28, 1026, 1972.

576. **Valcinkas, J. A., Lilis, R., Singer, R. M., Glickman, L., and Nicholson, W. J.,** Neurobehavioral changes among shipyard painters exposed to solvents, *Arch. Environ. Health*, 40, 47, 1985.

577. **Vanherweghem, J., Linkowski, P., and Mendlewicz, J.,** Hemodialysis in schizophrenics, *Arch. Gen. Psychiatry*, 40, 211, 1983.

578. **Van Heyningen, W. E. and Mellanby, J.,** Tetanus toxin, in *Microbial Toxins*, Vol. IIA, Kadis, S., Montie, T. C., and Ajl, S. J., Eds., Academic Press, New York, 1971.

579. **Van Itallie, T. B. and Follis, R. H.,** Thiamine deficiency, ariboflavinosis and vitamin B_6 deficiency, in *Harrison's Principles of Internal Medicine*, McGraw-Hill, New York, 1974, chap. 78.

580. **Van Praag, H. M.,** Significance of biochemical parameters in the diagnosis, treatment and prevention of depressive disorders, *Biol. Psychiatry*, 12, 101, 1977.

581. **Van Praag, H. M.,** The significance of dopamine for the mode of neuroleptics and the pathogenesis of schizophrenia, *Br. J. Psychiatry*, 130, 463, 1977.

582. **Van Praag, H. M., Verhoeven, W., van Ree, S., and de Wied, D.,** The treatment of schizophrenic psychoses with γ-type endorphins, *Biol. Psychiatry*, 17, 83, 1982.

583. **Van Sande, M., Mardens, Y., Adriaenssens, K., and Lowenthal, A.,** The free amino acids in human cerebrospinal fluid, *J. Neurochem.*, 17, 125, 1970.

584. **Victor, M.,** Alcoholism, in *Clinical Neurology*, Baker, A. B. and Baker, L. H., Eds., Harper & Row, New York, 1978, 1084—1129.

585. **Victor, M., Adams, R. D., and Collins, G. A.,** *The Wernicke-Korsakoff Syndrome*, Davis, Philadelphia, 1971.

586. **Vilter, R. W., Mueller, J. E., Glazer, H. S., Jarrold, A. J., Thompson, C., and Hawkins, V. R.,** The effect of vitamin B_6 deficiency produced by desoxypyridoxine in human beings, *J. Lab. Clin. Med.*, 42, 335, 1963.

587. **Vroom, F. Q. and Greer, M.,** Mercury vapour intoxication, *Brain*, 95, 305, 1972.

588. **Waksman, B. H.,** Immunity and the nervous system: basic tenets, *Ann. Neurol.*, 13, 587, 1983.

589. **Wallace, J. F.,** Disorders caused by venoms, bites and stings, in *Harrison's Principles of Internal Medicine*, Thorn, G. W., Adams, R. D., Braunwald, E., Isselbacher, K. I., and Petersdorf, R. G., Eds., McGraw-Hill, New York, 1977, 732—740.

590. **Walsh, J. C. and McLeod, J.,** Alcoholic neuropathy — an electrophysiological and histological study, *J. Neurol. Sci.*, 10, 457, 1970.

591. **Walsh, T. J., Schulz, D. W., Tilson, H. A., and Dehaven, D. L.,** Acute exposure to triethyl lead enhances the behavioral effects of dopaminergic agonists: involvement of brain dopamine in organolead neurotoxicity, *Brain Res.*, 363, 222, 1986.

592. **Walshe, J. M.,** The physiology of copper in man and its relation to Wilson's disease, *Brain*, 90, 149, 1967.

593. **Watanabe, Y., Tokomuto, H., Yamashita, A., Narumiya, S., Orizumo, N., and Hayishi, O.,** Specific binding of prostaglandin D2, E2 and F2 alpha in postmortem human brain, *Brain Res.*, 342, 110, 1985.

594. **Weaver, A. L.,** Lathyrism: a review, *Arthritis Rheum.*, 10, 470, 1967.

595. **Weiner, H. L. and Hauser, S. L.,** Neuroimmunology. I. Immunoregulation in neurological disease, *Ann. Neurol.*, 11, 437, 1982.

596. **Weiner, H. L. and Hauser, S. L.,** Neuroimmunology. II. Antigenic specificity of the nervous system, *Ann. Neurol.*, 12, 499, 1982.

597. **Weinstein, L.,** Diphtheria, in *Harrison's Principles of Internal Medicine*, Thorn, G. W., Adams, R. D., Braunwald, E., Isselbacher, K. E., and Petersdorf, R. G., Eds., McGraw-Hill, New York, 1977, 877—881.

598. **Werman, R.,** Criteria for identification of a central nervous system transmitter, *Comp. Biochem. Physiol.*, 18, 745, 1966.

599. **Wheatley, B., Barbeau, A., Clarkson, T. W., and Lapham, L. W.,** Methylmercury poisoning in Canadian Indians — the elusive diagnosis, *Can. J. Neurol. Sci.*, 6, 417, 1979.

600. **White, J. M. and Harney, D. R.,** Defective synthesis of alpha and beta chains in lead poisoning, *Nature (London)*, 236, 71, 1972.

601. **Whitfield, C. L., Ch'ien, L. T., and Whitehead, J. D.,** Lead encephalopathy in adults, *Am. J. Med.*, 52, 289, 1972.

602. **Wieloch, T.,** Neurochemical correlates to selective neuronal vulnerability, *Prog. Brain Res.*, 63, 69, 1985.

603. **Wilcock, A. R., Sharpe, D. M., and Goldberg, D. M.,** Kinetic similarity of enzymes in human blood serum and cerebrospinal fluid: aspartate aminotransferase and lactate dehydrogenase, *J. Neurol. Sci.,* 20, 97, 1973.

604. **Wilkins, J. N. and Gorelick, D. A.,** Clinical neuroendocrinology and neuropharmacology of alcohol withdrawal, *Rec. Dev. Alcohol.,* 4, 241, 1986.

605. **Williams, B.,** Cerebrospinal fluid pressure changes in response to coughing, *Brain,* 99, 331, 1976.

606. **Wilson, S. A. K.,** Progressive lenticular degeneration: a familial nervous disease associated with cirrhosis of the liver, *Brain,* 34, 295, 1911—12.

607. **Windle, W. F.,** Brain damage by asphyxia at birth, *Sci. Am.,* 220, 77, 1969.

608. **Winokur, A. and Utiger, R. D.,** Thyrotropin-releasing hormone: regional distribution in the rat brain, *Science,* 185, 265, 1974.

609. **Witt, E. D.,** Neuroanatomical consequences of thiamine deficiency: a comparative analysis, *Alcohol,* 20, 201, 1985.

610. **Wittels, B. and Bressler, R.,** Biochemical lesion of diphtheria toxin on the heart, *J. Clin. Invest.,* 43, 630, 1964.

611. **Wolff, J. R.,** The astrocyte as link between capillary and nerve cell, *Sandoz J. Med. Sci.,* 9, 153, 1970.

612. **Wood, J. D. and Peesker, S. J.,** Correlation between changes in GABA metabolism and isonicotinic hydrazide-induced seizures, *Brain Res.,* 45, 489, 1972.

613. **Wood, J. H.,** Neurochemical analysis of cerebrospinal fluid, *Neurology,* 30, 645, 1980.

614. Workshop on neurotoxicity testing in human populations, Rougemont, North Carolina, October 14—16, 1983, *Neurobehav. Toxicol. Teratol.,* 7, 283, 1985.

615. **Wright, G. P.,** The results of direct injections of botulinum toxin into the central nervous system of rabbits, *J. Physiol.,* 120, 618, 1953.

616. **Wurtman, R. J.,** Catecholamines, *N. Engl. J. Med.,* 273, 637, 1965.

617. **Wurtman, R. J.,** Catecholamines and neurologic diseases, *N. Engl. J. Med.,* 282, 45, 1970.

618. **Wurtman, R. J., Rose, C. M., and Chou, C.,** Daily rhythms in the concentrations of various amino acids in human plasma, *N. Engl. J. Med.,* 270, 171, 1968.

619. **Yang, H. Y., Goridis, C., and Neff, N. H.,** Properties of monoamine oxidases in sympathetic nerve and pineal gland, *J. Neurochem.,* 19, 1241, 1972.

620. **Yang, H. Y. and Neff, H. H.,** Distribution and properties of angiotensin converting enzyme of rat brain, *J. Neurochem.,* 19, 2443, 1972.

621. **Yates, C. M., Simpson, J., and Gordon, A.,** Regional brain 5-hydroxytryptamine levels are reduced in senile Down's syndrome as in Alzheimer's disease, *Neurosci. Lett.,* 65, 189, 1986.

622. **Yong, V. W. and Perry, T. L.,** Monoamine oxidase B, smoking and Parkinson's diseae, *J. Neurol. Sci.,* 72, 265, 1986.

623. **Youatt, J.,** A review of the action of isoniazid, *Am. Rev. Resp. Dis.,* 99, 729, 1969.

624. **Zilkha, K. J. and McArdle, B.,** The phospholipid composition of cerebrospinal fluid in diseases associated with demyelination, *Q. J., Med.,* 32, 79, 1963.

625. **Zippel, H. P. and Domagk, G. F.,** Versuche zur chemischen Gedachtnisübertragung von farbdressierten Goldfischen auf undressierte Tiere, *Experientia,* 25, 938, 1969.

626. **Zubenko, G. S., Volicer, L., Direnfeld, L. K., Freeman, M., Langlais, P. M., and Nixon, R. A.,** Cerebrospinal fluid levels of angiotensin-convering enzyme in Alzheimer's disease, Parkinson's disease and progressive supranuclear palsy, *Brain Res.,* 328, 215, 1985.

627. **Van Keuren, M. L., Goldman, D., and Merril, C. R.,** Protein variations associated with Down's syndrome, chromosome 21 and Alzheimer's diseae, in *Alzheimer's Disease, Down's Syndrome and Aging,* Sinex, F. M. and Merril, C. R., Eds., *Ann. N.Y. Acad. Sci.,* 396, 55, 1982.

628. **Feuer, G. and Broadhurst, P. L.,** Thyroid function in rats selectively bred for emotional elimination. I. Differences in thyroid hormones, *J. Endocrinol.,* 24, 147, 1962.

629. **Feuer, G. and Broadhurst, P. L.,** Thyroid function in rats selectively bred for emotional elimination. II. Differences in thyroid activity, *J. Endocrinol.,* 24, 253, 1962.

630. **Feuer, G. and Broadhurst, P. L.,** Thyroid function in rats selectively bred for emotional elimination. III. Behavioral and physiological changes after treatment with drugs acting on the thyroid, *J. Endocrinol.,* 24, 385, 1962.

631. **Feuer, G.,** Differences in emotional behavior and in function of the endocrine system in genetically different strains of albino rats, in *Physiology and Pathology of Adaptation Mechanisms,* Bajusz, E., Ed., Pergamon Press, Oxford, 1969, 214—233.

FURTHER READINGS

Asbury, A. K., McKhann, G. M., and McDonald, W. I., *Diseases of the Nervous System: Clinical Neurobiology,* Ardmore Medical Books, Philadelphia, 1986.
Bachelard, H. S., Lunt, G. G., and Marsden, C. D., *Clinical Neurochemistry,* Vol. 1 and 2, Academic Press, London, 1986.
Biggio, G. and Costa, E., *The Neurochemistry and Neurophamacology of Schizophrenia,* Elsevier, Amsterdam, 1987.
Björklund, A. and Hökfelt, T., *GABA and Neuropeptides in the CNS,* Elsevier, Amsterdam, 1985.
Blackwood, W. and Corsellis, J. A. N., *Greenfield's Neuropathology,* Edward Arnold, Baltimore, 1976.
Blum, K. and Manzo, L., *Neurotoxicology,* Marcel Dekker, New York, 1985.
Boulton, A. A. and Hrdina, P. D., *Receptor Binding,* Humana Press, Clifton, 1986.
Caputto, R. and Marsan, C. A., *Neural Transmission, Learning and Memory,* Raven Press, New York, 1983.
Collu, R., *Brain Neurotransmitters and Hormones,* Raven Press, New York, 1982.
Cooper, J. R., Bloom, F. E., and Roth, R. H., *The Biochemical Basis of Neuropharmacology,* Oxford University Press, New York, 1986.
Davis, R. L. and Robertson, D. M., *Textbook of Neuropathology,* Williams & Wilkins, Baltimore, 1985.
Dyck, P. J., *Peripheral Neuropathy,* 2nd ed., W. B. Saunders, Philadelphia, 1984.
Goldberg, A. M. and Hanin, I., *Biology of Cholinergic Function,* Raven Press, New York,1976.
Henn, F. A. and DeLise, L. E., *The Neurochemistry and Neuropharmacology of Schizophrenia,* Elsevier, Amsterdam 1987.
Hughes, J., *Centrally Acting Peptides,* University Park Press, Baltimore, 1978.
Jenner, P., *Neurotoxins and Their Pharmacological Implications,* Raven Press, New York, 1987.
Kunos, G., *Adrenoreceptors and Catecholamine Action,* Wiley, Boston, 1981.
Lajtha, A., *Handbook of Neurochemistry,* 2nd ed., Plenum Press, New York,1982.
Martin, J. B., Reichlin, S., and Blick, K. L., *Neurosecretion and Brain Peptides: Implications for Brain Functions and Neurological Disease,* Raven Press, New York,1981.
McIlwain, H. and Bachelard, H. S., *Biochemistry and the Central Nervous System,* 5th ed., Churchill Livingstone, New York, 1985.
Nemeroff, C. and Dunn, A. J., *Peptides, Hormones and Behavior,* SP Medical & Scientific Books, New York, 1984.
Prasad, K. N. and Vernadakis, A., *Mechanisms of Actions of Neurotoxic Substances,* Raven Press, New York, 1982.
Riddell, R. H., *Pathology of Drug-Induced and Toxic Diseases,* Churchill Livingstone, New York, 1982.
Roberts, E., Chase, T. N., and Towes, D. B., *GABA in the Nervous System Function,* Raven Press, New York, 1976.
Roisin, L., Shivaki, H., and Grcevic, N., *Neurotoxicology,* Raven Press, New York, 1977.
Schroeder, S. R., *Toxic Substances and Mental Retardation: Neurobehavioral Toxicology and Teratology,* Am. Assoc. Mental Deficiency, Washington, D.C., 1987.
Sinex, E. M. and Merril, C. R., *Alzheimer's Disease, Down's Syndrome, and Aging,* Ann. N.Y. Acad. Sci. U.S.A., 396, 1982.
Wauguier, A., Monti, J. M., Gaillard, J. M., and Radulovacki, M., *Sleep: Neurotransmitters and Neuromodulators,* Raven Press, New York, 1985.
Willis, W. D., *The Pain System: The Neural Basis of Nociceptive Transmission in the Mammalian Nervous Systems,* S. Karger, Basel, 1985.

INDEX

A

G

H

I

J

K